Praise for *The Real Diana:*

'You've really caused a stir with this book!' - *Richard & Judy*

'Explosive ... The most sensational book of the year' – *Mail on Sunday*

'Startling new revelations from the woman who has written the headline-making biographies about Princess Diana-astonishing' – *Hello! Magazine*

'Britain is buzzing about The Real Diana' – *Victoria Mather, The Early Show, CBS News*

'Some Palace watchers note that she has an impressive roster of well-placed contacts and credit her with writing the most believable Diana biography' – *People Magazine*

'Lays bare the facts about Diana's affair with James Hewitt and the reasons for Diana's death in 1997' – *Evening Standard*

'Bombshell revelations by Lady Colin Campbell, the former wife of a cousin of the Queen of England' – *Ireland on Sunday*

'A tribute to a truly remarkable and outstanding woman' – *Later Living*

'Lady Colin Campbell is a highly successful and prolific author, most famous for her two biographies of Diana, Princess of Wales' – *Sarah Wicker, chatshow.com*

'If you are maintaining a Diana library, Lady Colin Campbell's books are now must haves' – *Royal Book News*

Daughter of Narcissus

Also by Lady Colin Campbell:

Lady Colin Campbell's Guide to being a Modern Lady
Diana in Private
The Royal Marriages
A Life Worth Living
The Real Diana
Empress Bianca

Daughter of Narcissus

A family's struggle to survive their mother's narcissistic personality disorder

Lady Colin Campbell

Dynasty Press

Dynasty Press
36 Ravensdon Street
London SE11 4AR

www.dynastypress.co.uk

First published in this version by Dynasty Press 2009

ISBN 978-0-9928161-8-6

Cover artwork by Two Associates

Photography by David Chambers

Typeset by Strange Attractor Press

Printed in the United Kingdom

Acknowledgements:

This book would not have been possible without the benevolence of my sisters Kitty and Libby, and I would like to take this opportunity to thank them for the support and encouragement they have given me during its writing, as well as throughout our almost unbelievable lives.

I owe a huge debt of gratitude to Dr Erika Freeman, whose idea it was. I can still hardly believe that a psychoanalyst of such eminence, with her links to the great Dr Theodore Reik and Dr Sigmund Freud, could have considered me equipped to write on such an important subject. I thank her from the bottom of my heart for both the idea and her belief in my ability to address it properly.

I would also like to thank the psychologist Gloria Seigert for her help and encouragement throughout this long and sometimes arduous process, and also for believing in my ability to do the subject justice.

Thanks also to Ken Hollings my editor and Tessa Forbes of Dynasty Press, who nursed this book throughout its final stages; Leila Dear and Mark Pilkington of Strange Attractor Press who typeset it; James Empringham of Two Associates who designed the cover, and David Chambers who photographed me for it; to Judy Ann MacMillan for supplying the photograph of our parents, and to Charles Hanna for getting his secretary to send it. Old friends really are the best.

Author's Note:

Where appropriate the spelling of certain individuals' names has been altered to protect their privacy.

This book is dedicated to the memory of my late brother Mickey and to my sisters Kitty and Libby, as well as to everyone else everywhere who has shared the incredibly bumpy journey of having to share life with a narcissist.

Chapter One

It's funny how the really important moments in one's life are always squeezed between the mundane ones. I had just taken my three Springer Spaniel bitches for a walk around the domain of our family chateau in South-Western France near the great Cathedral city of Albi, birthplace of the French artist Toulouse Lautrec. It was a typical Midi-Pyrenean afternoon: warm and sunny and at least five degrees centigrade hotter outside than it was inside, where the massive stone walls, a metre thick, provided an air-conditioning system nature had neglected to give the lush and majestic countryside.

The summer of 2004 was turning out to be unusually hot, and would get even hotter still. The dogs and I walked out of the park surrounding our French home, up the old avenue of elms planted in the time of Napoleon I and into the late-nineteenth century avenue of plane trees, before heading into the woodland. Maisie Carlotta, the eldest of the three generations running around me, was really beginning to suffer from the heat, so I cut the walk short and headed back to the house with my panting pack.

It was my intention to start cooking as soon as I returned. I had a friend coming over for dinner, and my two sons had requested that I cook one of their favourites: sea-snails in garlic butter sauce to start, followed by breast of duck braised in olive oil, salt, black pepper and garlic, and ending up with a fruit salad of mangoes, bananas, oranges, pineapple and apples. As I was walking up the steps to the massive oak double doors, the telephone in the entrance hall began to ring. I ran to get it before the answering machine picked it up; frustratingly, many English-speaking people failed to leave messages, seeming to think that because the standard France Telecom message was in French, they were obliged to leave their message in that language.

This time, however, I didn't need to worry. It was my sister Libby. The way she plunged right in, I knew she had something of significance to report.

'It's me,' she said, before pressing on without further ado, 'Mummy left yesterday. Kitty flew up day before yesterday to pick her up. She's with her tonight, and tomorrow she returns to Cayman.'

I remained silent, which my sister knew meant that I really wasn't very interested in hearing that our mother was flying with our younger sister from Boca Raton, where Kitty lived with her husband and seven-year-old daughter, back to her home on Grand Cayman.

'I'm phoning to tell you that Ben thinks Mummy doesn't have long to live,' Libby continued, referring to her husband, who is a well-known physician and diagnostician.

'You can let her run rings around you if you want,' I said impatiently. 'That bitch has had all the sympathy she's going to get out of me. Not for a second will I be falling for her latest act – whatever it is. Be her dupe if it makes you feel better, but I don't intend to be so gullible.'

All my life I had seen our mother, who had the constitution of an ox in the delicate casing of a beautiful petal, play the health card whenever it suited her purposes. Never would I forget the anxiety she had put the whole family through in October 1967, when she told all of us the doctor feared she might not have long to live as he was sure she had terminal cancer; then, when she had got Daddy to buy her the diamond ring upon which she had her heart set – and which he had hitherto refused to get her – the health threat disappeared into thin air. Well, I knew exactly where I was coming from and what she was all about. 'Dearest Mamma' – as I usually called her ironically – was an inveterate manipulator and anything but anyone's dearest anything. Indeed, she had never been anything like a mother at all to the four of us siblings, much less one to whom anyone could ascribe adjectives such as 'dear' or 'dearest', except when being sarcastic. Those words, said without side, were ones we had always reserved for her elder sister Marjorie, our beloved Auntie, who had died the year before and whose estate had been the source of Mummy's most inglorious moment in a lifetime full of inglorious moments.

'No,' Libby said. 'It's true. She's not the same person you saw last year when

Auntie died. She's not even the same person I saw in February.' That was when Libby had flown down from her house in the Midwest of America to straighten out the mess of our mother's creation surrounding Aunt Marjorie's estate. At the time, our mother had been seventy-five but with the looks of a sixty-year-old and the energy of a thirty-five-year-old on speed.

'She's aged twenty years in the last few months,' Libby insisted. 'I was really surprised when I saw her.'

'Oh, for God's sake,' I replied irritably. 'When are you going to learn that Dearest Mamma is a consummate actress and utterly ruthless with it. She'll do *anything* to prevail. When she can't win, as she hasn't in this instance, she then tries to snatch a victory of sorts out of the jaws of defeat by making everyone feel sorry for her. That way she remains the focus of all activity and thereby satisfies her lust for constant attention, which in her sick way of thinking, means her will is still prevailing. Well, I don't feel sorry for her, and I'm certainly not about to give her an opportunity to reinterpret her attempt to rip us off and her ignominious failure to carry it off as anything other than what it is: a low down, despicable act of treachery and one, moreover, which doesn't deserve anything but contempt.'

'I appreciate why you feel the way you do,' Libby said, 'but she really isn't faking it this time.'

I was anything but convinced by what Libby was saying because I knew where she was coming from too. She was so intent upon being seen to be fair and even-handed on all occasions, and had such convoluted issues with a mother who had been nothing short of abominably abusive towards her from her earliest childhood until her husband had made the fortune which he now had, that she frequently erred on the side of fuzziness. Well, I had seen too many people fall for too many of our mother's acts to fall into that trap.

Because Libby and I had different issues with Mummy, I could afford to call a spade a spade and usually did so. In my view, one of the reasons why individuals like Gloria got away with their behaviour was that most people, especially those closest to them, simply did not want to accurately define their conduct. It was as if they feared that by giving a label to the unvarnished facts, their whole world would come tumbling down. So they obfuscated, minimized, prevaricated and, in my experience, remained trapped in a game they neither liked nor wanted to play. Not for one second did it occur to me that I might be caught up as a living participant in the tale of the boy who cried wolf and that our mother was genuinely dying.

'I'm not buying that,' I said. 'This scenario is just typical of her. It has all the hallmarks of Mummy's *modus operandi*: screw people, then when it backfires on her, the very people she's screwed are to dance attendance on her with lashings of sympathy and attention. No, my dear, not for one nanosecond will I express sympathy I don't feel. If you must know, it's us I feel sorry for. I may not know why God, in His infinite wisdom, chose to inflict such a poisonous mother upon us, but I do know it's my duty, to myself as a human being and to my children as their mother, to make sure that Mummy doesn't get away with her antics. If you want to assume the role of sympathizer when it's us she's been abusing, you go right ahead and waste your sympathy on the undeserving. For my part, I have better things to do with my time and energy. She's damned lucky I'm speaking to her at all, after that little trick she tried to pull in January.'

'I appreciate what you're saying,' Libby replied, 'but it really isn't like that this time. Ben says she has twelve to eighteen months to live – twenty-four at the most.'

'We should be so lucky,' I said wryly, convinced this was one of those occasions upon which she, the inglorious Gloria, was intent upon avoiding the consequences of her actions when she couldn't enjoy the ill-gotten gains of yet another act of manipulation.

'No,' Libby continued, by now quite used to the invective our mother inspired. 'This time she isn't putting on an act. She's lost a tremendous amount of weight and has become a wizened old woman overnight. She can barely get around. You know how she loves flowers. Well, I took her to the botanical gardens in Kansas City with my grandchildren, and she was near to collapse after fifteen minutes. I promise you, it was an effort for her to walk anywhere. She isn't the dynamo you saw last year at Auntie's funeral. Ben was so concerned about her that he insisted on checking her out. He took her to the hospital and put her through a full battery of tests…all of which he paid for, of course. It emerges she's developed cirrhosis of the liver. He sat her down and had a long talk with her. You know how mean she can be with money. He even offered to pay for her to go into rehab, but she said she doesn't want to. She said she has nothing to live for and she doesn't see the point of giving up drinking to prolong a life that she doesn't want to live.'

'All I can say is, if I had three children who as a rule behaved towards me lovingly and who were even prepared to have me come and live with them, despite my despicable behaviour, as well as six grandchildren who were prepared to give me love, even after I abuse them, not to mention a legion of acquaintances and relations and friends and enough money to enjoy them all, I wouldn't say I had nothing to live for,' I replied, thinking to myself how counterproductive it was when people who had everything to be grateful for ignored what they had and focused on what they lacked. If there was one lesson I had learned from observing my mother, it was that happiness and fulfilment are not possible unless you can count your blessings and have a genuine appreciation for them.

'Maybe she's depressed,' Libby said, doing what dysfunctional families so often do. They alight upon the symptom, not the underlying cause, and try to explain everything away in innocuous, everyday terms. However, Gloria's lack of regard for us deserved recognition and attribution if ever we were to understand what she was all about and how that had affected us. Without that knowledge, we could never be truly free of her malign influence.

The fact was that, unless we were prepared to accurately and dispassionately stare the truth in the face and acknowledge it, no matter how ugly it was, we would remain hostages to time, trapped in the prison of misery she had constructed so ably for us since early childhood. Sure, much of the truth we had to face was disagreeable, and confronting it was painful; but some of it, I had come to realize, was actually positive. It was in our interest to face all the facts squarely, for only then could we appreciate the reality of what we had experienced – and continued to experience – at her hands. It really was a case of the truth setting us free, and I couldn't see how seeking refuge in superficially acceptable explanations could ever provide the freedom I sought from the tentacles of our vicious mother.

'Maybe she is depressed,' I agreed, seeing no merit in pointing out to my sister that I disagreed with her attempt at palliation. 'If I were as cretinous as she is, and hadn't been able to snatch all that lovely money out of the mouths of my daughters and grandchildren, I'd be depressed too.'

'Be that as it may,' Libby said in softer tones than usual, 'it really is going to be curtains for her if she doesn't give up drinking. Her liver is now severely damaged. As Ben explained to her, if she gives up now, it will regenerate. But if she continues for even another three months, it will be too late to reverse the damage, and she will die whether she then elects to take up his offer of rehab or not.'

'Have *you* tried to talk her into going into rehab?' I asked, knowing very well how unlikely it was that Libby would do any such thing: not when Mummy had set out, since Libby was three years old, to crush her.

'You know what she's like. No sooner did I try to broach the subject than she cut me off,' Libby responded, alluding to the frosty obstinacy which was so much a feature of our mother's character, along with her bright intuitiveness which ensured that she always knew what you were going to say before your lips formed the words. Moreover, Libby and I both knew from bitter experience that no conversation – not even ones which were ostensibly pleasant – between Gloria and any of her children ever took place without her getting in one of her favourite expressions as a reminder to us that she was intent on maintaining absolute control. '*It's my way or the highway*,' she would trill rather than speak, as if the world really were a stage, and she the star, director, and producer. Meanwhile we, her children – *mere* children, mark you, and therefore subservient in every way, despite now being in our fifties – were expected to defer to her greater authority. She always made it absolutely clear, both by what she said and by what she omitted to say, that she '*ruled the roost*' – another of her favourite expressions which was also trilled rather than said, the very sound of the words being as much a claxon as the words themselves.

Gloria made sure that she left us in no doubt that she expected us to adhere to our allotted role. And what was that role? The audience. And, as all well-rehearsed audiences knew, we were not to try to take over the production. Because we could not contribute to the script, we must sit appreciatively, waiting for the cues the play offered: to laugh, to cry, to be sad, to be happy – but always following the lead of the playwright and, at the end of it all, showing one's appreciation with the applause that is the due of every great playwright. In Gloria's world, there was no room for Italian audiences, who booed and generally showed their displeasure whenever their vision did not accord with the playwright's. No. Gloria's audience was to be properly Anglo-Saxon in demeanour. It was to approve, and if it didn't, it was to stifle its disapproval and direct no trace of such unwelcome sentiments to the far more important arena of the stage, where she reposed with the absolute certainty that the world existed for her convenience and enjoyment.

'Yes, I know,' I said, sympathizing with my sister's lot. 'But you can't help people who don't want to help themselves. As Mummy herself is so fond of saying, *you can take a horse to the water, but you can't force it to drink.* And *a man convinced against his will is of the same opinion still.* I think it's important that we respect her right to make her own choices. She's always been excessively self-willed, and if her failings are catching up with her now, and she's going to have to pay the price, all I can say is that seventy-five years of getting away with murder isn't a bad innings. Most people can't ever escape the consequences of their actions for hours, much less decades. So on some level she's way ahead of the game.'

'You were always her favourite child. Maybe you should say something to her,' Libby suggested.

'No, no, absolutely not. Do you remember in 1976, when I introduced Brian Cox, that army officer who was a recovered alcoholic, to her? How she turned on me and spent the next several years going at me hell for leather? "Georgie is a little stinker who set Alcoholics Anonymous on me," she kept on saying to anyone who would listen. "And I'm going to make her pay." How she did! Oh, how she did! One malicious scheme after another. As if trying to get her into treatment was a crime. There's no way I'm running the risk of a repetition of *that*,' I said emphatically.

'I just thought that now that Daddy and Mickey are dead, maybe you could get her treatment the way they did.'

'I don't think so. In 1996, Mummy issued me with a stern warning, and I've heeded it ever since. Moreover, I propose to continue doing so. I'm not you. I don't have a rich husband to support me. And I have my two eleven-year-old children to think of. I need every penny of the money she inherited from Daddy, our brother Mickey, Grandma, and Auntie. You know how she's always threatening to leave everything to "a puss or dog charity" if we don't do exactly what she wants. She told me in no uncertain terms in 1996, and I quote: "I'm a big woman. Older than all of you, because I gave birth to you. I intend to continue drinking, and I don't want any interference out of any of you. Do I make myself clear?" I remember as if it were yesterday exactly what I replied. Although I felt like responding in kind and making the acid observation that she'd made herself only too clear, since we'd been getting on better than we had for twenty-five years, instead I said, "You've touched upon an important philosophic point. You're telling me you have an absolute right to do whatever it is you wish with yourself because you are an adult. I agree with you. I shall respect your decision in that regard until such time as you indicate to me that you wish to change it. If, indeed, you ever do." "Good," she said with rather more pleasure than one usually hears her employ when expressing herself. I meant what I said then, and I mean it now. I will never try to get her to stop drinking unless she indicates to me that she wants me to do so.'

'But you're the only one left who might have some influence with her,' Libby persisted, as if I had ever had any influence with our mother when it had come to anything of any consequence. She was clearly confusing teenage events – such as the times I approached Gloria to get us permission to go to the cinema or to a party when Daddy had told us we could not – with something of greater significance.

'Shall I tell you the truth?' I said, chary of being roped into a situation not of my own making, which could have adverse financial consequences for me and mine. 'It's her life, and if she wants to destroy it, she can do so. Moreover, I dispute the fact that I'm her favourite. If anyone is, it's you, because you're the only one to whom she ever accords even a modicum of respect. She has absolutely no respect for either Kitty or me, doubtless because we don't have the money you do. I agree it would be good if someone could get her to stop drinking, but I really think you're better situated than either Kitty or me to do so.'

'If Ben had no success, I won't either,' Libby sensibly observed. Gloria was always open about preferring men to women, and her son-in-law to her own daughter. 'You know how rabidly protective she is of her drinking.'

I remembered only too well the last time the subject of Gloria's drinking, which had been a major problem for all of us siblings since our teenage years, had come up. It was May 2001. We had been at Libby's house, where Gloria was staying for the wedding of Libby's elder daughter, who was marrying into one of America's great political dynasties

Elizabeth, the bride-to-be, and I pulled up into the forecourt of her parents' paean to the American dream; a spanking new custom-built house with several thousand square feet of superfluous living space situated in prime position on an exclusive golf and country club, whose membership seemed peculiarly representative of the *status quo* when Eisenhower was still president. If the tone of Libby's neighbourhood was pre-Kennedy in attitude, the services she and her kind availed themselves of were definitely Clintonesque. Thanks, therefore, to the effective deployment of the instrument of communication my sister and niece called a 'cell' – and I called a 'mobile' – Libby was standing in the forecourt to witness our arrival as I turned my rented car up the driveway of the house I had never seen before.

In books or films, sisters who have not seen one another for two years embrace and exchange niceties before plunging into the maelstrom of family problems, but this did not happen.

'Mummy's been knocking back straight scotch by the glassful from ten o'clock in the morning since she came last week,' Libby said with an intensity I recognized only too well, before I had even managed to swing my foot out of the car and place it on the smooth surface of her forecourt. 'I've been so concerned that I just had to say something. I told her you're upset with her. Just so you know.'

'I'm not sure I'm following you,' I replied, taken aback by this development. It was one thing to have to deal with a mother who was perpetually three sheets to the wind, with all the attendant turmoil and malice, but quite another to be dropped into that particular cauldron when I had been determined to avoid it at all costs.

'Scotch is so bad for her that I just had to say something. And I thought, since you're her favourite, she'd be more open to your disapproval than to mine.'

As invariably happens in families, dysfunctional or not, there were wheels within wheels. This meant that one either went along with the flow and accepted a situation one found unacceptable, usually with a whole unforeseen and undeserved set of consequences; or one stood one's ground and hopefully managed to avoid triggering one of the explosions characteristic of people with too much will and too little sense of how life should be lived.

Libby did not need to tell me that our mother drinking straight scotch was an undesirable development. Nor did she need to tell me that it was as much a shock to her as it was to me. We had all thought that Gloria had been drinking white wine and champagne since her return to the bottle in the late 1980s after ten years on the wagon. Giving voice to the comfort we took from the switch she had made from her previous practice of consuming a bottle of gin and a bottle of port a day in the 1960s and 1970s, she herself used to say: 'I don't drink alcohol. Only a little white wine or champagne. And you can't really class those as alcohol, for they're effectively fortified grape juice.'

To an uninitiated bystander, the scenario as it was evolving might well have seemed preposterous: a middle-aged woman firing information at a machine-gun rate about her mother's drinking to her elder sister, who had just flown halfway around the world, and doing so before she even had the opportunity to ask how her flight was. However, anyone who has had to cope with alcoholism will know only too well how the disease distorts the behaviour of everyone it touches, so that what is extraordinary in another situation is typical in the alcoholic's context. Furthermore, Gloria was not your typical alcoholic. Whether drunk or sober, drinking or dry, she was a forceful dynamo of unpredictability and outspokenness who brooked no opposition to the implementation of her will. To know her was to be in terror, if not of her then of what she could do. It was the feeling that you could never be adequately prepared for what she might come up with next that unsettled practically everyone who knew her well.

If Libby had hoped to give me ample warning of what awaited me before our mother wrested the reins back into her own hands, Gloria disappointed her. Clearly she must have heard the car for she now opened the front door with as much self-possession as if Libby and I were both guests – and unwanted ones at that – in her house, even though she was Libby's guest. She calmly cast her eyes over the scene of her two daughters and granddaughter huddled in a mass, patently talking about a forbidden subject, and without more ado literally hissed like a viper, turned on her heels in high dudgeon and sailed back inside like a stately galleon which did not condescend to acknowledge either the wave or the mess floating upon the sea.

'But I never said any such thing!' I protested, taken aback that Libby could have embroiled me in what was developing into yet another of the messes which had made life in our family something to dread rather than enjoy. 'How could I when I didn't even know she drank scotch? I thought it was a drink she never liked.'

'Well, she likes it now, that's for sure,' Libby retorted, pursuing her lips to indicate how rattled she was by Gloria having just shown up the way she had. 'I haven't even counted the quantity she'd got through. But you can depend on it: it will be quite a few bottles.'

'Listen,' I said, trying to be as supportive as possible. 'I appreciate what you've tried to do. But I have to tell you, you must keep my name out of your rescue attempts in future.'

With that, I headed straight into a house I did not know, walked from the entrance hall past the drawing room into the family room, where Gloria was sitting with haughty disdain, watching television and nursing a tumbler full of scotch.

Over the years I had learned how to deal with my mother. Of all her close relations and friends, I was the only one who was not afraid of her. I refused to take her rubbish while still maintaining the semblance of a pleasant, if sporadic, relationship. Dealing with her wasn't easy. Sometimes it was downright tiresome, but I was resolved to have as 'good and as happy a relationship' with her as I could: a refrain I did not shy away from reminding her of when it was necessary or desirable.

This was one of those occasions. The only way to defuse the situation was to grasp the bull by the horns and look him in the eye. So, without further ado, I bent over and brushed cheeks with her in salutation as she sat on the sofa studiously ignoring me.

'I want you to know,' I said in a normal tone of voice, free of either resentment or fear, 'that I never said anything to Libby about your drinking scotch. She's concerned that if you drink spirits, you'll do yourself more harm than if you drink wine or champagne. I happen to agree with her and think you ought to be made aware of the dangers. But, as I told you when you were taking me to Palisadoes in 1996, I respect your right to drink, and more than pointing out to you that wine is easier on the body than spirits, I have nothing to say on the subject. Frankly, I resent my name having been brought into it at all.'

'I'm glad to hear it,' she said coolly without bothering to look up from the television.

To an onlooker, the very indirectness of this exchange might have indicated that she was still upset with me, but I knew otherwise. She was not conveying displeasure. She was communicating assent. The great Gloria had condescended to let insignificant little me off the hook this time. In her scheme of things, if she had given a more overt response, she would have been endowing me with greater significance than she wished to convey. She intended me to discern that I was too insignificant to warrant anything but the most tepid of responses.

Was I grateful? Absolutely not. Was I relieved? Only slightly. Was I resentful? Not at all. What is the point of resenting the fact that the alligator has a rough hide and sharp teeth and will devour you if you get too close to it, or that the fire will burn you if you put your hand into it? The alligator and fire are as much facts of life as you or I; and it is up to us to deal with them appropriately. If there was one thing I had learned about handling my mother, it was that she was every bit as dangerous as an alligator or a fire, and it was far easier to acknowledge her for what she was and deal with it, than it was to deny it and run the risk of suffering the consequences of that failure.

Yet Gloria still remained my mother, and my goal was to have as good and as positive a relationship with her as possible. So, after I put away my luggage, I returned to the family room, where she was still sitting, and sat in the wing-backed armchair opposite her.

'Come and sit with me,' she said. 'And turn off that television. I can barely hear myself think with it on, much less talk to you.'

'I don't know how to turn it off,' I said.

'Libby, come here and turn this blasted racket off,' Gloria ordered without even bothering to look up to see where her other daughter – and hostess – was. Libby, however, was quite sensibly absenting herself from the maternal presence, so I had to go in search of her.

The television, it emerged, was one of those super-sophisticated systems that only a rocket scientist or a child of seven could work without studying the manual. So Libby came back with me, turned it off then fled back to another part of the house, the fact that it was her house making not one scrap of difference to the discomfort she was being made to endure by our mother. Of course, I could not help but recognize how ludicrous it was that a woman in her fifties would have to seek refuge from a guest in her own house, but this was a pattern that had been set decades before. As Libby scurried out of the room, I smiled to myself, thinking how very fortunate it was for us as a family that we had always been able to live in places that afforded us the protection of size. Could one have survived a mother such as ours at closer quarters? I doubted it.

With the television off, I now had to focus on attentiveness rather than escape. Gloria, fortunately, always made it easy for each of us, in one respect if in no other. She was such a compulsive chatterbox that she only ever asked the most cursory of questions, as good manners decreed, before plunging right into her latest preoccupation. And so it was this time. After asking me about my flight and hearing that it was uneventful, then asking whether the children were well and hearing that they were – all of which took no more than ninety seconds – she was off and running. She had recently left Jamaica to move to Grand Cayman, and she was full of what she was up to, including her incipient romance with her sister's brother-in-law, Anthony.

For the remainder of that visit, Gloria was on her best behaviour and was actually as much of a pleasure to be with as it was possible for her to be. Her rampant egotism and incessant need to dominate seemed to have evaporated along with the scotch she had ceased to drink. I actually got a glimpse of what a joy it could be to have a mother who was somewhat kindly, cooperative, pleasant and, above all, one of the gang rather than ganging up against everyone else. Whether this new attitude was because she was distracted by the hope of her budding romance or because her favourite granddaughter was getting married to someone of whom she approved – Quince was the descendant of two American presidents on his father's side and a member of one of Virginia's oldest and grandest families on his mother's – or whether it was because she was mellowing and making a greater effort to enjoy her children and grandchildren, I could not say. Nor did I care what the reason was. I was just happy to have happy memories and grateful for the occasion which provided them.

With the benefit of hindsight, I can see that Anthony was most likely the immediate reason for Gloria's good behaviour and positive attitude, just as the very hopes he instilled in her would provide the catalyst for her subsequent betrayal of her daughters.

This, however, was still in the future, as indeed was Libby's telephone call, which I was taking this June afternoon of 2004.

'So, you're telling me, this really is crunch time. It isn't another of Mummy's diabolical games,' I said to Libby.

'This is it. Unless she gives up drinking, which we all know she's never going to do voluntarily, she'll be dead in twenty-four months tops. And it could be much sooner if she gets flu or something like that. She's so thin that she won't have the resistance to fight off a strong virus or infection. She can't weigh a pound over one hundred.'

Suddenly I felt as if someone had deflated my balloon and released all the anger that I had been feeling towards my mother. Could it really be that this force of nature would actually die? Would she really leave us – dare I say it, release us? God knows, there had been ample times over the past forty-four years when I had wished that I could be rid of her. Yet now that the time had actually come, now that the countdown to death was beginning, I felt neither relief nor elation nor any of the other things one is expected to feel when a millstone begins to be lifted from around one's neck. What I felt was regret. Regret that it had come to this. Regret that we had so little to show or share in the way of positive memories of a woman who had occupied the most important role a woman can in the life of her daughters. She was still my mother. One could take a perfunctory view, the way so many people do nowadays, or one could take a spiritual view, which I preferred. I genuinely believed then, and still believe now, that the relationship between a parent and a child is sacred. I believe it is ordained by God and that we are put on this earth to fulfil a destiny which we can only ever partly understand but which, in its entirety, is one of our real purposes on this earth.

As far as I am concerned, this life is merely the first phase of life. In this, our earthly incarnation, we are bound by time, but upon death we are released into another dimension, which is timeless. It is therefore important for each of us to get our relationships and our souls into good order, as we will be stuck with the consequences of our choices not only for now but for all eternity. I do not take the view that what happens today doesn't matter tomorrow, or the day after tomorrow, because the past is the past and will never return. I think the past never leaves us. Nor do I believe that our time on this earth, short as it is, is relatively unimportant. On the contrary, I think that our every action and choice is of utmost importance; for what we are today, what we choose today, is a result of our choices and beliefs from yesterday and all our other yesterdays, and they will be with us not only for today and tomorrow but for all eternity.

Each of us has a system, priorities and a scale of values. Mine are relatively simple. I have always valued the people in my life above all else. Believing as I do, I had little choice but to confront my mother's mortality in as spiritual a way possible.

Although I did not know it at the time, by taking this approach I also gave myself the opportunity to find out what had really been wrong with our mother. The root of her problem had never been alcoholism, although her alcoholism had compounded the underlying problems. In my quest to discover what had motivated her, I would end up doing myself a huge favour, for there is no surer way of killing the ghosts of the past than by shining daylight upon them.

'I'll telephone her when she gets back to Cayman and arrange to take the children to see her,' I said. 'If she really is going to die, I'll do everything in my power to see her out with as much love and affection and kindness as I can summon up.'

'I understand,' Libby said.

Chapter Two

It would be wonderful if families really were the way Hollywood depicted them, with the mother being good-looking, well-groomed, sweet, loving, family-orientated and content to while away her day baking cookies and innocently gossiping with friends, while the father – a handsome hunk with fabulous pecs, a great income and a sense of moral rectitude that would put Clarence Darrow to shame – comes home from a challenging day at the office to enjoy his wife and children, all of whom live happily ever after in this haven against the world at large.

As we all know, real life in not like that. Few families live up to the ideal. Not even physically. Ours, however, was a family that, from the outside looking in, seemed to be a realization of the dream. To begin with, my parents were renowned in social circles as a good-looking and glamorous couple. My father Michael was tall, dark, slim and handsome in the Cary Grant mould, while Gloria, with her huge brown eyes, auburn hair, straight nose, fine bones and well-formed mouth, had a regularity of feature allied to an exoticism which ensured that she looked like no one else. Her figure was perfect for the fashions of the day, and she ensured that her clothes, which were usually couture, showed off her generous bust, small waist and slender hips to advantage. In the 1950s and 1960s, masculinity and femininity were highly prized commodities, and the eight-inch difference in height between Michael and Gloria emphasized how masculine and feminine they both were.

Aside from their physical attractiveness, they had worldly attributes which were fundamental to their social reputation. Michael's family was a household name, largely through their ownership of department stores and racehorses. The name Ziadie evoked money. Gloria's family did not have a name that would have been recognisable to the man in the street, but the Smedmore family on her father's side was English top-drawer, while the Burke family on her mother's was part of an eminent Irish dynasty that produced a variety of earls as well as the last Governor-General and first Viceroy of India. While the Smedmores had no money but a plethora of breeding, the Burkes had both, though in the rating of the day, the fact that they were Irish as opposed to English meant that they were not quite as eminent socially.

The problems that would ultimately play havoc with our lives were definitely not of the superficial variety. Indeed, a part of the problem would always be that the surface seemed so appealing that people either couldn't, or wouldn't, allow themselves to accept that any degree of misery could lurk beneath the magnificently veneered gloss of the perfectly good-looking, glamorous and socially desirable couple.

Michael and Gloria's relationship was supposedly a fabulous love story. They had met by accident when he was twenty-six and she fifteen. She was at the house of some friends when her maternal uncle John showed up unexpectedly with his good friend Michael Ziadie in tow. The effect she had upon him was instantaneous, as Michael told me shortly before he died. 'I fell in love with your mother the moment I saw her. She was beautiful and captivating. She was only fifteen, but I can tell you, she was no little girl. Even at that tender age she was dynamite.'

In those days, well-bred girls of fifteen were about to enter the marriage market and were considerably more advanced and grown-up than girls of the same age are today. This, remember, was at a time when the concept of the teenager had not yet been thought of. You were either a child or an adult, and fifteen-year-old girls who were as physically well developed as Gloria were regarded as young women. Gloria, by her own account, was already a practised vamp who exuded sex-appeal from every pore and had to be fighting off the boys. 'More than once I had to box one across the face when he tried to be over-familiar,' she would later recall.

One boy whose face this young Society vamp did not box, however, was the tall, slim, good-looking and sexually-appealing Michael Manley, who would later become prime minister of Jamaica three times and develop a reputation as a lady-killer, marrying five times and having countless mistresses. His father, Norman Washington Manley, was premier of Jamaica at the time and leader of the People's National Party. Although Gloria's father, Lucius Dey Smedmore, was a great admirer of Norman Manley's politics and professional accomplishments as Jamaica's leading barrister, both he and his wife May were aghast at the prospect of the relationship. In those days, white, upper-class Jamaicans practised a colour bar that was every bit as rigid as South Africa's, and the fact that Norman Manley was half-black rendered the match unacceptable. Tellingly, however, they did not seek to break it up directly, preferring instead to convey their disapproval subtly in the hope that time would do the trick. And it did. Michael Manley, who Gloria always said 'was the sweetest kisser', went away to fight against Hitler; and Michael Ziadie, whose kisses were never mentioned once throughout her entire life, came onto the scene.

Having seen off one Michael of whom he disapproved, Lucius Smedmore hoped to see off the second as well. As far as he was concerned, Michael Ziadie was simply not good enough for his daughter. The Ziadies were émigrés with money and, though descendants of the Emperor Charlemagne and European kings such as William the Conqueror, were not yet members of 'Society' in their new homeland; and the one thing Lucius Smedmore relished along with his Anglican faith was his place in Society. It was a source of some distress to him that his daughter could associate with anyone who was not in Society.

Society was then a hallowed place to many of those who occupied it. The prospect of his treasured Gloria having a romance with a man from outside Society was a catastrophe, but several things hampered him from preventing the relationship flowering into a marital union. Firstly, Michael Ziadie had no African blood, so he could not complain along those lines the way he did about Michael Manley. Secondly, Michael Ziadie was a successful businessman of considerable financial worth. These were formidable attributes which mattered greatly to both his wife and his daughter, even though money had never been of importance to him. Last but not least, he had always indulged Baby Gloria and couldn't summon up the gumption to change the habit of a lifetime. He therefore found himself fighting a losing battle with his wilful daughter, who continued to see Michael despite his disapproval, confident that she had the approval of the more powerful of her two parents. Her mother had a healthy respect for Michael for several reasons, chief amongst which were his bank account, his good-looks and his amenable character.

Although Lucius had no intention of encouraging the young lovers, by disapproving of the union without providing any real threat to it, he actually gave it the romanticism that parental opposition so often has. Then, after Gloria accepted Michael's proposal, but before the engagement was announced, he showed just how ineffectual he was in achieving his objective, by setting up his brother Julian to make fine fools of them both. Unrealistically hoping that the fact that he had spoiled Gloria all her life would somehow influence her into changing her mind from proceeding with what he regarded as a socially undesirable misalliance, Lucius persuaded Julian to convey Smedmore disapproval by refusing to shake Michael's hand when they were introduced. This petty snub caused a frisson of excitement at the time, but Lucius was clearly out of his depth, for neither Gloria nor Michael was in the least perturbed by the disapproval of his brother Julian or, indeed, by Lucius's own covert disapproval. Furthermore, knowing my parents as I do, I doubt whether a more pungent gesture would have moved them in the slightest either. The issue was never put to the test, for the remainder of Gloria's family approved of the match, and with time Lucius fell into line and had to accept the marriage.

Tellingly, Michael never held Julian's snub against him. In the years to come, they became firm friends, though Gloria never missed an opportunity to decry her uncle. She made no secret of despising him, calling him a penniless ne'er-do-well, and never allowed anyone to forget how he had snubbed Michael, though she paradoxically never held Lucius accountable for his part in the farce.

The wedding duly took place at Kingston's Roman Catholic Cathedral on September 11 1946, followed by a reception at the bride's parents' house on fashionable Fairway Avenue. Having started out with the right amount of drama for a love story, Gloria and Michael's marriage was known to one and all as a grand passion. They were supposed to be madly in love and to have a most torrid time between the sheets. After my parents' deaths, more than one cousin from both sides of the family asked the same question: 'Did your parents really have the fantastic passion which we were all led to believe they possessed?'

It was interesting for me, as their child, to be asked that question, for I had not been aware that theirs was supposed to be a great love-story. This was partly because sex was not a subject which was discussed in front of children in the 1950s, but there was also another reason. I saw precious little evidence of what I would call love, though I certainly saw a lot of fire and fury. When I was a teenager and my father took me to see Elizabeth Taylor and Richard Burton in *Who's Afraid of Virginia Woolf?* my comment afterwards was that it was 'tame stuff' and that if the producers had really wanted to know what marital fireworks were about, they should have consulted my parents.

Aside from being this good-looking and glamorous couple who were living out this supposed love story, Michael and Gloria were prosperous. Very prosperous. My father was a merchant by trade who owned a thriving business as well as a piece of several other businesses. We lived in a house of ambassadorial proportions, surrounded by grounds that would ultimately become renowned in horticultural circles for being one of the largest and most sumptuous orchid gardens anywhere in the world. In my parents' heyday, even the country in which they resided was regarded as one of the most glamorous places on earth: Jamaica in the 1950s and 1960s was the spot where the richest, grandest, most elegant and successful people in the world wintered. These sometime-residents were a veritable roll-call of the leading lights of American industry, the Social Register, Burke's Peerage and the pan-European Almanach de Gotha, with a hefty sprinkling of Hollywood stars thrown in for good measure. The world's most famous banking family, the J P Morgans; the world's most successful television tycoon, Bill Paley, with his wife Babe, renowned as the Best Dressed Woman in the World at a time when women lived by and died for the Best Dressed List; the world-famous composer of musicals, Oscar Hammerstein, and his wife Mary; the vastly rich German steel magnate Baron Heini Thyssen-Bornemisza and his latest Baroness (from Nina through Fiona to Denise), along with his children Lorne and Francesca; the Aga Khan's son (and present Aga Khan's uncle) Prince Saddrudin Aga Khan and the wife he shared with Heini Thyssen, Nina Dyer, who would actually take her life in Jamaica in 1962; the Duke of Marlborough and his daughter Lady Sarah Spencer-Churchill, who had been the primary recipient of the will of her fabulously rich grandmother Consuelo Vanderbilt, renowned in the late nineteenth century as the greatest heiress on earth; Errol Flynn and his final wife Patrice Wymore, along with their daughter Arnella; Noel Coward; Ian Fleming, the author of the James Bond books (and our North Coast neighbour) as well as his wife Anne, the former Viscountess Rothermere; Lord Beaverbrook, the famous newspaper baron, and his granddaughter Lady Jean Campbell, who would marry the American author Norman Mailer; Sir Jock Buchanan-Jardine, the former Taipan of Jardine-Matheson, the greatest Hong Kong trading company of all, and his wife Pru all wintered in Jamaica along with guests like Sir Winston Churchill; Elizabeth Taylor and her husband of the time; Senator Jack Kennedy and his wife Jackie, as well as her sister Lee, whose husband, Prince Stanislaus Radziwill, was a great favourite of everyone because of his erudition and charm; and indeed virtually everyone else in Europe or America who bore a recognized or recognisable name.

Then there were the new crop of permanent residents, such as the Duke of Montrose's brother Lord Ronald Graham, or Lord Methuen, whose father had been one of the most famous artists of the first half of the twentieth century, or Gay, Lady Avebury, whose ex-husband was the head of the Liberal Party in the House of Lords. These people were swelling the aristocratic ranks already resident in Jamaica, some for centuries, from whom many Jamaican families were descended, my own mother's included.

It is fair to say that you only needed to remain long enough on your back or front veranda, or be lolling about by your swimming pool, for some friend of yours to drop in unannounced with a world-famous personage in tow.

Nor were the moneyed winter guests or permanent residents the only foreign élite that found its way to Jamaica in the 1950s and 1960s. Dudley MacMillan, who owned Jamaica's leading advertising agency and became the island's foremost impresario by accident (he started it as a hobby), managed to import every artiste of any renown to perform in Kingston at the State Theatre, which he owned. Everyone from Arthur Rubinstein to Nat King Cole graced his stage and the attendant receptions which he and his wife Vida hosted at their Central Avenue residence for the visiting dignitaries and their glamorous circle of friends. According to his daughter Judy Ann, 'Daddy said it was easy to book the greats of the entertainment world." Those were the days when all popular *artistes* toured, and, because Jamaica was ideally situated to begin or end a tour of South or Central America, and because it had an international reputation for beautiful sand, sea and sun, as well as its amazing array of world-famous residents, everyone wanted to visit this paradise they'd heard so much about. Adding a dash of celebrities to a generous helping of glamorous Society figures made Dudley and Vida MacMillan's parties legendary, and my parents were at each and every one, because Vida and Gloria were best friends.

It is not an exaggeration to say that it was virtually impossible for anyone moving in Jamaica's social circles to avoid the international *crème de la crème* of the day. The Jamaican way of life was geared towards hospitality; and new blood, whether blue or red, was always treated in an equally welcome manner. These were the days before television came to the island in 1962, when people had to occupy themselves. As no ladies worked, and everyone had servants, the custom of dropping in had evolved over the centuries into a cure for boredom but also for predictability. Because employing servants was not only a necessary part of gracious living but also the Haves' way of relieving the penury of the Have-nots, most people had several servants, 'even though they spent their whole time chatting to or tripping over each other instead of working', as Gloria put it.

One way of keeping the servants occupied was to entertain, for entertaining involved a host of subsidiary actions which meant that the cook cooked more food than she otherwise would have done for just the family, while the housemaids had to clean up more as well, and even the gardeners could not let that overgrown patch of grass at the bottom of the lawn remain un-mowed, just in case his Massa or his Missus took the guests on a guided tour.

The one thing the domestic staff could not afford to do was let the standards of their employers' household slip, for upper class Jamaicans had very exacting standards. Nor was the way they had their servants keep their houses the only standard to maintain. All women were expected to be well-groomed. Unlike their English counterparts, who took a positive pride in being as plainly attired as possible, Jamaican ladies were expected to be clothed in the latest fashions, with hair and make-up to match; and by the time she was twenty-four years old, Gloria had a reputation for being one of the most glamorous beauties on the social scene.

The emphasis placed on grooming extended even to children. Although we were all given licence during the day to run around in simple clothes, we were nevertheless expected to be well turned out after our afternoon baths, when we would be taken for walks in the neighbouring streets, past vast stretches of open land, by our nannies, who used the occasion to link up with other nannies whose charges were turned out in equally smart fashion.

Only the men, in the tradition of English gentlemen, were expected to be plainly and conservatively dressed at all times, for it was considered vulgar and common for men to be flashy, and effeminate to be dapper.

This awareness of high standards had its roots in Jamaica's past, when that tiny island had been the jewel in the British Empire's crown, more valuable than all of British India or the thirteen American colonies. What fuelled the social imperative was the awareness that the Old Families maintained of their heritage. While the rest of the world might have forgotten that Jamaica had once been the richest country per capita on earth and therefore preeminent in terms of economic and social influence, Jamaicans had not. One only needed to read *Jane Eyre* and see how the mad Mrs Rochester was described – 'a Jamaican heiress' – to appreciate why her latter-day descendants had an ingrained sense of being the inheritors of a gracious past. In terms of wealth, Jamaica's glory days might have ended with the abolition of slavery in 1838, but to the descendants of those oligarchs, who had been the equivalent of today's computer billionaires, their heritage gave them a self-worth and self-belief that allowed them to feel entitled to a seat at any top table. The social confidence of people like Gloria was only one of the many welcome effects of such a heritage.

Not that my mother or her peer group relied exclusively on heritage, for they did not. Upper-class Jamaicans were raised from infancy to be gracious, hospitable, generous and kind. Gloria was superficially all of those, and she moreover shared the social conscientiousness so typical of her class. To them, patrician was not a meaningless word but a state of being to live out on an everyday basis. All married ladies were expected to dedicate a percentage of their time to 'social work', as charity work was called by them. It mattered little whether they had been married three weeks, three years or three decades. Once their honeymoon was over, they were supposed to volunteer for some of the worthy causes, such as the Wortley Home for Children (usually abandoned or orphaned non-blacks), which is what Gloria did. To people like her, *noblesse oblige* was not a tacky book with silly ideas about being superior to everyone else because you spoke in a certain way or said (and did not say) certain things, as Nancy Mitford and Evelyn Waugh would have had you believe. *Noblesse oblige* was a concept that required you, on pain of being revealed to be an inferior person, not only to help the disadvantaged of society but also to speak to them, and indeed everyone who crossed your path, from the Queen of England to the washerwoman, in the exact same way: namely, with identical courtesy and respect.

Admittedly, there were those of the new, up-and-coming order who criticized such a uniform way of speaking to people of all classes. They felt that the upper-class easiness of manner was not an attribute but an irritating manifestation of superiority, and that one should not treat everyone so uniformly. As far as I could tell, the true objection these *arrivistes* had to such a singular way of address was that it denied its practitioners the opportunity to make people feel inferior by the deployment of a lofty tone while also preventing them from sucking up to those they regarded as superiors.

Gloria herself used to mock those *arrivistes* who talked down to their supposed inferiors by saying, in a wickedly acerbic commentary of their pretentiousness: 'They have not arrived, my dear. They have *arriven*, and they're making all of us painfully aware of it.' This comment always provoked a laugh for her audience invariably appreciated that *arriven* is not actually a word but a state of being occupied by the pretentious. Of course, people who give themselves airs and graces have always been an easy target for the more naturally poised; and Gloria, who was genuinely witty and lacking in pomposity, never missed an opportunity to deflate them. Those who put on affectedly 'grand' accents were invariably mimicked and labelled 'speakey-spokey'. She once took off the way the mother of one of my sister Kitty's friends spoke so accurately – very affectedly even though she was from a perfectly good family and should have known better – that Gloria had everyone in stitches. Her impeccable timing came to the fore when she issued the *coup de grace* by saying: 'If you didn't know better, you'd think her mouth was full of stewed prunes.' From that point on the unfortunate woman has been known behind her back as 'Stewed Prunes.'

If the naturalness of Gloria and her circle jarred with the up-and-coming, it was a balm to the doubting soul of the super-rich Winter Colony, some of whom spent their whole lives wondering whether people wanted them for themselves or their worldly goods. Even the less paranoid wanted to be liked for themselves; and as they observed Gloria and other socialites of their host nation treating one and all with uniformity, they could see that the charm wasn't laid on for their benefit but sprang from a deeper well. One of the J P Morgan family summed it up best when he said: 'It's such a pleasure to meet people who don't want anything out of me except to entertain me in the most charming manner possible.'

Nor were upper-class Jamaicans the only ones who enveloped others with warmth and charm. With few exceptions, Jamaicans of all classes were warm and welcoming to both strangers and friends. Respect was not a meaningless utterance but a viable, vibrant concept. '*Respec'* was a word you heard then and even moreso now. Indeed, it has become such a part of contemporary youth culture that even Queen Elizabeth the Queen Mother used to say 'Respec' to her grandchildren in the style forged by humble Jamaicans.

It is a fact that much of Jamaica is a magical country and most of its people truly jolly, upbeat and humorous. The result was that foreign residents were often as seduced by the charms of their staff as they were by the charms of the upper classes. Mixing with the Winter Colony, however, was only a part of the social life of upper-class Jamaicans, and by and large not even the main part. To socialize excessively with the Winter Colony was frowned upon because it gave out the message that one's social position might not be by virtue of who one was, but was due to the foreigners with whom one mixed. As such conduct was considered déclassé, only those Jamaicans with no social position to protect tilted the delicate balance between the habitual and the winter residents. All other socially-established Jamaicans spent most of their time living, socializing, working, playing, having affairs of a social or monetary nature and sometimes even dying together. They married one another and, if they did not, quickly absorbed outsiders so completely that within a few years you would have been hard put to differentiate between them from the born-and-bred patrician. The result was that upper-class Jamaicans as a group shared strong identifying characteristics, almost as if they were mirror images of one another. Aside from having similar values, lifestyles, expectations, hopes and dreams, they spoke with the same accent, used the same slang, had the same gracious manners and prejudices, which were reflective of their generation though today they would be characterized as unattractively racist and elitist.

It is, of course, a feature of all élites that they care more about one another than they do about anyone else, doubtless because it is in the eyes of their own group that their importance is recognized and reaffirmed. Upper-class Jamaica was no exception. While it provided a delightful frisson for a Jamaican patrician such as Blanche Blackwell (whose son Chris later founded Island Records) to have an affair with a famous foreigner like Ian Fleming, or to have Queen Victoria's granddaughter and Queen Mary's sister-in-law Princess Alice, Countess of Athlone (a habitual winter resident) to tea, real life in real Jamaica took place between real Jamaicans of real consequence, and that was the really important aspect of their lives.

It is almost impossible nowadays, in this age of social transience, instant celebrity and reality television, when 'background' is a word more frequently applied to a photographic shoot than to social antecedents, to make people whose families were not a part of Society appreciate how vitally important social position was in days gone by. People like my mother-in-law, Margaret Duchess of Argyll, Barbara Hutton, Marjorie Merriweather Post and Elsie Woodward lived for, and died with, the concept that life was only worth living within Society. There was a starry, almost magical, quality to Society figures in those days. They were commonly accepted by people outside of Society as being 'special', as being more glamorous, desirable, important, than ordinary people. And the truth is that they felt the same way about themselves. Gloria certainly did.

It is symptomatic of the way the world has changed that only weirdoes or the unimaginative think like that anymore. Nowadays nobody even uses the word 'Society'. We talk about 'Social Circles'. Or 'People Like Us'. Or 'Our Kind'. Anything to avoid the word 'Society'. That is because the world has moved on from elitism to egalitarianism and meritocracy, and Society really doesn't exist anymore as a truly desirable entity – at least, not Society as one's parents' generation understood it. Certainly, there are established families who still mix with and marry one another the way they used to; but nowadays only the most stuffy and unimaginative people within those circles would seriously wish to exclude any non-Society newcomers, if only because the breakdown of barriers has made social life far more interesting and colourful than it used to be, thanks to the New Blood.

When I was a child, and Gloria was enjoying being a celebrated socialite, her social life, although it revolved around Society, was more complex and varied than that of the cousins or friends she grew up with. Largely this was because she married out of the WASP world into which she was born. My father, despite having an ancient lineage and the money to back it up, was neither Anglo-Saxon nor Protestant, but of Lebanese and Russian extraction, with a dash of other European nationalities such as French and Frankish. Nor did he aspire to Society, which then functioned by arcane English notions of who and what were socially desirable. There was a strong racialist element to these notions. It did not matter a jot whether you were in England, Jamaica or anywhere else on the globe where the colour pink indicated that a third of the world's surface had once been a part of the British Empire. English and Protestant were best. Next came Celtic and Protestant: the Irish, the Scots, and the Welsh. They were definitely a poor second and were despised by some of the English as being insufferably second-rate, almost on a par with the way Germans viewed the Slavs prior to World War II. Next came the grand English Catholic families, whose taint of Popery rendered them unacceptable for marital purposes, even though they possessed some of the oldest names and grandest titles in the Aristocracy. 'Wogs', wags used to say, 'start at Calais'; and the prejudice behind this adage was borne out by the ranking of Continentals behind the English Catholics in the pecking order. In the late eighteenth and early nineteenth centuries, they had even been frequently categorized as 'coloured' though they were no more so than their Anglo-Saxon counterparts. Although the Protestant Germans had been exempt from such contemptuousness prior to the Great War, by the time Hitler did away with himself in that bunker beneath the Berlin Chancellery in 1945, not even their Protestant religion or their Anglo-Saxon genes could spare the Germans from being lumped with, if not below, Catholic Continentals – irrespective of how many schlosses or titles they had. Indeed, it was better to be a Catholic Polish Count of no account, with neither country nor estate, than to be a Protestant German Furst, unless he had three palaces and a large slice of the Black Forest. The Americans then got a tenuous look-in along with the Semites, the Jews rating above the Arabs, all of whom had to have a lot of money to be even considered socially, the thinking being that, since they couldn't possibly have background, they had to be rich. After them came the Indian maharajahs and Pakistani nawabs, whose socially rich backgrounds could not be denied, though these were ignored, their thrones and jewels being the only things that made them acceptable socially. As for those of African descent, they were tolerated rather than accepted, though only if they too could come up with vast amounts of money and the patina of an English gentleman and weren't too dark. It is no exaggeration to say that racism reigned supreme along with the English.

Because it wasn't possible in those days to become a part of Society except through birth, stardom or a propitious and enduring marriage, Society's very inaccessibility rendered it even more glamorous and desirable to outsiders than it was to insiders. There was one unwelcome side-effect to the fact that admission into these hallowed confines was based upon birth, background and breeding rather than accomplishment. This was that social life was much more boring and colourless than it is today.

Any student of the *ancien régime* will know that ennui and boredom have always been problems amongst élites throughout the world. This is because few men and no women worked. This would remain a real problem in privileged circles until the end of the twentieth century, when it became acceptable for all classes of people to work. Certainly in Gloria's youth, when the rhythm of life had still not changed from the eighteenth century, and there was no need for people like her to work for a living – and the obligation to keep house did not exist, owing to the army of servants maintaining it – ladies were free to do whatever they felt like doing – as long as it did not breach Society's unwritten codes of conduct. Although some took the illicit route and spiced up their lives with affairs, the only really acceptable form of occupation open to them was socializing.

While Society events were frequently written up in the media as glamorous and exciting affairs, I can vividly remember, as a teenager, wanting to scream from boredom, not only in Jamaica but also in the most elevated social circles in New York, where one went from one social occasion to another and everyone, who had seen everyone else three times that week, talked about nothing, because all subjects of conversation had long ago been exhausted owing to the same people being present day after day and night after night. Any new faces had no more conversation and were no more interesting than the old faces, because they too were cut from the same cloth and had the same attitudes, prejudices and values. To a miserable extent, A was interchangeable with B socially, and what a bore it was. That no longer happens, thank goodness, because few occasions are so exclusively Society-laden that there aren't a plethora of newcomers who might not know which fork to pick up first or how to make a proper introduction or indeed what topics of conversation to avoid or how to shock acceptably, but who at least bring two most welcome elements to the table: novelty and interest. I cannot tell you what a joy it is to sit beside some *arriviste* at dinner who talks about all the things better bred people shy away from. Even when they are not particularly interesting, the mere fact that they have expanded the boundaries makes conversation so much more interesting. The satisfaction one derives is akin to eating a substantial meal of meat and potatoes after a protracted diet of *boeuf bouillon*.

Of course, people who have always had to strive and struggle financially might consider a socialite's boredom, which results from the restrictive practices of her social world, somehow undeserving of sympathy. I do not. This is not just because I have experienced it personally, but because I have seen what a pernicious effect it can have on people. Boredom, believe me, is enervating. Whether the wasteland is in a poor project in Harlem or a rundown housing estate in Manchester or a social exchange that is stultifying to the point of ennui, a wasteland is a wasteland; and the boredom and ennui that result from it are equally impoverishing to the person suffering from them. I have had several decades to think about the realities of that fact, if only because boredom and ennui were a part of my mother's problem, and I made absolutely sure from an early age that they would not be a part of mine.

For all its limitations, Gloria was not about to give up her treasured social position. She was too canny to underestimate its value and she relished the glory it shone down upon her. In fairness, she also earned enough of that glory to appreciate the fruit of her labour. It was she who parlayed Michael's money and her social cachet into something exceptional. It was she who used her wit, energy, looks and background to make herself into a renowned hostess and celebrated beauty. Without her, they would have been just another attractive couple where the woman had looks and breeding and the man had looks and money. Instead she turned them into one of the most socially desirable couples of the time.

Gloria delighted in being 'special' and relished being celebrated socially. It was a bargaining chip, and believe me, she used it – not always positively – with everyone, even with her parents, her sister, her uncles, aunts and cousins, and especially with my father and his family. I can remember as a small child being aware that she considered herself much better than my father by virtue of being a Society figure by right, while he was one only through marrying her.

Michael's strength, however, was that he wasn't a snob and had no interest in shining within the narrow confines of that gilded world, though he never stood in his wife's way of doing so. He was a pragmatic man, and I have no doubt he appreciated that her social stature enhanced his own status in the eyes of those who mattered to him. Although these were not Society figures, they were serious players in the commercial life of the country and included his fellow businessmen, industrialists, family and friends. Certainly, having a wife who was frequently written up in the social columns and regarded as being one of the most fashionable, beautiful socialites of the day did neither his ego nor his worldly stock any harm.

Because Michael cared nothing about mixing in Society, Gloria was obliged to cast a wider net socially than she would otherwise have done. Like the wives of all prosperous men, she also knew she had better keep her husband happy or a hundred other women would jump into her shoes if she vacated them. This forced her to associate with people from a variety of walks of life. Indeed, as a result of Michael's influence, the world in which we children were brought up was far more in keeping with the world of today than that of the 1950s and 1960s. Certainly, there were the Society friends, but there were also Jewish garment manufacturers from New York, black professionals and politicians, representatives of all the important mercantile and industrial families, even priests. Indeed our circle welcomed anyone who either parent liked or found interesting, the one proviso being that they had the social skills to fit in.

Michael and Gloria had a justifiably deserved reputation for hospitality. Jamaica in its heyday had a tradition of dropping in uninvited, at which point you would be offered lunch, tea, dinner or drinks, depending on what was appropriate for the time of day. Michael and Gloria – Gloria really, Michael being as incidental to the proceedings as any occasional visitor – took it that step further. Word clearly spread among their friends and relations that they would always be accorded a warm welcome, together with an interesting time and a generous helping of food, drink and cigarettes. I can remember few evenings which were not shared with numerous uninvited guests. These ranged from people like Attorney General Victor Grant, through Chief of Staff of the Army Rudolph Green, to sundry relations and friends. An ordinary evening at home was having two extra for dinner, and there was nothing exceptional about having four or six extra uninvited guests.

During the day, while Michael was at work, Gloria was either out visiting friends and relations, attending one of the social functions that were such a feature of pre-feminist social life, gardening (which involved sitting down on a stool in the shade under a tree and ordering about Owen, the head gardener, or Leslie, the under-gardener, who did the actual work) or receiving whomever dropped in. Dropping in during the day, however, was not such a feature of life as dropping in during the evening. The friends who came for a swim or lunch or to *labrish* – that splendidly old-fashioned Jamaican word which meant chitchat about non-malicious matters – were frequently asked to do so by Gloria herself.

Michael and Gloria drew their friends from a variety of sources. First, there was a large pool of cousins and siblings with whom they were friendly. They were both from large families, and most of them were sociable. Michael was one of ten children and the nephew of three brothers, each of whom had had between eight and fifteen children apiece. Although not close to either his elder brother or eldest sister, he saw his eldest brother and all but two of his other sisters at least once or twice a week. He was also close to several of his first cousins, especially four of the sons of his uncle Tewfik, who were renowned 'turfites'.

Though one of only two children, Gloria had parents who were one of nine and fourteen children respectively. While she had only two first cousins on the paternal side, she had dozens of first cousins on the maternal side, as well as a variety of second cousins, several of whom she socialized with frequently.

Looking back, I can see that the socializing Gloria did with her side of the family was considerably more structured than that which she did with Michael's. This was partly a cultural difference, because Gloria's family were European in origin while Michael's were Lebanese and Russian; and if there is one thing that Middle Easterners take seriously, it is their tradition of hospitality. While her Brooks cousins had their large New Year's Eve party every year for the adults, and we were often taken to the children's parties of our cousins, and while various of her aunts, uncles and cousins would drop in occasionally – or she would drop in on them – and she and her parents and sister were in and out of one another's houses constantly, it is fair to say that the everyday socializing was largely done with Michael's brother Solomon and his extended family.

At least once or twice a week, there would be a poker game at our house or one of the other Ziadie houses. These would usually begin after dinner and last for several hours. They seldom took place without the presence of at least a brace of Seagas, another Lebanese family with whom they were very friendly which would produce a prime minister. Occasionally, Uncle Solomon would vary the game and have poker on the front veranda and blackjack on the back and occasionally even roulette, though I never saw anyone else do that but him. Although these games involved stakes, they were basically for fun, not to break anyone's bank, so the winnings and losses were never so large that they became destructive.

Where losses were less easily regulated was at the racetrack. The Ziadies were Jamaica's leading racing family and took the sport seriously. No race meeting ever took place at Knutsford Park, which was where the beautiful old English-style racecourse was located in what is now New Kingston, prior to 1960, or thereafter at Caymanas Park, the Americanized grandstand on the Caymanas Estate near Spanish Town, the old capital of Jamaica, without a liberal sprinkling of what was then a vast, cohesive family. Every Saturday afternoon Gloria could be seen sitting in the box marked 'Mrs M Ziadie' which she shared with Mrs Millard Ziadie, who lived in Jamaica while her husband lived in Venezuela, where he was that country's leading racehorse trainer. Gloria and Helen had a double bond: they were married to first cousins who were close friends, and they themselves had been close friends from childhood. Indeed, my mother chose to be married on September 11 1946 so that she could go to Helen's twenty-first birthday party on September 10.

Chapter Three

You would imagine that a woman who had as much as Gloria would have been satisfied. But you would be wrong.

I was born when my mother was three months shy of twenty-two, and my father nearly thirty-three. They had been married for two years and eleven months and already had a son, Michael Jr., who was born exactly a week after Gloria's twentieth birthday in 1947. According to Gloria's sister Marjorie and her mother Maisie, she made it abundantly clear to one and all that she preferred me to Mickey from soon after I was born. On the surface, this might have been surprising, because I was born with a birth defect and Mickey – as my elder brother was called to differentiate him from his father – was not only perfect and the first-born child as well as a son to boot, but he was also the first-born grandchild of his mother's parents and therefore the first child in our generation. Gloria's paternal family, the Smedmores, were notoriously unproductive after her grandparents produced nine children: a fact that would result in the name dying out with Gloria's death. Mickey was therefore the first Smedmore descendent of his generation. His arrival was evidently greeted with all the enthusiasm, excitement and pride that a family as emotionally expressive as ours had at their command. Thereafter he was treated very much like a little prince and the heir apparent to a minor dynasty.

Gloria, of course, came in for congratulations from all quarters for having produced this marvellous specimen of humanity known as an heir. Her expected reaction should have been delight in the attention his birth and babyhood generated. However, she displayed impatience and annoyance with the baby rather than love. My father's first cousin Toni remembers her feeding Mickey when he was about nine months old and shoving the food down his throat with such force that, when he would not eat it quickly enough to satisfy her requirements, he started to howl and had to be taken away by his nurse.

It has to be said in her defence that Gloria might well have had a partial excuse for her callous behaviour. While Toni certainly picked up on the underlying cruelty which was a feature of our mother's personality – even though she usually took care to conceal it from all except her innermost circle, namely her husband, children, parents, and sibling, as well, of course, as her staff – Gloria also had little experience in feeding any of her children once they were weaned after a few weeks of breast-feeding. She would only have been feeding Mickey to make a show of what an attentive mother she was when, in fact, she was anything but.

Gloria, it has to be said, was the consummate actress, very adept at playing to audiences. When the Ziadie, Smedmore and Burke relations or the friends were not around, she abandoned us to the nursery staff and went about her business as if she were childless.

The regimen for her four children varied not a jot from the birth of Mickey in 1947 to Kitty in 1955. As soon as Gloria was released from Nuttall Hospital, where we were born in the very building that had once been the Burke family great-house of Newington a century before, she turned us over to a maternity nurse called Starridge. It was Starridge who cared for us for the first few weeks of our lives, maternity nurses then being an absolute requirement for the mother of a newly born baby. 'It', as all babies were termed in such circles, could then be properly attended to while the mother recovered from the birth and the regular nurse was broken in or if she were already an employee, got used to 'it'. Starridge also taught Gloria to breastfeed, something she did for the first four or so weeks of the lives of all her children (Gloria couldn't have breastfeeding interrupt her social life) and incredibly, how to hold a baby. Maisie did not know how to hold babies, despite having had two children of her own: a fact I would learn when I was twenty-two and tried to hand her great-grandson Andrew to her. There was therefore no prospect of Gloria learning such maternal tasks from her own mother.

I remember Starridge well for one particular reason. She took dinner with Daddy and Mummy and was actually at the table with them when I, who always had a strongly developed maternal streak, took Libby out of her crib and, cradling her in my arms, walked with her into the breakfast porch, as we called the family dining room. Starridge and my parents nearly had a heart attack lest all two years and four months of little me should drop the new baby. The dramatics of the incident have always stayed with me, and, as I grew older, so did the relevance of Starridge dining *en famille*, for regular nurses did not eat at the same table as their employers. But maternity nurses, who were not of the servant class, did, so long as there was no formal dinner party in progress.

Starridge always left after four weeks, at which point breastfeeding was terminated and we were turned over to our regular nurses. These were akin to what is now called nannies, but in our childhood they were still referred to as nurses. They usually had some nursing training, as well as experience in being 'nannies'.

It was our nurses who gave us our bottles once we were off the breast or fed us baby food after we were weaned off the bottle. They bathed us, played with us and took care of us, and I can vividly remember as a four-year-old that Mickey, Libby and I – who were four years apart *in toto* – had two nurses between the three of us until shortly before our baby sister Kitty was born, at which point the nursery staff was reduced to one. Gloria deemed it unnecessary to have two nurses when the three elder children ranged in age from four to eight.

'The house was crawling with servants,' she reminisced years later. 'Between the housemaid, cook, butler, laundress and nannies – not to mention the two gardeners and the chauffeur – you couldn't breathe for servants. There were eight in all. The more servants you have, the more confusion. They will insist on fighting and squabbling and setting each other up against their employer, so that they can gain an ascendant position over the servant they're competing with – and if you don't watch out sharply, once they've succeeded in getting their competitor fired, they then turn their talent for scheming against their mistress as well, until they're ruling the roost and you're in the subservient position. Experience has taught me that the fewer servants one has, the more peaceable a household is.'

Being the eldest child, Mickey was something of a special case. This showed up in a multitude of ways, including who his nurse was. Nana Alice was a legendary figure in the Burke family. Her mother had been a slave of the family and, in the post-slave tradition then prevalent in the former slave-owning colonies, had only ever worked for the Burkes. By the time Mickey was born, she was a very old woman. Having nursed Maisie's youngest siblings, as well as her two daughters Marjorie and Gloria, and various other Burke progeny of my aunt and mother's generation, Nana Alice wanted to fulfil the ambition of nursing the third generation. So, in keeping with the *noblesse oblige* that was one of the guiding precepts by which people like Gloria lived their lives, she obliged her old nurse by employing her.

'Shortly after Starridge left,' Gloria was fond of reminiscing dramatically, 'I walked onto the back veranda, and what did I see but Nana Alice, who had the baby in her arms rocking it back and forth, nearly dropped it onto the marble tiles. I flew across the room, grabbed it out of her arms and promptly employed a young nursemaid to nurse both Mickey and Nana Alice.'

Mickey's arrival was certainly a big event in Gloria's family, especially with her mother and sister. My sisters and I grew up with the full knowledge that Mickey was streets ahead of us where Grandma and Auntie were concerned, but that was not something that bothered any of us so far as I am aware. He was loved, indeed adored, by both Marjorie and Maisie. Maisie couldn't ever refer to him in a normal tone of voice. The way she said 'Mickey' or 'my grandson' was so imbued with passion that we children used to laugh about it amongst ourselves and with her. Without exaggeration, she could not refer to him without almost lifting off her chair with passion. Marjorie also 'worshipped Mickey', as she herself put it. 'My son', as she called her nephew, was fated to remain on his throne as the divine ruler of her heart until his death nine years before her own. She never did have any children of her own, and even her husbands knew that 'there is no one on earth I love anywhere near as much as Mickey. I have worshipped the ground he walked on from before he could even crawl, from the moment of his birth.' Even after his death, she claimed to love him more than anyone else.

The overt adoration of Gloria's mother and sister for her son was, in my view, the main reason she took against Mickey. His very existence was causing too much of a stir and thereby stealing some of the thunder that she undoubtly felt was rightfully hers. The one thing Gloria could not abide, throughout the seventy-seven years of her life, was sharing attention with any other human being. The only time I ever saw her permit anyone else to have any attention was when it was to her personal advantage.

Because Mickey was two years older than me, I don't remember much about his upbringing until he was about six. Thereafter, my memories are of one long assault course that my unfortunate brother had to endure. Gloria was very keen on 'discipline', and she reserved that right for herself, at least at that stage of our lives. Mickey was constantly being flogged for doing absolutely nothing at all. If he didn't answer a question in exactly the tone of voice Gloria required at that particular moment – and you had to judge her mood very accurately, for what applied yesterday did not necessarily apply today. Indeed, what applied yesterday usually didn't apply today, for how else could she have you on the hop unless she constantly shifted the boundaries, thereby making you culpable not according to rhyme or reason but according to her whim? She would press the buzzer and ring for one of the two gardeners, Owen and Denzil, who would later on be replaced by Leslie, to 'get a switch.' They would then have to go into the garden, pick a fern leaf that was long enough and thick enough so that, after being shorn of its leaves, it would provide a strong and sharp instrument of punishment to be applied to Mickey's bottom with maximum painfulness.

Although Mickey was the usual recipient of Gloria's mania for 'discipline', each of us children had on occasion to endure the torment that switching involved. You had to stand up, absolutely still, for the ten or so minutes it took Owen or Denzil to be called, go outside, then pick and deliver the switch. The anticipation of what was coming was, believe me, every bit as painful as the switching itself, which was agony. The sharp stem of the fern would cut into your skin, stinging like you wouldn't believe.

Sometimes, Gloria felt that discipline required an even more painful punishment. At times like those, she would snarl, again mostly to Mickey: 'Go and get your father's belt.' This, of course, was a way of heightening the torture, for, in forcing her victim to fetch the instrument of his own punishment, she was knowingly increasing the distress he would suffer. If he refused to do so, he would be in for an even worse beating than he would have to suffer by bowing to his mother's will.

When Mickey cooperated in his beatings, she would lash away for all it was worth on his bottom. If he squirmed, she would beat him some more until he stopped squirming. She inevitably left huge welts where Daddy's leather belt had made contact with Mickey's young flesh. Sometimes, she would get carried away and actually draw blood, and I remember on one occasion she crossed the Rubicon and actually beat him with the metal buckle of the belt so badly that he looked as if he had been scourged prior to crucifixion, his back and bottom covered in torn flesh.

Although our father seldom involved himself in the disciplinary actions meted out by Gloria, when he came home after that scourging, even he could see that she had gone too far.

'Are you mad, woman?' I remember him saying angrily. 'You can't beat a child like that.'

'He was stinkingly rude to me, and he has to learn to have respect,' she replied as coolly as if she were commenting on the weather.

This time, however, the normally compliant Michael was having none of it. He had a quick and fearsome temper – at least, fearsome to everyone except Gloria.

'You will never beat any of my children like that ever again,' he rumbled like the voice of God, as one of our friends once described his deep voice. 'If you do, you will live to regret it. Do I make myself clear? You're nothing but a damned lunatic.'

I have no doubt that Michael felt some sympathy for his son, for he really was not a hardhearted person. He would also have known that this incident could not be kept secret, and that knowledge of it would slip out into Gloria's inner family-circle, as so many of her other abuses of Mickey had already done.

Because our father was away at work all day, and these incidents seldom took place when he was present, Gloria could – and did – complain that Mickey was a recalcitrant child who took delight in giving her a hard time. When she was not beating him for some minor infraction, she would entrap him verbally.

Gloria was predictable – as her niece by marriage, Cissy, observed – in everything except the triggers that would set her off. In a set tableau she would ask Mickey something that seemed innocent. He would reply nomally.

'I will not have you speaking to me in that tone of voice,' she would lash out. '*I* rule this roost,' she would say, emphasizing the 'I' to drive home the point of who was the dictator. 'If you don't like the way things are run here, get out.'

Mickey would then try to explain that he had not meant anything untoward or disrespectful.

'I will not have you denying the undeniable. You were purposely impertinent.'

'I really didn't mean to be, Mummy,' he would reply.

'How dare you contradict me? If *I* say you were being wilfully impertinent, you were being impertinent. You are a child, and I will not tolerate you arguing with me.'

'I didn't mean to,' he would say, trying to make things better but making them worse. The one thing Gloria could not cope with was anyone who disagreed with her. She had to be right at all times.

'You are being stinkingly impertinent,' she would rasp, the word 'stinkingly' being an indication that one had crossed the invisible line. '*I* have stated that you were being impertinent. If I say that you intended to be, you intended to be. I have had quite enough of your stinking impertinence. This is my house. *I* rule this roost. The great Mickey does not. You can pack your bags and leave right now,' she would add, using the dismissive tone of voice she employed when firing one of the servants, who would be left in no doubt that they were low and insignificant compared with the great Gloria.

'Please Mummy, I really didn't mean to,' Mickey would implore, his face a picture of genuine innocence and miscomprehension.

'Get out. Get out right now,' she would order, her eyes ablaze with fury.

This scenario was played out, time and again, with precious little variation until his teenage years. The little boy would be made to walk down to his grandmother or his aunt's house, several miles away, usually in the hot sun, though sometimes in the pouring rain as well. And, believe me, a tropical downpour is not something that anyone from the temperate world can imagine unless they have seen it. It is like thousands of buckets of water being poured on you at once for the duration of the downpour, in which visibility might be all of five feet in front of you.

It would never have occurred to Gloria to give her son taxi or even bus fare for the journey. Doubtless, in her mind, part of the punishment was that his little legs would have to be used to cover a distance that would take him well over an hour. Whether it occurred to her that lightning might strike and kill him is also not something that I know. I *do* know, however, that I would never allow my children outside in a tropical downpour, with the dangers that lightning and poor visibility can cause to life or limb.

At times like these, Grandma and Auntie would happily take Mickey in for days, sometimes weeks, at a time. To the best of my recollection, our father never once put his foot down to stop this nonsense. Whenever Maisie and Marjorie tried to intercede, Gloria would haughtily declare: 'He is my child. *I* gave birth to him and *I* will discipline him. If it weren't for the both of you filling his head with a lot of nonsense of how wonderful he is, *I* wouldn't have to put up with his stinking impertinence. It's all your fault. You've spoiled him rotten. It's your interference that has caused these problems. But he's *my* child, and there's not a damn thing you can do about that.'

At times like these, she would slam down the telephone on her mother and sister, march outside to the back or front veranda, depending on the time of day, and begin fulminating against them, saying over and over again that they were responsible for Mickey's bad behaviour. If there was no one else present to hear the tirade, I would have to listen to it. When Daddy came home from work, she would replay that tape, blaming all her problems with Mickey on Maisie and Marjorie.

Her father Lucius Smedmore invariably popped around two or three evenings a week. Nothing ever interrupted these visits, not even the problems with Mickey or the fact that relations would be strained between her and his wife and other daughter while Mickey was being 'harboured', as she used to put it, at their houses. Gloria would then replay the tape yet again of how it was their 'interference' that was causing her the problems.

As Lucius lived with Maisie until Mickey was eight and with Marjorie thereafter, there is no doubt that he had also got the other side of the story from Mickey, Grandma and Auntie before coming up to our house.

I cannot recall him remonstrating with Gloria even once. If he did, it was never within my earshot. Nevertheless, he always enjoyed a happy and close relationship with his grandson, so clearly he cannot have actually believed that Mickey was the tearaway that Gloria painted him. In fact, Mickey was an exemplary student at both his schools, having been made a monitor at De Cartaret Preparatory School and a prefect at Jamaica College. To one and all, save his mother, he was accepted as being a quiet, polite, well-mannered and well-behaved child.

Looking back, I suspect that Grandpa and Daddy were both weak men who had decided that surrender was an easier course of action with Gloria than resistance. Since Mickey did not get into trouble at school or elsewhere, they simply ignored what was going on at home.

My memory of Mickey's childhood is not only of the frequency with which he was chucked out and had to seek refuge with our grandmother and aunt, but also of the many other occasions upon which he 'ran away' to them. They lived a five-minute walk from each other; and the battle-scarred Mickey, well used to treading the miles to their houses whenever Mummy forced him to walk there, developed a tolerance for midday sun and pouring rain that truly astonished me, who loathed walking in the heat and wet. But physical discomfort never once deterred my brother.

Sometimes Mickey would leave, not because he had been told to, but because Gloria had ordered him to fetch the belt, and knowing what was coming, he sought to avoid the inevitable. Other times, it was because he had been beaten for no reason at all. Once it was even because Gloria locked him in our father's clothes cupboard – again for some nonsense infraction of her ever-more increasingly bizarre and intricate injunctions – then forgot him for hours.

At times like these, until things had calmed down, Grandma and Auntie would give Mickey the refuge that they always provided when he was chucked out of the house by Gloria. On these occasions, Daddy usually agreed that he could stay with them for a few days; and Gloria, who would shield herself behind his decision, would graciously 'allow' it, presenting herself as the noble victim of an ill-behaved child, an interfering mother and sister, and a Solomonian husband. Over and over again, she would complain bitterly about Marjorie and Maisie's 'interference' and always shift responsibility for Mickey's 'bad behaviour' on to the fact that her sister and mother 'spoil him rotten'. I was fully aware that she wanted my sympathy, and I suppose, looking back on it, that I was sufficiently in her thrall to provide her with it, though not so much that I actually ever felt that Mickey was in the wrong. For that I never did feel.

After one of Mickey's stays with our grandmother or aunt, he would return home to a few days' peace, so I suppose he did enjoy some slight benefit from 'running away'. Then the abuse would begin all over again. Initially, this always took a verbal form, for that is how Gloria would lay the ground before escalating to whatever heights she deemed desirable. Because she did not usually lose her temper and rant and rave or indeed raise her voice, her abusiveness was rarely noticed by onlookers, despite being as destructive as if it had been louder.

Everyone who knew her agreed that she had one of the strongest, most forceful and determined personalities of anyone you could meet. In the course of a long and varied life, in which I have met everyone from Pope John Paul II and the Queen of England to notorious criminals whom my brother's law firm represented such as the Mitcham Rapist, I can assure you that I have never met anyone who had a stronger personality than my mother. The word 'potent' could have been invented to describe her. The fact that this potency was made more palatable by charm and an aura of fun did not lessen it, especially as it was one of her favourite tricks, as Cissy said, 'to throw you zingers even as she was supposed to be having a good time with you. You wouldn't be able to put your finger on why or sometimes even how she had stung you. But you knew you'd been stung. Oh, did you know you'd been stung!'

Gloria would employ this tactic against Mickey. Then she would escalate it with sarcasm. Because she had wit and articulation, she could stop even self-confident and worldly adults in their tracks, much less young children. She would confine her acid at a 'civilized' tone of voice, and onlookers would pass it off as irritability or an allusion they knew nothing about and did not wish to pass judgement upon, thereby allowing her to get away with it.

This was also where her charm and sense of fun came to her rescue. Even at the moment she was being cruel or vicious, people were frequently so amused by her, or so unused to someone whose façade so contradicted their underlying message, that they would miss the sting in the tail. Certainly, observing her in action taught me at an early age that too many people 'buy the lie', for they fail to make the connection between what they see on the surface and what they should be sensing beneath it.

Gloria's specialty was that haughty way of silencing people with the disparaging word or dismissive sneer. Virtually nothing Mickey said or did was ever greeted by anything but the most withering comment from his mother. And she did not, I can assure you, steer away from silencing him in public any more than she did in private.

Mickey, being a quiet and thoughtful child, would seldom speak without thinking. One would have imagined that that was an attribute which any parent would cultivate. Not Gloria. Sometime when he was around ten, she raised a laugh at his expense when she quipped, 'Hamlet, oh Hamlet, why doth thou procrastinate so much?' Never one to let a good line go to waste, she thereafter continued to mockingly jump into the gap between his thought and his words, repeating the same line, year in, year out, and, in so doing, portraying herself as the long-suffering mother of a dim-witted procrastinator.

If Mickey had not even a moment's respite from his mother's regimen, he was not alone in that. None of the rest of us did either. Even I, who was shielded by the umbrella of being her favourite, had to be instantly available as and when she required. I would also have to be on my guard at all times, delivering the goods she required in the form of attention, approbation and cooperation. I remember once, when I was six years old and we were summering in Boscobel beside Ian Fleming's house Goldeneye, she asked me to walk up to the house to get her cigarettes, which she had forgotten to take down to the beach. Now the beach, which was carved out of rock on a cliff that rose sharply out of the sea for well over a hundred feet, had only one access point to the house. This was up steep and winding steps that had been cut into the rock-face. There were about two hundred steps in all, quite a trip for a six-year-old child.

I willingly set off to fetch her cigarettes. Up and up I trudged until I reached the house. I located the cigarettes and, noticing that she had a lighter beside them as well, brought that down too. I can still see her face as I handed them to her. Something flashed behind her eyes when she saw the lighter, for which she had not asked me.

'I didn't ask you to bring the lighter, child,' she said in her most acid tone. 'Lighters don't work properly in the wind. Every fool knows that. Go and get me some matches.'

I had the impression then that she was deliberately showing off her power over me to the friend who was with her. Fifty-three years later, I am even more convinced of how right I was than at the age of six.

Even when Gloria wasn't present, there was no escape from her dictates. Her eyes and ears were operational through the medium of the servants. They had strict instructions to report any infraction of her rules that we had committed in her absence, under pain of dismissal if she discovered that we had done something they had tried to keep from her. As the rules covered just about every aspect of our conduct, whenever she returned home from her socializing and partying, the servants would be there waiting with a long list of nonsense infractions covering everything from not saying 'please' and 'thank you' to snapping at each other. As a result, there was always something she could 'get' us for if she so desired – and while she sometimes didn't want to ruin her mood with 'disciplining' us and would ignore the servant's reports, on other occasions she was so eager to discipline us that she would announce, 'Don't even bother to tell me what they did,' before launching into a beating with such classic comments as 'I don't need to know what you did. I know you did something, and that's what you're being disciplined for.'

It is no exaggeration to say that the household was run along militaristic lines. Gloria was the Field Marshal and everyone else, Michael included, was of infinitely inferior rank. Anyone who stepped out of line could, depending upon her mood, be penalized. The status of us children, though superior to the servants, allowed us as little freedom as they had. As far as Gloria was concerned, servants were little better than slaves who were paid a minimal amount of money each week to wait upon her pleasure. They could make no noise when working. Even when they were washing up pots and pans in the kitchen, they had to do so in such a way that she couldn't hear the sounds of their labour. They were never allowed to speak to one another in her presence or within her earshot. If they spoke to each other, they had to do so quietly so that she could *never* overhear them. If they dared to raise their voices to even soft conversational levels, and she happened to be passing by while they were doing so, she would rasp, 'Scream down the house for the whole neighbourhood to hear' or, using the old Jamaican version for the more contemporary n-word: 'This is not a *nayger* crawl.' Occasionally she would even eavesdrop. God help them then if they had said anything that displeased her, for they would be dismissed instantly.

'Discipline, discipline,' was a refrain Gloria loved to trill, and I mean trill literally. She would sing the word as if she were Joan Sutherland on the stage of the Metropolitan Opera in New York, clearly enjoying the power she had over us as much as La Divina enjoyed reaching the rafters of the great concert halls of the world. Her purpose and message could not have been clearer. Sometimes she would even spell it out, not that we ever needed to hear the words to get the message: 'I have the whip and the whip hand. You'd better do as I say, or you're in for it. There's only one way, and it's my way.'

I grew to dread hearing the word 'discipline' pass her lips, for I could sense the sadism that lay behind what others misinterpreted as genuine correction. To me, the word 'discipline' symbolized the jackboot on the head of the victim. I also knew that Gloria's message also contained another warning: resist and things will be worse, succumb and life will be relatively easier.

I am sure that one of the reasons why I became Gloria's favourite was that I was the most obliging of her children. Mickey, on the other hand, had the belief in his own self-worth that all little princes possess. While any normal mother would have relished that quality in him, Gloria was not about to allow any child of hers the right to an opinion or even a mood that did not absolutely accord with her dictat that she was the centre of the universe as well as the only perfect person within it, and everyone must at all times acknowledge that and tailor themselves to her needs. To her, his more overt independence was not something that she should encourage. Rather, it was something she must crush. 'I gave you life, and you must give me everything else,' she would frequently say to us when we were older, and that, I fear, was the truth rearing its ugly head. As far as she was concerned, we had no right to existence save as candy jars for her to dip into as and when she felt the urge.

Gloria's world-view was really very simple. Everyone existed for her own delectation or convenience. 'The only person who has any rights in this house is me,' she used to say to us children, to our father and to the servants; and that bald statement pretty much summed up her philosophy.

In September 1967, she provided me with an explanation of sorts for why she had mistreated Mickey the way she did. We were in New York and she had been telling me how I had always been her favourite child.

'I couldn't stand Mickey from before he was born,' she suddenly said. 'While I was pregnant with him, I discovered your father was having an affair. We had the most terrible row, and I left him and returned to Mama's house. But he begged and pleaded with me to return, and I did.'

'What did Mickey have to do with that?' I said, failing to see the connection she was seeking to establish between that poor unloved baby and Daddy's philandering.

'I was pregnant with *him*,' she spat, indicating that she blamed his very existence for having provided Daddy with an incentive to stray.

I felt my blood run cold for my brother's sake, and of course never told him what she had said, because it would only have hurt him. But it provided an explanation of sorts for her attitude towards him, which, from my earliest memory, had been antagonistic in the extreme.

As I write this, I can see that her comments in New York might have contained a kernel of truth, but they were by no means the sole reason why she took against her first-born so violently. Although she sought to blame her rejection of him upon his very existence snatching away her husband's attention, I believe that what infuriated her with him and triggered her antipathy towards him was that he stole the attention and approbation that Grandma and Auntie – and indeed all her thrilled relations who had cooed and clucked so avidly over her production of the little prince – had previously reserved for her. She was not only an attention-seeker but also intensely jealous. The fact that she lost her antipathy for him when he became an adult supports this contention. She had by then put distance between herself and her family; and, no longer caring about their opinions to the extent she had when she was younger, she did not mind anymore that Mickey had eclipsed her in their eyes.

I know for a fact that Gloria never fully faced the reality of how or why she felt the way she did about her only son. Insight was a virtue she did not possess, as I would discover towards the end of her life. She was not prepared to consider, even as a remote possibility, the hypothesis that she might have been anything less than a perfect being who was perpetually worthy of only admiration, approbation and attention. The fact that we are all flawed and imperfect, that our motives are mixed even at the moment of our most noble acts, that we are insufficient even when we are functioning at our fullest capacities, was not something she could ever countenance as applying to herself, though she effortlessly made the leap where everyone else was concerned.

Until Mickey's advent, Gloria had been the undisputed star of her family's show. 'Aunt May made it clear that the sun shone on Gloria,' her cousin Joy would later reveal. 'I remember when Marjorie was getting married – I was her chief bridesmaid – and she was dressed and ready to leave for the church with Uncle Lucius. Your mother arrived to see how Marjorie looked. And what did Aunt May do? Instead of telling Marjorie how lovely she looked – for she did look lovely – she raved about how beautiful and elegant Gloria was. It was Gloria's hat this, Gloria's hair that, how wonderful her clothes were, on and on and on. I could hardly believe it. I know Aunt May didn't intend to hurt Marjorie, and your aunt was never the great beauty your mother was, but I was nevertheless astonished that she could be so tactless.'

Gloria had, in her mother's eyes at least, achieved the very pinnacle of worldly accomplishment. She was beautiful. She was well-dressed. She was glamorous. She had married money and a household name in their world. In so doing, she had not only succeeded in retaining her position in Society but had actually enhanced it.

There is no doubt in my mind that my grandmother, who was a wonderful woman but also a worldly one, enjoyed having such a successful daughter. Maisie was never one to hide her light, or the light of any of her descendants, under a bushel. If her comment about Mummy's appearance at Auntie's bridal leave-taking was tactless, it was also an accurate gauge of the way she felt. As Maisie was far more of a power in the family circle than her husband Lucius, it mattered less to all concerned that even he had by this time reconciled himself to Gloria's marriage and also took delight in her having become one of the country's leading socialites.

Early success can, of course, turn someone's head. In my opinion, any chance my mother had of growing into someone whose awareness extended past her own nose was undermined in her early twenties by her parents as well as by my father, who also – by her own account – 'spoiled' her. The dynamics of their relationship were set early. 'Uncle Mike adored Gloria,' his niece Audrey, recounted. 'Nothing was too good for her. Nothing was too much trouble for him to do for her. He deferred to her in all things. Whatever Gloria said, went. Whatever Gloria did was the way it should be done. For the first three years of their marriage, while they were building their house in Barbican, they lived with us at Daddy's house, so I got to know her well. They had their own wing, their own staff, their own everything. I saw a lot of her and grew to like her very much. I was a little girl of about ten. Daddy had custody of us after he and Mummy divorced. I can still see Gloria now: eating dinner as the butler – her butler – served her. She was so elegant and beautiful. Her manners were so impeccable. I thought what a great lady she was. And she was a great lady. Whatever her faults, she was the archetypal great lady.'

For the three years of her marriage that she spent living in her own wing of her brother-in-law's house, Gloria enjoyed the companionship of her husband's three nieces and nephew. Elaine, Cissy, Eddie and Audrey ranged in age from nine to fourteen. She struck up with all of them firm friendships that would weather many a storm. She was not much older than they and identified with them, for their fate as the children of an adulterous mother was one she had shared in part.

Both my grandmother Maisie and their mother Nellie had fallen in love with other men while married. Gloria was two years old when her mother's affair with Rafael Perez Guerrero ostensibly began, making her just a few years younger than Audrey had been when Aunt Nellie started her affair with Uncle Solomon's first cousin Vernon Ziadie. Maisie wanted to leave Lucius and marry Perez, but he refused to give her a divorce unless she relinquished custody of their two daughters, and she would not do so. She therefore moved her lover into the house, declared him to be the lodger – a *politesse* which fooled no one but nevertheless maintained enough decorum for everyone to turn a blind if knowing eye – and continued on her merry way until 1956, when she duly insisted Lucius file for divorce citing her adultery as the grounds. She was trying to do the decent thing, for he was deeply religious and she did not want him lying under oath for her sake. But what neither of them appreciated was that divorces were then heard in open court. The result was that all the tawdry details of Maisie's adultery were spread across the gutter press for all to see. 'Mama put a good face on it and pretended that she didn't mind,' Gloria recounted years after the event. 'But she did mind. She minded so much that she went down to Beeston Street, where her mother-in-law and brothers- and sisters-in-law lived, and bawled like a baby about how she hadn't intended to cause a scandal. And cause a scandal she did. It was terrible for Dada and your aunt and myself to have all that muck plastered across the pages of the *Star.* But what could we do but rise above it and act as if it didn't happen? But it did happen. And for that I have never been able to forgive your grandmother.'

Fortunately for Gloria, this scandal took place once she was already an adult. However, the scandal involving her Ziadie nephew and nieces by marriage took place while they were still children. It began when Uncle Solomon and Uncle Vernon got into a row which ended up in a serious physical brawl at the Carib Theatre – the country's leading theatre at the time – over the latter's involvement with the former's wife. All attempts to separate the cousins having failed, the police were called. They duly carted them off to the station until the two men cooled down. This was the start of a marital scandal that had the public both enthralled and horrified; not only was the Ziadie family one of the most successful and renowned mercantile families in the land and the leading racing family in a nation obsessed with horseracing, but Uncle Solomon was also known as the richest of the Ziadies and reputedly one of the richest men in Jamaica. The wealth and renown of the cousins, who shared not only the same surname but also the same woman, was guaranteed to scandalize.

Fortunately for my mother and cousins, the public's attention span is short where scandals are concerned, and once the sensation had died down, the children concerned resumed the even tenor of their lives. That is not to say, however, that they were unaffected by the drama or the events which caused it. Certainly, Gloria always maintained that her parents' eccentric marital arrangement caused her 'acute embarrassment' while she was growing up, but I don't believe it. Apart from the discomfort the unfavourable newspaper publicity generated at the time of the divorce, there is little doubt that she exaggerated her childhood feelings and created acute embarrassment where there was little or none just so she could get herself some of the sympathy she was always seeking.

Gloria was unfortunately prone to dramatizing everything to make herself the central figure in every storyline; and her choice of godfather for her firstborn illustrates the point aptly. It was she who decreed that Uncle Perez, then her mother's lover while Lucius and Maisie were still officially together, should become Mickey's godfather. It is highly unlikely that she would have awarded a position of such honour to someone whose very existence had made her suffer as much as she later claimed it did. Her own sister and cousins also remembered that, as a child, she was markedly fond of Perez and found ways to be in his company as much as she could engineer. This took a variety of forms, from 'helping him with his English' to partnering him at tennis on the family's grass court.

I suspect that Gloria's discovery of the 'acute embarrassment' late in life was more a way of distancing herself from Perez once she realized that people close to the family were openly questioning her paternity, rather than anything she actually experienced while growing up.

While there had doubtless been speculation as to whether Lucius was her biological father once Maisie moved Perez into the family home as the 'lodger' when Gloria was two, it had been not been deemed a fit subject for open conversation until the Sexual Revolution of the early 1960s opened it up for inspection. Thereafter, the touchy question of her true paternity seems to have been aired enough for not only her but all of us children to get wind of it by the time we were teenagers.

For her, this must have been an acutely embarrassing subject. A large part of her identity was caught up with being a Smedmore, her social superiority based upon being a scion of that English family. Although in Society there was never any disgrace in having a natural father as well as a legitimate one – the celebrated beauty Lady Diana Cooper was not actually the Duke of Rutland's biological daughter, nor was Lady Cosima Somerset the Marquis of Londonderry's, to name but two examples – there is no doubt in my mind that Gloria would never have willingly swapped being English for Spanish at a time when being English was infinitely more socially desirable than Spanish.

I was in my mid-twenties when I broached the subject with my grandmother. She said that there was no doubt in her mind that Gloria was Lucius's daughter. As Alex, Marjorie's second husband said, when I told him and Marjorie what her response had been, 'She would, wouldn't she?'

Marjorie sensibly made the point that it mattered not a jot who Gloria's biological father had been, for Lucius had regarded her as his own daughter and proved beyond the shadow of a doubt the extent of his acceptance by spoiling her rotten. All the Smedmores had also unreservedly accepted her and loved her as being one of their own and had indeed gone on to accept the four of us children as members of the family.

Thereafter, all of us in the family turned the doubts about Gloria's paternity into a huge joke, to such an extent that Alex once even wrote her a letter addressed to: 'Dona Gloria Perez Guerrero Burke de Ziadie'. To her credit, Gloria responded with a half-hearted laugh, even though she could never quite bring herself to think the whole thing a hoot the way the rest of us did.

Hereafter, in keeping with settled practice in such situations, whenever I refer to Gloria's father, I mean Lucius. If ever a man earned the right to being acknowledged as such, owing to the love and care he lavished upon a child, it is Lucius Dey Smedmore. He was also the most wonderful grandfather to us children, and fair play requires that his role be acknowledged as such.

I have no doubt that it was through her parents' *ménage-a-trois* that Gloria learned the lesson early in life about how easy it is to bend the rules and get what you want, as long as you are decorous enough to pay lip service to appearances. This disparity between appearance and reality is a state which Gloria exploited throughout her own life with a ruthlessness which was as damaging to her family's happiness as it was unconscionable. I have no doubt that the six-year-old child who was bright enough to see through her parents' charade was also astute enough to see how invaluable hypocrisy and insincerity could be as technical tools in manipulating people and their opinions, if you simply presented masks of innocence and sincerity appropriate to the occasion. It is difficult to see where else she could have acquired both her lack of scruple and the manipulative skills which were clearly developed from an early age. Her father was not manipulative and was a gentleman of the highest scruple; and her mother, who was actually a lady of tremendous honour and rectitude in all matters save the sexual, was also extremely scrupulous.

From whatever source Gloria got her libertine attitude towards truth, sincerity and scruple, she certainly had it in spades. I was aware of this fact from earliest childhood. I was born with an excellent memory and can remember back to the afternoon of my second birthday, when my birthday party had to be wound up early because Hurricane Charlie was hitting Jamaica. I vividly remember the morning after the hurricane and even more vividly, my mother at the age of twenty-four and twenty-five. I can still see her, walking up the passage past my bedroom on the way to her own, in her finery as she returned from a tea party in her hat, gloves and crinolined skirt heavily appliquéd. I close my eyes and see myself on her bed keeping her company as she dresses for one of the many parties she went to. She is sitting at her dressing table putting on her make-up while my father reads in another bedroom. She is chattering away animatedly. She looks beautiful and smells luxuriantly of the powder she uses to dust herself down with after each of the two or three baths a day she takes, powder which she then overlays with lashings of the Chanel Number 5, which for a time was her favourite scent. But what springs out at me even now is not how beautiful she was, or how deliciously she smelled, even though both are true, but of her animation. Her energy and her vivacity were truly remarkable, and people frequently remarked upon them.

Unlike many beautiful women who trade upon their looks – which

Gloria most definitely did – she also had a captivating personality. Upon reflection, I would go as far as saying that her personality was even more enchanting than her looks. These were stunning, believe me, for she was never photogenic, and every photograph taken is a pale imitation of the reality that was Gloria.

'Gloria had a great sense of humour,' Cissy remembered. 'I have fond memories of the days spent sitting around the swimming pool at Gloria and Uncle Mike's house, laughing about everything and nothing. She could make you laugh about anything. It didn't matter whether it was funny, serious, sad or terrible. When she wanted to make you laugh, she made you laugh. Sometimes she made you laugh so hard the tears would stream down your cheeks. She really had one of the best senses of humour I've ever known.' Madge Seaga, a friend of hers throughout her adult life, also remembered what fun she could be: 'She was always fun and ready for a good laugh. And she made everyone else laugh with her.'

As with many genuinely funny and fun-loving people, it wasn't so much what she said as how and when she said it that brought the smile to one's lips. She had vivacity, intensity and such tremendous charm that when she turned it on, she could envelop you in something which many people mistook for warmth but which actually was not. Rather, it was charisma: something that seduces and bedazzles and sweeps one up in its wake but is ultimately, for all its superficial attractiveness, considerably harsher and less comforting than warmth.

Superficially Gloria was appealing, and at no time more so than when she was in her twenties and thirties. I remember Helen Duncan, a socialite friend of hers, saying, 'Everyone loves Gloria.' In those days, 'everyone' did. One of the endearing things she did – and would continue to do throughout her life – was give a nickname to everyone and everything. In so doing, she made them all peculiarly her own. Some of her nicknames might have seemed meaningless or abstruse on first rendering, but with repetition they invariably assumed a character of their own and always raised a chuckle. One such example was the nickname she gave her great-nephew by marriage, who was always 'Oh Toothless One', possibly because he had a mouth full of perfect teeth in the days before the current mania for orthodonture when perfect smiles were a rarity. The Australian classical pianist Brian Michell, mild-mannered to a fault, was 'Brian the Lion'. Her son-in-law Ben, the archetypal

Alpha Male, was 'Ben the Hen'.

Gloria even managed to turn the use of the word 'no' into a medium for stamping her individuality onto occasions. Rather than decline anything, she would say: 'That will be when apples grow on a lilac tree.'

Of Gloria's four children, I profited the most from the winning aspects of her personality, for I was the one closest to her. She was the sort of person who thrived on company. If she did not have adult companionship, she would scoop me up and take me wherever it was she was going, as long as it was somewhere that children were accepted and acceptable, for she functioned by the Victorian maxim, which she repeated *ad nauseum*, that 'children are to be seen and not heard.

In those days before supermarkets, meat came from the butcher, chickens were a rarity few people could afford (but we had plenty, having incubators and a large chicken shed tucked away in the grounds at the back of the house), and the purchasing of fresh produce was usually done once a week at Constant Spring market by ladies with the assistance of their houseboys or gardenboys. They carried the wicker market baskets laden with fresh fruit and vegetables. While Gloria's mother Maisie went 'marketing' religiously throughout her life – and enjoyed it – her daughter was already displaying the contempt for custom and responsibility which would only worsen with the passage of time. She would go 'marketing' only when she was having an important party. She regularly mocked her mother for making extra work for herself, and I regretted this attitude, as I loved going with Gloria to the market. With its hustle and bustle and the colourful market women, who were invariably warm and effusive towards all white children, I always wished that marketing would graduate from a treat into a habit, but it never did.

Being Gloria's favourite was not all my brother and sister would later seemed to think it was. I too was hemmed in by restrictions, though at least I was spared the more overt abusiveness with which she targeted them. I had to be absolutely still and quiet at all times. 'Be still, child,' she would snap if I so much as shook my foot. 'My nerves can't stand the constant movement.' Occasionally she would take refuge in my bed after a particularly bad row with Daddy. He would never disturb any of us when we were supposed to be sleeping, especially if there was school the following day, so she could be sure of avoiding the whirlwind after she had sown the wind by retreating to my bed. How I dreaded those occasions. I can still see her at the opposite end of the bed: she had a thing about sleeping at the opposite end of the bed, even with our father. 'Will you stop tossing and turning and squirming!' she would spit out. 'I'm trying to sleep.' For the rest of the night, I would be frozen to the spot, too keyed up to fall asleep until exhaustion overtook me, usually as the sun was rising - so fearful of disobeying my mother that I would willingly suffer anything rather than turn even slightly.

Worse than that, however, was Gloria's predilection for using me as her psychological dumping ground. Although she and her in-laws were constantly in and out of each other's houses, and although she would acknowledge just before she died how 'wonderful it was to be a part of three big families – the Ziadies, the Burkes, and the Smedmores', in those days she never had a kind word to say about any Ziadies. She spared a smattering of them, whose number always remained the same: her two brothers-in-law Solomon and Elias; Uncle Solomon's children; Uncle Wesley and Aunt Eily; his brothers Joe Joe and Millard and their wives Dorothy and Helen; their sister Toni; and cousin Ferris and his wife Gloria. Everyone else was a target for her free-flowing venom. Quite oblivious to the fact that she was speaking to Ziadie progeny, she would bang on and on about how lucky they were to have her in their family; how she had elevated them; how fortunate Daddy was to have married her; how fortunate we were to have her blood flowing in our veins; how they didn't 'know how to behave'; how, like all Catholics, they had preposterous ideas; how sick she was of hearing about the 'blasted Poop of Rome'. The greatest venom was reserved for the two sisters my father saw the most of: Doris and Juliette. Usually one was in favour while the other was out. For no discernable reason, their positions would be reversed, and the favoured one would suddenly and inexplicably become the object of contumely.

'Your Aunt Doris is nothing but a contentious bitch,' Gloria would say before recounting an incident that certainly did not put her in the right. 'Your Aunt Doris is an interfering busybody.' She would also assert when nothing could have been further from the truth, 'She's always poking her nose into my business.'

Poor Aunt Juliette, who was the archetypal devoted wife and mother, was a 'fool – dedicating her life to a man and children'. She would later die of a brain tumour in 1961 at the age of forty-one, leaving eight children. Occasionally Gloria would accuse Aunt Juliette of being a bitch as well, but even she knew that this particular accusation was hardly liable to fly no matter how many wings she pasted onto it. Aunt Juliette was such a sweet-natured and inoffensive person, which, of course, was the problem. She knew that Aunt Juliette's devotion to husband and children showed up her own selfishness and irresponsibility, hence the relish with which she would flounder around trying to come up with a valid criticism of her saintly sister-in-law.

'They're jealous of me,' was Gloria's refrain, and with hindsight I suspect she was jealous of the fact that Daddy loved them as much as he did. Jealousy was an ever-recurring theme with Gloria. Not only did she accuse most of the Ziadie family of it, but also anyone else she decided had not acknowledged her own greatness relative to their ordinariness. While it would have made sense for the poor to be jealous of someone as overtly privileged as Gloria, it wasn't them she was accusing of jealousy, but people who were on a par with her – or so it seemed to me. I therefore struggled to comprehend what she meant. I wanted to be fair, and I couldn't be unless I genuinely could get to the bottom of her comments and assess them for myself.

On the surface, it didn't seem that so many of her peers could be as jealous of my mother as she claimed. Admittedly she could be wonderful company. Admittedly she had charisma. Admittedly she was one of the stars of the social constellation. Admittedly most of the Ziadies weren't. But then, they had no desire to be. Why would anyone be jealous of someone who had something they didn't want? It simply didn't make sense. Why, especially, would Aunt Doris and Aunt Juliette, who both led full and fulfilled lives, be jealous of her? They didn't seem to be in competition with, or in awe of, her. Why indeed would half the people she accused of jealousy be jealous of her? It seemed to me either I was missing something or Gloria was misattributing motives which simply weren't there. In the absence of any concrete information necessary for arriving at an accurate assessment, I left the question open. In so doing, I was already gaining firm and reasonable doubt about her perspective on life, which was something that would stand me in good stead in the years to come.

In the meantime, my position as favourite forced me into being the dumping ground for my mother's resentments. And believe me: she harboured a wealth of them. Anyone and anything who did not bow down before her, or at the very least pay her court, was, in her mind's eye, a valid target. I hated it when she sat me down *à deux* and disparaged people I loved or liked. I really didn't want to hear her catalogue of petty complaints, most of which were, in my view, unwarranted. Unlike Mickey, who would be quite frank about where he stood and would defend his opinion when she sought to knock it down, I was far more tactful. I would swallow, swallow, swallow. My stomach would go into knots. I would curl over it, trying to protect myself against the onslaught of venom, trying not to absorb it, until she would say, as she invariably did, 'Sit up straight, child. You're not a snake. How do you manage to contort yourself into such positions?' Then I would straighten up and try to breathe as little as possible, hoping that, by so doing, I would somehow avoid sucking in the poison that filled the room in which we were sitting. Occasionally, I would not be able to remain silent any longer. Then I would try to give Gloria a new and less disparaging perspective about the loved one presently under attack. However, I quickly learned that she would never countenance any other opinion but hers, so I would back off and try to throw up my spiritual guard so that her venom wouldn't sully my soul.

In the midst of all of this, I was actually learning an invaluable lesson: how difficult it is for the weak to stand up for right against the strong. But also how necessary it is to do so, even if you do so in only a limited way. Nevertheless, I was already too canny to fall into the trap of joining my brother and sister as another of her victims. I was therefore always careful to drop my defence of her latest target before I raised her ire. I would then be trapped with her until she presented me with a moment at which I could extricate myself. This, however, was always easier said than done. No one ever took social leave of Gloria without her trying to prolong the encounter.

Included among the dozen or so variations on the leave-taking theme which she employed over her lifetime to prevent her audience wending its way out of the theatre of her company back into the safe harbour of its own life were: 'Stay, I'm enjoying you so much': 'Don't leave. We're having such a good time': 'I'm just beginning to enjoy myself' and even: 'You can't leave yet. I'm just starting to like you.'

On a primeval level, I appreciated the realities of my situation. In such a viciously dysfunctional family as ours, I could not afford to lose the protection that my position as Gloria's favourite assured me, no matter how odious I found it to be her dumping ground. It wasn't only protection against the more damaging and destructive aspects of her unconscionable and ruthless character that one had to consider. There was also the fact that our father seldom stood up for any of us against her cruelty. Largely because I had learned the art of agreement, my position as Gloria's favourite was never threatened. It remained intact even when she produced two other children after me.

Two years and four months after my birth, Gloria gave birth to Libby. If anything, her arrival solidified my position as favourite, because Libby was a beautiful little girl, and acknowledged as such by everyone who saw her. This, in my opinion, lay at the heart of Gloria's antagonism towards her. The one thing Gloria could not abide was competition. She had to be the centre of attraction at all times, and if anyone or anything deflected attention away from her, that person or thing would activate her 'seek and destroy' mechanism. Libby garnered attention wherever she went, even as a little girl, because she was so beautiful. As she grew older and started to get invitations to model at Society fashion shows and to be a flower girl or bridesmaid at the weddings of friends and relations, Gloria, whose public face was then one of gracious accommodation, would invariably accede to the request and would seemingly glow with maternal pride as people raved about Libby's beauty. The fact that she looked somewhat like Gloria mattered not a jot, for the one thing Gloria was not about to do was enjoy any child's reflected glory – not even when it reflected well on her. So Gloria made Libby pay privately for her public glory by treating her callously and cruelly when no one was around to see her in action.

No matter what Libby said or did, Gloria sniped or snapped at her in much the same way as she sniped and snapped at Mickey. If Libby asked for something, she would accuse her of being needy and greedy. When Libby understandably reacted adversely to such undermining, either by protesting her innocence or with tears, Gloria would mock her for being a 'Jezebel' or 'Miss Misery': two monikers she stuck her with for years.

By the time Libby was five or six, Gloria had so established the regimen of abusiveness, which was in many ways a repetition of her relationship with Mickey, that she felt able to go public with it, albeit in as limited a way as she publicized her disparagement of her son. Every word out of Libby's mouth, when uttered in the presence of any visitor, friend or relation, was greeted by her mother with disdain covered in vicious but nevertheless humorous mockery. 'Yes, Jezzy, what is it this time?' Gloria would ask, exaggerating Libby's discomfited tone of voice so that it appeared as if her daughter were congenitally incapable of ever behaving in anything but an obstreperous manner – a failing which she, Gloria, was nevertheless handling bravely and humorously. However, it was Gloria who was actually manipulating Libby into appearing less obliging than she was inclined to be.

Naturally, any child, knowing that its needs, desires, comments or opinions will be denigrated so cruelly, is bound to express the discomfort it knows is an inevitable part of making itself heard. However, Gloria was already a past-mistress at the art of turning the tables on others, and turn them on Libby she did until poor Libby closed in on herself and became more withdrawn than her earlier outgoingness indicated her true nature to be. Thereafter, it wasn't only Mickey who regularly and frequently sought refuge with our grandmother or maternal aunt. Libby could now frequently be found at Grandma's or Auntie's, 'staying' for weeks on end during the holidays to escape from the cruelty of her mother.

This cruelty was usually verbal rather than physical, for while Michael allowed Gloria to get away with physically abusing his son, he did not allow it with his daughter. The turning point came when Libby was about five. Gloria beat her for something. I should say at this point that Jamaica in those days was very much a 'spare the rod, spoil the child' culture. All classes were heavily into corporal punishment. But while it was acceptable to beat a child with a switch or belt on its bottom and even to leave marks, it was not acceptable to draw blood. And under no circumstances was it tolerable to beat a child on its naked bottom with a belt buckle, which is what Gloria did with Libby – until she drew blood. When Daddy came home and saw the state of Libby's bottom he erupted. 'Are you mad, woman? Look at what you've done to the child? If you ever touch her like that again, I will divorce you. Do you hear me? Divorce you. Damned madwoman.'

That preserved Libby from the physical abuse but not from the verbal.

If Gloria had it in for Libby from early on, at least she received love from our father, whose favourite she was – in early childhood at least. Libby, however, would turn out to be less lucky than me, for while my reign as maternal favourite would last for twenty-one years, hers as paternal favourite would prove to be much more short-lived. I can remember as if it were yesterday the brutal way it came to an end. It was the morning of Monday, September 13 1955. Mickey, Libby, Daddy and I were sitting around the breakfast table. Daddy was served his bacon and eggs, and Libby did what she had done every morning since she had been eating breakfast with our father: she reached in with her little fingers to take a strip of his bacon. Michael covered her hand with his and pushed it away. 'You can't do that anymore,' he said. 'There's a new baby now.' Libby's eyes opened wide, and you could see that she was shocked; but we had been brought up to behave well, so she did not react with tears or tantrums or any of the things that modern children might do, nor did she backchat. You could tell, however, that she knew it was a decisive moment. Poor Libby had been dethroned in the most direct and unceremonious manner possible.

Kitty, the new baby, had become Michael's favourite, a position she would retain until his death. 'Your father always favoured the baby,' our maternal grandmother told us in 1972. 'If your mother had had another child after Kitty, you can depend upon it, Michael would have transferred his affection to it.'

While he might well have replicated the bond he had with Kitty with another daughter, I suspect he would not have loved a son as much as he loved Kitty, unless that son shared his interest in sport, horses, poker and dominoes. Mickey liked none of them, so had nothing in common with him. Michael made it only too plain that he much preferred his nephews and great-nephews, who were as obsessed with sport and games of chance as he was.

All her life Kitty would remain Daddy's favourite. She was the only child allowed to sit on his lap. Whatever she wanted, she got from him. She only needed to ask, and it was hers. Mickey, Libby and I would look on transfixed. Yet we were never jealous. We were always happy for Kitty, even if we might, occasionally, have wished that some of Daddy's largesse could wend its way in our direction.

Quite how Gloria felt about Kitty was a mystery. She had absolutely no relationship with her once she weaned her off the breast. She made no show of loving her, liking her, disliking her or loathing her. In fact, she paid her absolutely no attention at all.

This total disinterest started shortly after Kitty's birth. Gloria didn't even bother to attend her christening. This, of course, caused consternation in all branches of the family. The Ziadies, being Lebanese and Russian; and the Burkes being Irish and French as well as partly Jewish, all loved children. Even the Smedmores were very family-orientated, despite being English, and couldn't comprehend a mother failing to attend her own daughter's christening. But Gloria didn't.

'I didn't have a conversation with Mummy until I was in my thirties,' Kitty says; and that, I fear, is the truth. 'She dropped kid. And dropped the kid,' I used to quip, seeking to make sense of Gloria's completely unnatural reaction to her youngest daughter's existence. It wasn't that she even disliked her. She simply had nothing to do with her.

Occasionally, of course, mother and daughter would be thrown together by circumstance. Then, Kitty would experience how fortunate she was to be ignored. One such incident occurred when she was a year and three months old. It was her first Christmas as a toddler. Gloria was dressing the tree as we children entered into the spirit of things and passed her ornaments and otherwise generally partook of the fun. Christmas was a big thing in Jamaica generally, and in our family in particular. Gloria loved it especially. She encouraged Michael to give us generous allowances so that we could buy presents for all our friends and relations. We children would be taken down by one of our father's floorwalkers to Hanna's Wholesale, a vast emporium which supplied many of the chains of stores throughout the island with merchandise, where one of the senior executives would accompany us as we made our selection of gifts. These would then be delivered to our father's store and brought home for us to wrap. Wrapping Christmas presents with Mummy was one of the only activities we ever shared – that and dressing the Christmas tree. They were fun and gave us a glimpse of what life could have been like had our mother been more interested in her children.

We were all having a wonderful time that Christmas of 1956. Gloria's charm and fun-lovingness were in full flow. There were high spirits all around. We finished dressing the tree, and Gloria instructed one of the servants to plug in the lights. The tree glittered and glowed brilliantly. Kitty, caught up in the magic of the moment, did what any one-year old would do. She crawled over to the tree to touch the lights.

Quick as a flash, Gloria said: 'Pretty, pretty. Yes, Kitty, pretty, pretty.' Kitty crawled towards her, a huge smile lighting up her little face. 'Come Kitty,' Gloria said, and taking the baby in her arms, instructed the servant to remove one of the bulbs from its socket. When he did so, she said, 'You see, Kitty, pretty. Lights are pretty. But you mustn't touch them.' Then she pushed Kitty's finger in the socket and the baby gave out an almighty howl as the electricity coursed through her body.

Michael was in his bedroom reading when he heard what was clearly a cry of anguish. All parents know their babies have different cries for different things, and this one was indicative of something serious. So he rushed into the drawing room to see what was happening, only to be told by his wife: 'Kitty pushed her finger in the socket and got a shock. She won't be doing that again in a hurry.'

To this day, I do not know if Michael ever realized what Gloria had done. But I do know of two other incidents involving Kitty where he was certainly privy to her cruelty. In the first, Kitty was about three. Gloria directed her to do something. She did not. 'Get into punishment,' she commanded, which meant that Kitty was to go into the study for what is now called 'timeout'. But Gloria's timeout wasn't like timeout today, when the punishment is determined in minutes equivalent to the age of the child. If she were in a good mood, you might spend twenty or thirty minutes in Coventry, but if she was in a bad mood, she could keep you there for hours. Once, she forgot Mickey for a whole day; and he, knowing that a reminder would result in the punishment being perpetuated, said nothing until dinner time rolled around and his absence was noted.

Faced with the prospect of an open-ended punishment that could last for what is, to a child, an unendurable length of time, and knowing that her adored father had just returned home, Kitty refused when Gloria demanded that she obey her.

Before the words were out of Kitty's mouth, Gloria grabbed her by her hair and, lifting her off the ground, marched the dangling child into the house through the back door. I couldn't help following them into the kitchen, through the breakfast porch, into the dining room, where they nearly collided with Daddy, who had heard the commotion and was coming out to see what was happening.

'What are you doing?' he demanded, his face the embodiment of disapproval.

'What does it look like? Kitty's been stinkingly rude, and I will not have it. Since she won't go into punishment voluntarily, I'm taking her.'

'Not like that, you're not,' he thundered. 'I will not have you mistreating my children. Do you understand me, woman? No sane person treats a child like that. Let her go immediately. Are you mad or what?'

'She will do as I say,' Gloria persisted as she continued dangling the screaming Kitty by her hair.

'Put her down this instant, before I make you,' Michael bellowed.

Gloria dropped Kitty, who fled to Daddy.

'Did you not do what your Mummy told you to?' he asked, lifting her into his arms.

Kitty's howls turned to sobs.

'If I go, she'll forget me.'

'You see what your nonsense causes?' he asked Gloria. 'The child is terrified of your punishment.'

'Join Mama and Marjorie. Let the monsters run wild. Undermine my authority. I try to discipline them so that they grow up to be civilized human beings, instead of savages like half your family. Well, let me tell you something: if you succeed, you'll pay the piper. I'll divorce you and take you to the cleaners. Then let's see how you handle those wild animals you call your children.'

'Say sorry to Mummy, Kitty,' Michael said.

'Sorry, Mummy,' Kitty gasped between sobs.

'You're on very thin ice,' Gloria warned Michael.

'You're on even thinner ice if you ever do anything like that again to one of my children. No civilized person carries a child by its hair,' he riposted before taking Kitty into his bedroom, where he read while she cuddled with him.

On the second occasion, the five-year-old Kitty continued to talk when Gloria instructed her to be quiet. We were on our way home from lunch. Without another word, Gloria brought the car to a screeching halt by slamming her foot on the brakes, 'You may get out and walk home, Kitty,' she said in that cool way she had when asserting her authority. When Kitty refused to leave the vehicle, she pulled her out and left her standing on the side of the road at Donhead Avenue. This was a good mile and a half from our house, and Kitty of course was too young to know her way home. But that didn't stop our authoritarian mother from depositing her youngest daughter on the sidewalk, crying hysterically as the car receded into the distance.

On this occasion, even we children couldn't remain silent; and as Gloria put her foot down on the accelerator, we begged and pleaded with her to go back for Kitty. She refused to do so. 'You can go and pick up your daughter,' she calmly informed Michael, who had got back before us, when we were home.

'She's on Donhead Avenue near where Joe Joe and Dorothy used to live.'

Not even his explosion could rock her indifference to the wrong she had committed. As far as Gloria was concerned, she was right – as usual. Anything Michael or anyone else said to the contrary was simply so much noise. However, he would not back down, and when he had finally threatened to take his belt to her, she must have realized that he really meant business, for she never did anything like that to Kitty ever again.

Chapter Four

Despite Gloria's cruelty, our childhood was not one long saga of pain and misery. On many levels, it was happy, indeed magical. One virtue of being so well-off was that we had a luxurious way of life. Having highly social and socialized parents meant that we were always surrounded by people, both adults and children; and, this being Jamaica where most blacks and many whites had a far greater regard for children than their English counterparts, we knew from an early age what it was to be relished. Being members of three big and close families, all of whom were loving and geared towards making children feel appreciated, we were never at a loss for adults to give us love and attention or for children to play with. Because we were well behaved and well mannered, all the adults liked us and seldom had cause to correct us for any transgressions. Because we were good sports, we were also popular with the other children. We had a multitude of cousins of our own ages, with whom we were close, as well as many friends. With no chores whatsoever to do, the servants taking care of the day-to-day mechanics of living, life was frequently full and jolly. Indeed, looking back on it, life was filled with innocent but enriching activities, from picnics and days at the beach to riding our bicycles with friends.

Libby was a tomboy. She and Mickey were forever climbing trees and having bicycle races with Michael and Peter, the grandchildren of our immediate neighbour, while I was always arranging parties for my collection of dolls. At these I would serve diluted port wine in Gloria's silver goblets, decorating the doll's house with masses of flowers picked from the garden, which was already noted as being one of the most beautiful in Jamaica, and would in years to be recognized worldwide when Gloria turned much of it into a vast orchid garden. Then there were the children's parties which we either hosted or attended. Having so many cousins of our own age, as well as a multitude of friends from our parents' social circle, we seemed to be forever attending one party or another when Gloria wasn't throwing her annual extravaganzas for each of our birthdays. At these, there were frequently things like clowns and donkey rides. Once, for Libby's fifth birthday party, Gloria outdid herself by getting Adassa, a market-woman who used to come to the neighbourhood once a week with her donkey-cart to sell fruit and vegetables, to clean it out and take the children for rides. I don't know whether it sounds like fun to adults, but I can assure you that it was great fun for children – especially white children in class-stratified Jamaica, for it was unprecedented for upper-class Jamaicans to ever do anything that the lower classes did. Doubtless, the fact that we were consuming forbidden fruit made it all the sweeter to us children.

In the 1950s and well into the 1960s, precocious children were highly regarded. The film star James Mason's son Morgan and daughter Portland were regular features on the Jack Parr and Johnny Carson talk shows in the US, regaling an entranced public with tales of smoking cigarettes from the age of eight and attending grown-up parties with the approval of their parents. The Mason children had nothing on Gloria's brood, save attending adult social events. Otherwise, Gloria saw no reason why her children – indeed, any children – should not be as worldly, accomplished and sophisticated as the adults around them. She despised childish children and never missed an opportunity to mock them as imbeciles and their parents as idiots for having rearing them to be 'fools'.

'Never make the mistake of speaking down to children, as if they're idiots who can't understand you just because you're four feet taller than them,' Gloria warned each of us when we had our own children, hoping that we would repeat the process by which she had reared us to be articulate, socialized mini-people. 'The only way to have intelligent children is to speak to them as if they're intelligent. That means no baby talk. Never speak to them any differently than you would to a grownup, unless you want them to grow up to be tongue-tied fools.' We all did, with the result that her six grandchildren were all extremely articulate and sophisticated from toddlerhood.

Gloria being Gloria, however, she was not content to stop at instilling a heightened sociability in her progeny. I suspect she regarded Mickey, Libby and me as being very special, indeed superior, not only because we were all academically and socially advanced but because we were her – the great Gloria's – children. This could have entertaining results, such as the Sunday afternoon in 1956 when she decided to teach the three of us to drive.

Daddy had recently bought a green Morris Minor car for himself as a run-around following Gloria's refusal to employ another chauffeur after she had dismissed the last one. The inconvenience of the big American car always being on the road ferrying his wife and children everywhere meant that sometimes Daddy would have to wait to be picked up. However, the one thing Michael never had was patience. If he didn't receive instant gratification of his wishes, you could depend on Mount Vesuvius erupting. So he solved the problem by getting himself a little car.

His choice might have surprised many of my parent's friends, but it was also revealing of the type of man he was. When he bought the Morris Minor, a friend asked Gloria why hadn't he bought a better car.

'It's a family tradition,' she said wittily, refusing to let a good opportunity slip by for one of her zingers. 'He and his brother Solomon believe in cars with a top speed of twenty miles an hour. That's why I have an eight-cylinder vehicle, and he has that metallic snail. God forbid that he or Solomon should *approach* the speed limit, much less exceed it.'

There was more than an element of truth to that statement, though Uncle Solomon would later provide me with another explanation when, at the age of seventeen, I asked him why he always bought Renault Dauphins when he could have any car he wanted. 'To me, cars are a method of transportation, nothing more, nothing less,' replied this uncle of mine, who was renowned as one of the richest men in Jamaica. 'I know some people regard them as status symbols and announce their wealth to every passer-by on the road by driving a Mercedes or Lincoln or Cadillac or one of those other hearses people call cars. But I have no need of that.' I would come to realize that those were sentiments my father shared, even if my mother did not until 'Democratic Socialism' and the threats it presented to the upper classes forced a change in her habits.

We children also had reason to be grateful for the metallic snail's acquisition when Gloria asked us at Sunday lunch shortly after the car arrived early in 1956 whether we would like to learn to drive.

'Yes,' we chorused.

'Good, I'll teach you on Scrammy,' she said, using the nickname she'd bestowed upon Daddy's car.

'Don't you think the children are a little young to learn to drive?' Michael said.

'Of course not. Mickey's eight. Georgie's six. And Libby's four. They're not fools, you know.'

As soon as the butler had cleared the pudding dishes, Gloria and the three of us children were excitedly off on what was a true adventure for us.

First up was Mickey, to be followed by me, then Libby. She started by teaching us to change the gears. Once we had the hang of neutral, first, second, third, fourth and reverse, all of which had to be managed with the clutch, she taught us, clouds of her DuMaurier cigarettes enveloping us, how to start the car. 'Look at what I'm doing, then do *exactly* the same thing,' she said, her long, painted fingernails turning the key to the right before she released it, dramatically opening up her hands so that we would understand precisely what was required of us. 'First you must put the car in neutral before starting it. That will save you having to use the clutch. Then, turn the key gently to the right, and, *as soon as* the engine fires up, *let go* of the key, *otherwise you can break the starter.*'

Having taught us how to change the gears and to start the car, Gloria rubbed her hands with glee. 'Now for driving itself,' she announced. We all knew that she was a superb driver. She often drove us to the country herself, zipping around the winding mountain roads with aplomb and ability, always speedily but never carelessly, quite unlike our father, who was a Nervous Nellie behind the wheel and 'crawled like a snail', to quote her. 'Put your damned foot down and let's reach our destination before Christmas comes,' she used to say to him. 'What's the point of having an eight-cylinder car, if you won't give it any gas? The car won't go on its own, you know.'

This Sunday afternoon in 1956, our father's loathing of speed was proving handy as Gloria sat first Mickey, then me, then Libby behind the wheel of the Morris Minor. Having taught us the intricacies of changing the gears and starting the car, she now showed us how to co-ordinate those lessons with putting our foot down on the accelerator and 'gassing the car'.

Mickey quickly got the hang of the lesson, though he was inclined to take his foot off the clutch too quickly, with the result that Scrammy lurched as he drove up the driveway to the top gate. Once there, he either had to drive into the street, which was of course against the law, or learn to reverse. As Gloria was not about to allow us to flout the law, she ended his first driving lesson by teaching him to reverse, which he actually did more smoothly than driving forward.

Next up was me. I took to driving like the proverbial duck to water. I loved it from the moment I slid into the driver's seat: a sentiment that has remained unchanged for the fifty-three years since that first lesson. I too proved to be a quick learner; and even on that first occasion, I was aware of the glorious sense of liberty that getting behind the wheel provided for me.

This, however, was not a sensation Libby would enjoy for many years to come. That Sunday afternoon in 1956, the four-year-old Libby simply couldn't get the hang of driving. This should hardly be surprising to anyone but clearly wasn't to her mother, who simply ignored Libby's struggle to reach the accelerator with her toes while perched on the edge of the seat so that she might see over the dashboard while steering the car. 'Christ, child,' Gloria finally rasped after Libby's umpteenth attempt to move Scrammy forwards without stalling her. 'You're exasperating me. My nerves can't stand any more of this. Enough for one day. At least Mickey and Georgie can now drive.'

After that, I was forever asking Daddy if I could 'practise my driving' in the driveway, something which he frequently allowed Mickey and me to do on Scrammy, so that we were fully proficient behind a wheel long before we were old enough to qualify for our driving licences.

Nor was this the only fun we children had. At the start of the summer holidays in 1958, Gloria announced to Mickey and me that we were to accompany her and Lucius on a cruise. 'The *Evangeline* is owned by the Frasers,' she informed us, describing the luxurious ship belonging to Maisie's neighbours and friends of the family, which was large enough to be grand but small enough to be personable . 'We're going to Santo Domingo, Puerto Rico, St Thomas in the American Virgin Islands, Cuba, and Miami, where we'll meet up with Jean and Ronnie before steaming back to Jamaica.' Jean was her mother's niece and Ronnie was Jean's only son, a year younger than Mickey.

I cannot convey the excitement I felt as we boarded the ocean liner in Kingston Harbour late at night that July. Kingston had the sixth best natural harbour in the world, and I can still smell its scents: the salt of the sea water, the oil from the ships and boats, the sweat of the dockers. The sounds have also stayed with me – the horns of the seafaring vessels in the distance as the larger ships were being towed out to sea; the engines of the launches ferrying passengers from the dock to an even larger ship which couldn't dock at the wharf; the shouts of the porters; the goodbyes, some excited, some sad.

Only too soon Michael was leading his wife, father-in-law and children up the gangplank, which, to my child's eye, was a precarious bridge running from the dock to a deck in the side of the ship way below its upper decks. Then we were on board, being met by the purser and taken to our staterooms by the stewards. It was all riveting stuff for an eight-year-old. For the first time in my life I was glad that my mother, whose peregrinations had started before her marriage and continued throughout it, loved to travel.

Prior to this, we children had hated it when Gloria was abroad because her Aunt Elma stayed with us, our nurses being deemed insufficiently responsible to actually take care of us unless they were supervised by a female family member. Aunt Elma was one of the Smedmore spinster sisters of our grandfather: very English in her (mis)treatment of children. Not for her any of the kindness, tolerance, understanding, warmth, or humour of our Russo-Lebanese Ziadie or Franco-Irish-Jewish Burke relations. To Aunt Elma, children had no feelings. Nor, in her eyes, were we mere children. We were disobedient and untruthful and needed to be curbed.

I can now see that our relationship with Aunt Elma was bad owing to a misunderstanding that was never cleared up due to a lack of communication. It arose because one of our favourite play areas was in the grounds behind the house on a plot of land that lay behind a hedge beside the summer house. Aunt Elma would chase after us, declaring that we were on 'open land' just because a hedge separated it from the rest of the grounds. She would yank us back to that part of the grounds which she had decreed was ours. When we protested, as we always did, that it was our land too, she would reprimand us for lying and give us sermons on the need to tell the truth. Peculiarly enough, she never once asked Daddy or Mummy if the land was ours; and I suspect now that the reason why she did not do so was that she did not want to get us into trouble.

She could also, of course, have asked the servants whose land it was, but I daresay such a course of action would never have occurred to a West Indian patrician, servants being there for the sole function of serving. I am sure in Aunt Elma's scheme of things it would have been inappropriate for someone like her to consult a servant about anything as material as land ownership. To do so would overstep one of the many invisible lines separating servant from master, endowing the individual consulted with an importance that would be deemed threatening to the very fabric of society, giving him or her ideas above his or her station and thereby contributing to the erosion of the social order. Already everyone in upper- and middle-class circles was worried about what would happen if the rumours of the English pulling out and giving their colonies independence were true. 'Revolution' was a word whispered late at night on front or back verandas after the servants had gone to bed, so people like Aunt Elma were hyper-vigilant about what they said or did lest they inadvertently contributed to threats they hoped to avoid. Such were the values and the ethos of that age.

I no longer remember if Aunt Elma stayed with Libby and Kitty while Mickey and I were cruising in the Caribbean Sea with our mother and grandfather. What I do remember is having the time of my life as we did so. Mickey and I were given the run of the vessel by Gloria, who knew that we could be trusted to behave responsibly and not endanger our lives or those of our playmates. Like all young children, we struck up firm – if transient – friendships with some of the other children on board. We swam in the pool, having been taught to swim from an early age by Auntie's husband Uncle Ric. We went on tours whenever the ship docked at one of the ports of call. We were especially thrilled to be taken to Bluebeard's Castle and to Christopher Columbus's house. We even turned the life drill into an adventure, when everyone was called to their stations and we rehearsed what to do in the unlikely event that the ship was sinking. Ironically, it would sink about twelve years later, with considerable loss of life. I discovered a wonderful plaything called the slot machine, and being a member of the Ziadie family to whom gambling came a close second after the twin gods of religion and sex, I was allowed to play it endlessly. I loved the roll of the scroll, whether I won or lost, though I must admit I liked it more when coins clattered out, as they did periodically. This saved me the necessity of having to go in search of Gloria to ask her for some more money to feed the machine. I was always mindful that she didn't like being interrupted and that she was also ordinarily thrifty with us – 'Wilful waste, woeful want' being one of the mantras she was intent upon instilling in us – but, surrounded by her friends and father, with whom she was invariably drinking gin and tonic and shooting the breeze, she had a largesse she lacked at home when I was negotiating for a doll or some such toy. So I always got the money I wanted with a surprising lack of difficulty. Once I even hit the jackpot, American quarters pouring from the slot like manna from heaven, which thrilled me no end, not because I had anything I wanted to buy with the money but because I would now be spared the necessity of asking Mummy for money for the slot machine for quite a while.

I had a little American friend, whom I had made on board the ship, who was endlessly surprised that I was allowed to play the slot machine. I couldn't understand why his parents wouldn't allow him a similar liberty. Not even after he explained to me that gambling was illegal in America except in a desert called Nevada, did their interdict make any sense. We, after all, had been going to the race track since the age of three or four; and Gloria and Michael had already taught me to play poker and dominoes respectively. How could people be so stuffy as to disapprove of gambling? It was fun, for goodness sake, sport: something to be enjoyed, not something to take seriously and certainly nothing about which to be sanctimonious. I remember evincing sympathy for my friend's deprivation. 'I'm just glad my parents aren't stuffed-shirts,' I said, giving him some quarters to play with. As luck would have it, who should happen along just as he was pulling down the lever but his mother? She made an almighty fuss, dragged him away, found Gloria and complained about me allowing her precious little angel to gamble, the implication being that I was corrupting him. Although Gloria was often reading us the riot act over nothing, on this occasion, she did not do so. She simply explained to me that not everyone was as fortunate as we were to have enlightened parents. In future I was to ensure that I never gave any money to any child to gamble with, our relations excepted – and especially not to an American child. 'Those Americans have the most unsophisticated approach to pleasure,' she declared. 'Everything is against the law. Not that you broke the law. We're on the high seas, and American law doesn't apply to a Panamian-registered ship. Silly woman, making such a fuss about nothing. I wouldn't be surprised if her child ends up a hopeless mess with an attitude like hers.'

I did so love it when Gloria went on like that. It was such fun. She could be so daring. So wonderful. I absolutely adored her at times like that. She made everything seem so right, so appropriate. Life for us could be so much better than for other people. The only pity was that the good times seldom lasted for long.

It was also while I was on the *Evangeline* that I witnessed for the first, and indeed the only, time Gloria being sick from drink. Every night Mickey and I would dine with her and Grandpa, after which we would kiss them goodnight and retire to our respective staterooms. One night I was fast asleep when I was awakened by Gloria being sick in the bathroom. I got out of bed and went next door, where I saw her bent over the lavatory. 'Do you want me to fetch you some proof rum?' I asked.

Appleton overproof rum, known to one and all in Jamaica as 'proof rum', was the national panacea for all ills. It was utilized with equal relish by patricians, peasants and everyone in between. At the first sign of a headache, they would wash their faces with it, then douse a handkerchief and tie it over their forehead prior to taking to bed. If they had a fever, they would 'rub themselves down' with it to bring the fever down. If they had a chill, they would 'rub themselves up' with it to elevate their body temperature. If Gloria had an upset stomach, as I assumed she did, she would need me to rub her forehead with some proof rum prior to soaking a handkerchief with it so that she could sniff it. This would doubtless settle her stomach.

'I'll be okay,' she said. 'Go back to bed. It must be the lobster I had for dinner.'

Believing her diagnosis to be accurate, I went back to bed. Only in years to come, when her drinking became a real problem for us as a family, did I realize that I had been privy to an early episode which was a harbinger of the difficulties alcohol would trigger.

A few days later, the ship docked in Havana Harbour and we set off on a tour of the Cuban capital. Afterwards, we were taken to a sugar cane factory, where we were shown how the Cubans made sugar, which was the same way we did in Jamaica. At the end of the tour, frozen banana daiquiris made with rum were offered by the factory to anyone who wanted them. Fortunately, the Cubans had a similar attitude towards the consumption of alcohol by minors as Gloria, who had reared us from an early age to drink champagne or rum punch and wine at celebratory moments. Since neither Mickey nor I had tasted a frozen daiquiri before, and 'since it's mostly ice in any case, Dada', as she observed to our grandfather, we were allowed to try this exotic new drink. I liked it so much that I contrived to walk off and down two more. By the time we got back to the ship, I was feeling very much as if I had too had eaten some of the lobster that had so upset Mummy's tummy.

Failing to be limited by any boundaries but her own was something that Gloria would do all her life. Sometimes, as with Adassa and the donkey cart, learning to drive in early childhood or drinking banana daiquiris and playing the slot machine, it was great, but there were times when the effect was rather more dubious. One universal boundary which she resolutely refused to acknowledge was that which demarcated where her responsibilities as a mother lay. While she was up and running for anything that was fun or that she could turn to her own advantage, responsibility was something she was intent on avoiding. Doctors and dental appointments were a case in point. While all other mothers of her peer group took their children to the doctor or the dentist, Gloria only ever did so once that I can recall. That was when I was six. She made back-to-back doctor's and dentist's appointments for us. First she took Mickey, Libby and me to Dr Hollar, who had been the Smedmore dentist for years. Prior to that, Marjorie had always taken us to the dentist or the doctor. Auntie would follow us into the dentist's surgery and stand beside the chair holding our little hands as Dr Hollar drilled away. Those were the days before fast drills with thin points, when local anaesthetic was administered with thick needles only if you were having a tooth extracted. As the thick, slow point of the drill ground its way inexorably into our cavities, we felt each and every twinge of pain and howled accordingly. 'I know it hurts, darling,' Auntie would say while we were suffering, 'but you've got to be brave. It will soon be over, and then I'll take you to Justin McCarthey's,' referring to the best toy store in town, 'and you can have something as a reward for being good.'

Gloria's approach, however, was entirely different. The only thing the two sisters had in common, aside from smoking Du Maurier cigarettes, was that they were both pictures of elegance even when they were taking us to the doctor or the dentist. Mickey was called in first by Dr Hollar, who greeted Gloria warmly and asked her if she wanted to come in while he treated her son. 'My nerves can't stand the drama,' she said and lit up a cigarette as Mickey's eyes opened wide and he had to face the hangman's noose on his own. Next up was me. When Mickey stepped out of the surgery into the waiting room, his face ashen, I wondered whether my mother would bestir herself for her favourite. 'Make sure you don't make an exhibition of yourself the way your brother just did,' came her remark, cool as ever. 'My nerves can't stand all that caterwauling.'

I tried to be as quiet as possible, but I can still vividly remember the drone of the drill and the agony as Dr Hollar ground away at my cavity. Of course I disgraced myself by crying out loud. Bad as it was for Mickey and me, it must have been immeasurably worse for Libby. Not only was she the youngest, but she had also had to sit down quietly and listen to the pained sounds of her two siblings in the room next door. When it was her turn to go into Dr Hollar's chair, do you think Gloria softened and went in with her little girl? As she herself would put it: do you think apples grow on lilac trees?

Although Dr Hollar's surgery was only about a block and a half away from 'Uncle' Tony's – as we children were made to call the man who was now our family doctor and who, I would later learn, was the object of my mother's desire – we duly trooped into the car for the short drive from one to the other. Once there, Gloria announced herself to the nurse, and we sat down in the waiting room until 'Uncle' Tony was finished with the patient he was seeing. He then came out to greet us. We children, who knew him well and liked him, duly gave him kisses. He indicated to us that he was ready for us, and to our surprise, who should jump up to accompany us but Gloria?

While 'Uncle' Tony examined our throats and ears with his light-bearing instruments, Dearest Mamma stood beside us, holding our hands and cooing words of reassurance so that 'Uncle' Tony could see what a loving and devoted mother she was. Then she agreed with 'Uncle' Tony that it would be best if Mickey and I had our tonsils and adenoids out, but that he should leave Libby's in, since they weren't giving her any trouble and she was still so young.

Even though I was only six, I was struck by how differently Gloria had behaved towards us at Dr Hollar's and 'Uncle' Tony's respective surgeries. There was, of course, an explanation, but I didn't know what it was then. It would take over thirty years for me to hear it. But hear it I would, and from a most unexpected source.

Vida MacMillan, Gloria's best friend throughout our childhood until they had a massive bust-up in 1958, was in London. I had always been fond of her, and she of me, so of course I asked her around for dinner. We were reminiscing about the past when she said: 'You know your mother was desperately in love with Tony Feanny.'

Gloria had always told everyone how desperately in love Tony Feanny had been with her prior to leaving Jamaica to study medicine in the US. This was while Michael was courting her. Daddy certainly knew about Tony's love for his wife prior to their marriage and had never allowed it to interfere with their friendship. Now I was hearing something that was filling in a lot of the gaps in my childhood perceptions.

'When Tony returned to Jamaica from America, your mother would have loved to marry him,' Vida continued.

'Did she tell you this?' I asked.

'Of course. We were best friends for years. You ought to remember that.'

'I do.'

'I felt very sorry for her. She was so in love with Tony, but marriage wasn't on the cards. She was already married with four children, and Tony was a devout Catholic who would never have given up his religion for any woman.'

As Vida spoke, I well remembered how devout a Catholic 'Uncle' Tony was. Gloria had been very publicly married according to the rites of the Catholic Church by Catholic clergy in the only Roman Catholic Cathedral in Jamaica, to the scion of another well known Catholic family. Indeed, Michael was the brother of a nun and the nephew of an Archbishop. There was therefore no prospect of the lovebirds ever obtaining permission from Rome to marry. Annulment was the only option the Sacred Rota could exercise in dissolving the marriage of Michael and Gloria, but their marriage was patently valid according to Church law.

Prior to her marriage, Gloria had been made to sign a variety of documents, including one guaranteeing that any children of the marriage would be raised as Catholics, another being that she understood that her marriage was a Catholic marriage bound by Catholic rules and subject to Church law. It should also be remembered at this juncture that the Pope is not only head of the Church but also Sovereign of the Secular Papal State, so any issue involving Catholic law has the double dimension of the religious as well as the secular. If Tony and Gloria wanted to marry, they therefore had only one course of action open to them: to violate the teachings of the Church and marry civilly after she had obtained a civil divorce, thereby 'living in sin', as the Church put it. This, however, was always going to be anathema to any practicing Catholic. If 'Uncle' Tony had done it, he would have been excommunicated as soon as he put the ring on Gloria's finger. Thereafter, he would never have been able to partake of any of the sacraments, especially Holy Communion, unless or until he turned his back on a marriage his Church regarded as nonexistent. If he died while living in sin with Gloria, he would go straight to Hell and his soul would be damned for all eternity. Not even Gloria's charms could outshine the glow of hellfire, and she was therefore condemned to being in love with one man while being married to another.

This period of her life must have been torture for her. Michael was, by her account, an extremely highly-sexed man, which made him a sexually demanding husband. No matter what happened, she had to perform, and perform well, if she wanted her marriage to continue successfully. She therefore had to continue fulfilling her conjugal duties with a show of enthusiasm she could no longer have felt, if indeed she had ever felt it. The one thing Gloria preached to Libby, Kitty and me from an early age was that 'sex isn't all it's cooked up to be. In fact, one might enjoy it once in ten times if one's lucky.' What she did not spell out, but we nevertheless understood only too well from the way she spoke, was that a woman had to give a convincing performance of enjoyment even when it left her cold, for in that lay her hold over the animal called a husband.

Everything about Gloria's demeanour with Michael pointed to the fact that she had based a large part of her allure for him on being sexually desirable. The official line was that they were madly in love and had such a torrid sex life that they could barely keep their hands off each other. This version of the facts was repeated time and again to everyone who came to the house to visit. What we children saw and heard didn't always accord with the official line. Michael and Gloria rowed with vicious and disturbing frequency. They were two strong-willed, spoiled brats who each wanted his or her own way and would give no quarter. There was practically never any visible sign of affection between them. Of course, we were never present when anything sexual took place; and Gloria had not yet confided her distaste for Michael's constant physical attentions to any of us, so we were left with the dichotomy of great lovers who seldom showed each other any affection. I don't know whether

Gloria confided in her mother and sister as she did in her daughters, but if she did, they were as careful as we were to toe the party line. Certainly the one person who did not appreciate how uninterested she was in sex was Michael. It was obvious even to us children that she had him absolutely convinced that she was the hot little number she pretended to be to everyone else as well.

Aside from assuaging lust, Gloria had strengthened her hold over the highly sexual but moralistic Michael by being sexually pure prior to marriage. 'You married a virgin,' she would remind him every time they had a row, knowing that that would provide her with leverage. The one thing that mattered to him above all else, as it did to all of the other men of his background, was the sexual purity of his wife. 'I would never have married your mother if she had put out before marriage,' he used to tell us when we were older. 'If I'd been able to convince her to deliver the goods, so could another man. Remember, no man buys the cow if he can get the milk free. Soiled goods have no value. The only goods that are of value are pure goods. Any man who finds that his wife has betrayed him must get rid of her. Instantly. Even if everything else might be forgivable, that is not. '

With an attitude like that, frequently articulated to his flirtatious wife and to all and sundry so that the warning was unmistakable, Michael had laid down the one boundary which Gloria dared not push against. To give my mother her due, she made sure that this was the one boundary she claimed never to have strayed over. 'Your father is the only man I ever slept with,' she would maintain until she died.

This disclaimer did not gel with what Vida MacMillan and other of her friends said. It did not gel with our perceptions of her conduct either. When we were children, she was always going out on secret assignations. Whenever we asked her where she was going, she would say: 'To see a man about a dog.' Whenever she returned and we asked her where she had been, she'd again say: 'To see a man about a dog.'

'Why did you always tell us you were going to see a man about a dog?' Libby asked towards the end of her life. 'Surely you must have realized how cruel it was? You knew we wanted a dog. Didn't it occur to you that you were keeping us dangling unconscionably? That you were building up our hopes each time you said it? Then you were dashing them?'

'It was just an expression,' Gloria replied rather lamely, but I knew it was a lot more than that. It was her way of obtaining our silent collusion in her secret activities. As long as we had hope of her getting us a dog, we would accept her comings and goings without comment. But, if we had no hope, we might well open up our mouths and say something to Daddy which would have triggered his suspicions. It was heartless, yes; but it was also clever. We never once let the cat out of the bag, if I may mix the metaphor.

Gloria's need for secrecy was doubtless what also triggered her refusal to employ another fulltime chauffeur. I remember well the incident she used to drop the axe. This she fabricated out of nothing. She was pregnant with Kitty. It was about eleven o'clock in the morning. She was standing in the back passage that ran from the side of the kitchen to the garage, waiting for the chauffeur, whose name I no longer remember. George, our long-time driver and favourite, had been pinched the year before by our friends and neighbours Michael and Peter's grandfather, after which none lasted very long. It was rare for Gloria to stand and wait for anyone and never for a servant, so that in itself made the event memorable. We children knew that the reason she was doing so was that she was after blood or, as she herself used to put it: 'waiting for him to fall into my wasp's nest'. I can still see her, dressed in a black hobble skirt and yellow, short-sleeved, scoop-necked maternity top, her face a mask of determination. She was going on and on about him being late, but his time-keeping didn't seem to be any different from the past. Then we heard the car turn into the driveway and go into the garage. The engine fell silent. I half expected Gloria to storm off in the direction of the garage, but she provided a lesson in tactics by holding her ground. A few seconds later, the driver emerged into the passage from the doorway leading to the garage.

'Is this the time you've come to pick me up?' she demanded.

'W'a' 'appen, ma'am?' the surprised driver asked, in a tone of voice I took to be genuine innocence.

'W'a' 'appen, indeed,' Gloria said, mimicking him with such acerbity that we children couldn't help laughing out loud, as she shifted gears and accused him of using the car as a taxi. In fairness to her, it should be noted that this was a scam frequently practised by chauffeurs, though I very much doubt any of ours would have had the opportunity – not when Gloria almost regulated the number of breaths everyone in the household took. She kept them on such a tight rein that they only had time to travel from one designated point to another.

'No, ma'am, I would never do somet'ing like dat. Mis'er Ziadie tell me to drop somet'ing off at Kensington Crescent. Das all I do.'

'That would have taken you no more than five minutes,' Gloria observed in a tone of voice which made it plain that she believed him to be lying.

'I stop to talk to Miss Edit',' he said. Edith was the most venerable of Daddy's branch of the Ziadie family's female servants.

'You mean Edith,' Gloria said. Although he didn't know it, we children knew she had laid the trap for him and was now springing it.

'Yes, ma'am. Miss Edit'. Das what I say.'

'No, you didn't. You said Miss Edit', not Edith.'

'Yes, ma'am. Das what I say,' the poor man said, missing the nuances and clearly not comprehending what was going on.

'That is *not* what you said,' Gloria snapped. 'You said what I said you said, not what you've just said you said. How dare you contradict me?'

'But, ma'am, I don't contradic' you. I agree wid you.'

'So now you're accusing me of being a liar?'

'No, ma'am,'

'Yes, you are. If I say you are, you are.'

'But what 'appenin' 'ere? Miz Ziadie Ma'am, I don't know what you is sayin', ma'am, but whatever it is, I didn't do nothin', ma'am.'

'I will not have you contradict me and denying that you did it. You are stinkingly impertinent. I will not have it. You can pack your bags and leave this instant.'

'But what me do, ma'am?' the befuddled man asked, clearly needing to understand what was happening.

'What you "do",' she spat, mimicking his way of speech, 'is contradict me and be damned impertinent.'

'You really goin' fire me over this?' he asked, perplexed.

I can tell you, by this time, we children had seen so many variations on this theme that we were anything but perplexed. He was only the latest in a long line of servants to be sent packing for reasons beyond their comprehension over offences which Gloria had trumped up so that she could drop the axe.

'That's right. Now pack your little knapsack and be off these premises in ten minutes sharp,' she ordered.

'What about me two weeks' pay?' he asked. All servants were entitled to two weeks' severance wages if summarily dismissed.

'What about it? Have you worked for it? Have you done anything at all except use my vehicle as a taxi and speak to servants whom you were impertinent enough to address as "Miss" to me?'

'You mean you don' give me me two weeks' pay?'

'You're a bright one, aren't you?' she said sarcastically.

'You white rass,' he screamed at her – 'rass' being the worst swearword in Jamaica. 'Dat is my money and you better give it to me!'

'And what are you going to do when I don't, you ugly nigger?' she mocked as she walked off.

He kicked out at Gloria, missing her protruding belly by a comfortable margin but nevertheless making the point that he too had resources he could utilize.

'Owen! Denzil!' she screamed. 'Come here this instant.'

'You is a mad rass,' the driver said, stomping off in the direction of his room before the gardeners could come. By the time they reached the house, Gloria was inside, telephoning the police. We children knew the form only too well even before the police arrived in their Black Maria. Three policemen would come from Mathilda's Corner Police Station. They would be ushered by the butler into the house. They were always offered something to eat and drink: an invitation they seldom declined, for when they said they were on duty and really shouldn't, Gloria invariably told them it was perfectly all right and she would clear it with the Commissioner of Police if that made them feel better. She never needed to do so, and in being ostensibly gracious she was also cleverly delivering a double message: firstly that she was influential enough to waive rules that applied to more ordinary people, and secondly that she was charm itself to them. On this occasion, as on all others, they listened to Gloria's latest tale of woe. This being Jamaica in 1956, they were firmly on her side – or, at any rate, they made a fine show of being so. They duly reprimanded the chauffeur, telling him he was an 'ungrateful wretch. Don't you know how lucky you is to 'ave a job with a fine lady like Miz Ziadie?' When the unfortunate driver brought up the subject of his severance pay, she mockingly said 'Sue me', as they grabbed him under his arms and manhandled him out from the back veranda, where this was taking place, into the back of the Black Maria, pouring scorn on his presumption for demanding what was his by law and right, while Gloria calmly sat down, graciously thanking the senior officer for their assistance.

Thereafter, she resolutely refused to employ another chauffeur for nearly a decade, the reasons for which, I would come to realize years later, dovetailed with Diana, Princess of Wales's reasons for getting rid of her police protection officers. Wives who want to keep their activities secret from either their husbands or the rest of the world cannot afford to be observed by drivers or security officers.

Faced with his wife's intransigent refusal to employ another driver, Michael bought himself the Morris Minor that became Scrammy shortly after Kitty's birth so that Gloria could have exclusive use of the smart American saloon which they had hitherto been able to share, thanks to the services of the chauffeur.

With hindsight, I can see that Gloria was wise to be careful. Not only did she take the most sensible step possible to ensure that no one would actually acquire knowledge that they could then use against her, but she also countered the gossip that was, by this time, rife about her activities. How she defused it was a study in holding your nerve. 'Everyone is always saying that all my children except Mickey have fathers who aren't Michael,' she would announce to all and sundry in her husband's and children's presence. 'Georgie is supposed to be Basil's, Libby is Bernie's, and Kitty is Ric's. If I had had one tenth the affairs that the general public have ascribed to me, I wouldn't have had time to get out of bed, much less give birth. Women can be so jealous of other women. They have nothing better to do with their time than trying to destroy the life of someone they're jealous of. That's why I prefer the company of men.'

As a way of shifting the blame for her clouded reputation from her own activities onto the malicious and competitive motives of peers who were less attractive and less-privileged than she was, Gloria's technique could not be bettered. And it worked. Michael accepted that there was talk, but that it was motivated by jealousy. So Gloria didn't need to worry that stories would get back to him which could undermine her position, by being the person who brought them out into the open.

Only once did she suffer a real threat from gossip and that, according to her, was when her own mother was indiscreet enough to contribute to the chatter. In 1996, Gloria brought up the subject herself when we were speaking about her relationship with Maisie, which had been, from my perception, warm until Gloria's thirties. Indeed, as teenagers we children used to laugh and say: 'Mummy's rebelling as a big woman instead of in her teens like everyone else.' However, Gloria came up with another explanation for her antipathy in 1996. 'Your grandmother went around telling everyone that I was having an affair with Tony Feanny. She couldn't see any harm in reducing me to her status of flagrant adulteress. She jeopardized my marriage with her idle talk. I never forgave her for that.'

I knew only too well that if Grandma had indeed been so indiscreet – and, I have to say, it might well have been possible, for she saw nothing wrong with ladies seeking their pleasure elsewhere after they had fulfilled their duty and provided their husbands with progeny, – she was indeed jeopardizing her daughter's position as a wife. Had word got back to my father of what his mother-in-law was saying, he would have divorced Gloria instantly.

However, circumstances had changed by 1996. Michael was now dead. Tony Feanny had been married for decades and was an old man living in the United States. It was perfectly safe to come clean and end the once-clever game of denial. So I told her what Vida had said, giving her the ideal opening to confirm what she, by her own admission, was stating her own mother had accused her of.

'Vida was imagining things,' she said.

'And Grandma?' I asked.

'Do you know why I have never worn red in my life?' she said pointedly, and I waited for what she had to say, knowing that this was her way of providing an answer in a roundabout way. 'Because I was the daughter of a scarlet woman who was so proud of what she was that she even announced it to all and sundry by always wearing red.'

That wasn't actually an answer to my question, and I wasn't about to let her off the hook any more than I had been prepared to let off the subjects I wrote about in my biographies. I had learned from Gloria how people slide away from the truth with non-answers, so I put on my biographical cap.

'I accept that you didn't want to announce to the world that you might be having an affair with Tony Feanny,' I said, 'but now that Daddy's dead, admitting it won't undermine your interests. Indeed, it might even shore them up.'

'And how would that be?' she asked coolly.

'Well, it would give us children a deeper appreciation of the sacrifices you had to make to remain married to Daddy.'

'I've only ever known one man in my life, and that man was your father,' she said coldly, trying to bring the subject to a close.

I, however, hadn't become a successful writer by being so easily fobbed off.

'So you're saying that both Grandma and Vida were lying,' I said.

'You said it, not me,' she retorted.

'And why would they have done that?'

'You'd better ask them, not me,' she said, only too aware the dead have no voice.

I must confess I was disappointed in Gloria for not seizing the moment to become more intimate with one of her children. I felt it was a great pity that, even at that stage of her life, she could not and would not drop the façade of impervious perfection that prevented any real human interchange. Even though I regretted her choice, I nevertheless respected it. It also drove home the point to me yet again how futile it was to try to build bridges with her. Although she was always moaning about feeling lonely and isolated, she had always made her true self inaccessible and must therefore pay the inevitable price for such disconnectedness. It was depressing to think that someone could claim to want human companionship then cut themselves off from the substance of it. Moreover, it was depressing as well to think that I could not actually rely upon her claim that Maisie had actually been gossiping about her. False accusations were an integral part of Gloria's *modus operandi* and it was, I knew from experience, as likely – possibly even more likely – that she was inventing the whole sorry scenario to justify the way she had mistreated her mother for the last twenty years of her life.

Nor was Gloria's motivation so hard to see. She was intensely competitive and felt the need to place everyone in her shade. But the one person she would never nudge there was her gloriously indomitable mother. Not only was Maisie Gloria's equal in terms of strength of character and as a *femme fatale*, but she was also her superior in worldly accomplishments. She was a successful businesswoman in her own right, with a considerable property portfolio all of which she had acquired through her own initiative, at a time when such activities were truly exceptional. And the one thing the Glorias of this world cannot cope with is people who are not subservient.

If I cannot rule out the possibility that Gloria felt no compunction about coming up with a base lie to discredit the mother she could not eclipse, that is only because of her disregard for the rights and wrongs governing her own general behaviour. Her attitude bespoke not so much arrogance as a genuine belief that anything she did was all right, even though that same conduct would be wrong when indulged in by any other human being. In her mind's eye, the rules governing other mortals simply didn't apply to her. It's not that she denied the existence of right and wrong, nor that she was blind to where duties and responsibilities ordinarily lay. She was the first to criticize anyone who deviated from the highest standards of behaviour, so she cannot have been unaware of what those standards, or their ethical underpinnings, were. She simply had one set of rules for herself and another set for everyone else; and the former gave her absolute licence to say or do exactly as she pleased at any time and under any circumstance.

An illustration of this attitude took place early in the evening of the 3rd of October 1957. I was sitting semi-recumbent on my parent's bed, staying with Gloria while she was dressing to go out. Libby and I had just returned from a friend's birthday party and, having gorged ourselves on cake, ice-cream and candy, had been allowed to skip dinner. One of Gloria's rules, and a sensible one at that, was that our nurse could not force us to eat anything we did not want. Libby was in her bedroom with Michael, who was indulging in his usual pastime of reading until just before his wife had finished beautifying herself, at which point he would then get dressed in the five minutes it took her to finish off what she was doing.

By this time, Michael and Gloria had been married for eleven years, and they knew each other's habits so well that he always seemed to time the moment for attiring himself magically. There was never any direct communication between them as to when he should start dressing. Since neither of them could tolerate waiting for anyone, even for two minutes, he needed to judge that particular moment carefully otherwise either he or she would keep the other waiting.

When Michael entered the marital bedroom, Gloria had already put on her clothes and was fussing with her hair. I can still see her sitting on the stool at her dressing table, her tail comb in hand, messing with her pony tail. Pony tails, pedal pushers and mules were then in vogue; and she, naturally, was sporting all three as all other women on the cutting edge of fashion then were.

'Where's the shirt I got from Bernie's?' Michael asked, opening drawer after drawer of his chest of drawers.

'How would I know?' Gloria replied in the haughty tone she frequently employed with him and with everyone else.

'You should know. It's your duty to know.'

'Why? Do I look like a laundress to you?'

'Woman,' Michael erupted, 'I spend half my life breaking my back to keep you in luxury. The least you can do is make sure that the servants under your command are doing their jobs properly. I want my shirt, and I want it now.'

Coolly, so that the contrast between her lack of emotion and his expression of it was all the more apparent, Gloria said in her best mocking tone, 'Well, my dear man, if you want it you'll just have to go outside to the laundry and find out where it is.'

'No. You will go and find out where it is. It is your duty as a wife to take care of this sort of thing. You will go,' Michael bellowed.

Quick as a flash, Gloria jumped up.

'I'm not one of the niggers you employ,' she declared. 'How dare you speak to me like that?'

'You think you're better than them, but you're not. They work for a living. They fulfil their duties, which is more than I can say for you.'

While Michael was speaking the unvarnished truth, Gloria, standing no more than eighteen inches from him, slipped her hand down the side of her body towards her right foot, which she had bent upwards towards her bottom, to make her shoe accessible. She quietly took off the mule, and in one fell swoop cracked Michael on the forehead with its heel before he even knew what was happening. Blood gushed from the wound. I, sitting on the bed, was transfixed, too horrified to move, too curious to run away from the first real row I had ever witnessed in its entirety. Up to then, I had only heard or seen snippets.

'You must be mad,' the inarticulate Michael, who ordinarily stammered except when he was angry, said. Then, in a ploy which I recognized, even at the age of eight, was masterful, he turned, opened one of Gloria's drawers and removed the first article of clothing he could lay his hands on to use as a mop. It happened to be a white, heavily embroidered stole she had recently brought back from Mexico.

'Mad or not, you're going to learn it's easier to love me than to master me,' Gloria retorted. 'Do you think I'll ever forget when we were first married how you had the gall to say to one and all, "I married a young girl so that I could bend her to my ways while she's still young enough to learn." Bend me to your ways, indeed! The only bending that is ever going to be done around here is by you, you stinking Syrian shit.'

'You really must be mad. Sane people don't behave like you,' Michael repeated, his usual riposte during one of their rows.

'If I'm mad, it's because you've driven me to it. You didn't pick me up off the street. You took me from my parents' house, a young virgin. I should have listened to Dada and never married you. You're the one who's mad. You're erratic and cannot control your temper. Well, you can bully all the niggers you employ, but you won't be bullying me. I am here to tell you that you'll find it a lot cheaper to love me than the alternative. I'll take you to the cleaners and strip you of every one of those precious pounds you're always going on about working so hard to acquire, unless you treat me the way I expect. Do I make myself clear?'

'You're mad.'

'Whether I'm mad or not is immaterial. All that you need to concern yourself with is keeping me sweet. Now throw my stole in the wastepaper basket and not the laundry box. And be quick about it, because, thanks to your lunacy, you've now made us late,' Gloria said, sweeping out of the bedroom.

Michael was muttering to himself about what a lunatic his wife was when I heard her shout: 'Georgie, it's time for bed.'

Reeling from the shock of what I had witnessed, I went into the drawing room, where Gloria was sitting, drinking a glass of sherry from a silver goblet, to tell her goodnight. She looked surprisingly calm and composed after a scene that had shaken both my father and me. Indeed, if I hadn't been privy to it, I would never have believed that she had taken part in it. She seemed so unscathed, unaffected, unmoved.

But Michael would bear the scar from that attack, just above and between his eyebrows, for the rest of his life. It might have been obscured by the lines on his forehead, but it remained visible, proof that Gloria didn't need rhyme or reason to strike out.

Chapter Five

The 1950s would turn out to be the decade when the British Empire, and the way of life it had fostered for the past three centuries, experienced its swansong. It was a decade in which the old ways still flourished. Traditional values still held true. The rich man truly was in his castle, the poor man at his gate, the world perfectly ordered according to long-standing English values.

The 1960s, by contrast, were the decade which saw the dismantling not only of the British Empire but also of its mores, traditions and way of life. Everyone was affected: the rich man in his castle, mostly by fear, misgivings, unease over what the future might hold; the poor man at his gate, mostly by hope, frustration, expectation of the liberties and prosperity that Independence would bring; and everyone by thoughts of what they could gain or lose.

As far as the colonial upper classes were concerned, Independence was not without its drawbacks. All over the Empire, the white ruling classes were only too aware that they were a tiny minority in countries with largely black populations. There was a genuine fear of revolution when the British withdrew, leaving a power vacuum which would have to be filled largely by dark-skinned citizens who might well have grouses – and valid ones at that – against their white former rulers.

For too long the white man had reigned supreme, and there was a fear that Independence would bring with it a day of reckoning for the many injustices of the past. I remember my parents and their friends having many a conversation on the front veranda (the back veranda was too close to the servants' quarters to take the chance of being overheard) after the staff were in bed. Everyone bitterly condemned the English. 'Now that they can't milk any more profits out of us, they're going to abandon us to old *nayger*,' was the oft-repeated comment. 'So much for the great Mother Country, for which people willingly gave their lives in two World Wars! Not to mention all the centuries of enriching England!'

This feeling of abandonment, of being used then discarded now that the colonies were no longer the money-spinners they had been over the previous three centuries, had one immediate and dramatic effect. Once the date of Independence was announced, and everyone realized that the British really were going to leave us all – rich and poor, white and black – to our respective fates the way Pontius Pilate had left Jesus Christ to fend for himself, the reverence with which the English had been regarded for centuries literally evaporated overnight. It was quite extraordinary to witness how one day everything English was the best and most desirable, then a week later people, including English families like the Smedmores, were vociferously distancing themselves from that which had been respected for so long. It was as if the scales fell off everyone's eyes at the same moment, and people realized that the oasis of safety, security and care, which the English had peddled for three centuries as the basis for their imperial ambitions, was nothing but a mirage of disinterest and self-interest. 'Hypocrites', 'con-artists', 'deceivers', 'parasites' and 'leeches' were only a few of the words everyone now started to use when speaking about the British; and as resentment and feelings of betrayal replaced the respect which had proliferated for centuries, most English families started to downplay their heritage.

I remember when the subject of the family's citizenship first came up. My parents and Lucius were discussing the matter over dinner prior to Independence. My father, having been born in Jamaica of parents of Ottoman citizenship at a time when all wives took their husbands' nationality and automatically lost their own upon marriage, was entitled to choose between British and Jamaican as well as Lebanese citizenship. My mother, with her paternal English and maternal Irish heritages, had the choice of retaining a British passport or opting for a Jamaican one. Grandpa, always so English until then, thought the English had behaved shockingly and said he would turn in his British passport for a Jamaican one at the first opportunity.

'I am Jamaican born and bred, and Jamaican I intend to die,' said Michael.

'This is our country,' Gloria said, 'England is not our country. Why would I want a British passport when I can have a Jamaican one? The Mother Country indeed! Motherfucker, more like it.'

'Language, Glory dear,' Lucius said, raising his finger to his lips.

'I'm sorry, Dada, but it's absolutely true.'

'Nevertheless, you are a lady and one simply does not use language like that.'

'All of that nonsense is going to be consigned to the rubbish heap along with the Union Jack,' Gloria said with a prescience which time would bear out.

Independence Day was Sunday, August 5 1962. Mickey, Libby and I attended the ceremony with Lucius at the recently constructed Stadium in the presence of Princess Margaret, who, together with her husband Anthony Armstrong-Jones, represented the Queen. I can still see PM, dressed in a white evening dress wearing the Politmore tiara. She really was ravishing and made more of an impression upon us children than the whole business of lowering the Union Jack and raising the green, gold and black flag of the newly independent Jamaica. Afterwards there was a fireworks display, but we watched it with interest rather than joy. The mood in families like ours was sombre, with people recognizing that we were now entering uncharted territory, and only a fool would expect all the inevitable changes to be improvements.

What also put a damper on us children's perception of the Independence celebrations was Marilyn Monroe's death. Her body was discovered the morning of Jamaica's Independence. As she was our favourite movie star, we were glued to the television set when the news was announced. Jamaica had got its first television channel only a few weeks previously, and we children were having an early supper prior to going to the Independence ceremony when the announcement of her death was made. It was as if the world we had known was being changed left, right and centre, which indeed it was. Even the advent of television would prove to be a lasting change, for thereafter one did not have to be as reliant on people for companionship as one had previously been.

Independence brought with it a fierce pride in our new nation. The national motto symbolized the racial multiplicity of Jamaica: 'Out of many, one people.' Early representations showed citizens of every shade and degree of colour, from white to black, with lashings of yellow and brown filling out the spectrum. Jamaica was promoting itself as an island paradise where racial harmony was a reality, not a goal; and that, to an extent, was the truth. While there were inequities – and while class and colour coincided – generally speaking, it was a lot less colour-prejudiced than most other places. Indeed, in Florida – then a Southern state with the colour bar in force – people used to say they could always tell when passers-by were Jamaican, for the only racially mixed groups were Jamaican visitors.

Also, in Jamaica itself, 'everyone' mixed socially – 'everyone', that is, who was not a part of Society, where exclusivity still reigned supreme. If you went to any non-Society Establishment gathering, you would see whites, coloureds, Chinese, Indians and the occasional 'dark'. If black people were still not generally seen except in servile positions, this was because they were still less prosperous and less well-educated than their richer brothers of colour. While one could have said that blacks were still generally excluded, the fact is, people of colour no longer were.

This was more than could be said for just about every other country on earth, where no distinction was made between black or brown; and everyone of African ancestry was lumped together and excluded.

Though not yet Nirvana for uneducated blacks, Jamaica was nevertheless within its rights to lay claim to being a truly interracial society where exclusion was due more to socioeconomic factors than to colour.

The shake-up that Independence brought also extended to Society. Families like my father's, which only a few years before had been on the periphery of Society – admitted out of sufferance, if at all – suddenly found themselves catapulted to positions of respect as a result of the vacuum created by the loss of respect for the British. A host of non-WASP names, which had once typified wealth alone, now represented social kudos as well, while Anglo-Saxon families like the Smedmores suddenly found themselves associated with an order that was discredited and therefore no longer desirable.

To people like my grandfather Lucius Smedmore, these changes were discomfiting as well as ominous. I remember Grandpa sitting on the front veranda one evening holding forth about Marcus Garvey, the civil rights pioneer who had been voted a National Hero of the new Jamaica. 'This is insanity,' he declared. 'The man was a scamp. He set up a company called the Black Star Line, ostensibly to take black people back to Africa, in a boat that had more holes than a sieve. Back to Africa indeed! He lost them their life's savings. The man was a scamp, I tell you. Depriving all those poor, innocent, gullible people of their worldly goods. His memory should be reviled, instead of which they're rehabilitating his reputation and making him into a National Hero.'

I was far too young to know whether Marcus Garvey was a scamp or a hero but not so young that I could not see – and enjoy – the justice of some of the changes. Despite being a genuinely decent and God-fearing man who was a pillar not only of Society but also of the Anglican Church, Grandpa was an insufferable snob who was always going on and on that 'everyone may be nice, but not everyone is your social equal'. He was always preventing me from mixing with school friends on the grounds that they were not 'suitable'. More dangerously, he was always supporting Gloria in her never-ending complaints about her husband, failing to see that his precious daughter might be in the wrong. Instead, he criticized his son-in-law along snobbish lines, even saying to us things like, 'Your father just doesn't know how to behave,' and 'I always knew your mother would have a hard time with a man like your father. He can't help it. He just doesn't have the right sort of background.' I am sure he said far worse to Gloria herself.

Lucius never missed an opportunity to deliver the message to his grandchildren that our Smedmore blood (if indeed we had any) was superior to our Ziadie blood, and that it was our Smedmore manners that set us apart, not only from the common herd but also from the Ziadie family.

Over three decades after his death, while clearing out my brother Mickey's papers after his death in 1994, I would run across a note Grandpa had made as Secretary of the DeCartaret Ball in 1960. DeCartaret was then a leading prep school, and Gloria was chairing a fundraising ball. Grandpa's note revealed the full extent of his antiquated, arcane but oh-so-English social prejudices: in the list of attendees, he listed himself as 'Lucius Smedmore Esq.' – namely a gentleman. Meanwhile he listed Alec Durie – the scion of an old, good and rich mercantile family who was heir to one of Kingston's greatest great houses, Cherry Gardens, and certainly every bit Lucius's social equal – as Mr Alec Durie: in other words, not quite a gentleman because he was in trade and therefore inferior socially.

'Oh Grandpa, how could you?' was my initial reaction. Everyone knew that King George V's daughter Princess Mary, the Princess Royal, had married Viscount Lascelles, later the Earl of Harewood and that the family's wealth originated right in Jamaica from the mercantile group Lascelles de Mercado.

Surely if mercantile families were good enough for the King of England, they should have been good enough for Lucius Smedmore. Evidently not.

If I felt a certain amount of distaste for my grandfather's stance as an adult, it was nothing compared with what I felt as a child. Possibly I might have been more receptive to his snobbery had he not interfered with friendships I wished to pursue. I can vividly remember how turned off I was every time he or my mother launched into another of the diatribes to which they were wont, about the Smedmore family history. To me, it was bad enough that their snobbery was placing unnecessary limits upon my friendships, but the fact that it was boring as well made it doubly unacceptable. It created a distaste in me for snobbishness which has never left me.

As a result, I was secretly delighted when Independence brought an immediate diminution in the stature of the Smedmore family and an immediate increase in the Ziadies'. While Grandpa still persisted in affirming the Smedmore family's superiority at every opportunity, I – and I felt sure, just about everyone else – could see that the validity for making such claims had been exposed as the emperor's new clothes.

Without the link to the English master race to prop up claims to ascendency, the Smedmores were just another well-bred family amongst a host of other well-bred families of equal stature and pretensions: in other words, well mannered but in no other way special and therefore not particularly superior.

The Ziadies, on the other hand, had more energy and greater dynamism. They were a more intelligent family and far better-looking. They were more successful and more accomplished. In my view, they were therefore the Smedmores' natural superiors, and I considered it entirely fitting that the new values of the new nation were rectifying the errors of the old English order, based as it had been upon the fallacy that British was best, even when it was patently not. Indeed, the new order was truer and healthier.

The social changes taking place in the country were not limited to drawing rooms. Arguably, the most profound of them were taking place at grass-roots level. The people saw Independence come and go, and the improvement in their lives – which the politicians of both parties had promised, as a natural effect of voting for one party or the other – did not take place. This bred a dissatisfaction which would see a rise in crime, as people now felt entitled to take, by stealth or by force if necessary, what they had been promised.

Up to that time, Jamaica was a relatively crime-free country. There were thefts and burglaries and petty crime, all that one would expect from people in need, but it was not a violent society. Such violence as there was usually took place within and amongst the lower classes. It was virtually unheard of for the upper or middle classes to be murdered. When they were, it was usually an in-house killing.

There had been only two murders resulting in white men being killed in the previous forty or so years. One was the Alexander murder case, in which Mrs Alexander and her lover were tried and found not guilty of murdering her husband, though it was commonly accepted that they were guilty. The other involved the lover of a prominent mercantile family, a distant cousin of my father's, which in part inspired my novel *Empress Bianca*. While she was never charged or tried, it was commonly believed that the lady in question had blasted her lover through the head after they had made love, because he was going to abandon her. Unfortunately for her, the bullet passed through his skull and entered her hip, thereby linking her forever to the crime. Her story, of a gunman coming upon them and shooting him while his head was in her lap, was implausible in the extreme and easily disproved.

Then, on the night of May 18 1963, an event took place which would precipitate a trend that ultimately shook Jamaica to its foundations, resulting, in a matter of years, in the country acquiring a reputation as one of the most violent and dangerous places on earth. For the first time in living memory, a white man was killed by a black man to whom he had no connection. The murder was gory and gruesome, the violence gratuitous. The victim literally had thousands of lacerations, bruises and cuts; and he had been hacked to death in the most brutal manner. It was a crime not only of violence but also of passion and bespoke the many other murders that followed where the level of violence indicated 'score settling'. The first instrument the murderer used was a plank of wood studded with nails. This he beat his victim with, hoping to batter him into submission, but that failed; and the older victim, sixty-three to the murderer's twenty-something, fought back in a desperate struggle to keep alive. So the murderer switched to a machete. He used this to chop the unfortunate older man, who continued to fight furiously for his life. He managed to wrest the machete from his killer's hands and push him out of the house. Regrettably, he neglected to lock the front door, and the murderer came back with a flower pot, which he crashed over his victim's head, spilling his brains onto the floor and finally killing him.

The victim was my grandfather, Lucius Smedmore; and his murder was truly one of the most shocking events to have happened in Jamaica up to that time. Although it would turn out to be a robbery gone wrong, no one knew it at first. The upper classes, always so prone to expect the 'revolution', openly questioned whether it had now arrived. Sir Alexander Bustamante, the prime minister, was on his way home from church when he heard the news on his car radio. He promptly instructed his driver to turn around and head towards Trafalgar Road, the site of the murder, where Lucius's body still lay.

When Busta arrived, it was to find my parents and grandmother there and the place crawling with the police. They were combing the property looking for the murder weapons, while Roy, the gardener, who had discovered Grandpa's body, stood by and recounted how he had climbed up a ladder and looked into Lucius's bedroom to see a bloody shirt on the bed, alerting him to the fact that something was amiss when he could not rouse Grandpa to let him into the house. He then went next door, to the neighbour's house, and she telephoned the police as well as Maisie and Daddy to tell them that something was obviously very wrong.

First on the scene was the local police, who entered the house to find Lucius dead, sitting upright in a chair in the drawing room, his head thrown back, his brains having trickled down the back of the chair onto the floor. A 33 rpm record of Stainer's *Crucifixion* was still spinning on the turntable of the gramophone. Clearly visible from the death chair was the dining room, where the murder had actually occurred. Blood was splattered all over the wall and up onto the ceiling. It is a peculiarity of murder seldom appreciated by the general public or the entertainment industry that the blood of the victim splatters over a distance of several feet; the pumping heart of someone who is still alive is like a fire hydrant which gushes away once the pressure is released.

Maisie never got any further than the drawing room. She took one look at her ex-husband, with whom she had had lunch the day before, and promptly went into shock. When Michael and Gloria arrived at the house a few minutes later, the former had to arrange with Perez, the cause of her divorce, to come and pick my grandmother up and take her home. Once there, the doctor came to sedate her, and for the next three weeks, she remained in bed, either sedated or a jabbering, semi-hysterical wreck, when the medication wore off.

Gloria herself never entered the house. The police, seeing what had happened with Maisie, advised her not to look at her father but to remember him the way he had been. 'They told me if I saw him the way he was, I'd never get the image out of my mind. And I wanted to remember him the way he had been in life, not the mangled creature he had been reduced to. So I stayed outside,' she said.

Busta's visit picked them up somewhat. It is incredible how the unexpected kindness of others helps at moments of tragedy, and both Gloria and Michael were appreciative of the prime minister's gesture. Although our family were staunch supporters of his party, my parents were not his close personal friends, so his action was all the more gratifying for its unexpectedness. It also demonstrated how the murder of one white man was still a remarkable event. Within a few years, such an occurrence would be commonplace, and prime ministers no longer called in on death scenes, no matter how eminent the family was or how close they had been to them.

By the time Busta departed, the hearse had arrived to collect Lucius's body. So that Gloria would not see her father's body being removed from the house, she was taken next door to the neighbour's house. She remained there while Michael went downtown to the morgue to identify officially his father-in-law's remains. Until his dying day, he found what he had seen so distressing that he could never talk about it. There really are some sights that are so awful that one simply can never recover from them; and this, unfortunately, was one of them. Having identified Lucius, Michael returned uptown, picked up Gloria and took her around to Tony Feanny, who lived nearby, where he medicated her, then brought her home.

Death in Jamaica, like in many Third-World and Mediterranean countries, is an intensely sociable time. From the minute people hear of a death until after the funeral, all and sundry drop in to offer their condolences. There is an appreciation of the fact that the grieving cope best if they are emotionally supported by the care not only of close friends and relations but also by passing friends and acquaintances. I remember the constant stream of visitors from that Sunday morning of May 19 until after the funeral on the Tuesday afternoon of May 21.

The funeral itself was a massive affair. Held at Kingston Parish Church, the leading Anglican church in the country, where Grandpa had been one of the governors, it was packed to the rafters with friends and relations of all the various branches of our family as well as various representatives of official bodies such as the government and the police and Grandpa's Masonic lodges. There was also a large police presence inside and outside the church, for the authorities did not yet know who had killed Lucius or why, and on the supposition that it might be an assassination and the murderer or murderers could be after the rest of the family, the place was crawling with uniformed and plain-clothes officers, some of whom mingled with the crowd of several thousand spectators outside the church. Even Uncle Perez, who had displaced Grandpa in Grandma's affections so many years before, attended the funeral, sitting in the family pew between Marjorie, who had had to return from Mexico where she was on holiday, and Mickey. Maisie, however, did not attend. She was still too ill to leave her bed. Even if she had been well, however, she would not have been there. She didn't 'do' funerals, not even for her favourite brother, who was killed in a car crash while still in his thirties. She would actually only go to two in her whole life, those of her mother and father.

Inevitably, things quietened down after the funeral. They did not, however, return to normal. Firstly, it took nearly another month before the murderer was apprehended. In that interval, the family had to be hyper-vigilant in case we were also targets. Then, the murderer killed another member of the Establishment and was caught shortly thereafter when his girlfriend, worried about the level of violence lest it escalate to include her, turned him in.

It turned out that Clifton Eccleston's motive in killing both Lucius and Eric Clarke was robbery, but that this was coupled with a truly chilling lack of regard for their right to life. There was, indeed, an element of class-prejudice payback. In the years to come, as Jamaica underwent ever-increasing political turbulence, one would see, time and again, the vicious and gratuitous way in which the murderous element of the Have-nots, as they are called in Jamaica, would torment the Haves before killing them. Death was invariably a mercy, but one that arrived too late to spare the innocent the most appalling suffering.

To his credit, Clifton Eccleston had the decency to apologize to my grandmother at the time of his trial, which took place in 1964, a year after the murder. By then he had discovered that Lucius had been a genuinely kind person. 'Me come into the world like a wild beast, and me going leave like one,' he said to Maisie, knowing that he would be hanged for his crime. 'Me only regret is dat me kill your husband. Me hear him was a good man. Me sorry.'

The time between the crime and the apology was turbulent, to say the least, for the immediate family. Once Eccleston had been arrested and confessed, it emerged that he had targeted Lucius as a result of reading in the social columns that his daughter Marjorie and her husband Ric would be in Mexico visiting her maternal aunt Pauline. On hearing this, Gloria sensibly banned the social columnist, her friend Violetta, Contessa de Barovier-Riel, from writing about the family's forthcoming activities thereafter.

Eccleston had cased the joint for a few nights, noting the time the staff left to go home. Observing that only Lucius was in residence until the staff returned to work the following morning, Clifton Eccleston had found his window of opportunity.

On the Saturday evening, he made his move at around nine o'clock. Grandpa was alone, sitting in the chair where he was found in the drawing room, listening to Stainer's *Crucifixion*. The front door, leading from the drawing room to the front veranda, was open. Eccleston burst in and demanded all the money Lucius had in the house. Lucius opened his wallet, gave him the one five-shilling note he had, but this was not enough for Eccleston, who couldn't get his head around the idea that just because Lucius was white and lived in a good area, this didn't mean that Lucius was rich. As far as Eccleston was concerned, all white people were rich and therefore a 'rich white man' like Lucius would have a lot more money hidden in the house. Lucius tried to point out to him that that really was all the money he had, but this disclaimer enraged Eccleston, who was convinced that Lucius was holding out on him and taking him for a fool. Eccleston knew with the certainty of the ignorant that Lucius 'had a whole heap of money hidden in the house'. He had to. Hadn't Eccleston read about Marjorie and Ric in the social columns? You surely had to be rich as well as grand to be in those, so he set about battering Lucius in the certain knowledge that his brutality would yield up the secret of where the hoard was hidden.

When his physical abuse failed to produce dividends, Eccleston killed Lucius for no other reason than that a 'rich white man' who had caused him such trouble deserved to die.

When he had finished the job, he moved Lucius's body from the dining room, where he had killed him while Lucius was telephoning for help, to the drawing room. Then he removed his watch, which was one of a limited edition of twenty-five, and let himself out of the house. It was that watch that would seal Eccleston's fate, for when he was caught and tried to lie his way out of what he had done, he could not come up with a good enough story to explain away how he had come into possession of such a rare item.

Murder inevitably has a pronounced effect upon the family of the victim, as I suspect it also does upon the family of the perpetrator, especially when the death penalty is involved. Indeed, one could go as far as saying that the effect says a lot about the characters of the people affected. Marjorie and Ric couldn't quite forgive themselves for being abroad, blaming their absence for the tragedy. At first, they refused to return to the house, preferring to stay with Maisie, but a few months later, they bit the bullet and returned. This turned out to be a mistake, for they could not get what had happened out of their minds, not even after the bloodstains had been washed away and the walls repainted. Ric started to have heart attack after heart attack, and, realizing the futility of living there, with its constant and awful reminders, they built another house, which they moved to within a year. It was then, and only then, that they could somewhat resume the tenor of their lives. But the effect upon Ric would prove to be lasting, for the trauma had caused such a weakening of his heart that he would die three years later, aged forty-two.

Maisie also blamed herself for what had happened. She kept on saying that Lucius would not have been killed if they had not been divorced, but with the passage of time she realized that she was in no way responsible and resumed her life free of guilt, if a lot sadder than before. She had always looked remarkably young for her age until then; and the most pronounced residue of his murder was that she aged twenty years in as many days, losing her youthfulness forever.

In some ways Michael never recovered from the murder. Having seen his father-in-law's body, he appreciated, as none of us actually could, what Eccleston had done to Lucius and how he would have suffered as a result. Thereafter, he was preoccupied with the safety of his family. This was not in an unrealistic way, but with an understanding of the dangers we ran each and every time we came or went, day or night. It resulted in a wealth of restrictions placed upon our movements which, to young people, was frankly nothing but a major pain.

Gloria, however, was the person who seemed to be the most affected. 'All that morbid, excessive grief she displayed,' was how Mickey, who loved his grandfather and was very similar to him in manner and character, disapprovingly described her reaction in 1994. Although she and Michael quickly resumed their social lives, if Gloria was not going out, she would sit on the front veranda, night after night, with the lights turned out, Michael's revolver in her hand, bawling like a baby and pointing the gun in the direction of the street, shrieking, 'Come, you ugly niggers. Come and let me give you what you have coming to you.' These hyper-emotional dramatics went on for about a year, causing me to remark to Mickey after a few months that Mummy must now be eating her words about Aunt Doris.

Gloria, never the most compassionate of people, had mocked Aunt Doris's grief when Aunt Juliette died suddenly at the age of forty-one of a brain tumour two years before Lucius. 'Every night, when she doesn't have a poker game to go to, Doris sits on the front veranda at Tucker Avenue,' Gloria used to remark, referring to Aunt Juliette's house, 'rocking in a chair and mewling in the most disgusting fashion. My nerves can't take the histrionics. She clearly has forgotten she's not a Jewess at the Wailing Wall.'

Having made her disapproval of such displays of grief evident, Gloria was now doing the wailing, and for a lot longer than the six weeks indulged in by Aunt Doris. Never when there were visitors but always when she was alone with her children and husband.

After about a month, Michael started to duck out. If he was at home, he would go to bed as soon as the floodgates opened, but more usually he timed his escape so well that he would leave the house as soon as dinner was finished, usually going down to his brother Solomon's house to play cards. That meant that, during term time, I was left alone to sit with Gloria, for Libby and Kitty were safely at boarding school, and Mickey had also opted to start boarding again.

At first, I accepted at face value that Gloria was genuinely grief-stricken. With the passage of time, however, I came to realize that something more than grief was feeding this morbid flood of tears. Quite what it was, I couldn't put my finger on, but I knew that Lucius's death was simply the vehicle to which my mother had attached her emotional baggage. Of course, I had little doubt that Gloria had loved her father, and I knew that he had loved her; but even so, what was happening on a nightly basis, seemed way beyond what anyone could recognize as a genuine or acceptable expression of grief.

Later on, when I was old enough to have some experience of life, I would come to believe that Gloria had used her father's death as the cover to release emotions she had been otherwise bottling up. She was already on the way to being a very disenchanted person, and I suspect many of those tears were for her shattered illusions and the pain they were still causing her. Later on, I would also come to see that Gloria was your typical histrionic personality, whose emotions are as exaggerated as they are shallow. Such personalities utilize every experience they have to maximize every sensation they feel, not because they feel so much more than others, but because they feel so much less. While those of us with deeper, fuller and greater emotions struggle to contain or minimize feelings that might otherwise blow us away, people like Gloria whip themselves up into frenzies to escape from the reality of the emotional desert they occupy.

It is a feature of the histrionic personality that they must be the centre of all attention. No matter how great anyone else's happiness or suffering, theirs must be greater. That is the only way they can remain centre-stage and can keep the spotlight upon themselves. The irony is that people like that are as much their own audience as anyone else. They will happily spend two hours crying or uncomfortable just so that they can witness themselves as the stars of their own show. Of course, they usually make sure that there is someone else present to act as the audience, but the paradox of such personalities is that they do not always require third-party participation, for their whole lives are dramatic productions with themselves as the star; and even when the external audience is absent, the production – and the need for observation – persists. So they also watch themselves, valid enough participants in the drama to be both star and audience. It really is a case of the show going on irrespective of who is in the audience; in some ways, the histrionic personality's life is more a theatrical production than an actual life.

I can now see that Gloria was actually enjoying her surrender to grief. She was wallowing in it, in the certain knowledge that she was the star of a genuinely tragic show. It was too great a starring role to resist, and she dragged it out for as long as she could. Only after a year, when she had milked it of every advantage, of all attention, and had grown as bored by it as everyone else, did she move on. And when she did, it was with a finality that was absolute. Thereafter, she never once, insofar as I am aware, ever grieved for her father and never mentioned him in passing the way one does a departed loved one, though she would occasionally dredge him up to make the point that she was a Daddy's Girl, the implication being that she was a very special person who had always deserved to be spoiled. The affection she was alluding to, therefore, was all in one direction: towards her, and not from her.

This always struck me as odd, though it would only be after I had grown up and experienced grief for myself as an adult, when my brother died prematurely, that I could put my finger on what was wrong with her reaction. With most of us, grief follows a pattern that is more or less similar. It is intermittent, coming in great waves or little rushes, but not as regular and predictable as a theatrical production, nor of the same duration as a Broadway play. It doesn't last for two or three hours a night, and seldom strikes as regularly as clockwork. A great wave might take five or ten minutes, a little rush a matter of seconds. And grief lingers. One does not wake up one day, a year after someone one loves has died, dust oneself off and mentally decide: 'Okay, I've milked that event of every sensation it affords. Let's now see what other event I can exploit for some more attention and sensation.' Such opportunistic and self-aggrandizing exploitation of emotion is a sign of a very disordered personality and one, moreover, which is ultimately callous and uncaring of anyone and anything but itself.

Chapter Six

In many ways, Lucius's death marked a real crossroads for both my immediate family and for the island of Jamaica, which thereafter hurtled down a violent path that would ultimately lead to the destruction of its tourist industry, as the criminal element of the Have-nots waged deadly war against the Haves. Insofar as my own family was concerned, the heightened awareness of danger that was an inevitable result of the murder might have been a drag, but it had one unforeseen benefit. We finally got the dog for which we children had long been agitating.

Asocka Charuska was a German Shepherd puppy. The son of two world champions, he came to us when he was eight weeks old. As with just about everything in our life, it was through 'contacts' – in this case, Uncle Ric's brother-in-law, who was a great dog-lover and had imported some of the litter from England.

'I don't want that animal in my house,' Gloria informed us when the puppy arrived. 'He's not here as a pet. You know I can't stand puss or dog. He's here purely as a guard dog. To protect us. You know how terrified old *nayger* is of dogs. I don't want you children spoiling him and turning him into a pet, for then he'll be no use to us. Remember, he has a specific purpose: to tear to pieces any old *nayger* who comes here to harm us. Do I make myself clear?'

While we all nodded assent, I seized the moment and used my position as favourite to negotiate a better deal for the puppy and for ourselves. It was Gloria's intention to make the poor animal stay outside rain or shine, even during tropical downpours or when there was thunder and lightning. As anyone who has even the most rudimentary knowledge of animals knows, dogs are terrified of those elements, and moreover, he could easily get struck if he was stuck outside. 'Mummy, can you have him stay on the back veranda?' I suggested hopefully, swallowing the wave of anxiety I felt each time I was opposing, however subtly, my dominating mother's wishes. 'It's not inside the house. Then he can protect us while we're looking at television; and if it rains, he won't run the risk of being struck by lightning.'

To my delight, Gloria considered the idea. 'He can stay on the back veranda,' she consented, 'but he's not allowed to cross that threshold,' she added, pointing her engraved ivory cigarette holder, which Mickey had bought her for her thirty-fourth birthday, in the direction of the step dividing the back veranda from the interior of the house. 'We will start the way we intend to continue. He can spend the nights in the laundry until Clunis builds his house, and he can stay on the back veranda or in the grounds during the day.'

'Can the house be built on the back patio?' I asked, figuring that I might as well continue while I was on a roll.

'That's a very good place for it,' Gloria declared, to my surprise. 'Near enough to the house for our protection, but far enough away so that I don't have to contend with dog hairs.'

Because much of family life took place on the verandas, whether front or back, and because Sportie, as we kids nicknamed him, had not been excluded from them or from the pool house or the pool veranda, I had achieved something remarkable. Thereafter, we children could have the joy of a pet, while Sportie ostensibly remained a guard dog.

Sportie proved to be a captivating dog. Ravishingly beautiful, he was also bright and affectionate. Soon even Gloria liked him. 'I can't stand dogs,' she would say, 'but Sportie is the best of a bad bunch.' She was particularly entertained by the way he would greet her in the garage when she drove her car into it. 'What are you trying to tell me?' she would ask him, laughing and barking back at him in what became a set-piece.

'Life is so funny,' Gloria would frequently observe to whomever was present when she arrived home to Sportie's greeting. 'I can't stand dogs, but this animal loves me more than he loves anyone else in this family of animal-lovers. Now run along, Sportie, and keep watch,' she would say, taking care not to touch him.

As Sportie grew up and proved to be an excellent guard dog, it was a never-ending source of amusement – and something of a relief – to Gloria that he was a natural racist. 'Our lives certainly aren't in danger from other white people,' she said on many an occasion, pleased that Sportie had a natural antipathy to the very pool of the population whence burglars and thieving murderers customarily came. He never rushed whites who dropped in to visit, not even when they were strangers, but he was notorious for rushing people of very dark hue, even if he already knew them. On one notable occasion, he bit a peddler who made the mistake of entering the grounds unannounced and would have killed the man if Owen, the head gardener, hadn't managed to pull him off. On another occasion, Owen saved the life of the fishmonger with seconds to spare when Sportie had the man pinned down on the driveway and was getting ready to tear his face off, even though the dog knew him well. There were several lesser episodes like that, but the most embarrassing and potentially dangerous, from the family's point of view, was the night he lunged at the throat of Victor Grant, the attorney general.

Victor, who had become a good friend of my parents in the four or five years since becoming attorney general, was walking up from the driveway by way of the back passage to the back veranda when we heard the most ungodly growl followed immediately by a blood-curdling scream. By now Sportie's proclivities were well enough established for Michael to conclude that a friend rather than a thief or murderer was in difficulty, so he immediately jumped up. 'Don't move!' Gloria shouted out at the unseen victim. 'Whatever you do, don't move!' Michael rushed out to see Victor standing frozen to the spot as Sportie, on his hind legs, was dancing around his throat, inviting him to move so he could be justified in ripping out his windpipe.

All Daddy needed to do to stop Sportie was say: 'Enough, boy.' Sportie then returned, docile as a lamb, to the back veranda in front of Michael and a trembling Victor, whom Gloria received with a tinkling laugh, 'You'd better hoot your horn the next time you come,' she said lightly. 'The country needs you more than Sportie needs human flesh.' Then, before he had a chance to reply, she ordered the butler, who had come out of his room at the sound of the kerfuffle and was standing in the other back passage opposite the summer house: 'Get Mr Grant a *crème de menthe frappé* the way he likes it, Edward. He needs something to steady his nerves. You know how

Sportie inspires terror in one and all.'

In what I did not then recognize was a revealing vignette of Jamaican life, Edward went to the liquor cupboard and started muttering to himself. Thinking he was disaffected to be called out after he had gone off duty, I asked him what the trouble was. 'This damn house gone to the dogs. Is bad enough that me have to serve old *nayger* when him should be working beside me. But the damn man don't even know that what a proper *frappé* is. Who ever heard of *frappé* with ice cubes? I tell you, the world really is a mess when respectable people,' he went on, referring to himself, 'have to serve *buttu*,' using the term reserved for Jamaica's 'scum de la scum', 'who don't even know that them must either drink *crème de menthe* straight or then have it on a bed of crushed ice.'

I could scarcely believe my ears. Edward was not complaining about being called out of his quarters out of time, or of Sportie nearly killing the attorney general. Instead he was bemoaning Victor's lack of refinement and the fact that he should not have to serve someone of his calibre. I couldn't help laughing out aloud. 'Edward, you are such a snob.'

'All good butlers is snobs,' he said grandly and with more than a hint of truth. 'And me still say, this house go more and more to the dogs every day. All that is left is for a Rasta to come here and ask your mother to order me to fetch him him ganja tea.'

Edward had hit upon one of the welcome effects of our grandfather's death. Aside from bringing Sportie into our lives, almost overnight there was a marked decrease in the snobbish attitudes to which Gloria had hitherto clung. Lucius had been her most stalwart supporter where snobbishness was concerned, as well as a rigid policeman of the family's social circle; and with him gone, the barriers were to a large extent down.

Nor did Lucius restrict only our social circle. He was always backing Gloria up when she complained about our father, attributing the difficulties in their marriage to Michael not being Gloria's social equal. The possibility that the difficulties might well have had more to do with them both being spoiled brats, and she even more than he, seems not to have occurred to him. Certainly there were superficial differences in background and culture, but these were a lot less significant than a first glance might suggest. The Ziadies, despite being a mercantile family of Lebanese and Russian origin, would have been every bit the social equal of the Smedmores, had the politics of their native country not forced them out of it. Status, of course, doesn't travel well, as any Russian prince or Austrian archduke – or indeed the Duke of Edinburgh, who had personal experience of that fact when he was the exiled Prince Philip of Greece – can tell you. Nevertheless, a dispassionate examination of the facts indicated that the Ziadies had parity with the Smedmores because they had an equal background in their native land. They had been landowners as well as a prominent religious and intellectual family, which had produced two of the leading Middle Eastern writers of the twentieth century. The first was May Ziadeh – the family has six different ways of spelling its name, as there is no one equivalent transcription from the Arabic alphabet to the Latin, and various branches spell it according to their convenience. She is the Jane Austen of the Middle East, to this day the most eminent female writer in Arabic and French for the first half of the twentieth century. Then there was another cousin, Kahlil Gibran, who by the 1960s was one of the most popular *philosophes* in the Western World and indeed something of a favourite of Gloria's. She was always raiding his books, *The Prophet* and *The Wanderer*, for quotes when she had to make speeches to the various charitable organizations with which she was associated.

Such facts, however, would never have made any real difference to either Gloria or her father. They were intent on always being superior socially; and if they could have dragged a dead rat out of the cane field and used its existence to gain the ascendant position, they would have done so. With Lucius out of the picture, Gloria had no one to encourage her in the snobbish arcana. Gone was her main support, the man who had consistently and continuously fed her superior stance, as long as she took care to present her case to him in a ladylike manner. I cannot remember one occasion upon which Grandpa ever put his precious 'Glorydear' in the wrong unless she used foul language, which she, like all cutting-edge socialites of her generation, was starting to do occasionally.

My whole childhood is a haze of Gloria moaning and groaning about everyone and everything, but most especially Daddy and the Ziadies. Do you think it would ever have occurred to Lucius that maybe, just maybe, someone else had a point of view except Glorydear? Never. Absolutely never. Not even once. She used to whine and whinge, not just for Jamaica but for the whole British Empire. She had a real need to obtain sympathy at the very moment that she wanted your admiration. And Lucius supplied her with both – in equal and never-ending measure. And always, at the end of it, he had somehow spun it around so that Glorydear was suffering because she was better than everyone else, largely if not entirely because she had been born Gloria Dey Smedmore.

And yet, when I look back on one of Lucius's favourite comments, I wonder if the remote possibility does not exist that he was aware that maybe his Glorydear wasn't quite as perfect as he indicated. 'Gloria is younger than my four grandchildren,' he was always saying to her and to anyone who would listen when she was around – but never when she was not. He would say it with a laugh, but he repeated it so often that I now suspect he was trying to give her a message. And, because he knew she took pride in looking young, and in people saying how she didn't look old enough to have children our age, appearing more like our sister than our mother, he must have been hoping to deliver his message in a way that appealed to her vanity. I now suspect he was trying to say that Gloria was immature and needed to grow up. That, certainly, must have been the real meaning of his words, but they were couched in such terms that he was not criticizing, and might even have been praising, her. Lucius must have known what I, and many others, would discover in the years to come. While his daughter felt entitled to praise, criticism was not something she would ever countenance. And, because he loved her and was intent on keeping in her good books, he took care to drop his hint in a way she would find acceptable.

If he was trying to edge her towards the realization that she needed to mature, his actions were doomed to failure. 'Thank God Lucius died before he saw what Gloria turned into,' Grandma rightly used to say in the years to come. The problem was that his daughter's self-perception, as the only embodiment of perfection on earth, was so utterly ingrained that she had absolutely no insight. Without insight, she could therefore get no hint. Indeed, if you strayed from the soft option of hinting to the middle ground of factual declaration and made the dispassionate observation that she, like all human beings, had failings, the self-evident nature of what you were saying would be lost on her, because she truly believed that she was the yardstick by which perfection was measured. This made dealing with her extremely difficult; her self-belief left no room for any other opinion or consideration than her own. If, however, you went to the other extreme and clobbered her over the head with the fact that she was just as imperfect as anyone else and in fact a damned sight more so than many another person, she would think you were either mad or malicious. That you might be neither and were simply speaking the truth would never have entered her head.

It would take another twenty years from the time of Lucius's murder before I was presented with an explanation that actually made sense of what had started Gloria on the road to becoming the monstrous creature she grew into. It was an evening, like many another, early in 1973. I had dropped in on my grandmother and my step-grandfather. We were talking about Gloria and how unnecessarily offensive and cruel she had been to her mother in calling her an 'old whore' after Maisie had remonstrated with her for dropping in on her sister at eleven o'clock in the morning with a glass of gin in her hand. 'Life is very funny,' Perez said. 'Your grandmother has been such a good mother to your aunt and your mother, and look how they've turned out, your mother especially. Your parents have been abominable to you children, yet you've all turned out so well. I suspect the secret of child-rearing is that if you want to have nice children, treat them harshly instead of indulging them the way your grandmother and grandfather indulged your mother and your aunt.'

'That's not fair,' Maisie protested. 'We had no choice. You remember what Dr Mosley said. We had no choice. Gloria required special handling.'

'What are you talking about?' I asked, perplexed.

'When your mother was about three, there was an awful incident. We had to call Dr Mosley to come and see her. He gave us some advice, and we took it.'

'Details, Grandma, details,' I said. 'What incident? What advice?'

'You know how highly strung your mother is. She always was. Even as a little girl. If it's possible, she was even worse then. She used to give us the devil. One of the worst problems was in getting her to rest. Every afternoon Nana Alice would have the most terrible trouble with her. As soon as she put her down and left the bedroom, Baby Gloria would start to howl and scream. One afternoon I came home and she was demanding to be let out, saying that dogs were surrounding the crib and trying to bite her. I went into the bedroom and smacked her on her little bottom and told her she would have to rest quietly until it was time to get up. She became hysterical – literally hysterical. Nothing could quieten her. Nana Alice tried. I tried. Nothing worked. She was totally inconsolable. Finally, in desperation, I told Nana Alice to leave the room, then I shut the door and left her there. I was quite determined that she would not cry me into relenting, but a little later Nana Alice came to me. She'd looked in on your mother and couldn't believe what she saw. Gloria had bent the iron bars of the crib and had wriggled out onto the floor, where Nana Alice saw her sobbing and telling the imaginary dogs to go away. I telephoned your grandfather who told me to call Dr Mosley to come immediately and give the baby something to calm her nerves. She can't have been more than three at the time.

'Afterwards, he said to us, "Mr and Mrs Smedmore, Baby Gloria is very highly strung. She's not like other children. She needs special handling. You mustn't ever tell her no. If you do, you can tip her over the edge. You will have to find a way of dealing with her without ever telling her no."'

I could hardly believe what I was hearing. One look at the expression on my step-grandfather's face, however, told me that the unbelievable was true. 'You can't be seriously telling me that you and Grandpa never told Mummy no again?' I exploded.

'Dr Mosley told us we would do her irreparable harm if we did. She was too highly strung to be told no. We couldn't tell her no.'

'I can't believe I'm hearing this,' I said, making no attempt to mask my horror. 'Didn't you realize that that was a recipe for creating a monster?'

'We had no choice,' Maisie said doggedly. 'We couldn't run the risk of destroying her nervous system.'

'Meaning no offence, Grandma, I have to tell you, I've never heard such horseshit in my life.'

'Now, Granddaughter,' she scolded, 'you know I can't abide language like that.'

'I'm sorry, but it's true. How could two intelligent people like Grandpa and yourself have fallen for horse manure like that?'

'That's a bit better,' she relented.

'Surely you must have realized that a child who is never told no grows into an *enfant terrible*? No wonder Mummy is the monster she is. Anyone would be if they never heard the word "no" while they were growing up.'

'Don't misunderstand me,' Maisie said. 'She had discipline. She had to behave herself like a lady. We never had any trouble with her on that score… at least, until she started using foul language, which is a recent development and, I regret to say, something you children also use…you more than the others,' she quietly reprimanded.

'I happen to like cursing. It's emotionally expressive. My psychiatrist says it's good for one to express oneself. Everyone curses nowadays.'

'It's vulgar and common, and the only people who can be excused for using foul language are those who have a limited vocabulary. Which neither you nor your mother has.'

'Okay, okay, I won't curse for the rest of the evening,' I said, conceding the point.

Then Maisie said something else that took my breath away. 'Your mother always understood discipline, so Dr Mosley can't have been so wrong. Look at how she's disciplined all of you. Look at how she controls your father. And, much as I love my son-in-law, I have to acknowledge, controlling him hasn't always been an easy task. But she always had a natural aptitude for discipline, so I wasn't worried about not telling her no. I remember her very clearly as a little girl having her dolls lined up in a row. She used to love pretending to be a school mistress. And she would take out her ruler and smack them for being rude or turn them over on their stomachs and lower their little panties and beat them on their little bottoms for some imaginary infraction or other.'

'Good God, Grandma,' I spluttered. 'Can't you see that Mummy was always nothing but a punitive, sadistic bully?'

'But she could be so kind,' she said.

Perez looked at me, his blue eyes sparkling with approval that someone was finally seeing the light of day.

'I don't want you using words like that to describe your mother,' Maisie said, catching the look between us. 'She's still your mother, no matter what else she is.'

'I have to tell you, this conversation has been a real eye-opener. All I will say is that Dr Mosley has a lot to account for.'

I went back home with a greater appreciation of how my mother had been allowed to get away all her life with being a spoiled brat. So far as her parents were concerned, as long as she had the social graces which were a requirement of her class, she would remain unchecked while she said and did as she pleased.

Of course, once Gloria had grown up, things changed. Her cruelty towards Mickey and Libby had been unacceptable to both her mother and her sister; and their avid protection of her two children had doubtless been responsible, more than anything else, for the erosion of her relationship with both Maisie and Marjorie. If she hated hearing the word 'no', one does not need to imagine how she loathed the criticism implicit in their standing up for her abused son and daughter.

The fact that Gloria's relationship with Lucius remained as good as it did is a testament to his restraint and diplomatic skills. I remember him as being an openly loving and fair grandfather to all of us, but especially to Libby, who was his favourite, and to Mickey, who – being the grandson and the most 'Smedmore' of the four of us in interests and demeanour – was particularly close to him. He cannot have condoned her mistreatment of the grandchildren whom he made it only too clear he loved, though quite how he resolved batting for both Hitler and the Jews is something of which I have only a slight recollection. I suspect that he managed it because Lucius understood that Gloria respected him enough to want to retain his good opinion and that, as long as she sought that good opinion, he could pour oil on troubled water by 'massaging' situations. His technique was to jolly everyone along without attributing blame to one quarter or the other, interceding before a problem blew out of control or after it had done so but never during it, the way Maisie and Marjorie did. I cannot recall him once putting Mickey or Libby in the wrong, yet he somehow managed to keep in with Gloria in a way that neither Maisie nor Marjorie, who were more straightforward and strident, did. His very presence was therefore a moderating and restraining influence upon his recalcitrant daughter, and I suspect that it would have remained so as long as he played his part with the skill he deployed.

Lucius's death therefore had one particularly negative effect upon the family in that it removed the one source of restraint in Gloria's life. Thereafter, self-indulgence without restraint was the order of the day.

If Mickey's life had been torturous before, then it became far more so after 1963.

At the time of Lucius's murder, Mickey was a sixth-form student at Jamaica College. He had done his 'O' Level examinations the year before, sitting and passing them at the unusually young age of fourteen. One would have thought that that was all the evidence his parents needed to respect his intellectual abilities; few children before or since have completed high-school examinations at such an early age. Not Gloria and Michael, however. Although Michael was very much Mr Tag-Along, he nevertheless either sat by like a silent and passive blob while Gloria abused his son for being 'a fool' or would sing the chorus to her tune. Mickey was a born liberal politically, always espousing views that were centrist or left of centre politically, which was anathema to his ultra-right-wing parents, so they soon added the insult 'communist' to 'fool' every time he opened up his mouth to evince a political opinion.

In an attempt to escape from the constant stream of abuse which emanated from parental quarters, but largely from the maternal, Mickey sometimes opted to board at Jamaica College, using the excuse that he wanted to study without distractions. Even such a responsible choice was pounced on by Gloria, who used it as proof that his desire to study in peace was a sign of stupidity rather than good sense.

Mickey was now a very good-looking fifteen-year-old. Although not tall, he had a trim, muscular physique and the exotic looks of his father: regular nose, generous mouth, finely shaped face, noble brow and huge eyes of the palest, purest green, framed by the longest lashes anyone had ever seen. All his life his eyes and eyelashes inspired comment. 'A positive waste on a boy,' was the most common. They were truly remarkable, and even in the years to come, when I was being written about as a great beauty and people would remark on how beautiful my supposedly Garboesque eyes were, I would always say with more truth than modesty: 'If you think my eyes are beautiful, wait until you see my brother's. Mine are very commonplace beside his.'

He was also popular. Sociable by nature, with the impeccable manners of the Smedmores, allied to the charm of the Burkes and the largesse of the Ziadies, he made friends easily. He had a ready source of friends, whom our parents and our snobbish grandfather found suitable, because Jamaica College was where most of the scions of the good Protestant families went. This meant that prior to Grandpa's murder he could bring home school friends without Gloria or Lucius objecting to them the way my grandfather and mother had objected to my school friends.

Shortly after Grandpa's death, the swimming pool and pool house, which had been under construction, were completed. This, in my opinion, was the single most important factor which caused us to develop the tremendous social life we did. Ours was one of the few swimming pools in our circle of friends, pools then being still something of a rarity, even amongst the very rich. Because the pool and pool house were deliberately located well away from the main house – so that 'the noise won't disturb anyone in the house,' as Gloria put it – our parents could not see what was going on unless they actually went to the trouble of coming out to the pool, which was something they seldom did. This made our pool a lot more desirable than the pools other friends had, for theirs were too close to their houses and their parents were therefore always able to monitor what was going on. This degree of privacy, together with our parents' surprising leniency in allowing us visitors, without regard to their quantity so long as they approved of them, was responsible for turning our house into the main meeting point for our circle of friends during the holidays. During term time we could still have one or two friends up at the pool, about whom our parents wouldn't even know as long as we were discreet, so the pool house became the hub of much social activity.

I used to be perplexed by the apparent paradox of how, on the one hand, Gloria would be so generous in allowing our friends to use our home almost as a club and giving us extra money to go partying with friends from an early age while on the other, being so harsh and mean to Mickey and Libby when the guests had gone and we were on our own.

Even before Grandpa's death, relations between Gloria and Mickey had been building to a climax, but it was only after Lucius's death that they achieved it. Over the next three years, things went from bad to worse. Tension crackled in the air whenever mother and son were in the same room – not, I must say in my brother's defence, that it emanated from his quarter. He had the sort of personality that always believed the best of everyone, even when the evidence to the contrary was overwhelming. Each day he would bounce out of bed, full of the joys of life, happy to be alive and ready to like and love everyone and everything – including Gloria. Even after she had roundly abused him, he would always wipe the slate clean and act as if nothing untoward had ever happened. I remember when he bought her that ivory cigarette holder. It was a day or two after he had returned from one of his stays at Grandma's house. I would have sooner eaten grass than spend my saved-up pocket-money on such an expensive present for someone who had treated me so badly. But he headed downtown to the shop on King Street where he had seen it. He happily spent what was for him a small fortune and said, 'Isn't it beautiful? Mummy will love it.' And she did. Mickey's eight-inch cigarette holder became her trademark until she bit a hole into the ivory years later, rendering it unfit for further use. Not that the visible symbol of her son's good nature made any difference to the way she treated him.

As Gloria sucked smoke from her Du Maurier cigarettes into her lungs through Mickey's cigarette holder, you would have had to be blind, deaf and dumb to miss the degree of abusiveness which characterized her relations with a child who never initiated any of the hostilities that rained down upon his head.

A case in point was music. Gloria loved music, and so we had been brought up in a musical environment. She was always playing records; so from an early age, we were exposed to good classical music as well as popular music. Like all children of our background, we were also given piano lessons from about the age of five or six. While my sisters and I demonstrated a marked lack of talent, our brother displayed a considerable degree of it. Moreover, he had an unquenchable interest in the piano. Unlike most children, to whom practising is a chore, he was always eager to do his scales and perfect the pieces he was learning. It was his often-stated ambition, from an early age, to be a pianist one day. And when he wasn't practising or playing some piece by Brahms, Mozart, Chopin or Beethoven which he had learned, he was listening to gramophone recordings by the greats such as Claudio Arrau, Arthur Rubinstein, Shura Cherkassky and George Bolet, which he had bought with funds saved up out of his pocket money. He had been doing this since about the age of eight so there was no doubt that his love of music was both sincere and commendable; and, indeed, anyone who knew Mickey associated a love of music with him.

Most parents of musically gifted children encourage them when those children express a desire to practice. But Gloria was not like most people. Whenever Mickey was home from school, either during the holidays or when he was going through one of his non-boarding phases, he would want to practise in the afternoon. If Gloria was at home, she would prevent him as soon as he started. 'Not now. My nerves can't take the din,' was the phrase she often used. So Mickey would silently close the piano and, taking her words at face value, hope that he would get another opportunity later that day. I wish I had a pound for every time he opened up the piano after dinner and struck the first chords, only to be accompanied by Gloria's remark 'Night time is my time' which, we all knew, meant that he would have to desist.

The problem was that morning time was as much Gloria's time as night time or afternoon time. It was rare indeed for Mickey to open up the piano in the morning without Gloria stopping him with her morning variation of her nerves not being able to cope with the noise so early in the day. So Mickey would have to snatch practice sessions when Gloria was not at home. This was hardly an ideal way of perfecting his craft, but at least she was out often enough for him to achieve sufficient of his objective, though without the frequency that his talent needed if it was to mature and flourish.

And where was Michael while these blocking techniques were going on? Either at work or reading a book in his bedroom, his head buried in the sand like the proverbial ostrich. I can never recall him once calling his wife to order for preventing his son from doing something voluntarily that most other parents had to force their children to do. His prevailing stance was all about keeping the peace. Not that he kept it at any cost. If Gloria tried to curtail his activities, as she sometimes did, by accusing him of leaving her too often, he would immediately display the backbone which at all other times was absent. Then, he would fight her tooth and nail so that he could continue going to whatever outside activity he wished to indulge in. 'I love Daddy,' his favourite child Kitty once said, 'but he is the most selfish human being I have ever run across in the whole of my life.'

Mickey had not yet reached the age when his career had become a factor in his parents' thinking, but when it did, Michael must have been grateful to Gloria for having thwarted their son's musical talent at every turn. 'You cannot become a musician,' Michael said every time Mickey said he wanted to study music. 'Musicians don't make enough money unless they are at the very top. What guarantee do you have that you have enough talent to make it to there? No. You cannot become a musician. Music is a hobby, not a career. I'm not going to be supporting any child of mine once you're grown up, let me tell you. You'll do something that pays. Like medicine or dentistry.'

Meanwhile, Gloria remained intent on thwarting her son at every other turn as well. She used to take malicious delight in frustrating him, the piano being only one of the many forums she devised as a suitable place to exact her malice. Another venue was the dinner table, table manners being the pretext for spewing forth yet more venom. Every night, when the family was on its own, she would start in on Mickey and make us grateful for the fact that we seldom dined without guests. 'Where are you flying to?' she would mock, spreading her elbows and flapping them about in a gross exaggeration of the movement he would make as he used his knife and fork to cut his meat. Mickey would then tuck his arms closer to his side, only to be reprimanded two minutes later for the way he was holding his knife. 'Do you think you're digging a ditch?' she would say, stabbing her knife into the plate. Once or twice, she sent her food flying, which only resulted in her ringing the silver bell by her side for Edward, the butler, to come and clear up whatever now reposed on the Persian carpet beneath the table. By this time, there would be a blanket of silence enveloping us, only for it to be pierced a minute or so later by another of Gloria's catty observations about the way Mickey was now chewing. This would create another pregnant silence before she started mimicking him smacking his lips, when he had been doing no such thing.

By now my stomach would be in such knots that I could barely swallow my food. Which was just as well, for if it was not, and I was eating, she was liable to alight upon her supposed favourite with the withering remark: 'The food isn't running away from you. Stop cutting and swallowing.' Or she might sneer at me: 'Stop contorting yourself like a snake. Sit up straight when you eat. Your back should never touch the chair. When will you learn, child?'

I can now see that she, who had no interest in food, must have found it intensely annoying to have to witness others enjoying theirs. Daddy and I, who both loved our stomachs, were not only the most constant members of the family at the dinner table but also the two who were most overtly gourmet. We were always making comments about this meat or that vegetable or something else being particularly good, while she would either cut her eyes at us or sneer and say: 'Good food is not remarkable. It is to be expected. That's what we have a cook for.'

With Gloria setting the tone, conversation would be nonexistent when we dined *en famille*. Mickey, Libby, Kitty, Daddy and I always concentrated on getting through the meal without further vitriol from Gloria. You could hear a pin drop and each chew of whatever mouthful we had taken, as we sat speechless and withdrawn, hoping that by being silent and as near invisible as possible, we would be spared the next barrage of bile from this pillorying self-perceived paragon of perfection.

While Michael always ignored Gloria's ordinary acts of cruelty, sometimes her viciousness – invariably towards Mickey – would be so acute that even he could no longer stand by silently. 'Leave the child alone, for God's sake,' he would rumble - or some other variation on the same theme, which would always shut her up. This would lead me to wonder why he didn't intercede more often, but it taught me something useful about dealing with her, which I would utilize in the years to come.

One night, shortly after Grandpa's death, Mickey hit upon the perfect form of revenge. It was during the summer holidays of 1963, and Gloria had ruined just about every dinner we had sat down to *en famille* for the whole of the holidays with her vitriolic scapegoating of poor Mickey. In an attempt to deflect further abusiveness, Mickey said to Libby and me: 'Did I ever tell you the joke about the man in the London restaurant?'

'Not that corny joke,' Libby and I responded as one.

'It's not corny. Let me tell it to you again so that you can get the joke,' he said, launching into it with fervour: 'A man went into a London restaurant. He signalled to the waiter to come over to him. The waiter came over and said "Yes, sir. What is it?" The man said,' Mickey continued, lowering his voice to a rasping whisper, '"See that man over there? He's been dead for three days."'

Mickey, who had a 'haw-haw' sort of laugh, started to guffaw for all he was worth, killing himself with laughter at a joke that neither Libby nor I found in the slightest bit funny even after hearing it for a second time.

One look at our parents, however, was all we needed to get the real joke, which was their response to it. Michael, who had no sense of humour at all, was looking around, perplexed but relieved that something rather than Gloria's abusiveness was happening at the dinner table. At the same time Gloria, who had an excellent sense of humour, shot Mickey an icy stare down the length of the table and pursed her lips contemptuously, irritated that he had trumped her by embarking upon a distraction technique which made her sadism impossible, at least for the length of time it took him to tell the joke.

Gloria's look – so reminiscent of 'The Look' from our childhood, when it had taken only one glower to stop us dead in our tracks – was all the invitation Mickey needed. 'And have you ever heard the one about Christopher Columbus?' he went on.

'No, not Christopher Columbus,' Libby and I chorused, having also previously heard that non-joke and found it no funnier, though by now we were complicit in the game and hopeful that our response would make our brother continue.

'It's really very witty. Listen to it again. You're sure to get the humour this time.'

Libby and I groaned in mock horror, giggling delightedly as we exulted in our brother having stolen the floor from his tormentor.

'What did the Indians say when Columbus arrived in the Americas?' Mickey asked.

'What did they say?' asked Daddy, who had not yet heard the joke and was happy to join in anything that would avoid further unpleasantness.

'Columbus has arrived. At last we are discovered,' Libby and I chorused, pre-empting Mickey from recounting the punch line.

'Is that a joke?' Michael asked, while Libby, Mickey, Kitty and I started to howl with laughter.

'Huh,' Gloria spat out from under her breath, ringing the bell so that Edward would come to clear the meat course prior to serving the pudding, even though Mickey had still not finished his dinner.

'You can clear Mister Mickey first,' she declared imperiously as Edward entered the room. 'He's finished too.'

Even though Gloria snatched a measure of victory out of the mouth of defeat by preventing Mickey from finishing his dinner that evening, he had nevertheless succeeded in wresting control of the occasion from her. This set the scene in a wholly unexpected way for Mickey to turn the tables on our mother. The next time we were dining *en famille*, before Gloria had a chance to pick on Mickey, he launched into the London restaurant joke followed by the Christopher Columbus one. Libby, Kitty and I, relieved that we would not have to endure the agony of seeing our brother wriggling on the hook of our angler mother, came to his rescue by playing our parts to perfection. We could hardly have done better had we practised. We moaned and groaned in protest at having to listen to the joke yet again but remained vastly amused as he ploughed ahead, recounting it to his ostensibly-reluctant audience.

Mickey had found the way to break the cycle of Gloria's domination of the one meal a day we ate as a family. The next time we dined *en famille* and after she had launched into her usual attack on him, he waited a decent interval and piped up with, 'Have you ever heard the one about the man in the London restaurant?'

This was Libby's, Kitty's and my cue to protest, amidst gales of laughter, that we didn't want to hear the non-joke, which Mickey nevertheless recounted yet again. Then, in an absolute repeat of the two previous occasions, no sooner had he finished that joke than he regaled us, as if he had never told it before, with the one about Christopher Columbus.

By this time, Michael had also picked up on the joke, but Gloria was not amused and never would be. So the next time she criticized him, Mickey recounted both the jokes. By now, the recounting of the non-jokes was itself the joke; and we would each assume our allotted roles, Libby, Kitty and I protesting at having to hear them again while laughing nevertheless, as Mickey started in on yet another retelling, with Gloria's face assuming a more thunderous or icy expression than usual.

Although I suspect that we children were too young to fully appreciate what was going on, on an atavistic level we knew that Mickey had succeeded in turning the tables on our mother. He had made her the victim of his joke. Moreover, he had done it in such a way that she dared not unmask him, for to do so, she would have to acknowledge that he had turned her into the joke figure. Her overweening pride and sense of self made such an admission – indeed, even a hint of the existence of such a fact – unacceptable. So she had little option but to ignore what was going on, thereby allowing it to continue.

Only too soon, Mickey wasn't even waiting until Gloria attacked him. No sooner were our knives and forks poised to cut into the meat course, than he would introduce his set piece with the words: 'Have you heard the joke about the man in the London restaurant?' To howls of mock protest and barely suppressed giggles from the rest of us children, he would begin a faithful repetition of the same two jokes as Gloria shot daggers down the length of the table at him.

One night, after about two months of this, Gloria could stand it no longer. As soon as the words 'man in a London restaurant' were out of Mickey's mouth, she picked up her glass of water and sailed it down the length of the table at him.

'Stop it! Stop it!' she yelled. 'You little shit. Stop it right now. I've had enough of your nonsense. Get to your room this instant.'

'Are you mad?' Michael rumbled to his irate wife as he mopped up the drops that had landed on him. 'The children are only having a little fun. They mean no harm.'

Mickey started to mop his forehead with the linen napkin as Edward rushed in and brought a couple of kitchen towels to absorb whatever water remained on the table.

'Bring Mr Mickey some more dinner,' Michael ordered.

'Yes, sir,' Edward said.

The look on Gloria's face was a revelation. Fury was mixed with frustration as she realized she could not actually call time on the tune without embarrassing herself. So she pitched back her chair, sending it flying and leaving it for Edward to pick up as she dramatically departed, announcing to no one in particular that she was going to bed. 'I can no longer endure sitting with a bunch of morons,' she added.

Gloria had made a big mistake. Now that Mickey had absolute confirmation that he had really got her goat, he was encouraged to continue. When weeks had given way to months and Mickey was still telling those two same jokes each night at dinner, Libby and I started to count the number of times we had heard them. I gave up when the tally reached well into the hundreds. Night after night, year in and year out, over the next three years, until he left home to go to school in England, Mickey would recount those two same jokes. He had found a way to amuse himself and his siblings while at the same time tormenting his tormentor.

Gloria, who took pride in 'eating like a bird', would sit picking at her food and downing her drink, waiting for the joke period to end before she could resume taking pot shots at all and sundry.

Of course, while this set piece was going on, no one knew that Mickey would actually tell the same two jokes every night for years. I don't think it could have occurred to Gloria that her son would perpetuate the saga for the length of time he did. Certainly, neither Libby nor Kitty nor I thought he would. But when it had gone on for over two years, Gloria, who had the choice of ignoring what was going on or absenting herself from the table, started to have her dinner served on a free-standing tray while she sat on the back veranda and watched television. This was fine by me – as indeed it was by all of us. At least we would be spared the unpleasantness of our mother's presence while she spewed out nasty comments.

It was becoming obvious that, with Lucius out of the way, not only were the brakes off Gloria's tongue but they were also off any check in the amount of alcohol she consumed. Within two or three years of his death, she had taken to drinking a bottle of gin before sunset and a bottle of port thereafter. Owen, our head gardener, nicknamed her 'Gin and Tonic'; and, as her drinking got out of hand, so did the natural venom of a naturally acerbic and sarcastic woman. I cannot tell you the relief it was to see her sitting thirty feet away from us during dinner, instead of at the same table. When she dined with us, the tension was so intense that I was finding it more and more difficult to swallow my food.

If, however, I thought we were in for anything but a temporary respite, I was wrong. I had reckoned without Gloria's resourcefulness. Only too soon, she found an effective way of withdrawing from dining with us while retaining her ability to blight the occasion for us. For the first week or so, she sat in isolated but only-too-accessible splendour, the television set blaring so that we would have to compete with it while we conversedThen she started a running dialogue with the news, a practice which evoked nothing but laughter from us. This was a big mistake on our part, for we had thereby informed her that she could still provoke reactions from us. This precipitated the next and most enduring phase of the proceedings: until her death some forty years later, Gloria would never again as a practice dine *en famille* with us. Instead, she would sit next door, hurling comments and brickbats at us while we ate.

While I was a teenager and needed the protection my position as favourite afforded me, I would swallow the urge to ask her to please stop ruining our food. However, once I was an adult and my circumstances had changed sufficiently for me to be able to endanger my status as favourite, I did indeed start protesting. It did no good. She indulged her mood, irrespective of the negative effects.

Chapter Seven

If Gloria had ever shown any of the self-restraint that I believe she displayed while in her twenties and early thirties, she had cast such pedestrian behaviour aside by the time she was approaching her forties in the 1960s. It was as if she had decided that, now she had popularity in the bag, she could dispense with the seductive quality of charm and surrender to being the vicious bully that had always been lurking beneath the beautiful façade. All the world became her stage, and as far as she was concerned, she was the main player and the only person entitled to strut and fret her hour. 'I am the only person in this house who has any rights,' she would endlessly repeat to servants, children, sibling, mother and husband as she cut an aggressively self-centred swathe through life for no other reason than that she wanted to.

When she was in a good mood, she would bounce out of bed at about ten o'clock in the morning, put on one of the house coats she bought in America, where all Jamaicans of her kind shopped for their clothes, and sail down the passage lightly clapping her hands twice, saying as she did so: 'I'm ready for my breakfast, Edward.' She would never have dreamed of raising her voice and would actually have regarded it as *lèse majesté* on the part of the servants if they were not hovering, ready and waiting, for the moment when she required their attention. On the few occasions she had to ring for them, there would be all hell to pay. And God forbid if she had to go in search of an unresponsive servant. Such conduct was serious enough to warrant instant dismissal or, if she was in a particularly benevolent mood, a severe tongue-lashing. However, as she had them so whipped into shape, I can only think of one occasion upon which she ever had to go in search of anyone; and that was when she sent Owen to the drugstore to buy something then forgot that she had done so.

While Edward went into the kitchen to fetch Gloria's tumbler of freshly-squeezed orange juice, sachet of gelatine and cup of freshly brewed Blue Mountain coffee, she would glide onto the back veranda. Even when she was not aware of being observed, she walked as if she were on casters instead of feet. Having reached her chair, the only one she ever used in that room, she slid into it, her back erect, as if she were an empress on show before the whole court instead of a private individual sitting down at home. She would then stretch out onto the ottoman, her feet poised at an angle that bespoke elegance, even though Edward would then come out a minute or so later and have to move it so that he could place the standing-tray containing her breakfast in front of her.

Once Gloria had finished her breakfast, she would again lightly clap her hands twice. This was the signal for Edward to bring out her first drink of the day; a tumbler of Gordon's Gin over ice with a splash of tonic water. The ritual never varied. Day after day, he arrived with a gin and tonic on a silver tray for 'Gin and Tonic'. He would put it down on the mahogany side-table at the right-hand side of her chair, always taking care to put it on a coaster and to provide a napkin. Having executed that manoeuvre, he would then remove the breakfast tray, put it to one side, slip the ottoman back in front of Gloria's chair and take the standing-tray containing the breakfast dishes into the kitchen. Gloria would always thank Edward, and if she was in a good mood, which was quite usual in the morning, she would 'run a little joke' with him before turning her attention to whatever else was at hand.

Because she did not work, Gloria's life offered one endless prospect of doing as she wished. This was not quite the unexpurgated joy that people who have responsibilities and labours might think. As I often tell my children, they should use their grandmother as an awful warning of what life's true blessings are all about. If you have all your needs taken care of and have no real interest outside of yourself, even pleasure becomes hard work. On the other hand, if you find work you enjoy, that work becomes one of life's great pleasures.

Unfortunately for all concerned, work was not a part of Gloria's life. This was not entirely her own fault, for few women of her time and station actually worked, though many of them managed their privileged existence without developing into monsters. I remember in the early 1960s she said she would like to open up a flower shop and even bought some land from her stepfather in a shopping centre he was developing as a precursor. Gloria did genuinely love flowers and would ultimately become a highly-respected horticulturalist. Michael, however, refused to hear of it.

'I can't have my wife working,' he declared, only too aware that it would be *infra dig* to have a working wife. 'I can't afford it,' he'd then argue when Gloria persisted. 'It will have tax implications.' She pointed out that they both had pull with the tax authorities: she through her uncle by marriage, and he through his good friend 'Tecktime' Monroe. At this point the truth finally emerged. 'No sensible man allows his wife to become independent,' he declared.

So, there you had it. He was worried that she might leave him if the shop flourished and provided her with the means to do so: a worry, I daresay, that wasn't without foundation, for by this time she had left him on two separate occasions, though never for very long, and always with a view to bringing him to heel when he was resisting one of her demands.

If Gloria was a nightmare to live with, Michael was nohooley either. Although he had a reputation for being easygoing socially – and although he was far more easygoing than she was on a day-to-day basis – he was risk-averse to the point of it becoming a real problem. If he had done *it* before – whatever *it* was – there would be no problem in getting him to do it again. However, if *it* was something new, you could forget it. Then he had the strength of the weak and the stubbornness of the fearful. This applied across a whole range of issues, though the only one that seemed to matter to Gloria was travelling. To her credit, she was sick of doing so on her own or with relations. She wanted to travel with her husband, at least some of the time, but Michael would not hear of it. He had never been abroad and, if he could help it, he had no intention of ever going. It did not matter whether it was by boat or aeroplane. All that mattered was that she was asking him to substitute his accustomed environment for another one, and that he refused to do with a determination that indicated a real psychological problem.

Michael, however, had reckoned without the determination of his wife. For a period of about two years, she kept on floating ideas until even he could no longer refuse. That initiated the next phase. I remember many an occasion when Gloria would book overseas trips for them. Always, he would contrive to withdraw at the last minute. Sometimes, he would pick a row with her so that he could say he was not in the mood to go. Other times, he would discover some business reason which was plainly a concocted excuse but which he used to make his presence at home necessary. Then, in 1962, they were due to go to the races at Hialeah and he tried to back out yet again. 'I am going tomorrow, and if you aren't on that plane with me, I am going to divorce you,' she said, and picked up the telephone, calling his lawyer to inform him to draw up the papers.

I suspect that George Desnoes must have told Michael he'd better go, but, whoever waved the magic wand, he finally left Jamaican soil, though that didn't stop him, over the next two or three years, from still trying to stay at home every time Gloria made travel plans that included him. For instance, in 1964, the whole family was booked to go to America when he tried to back out on the very morning that we were due to depart. It was clear to me that his primary motivation was fear, and I was as perplexed then as I am now as to the reason. Gloria wasn't having any of it. She went to the cupboard where he kept his revolver, pulled it out and pointed it at him.

'If you don't get your backside into the bathroom and start to get yourself ready,' she said, 'I'll shoot off your goddamned cock.'

As his cock was the most precious thing to him – it certainly came in for wide use not only with her but elsewhere with a variety of women of all classes and colours; and as no one could ever tell whether she would actually do what she threatened to when she came out with statements of this kind – he scurried into the bathroom to shave and have his bath as we children excitedly had the servants load our suitcases into the car. Even then, we couldn't be sure that he would really go until we were actually on the plane. Only then did we know for a fact that we would have the pleasure of spending the next two weeks in the U S of A, shopping up a storm as well as seeing friends and relations.

The prospect of a cock-less existence must be what cured Michael of his aversion to travel, for thereafter, until he was too ill towards the end of his life, he never once tried to back out of another of the trips Gloria organized for them. However, he was only too happy to beg off at the arrangement stage whenever he could and send her to places like Peru and China without him.

His risk-aversion aside, two other aspects of Michael's personality would have made living with him a rough ride for any woman. Like all men of his station and background, he saw nothing wrong with availing himself of the plenitude of '*pum-pum*' – as Jamaicans called the female organ – which was always on offer. It is a fact of life that well-off men will always attract poorer girls, even if the men themselves are not sexually appealing – which Michael, according to just about every woman who knew him, was. It is also a fact of life that the wives of rich men know that there is a queue of hundreds, if not thousands, of girls who will happily jump into their shoes, if they should vacate the position of wife. The divorce laws in England and America have gone some way towards redressing the balance in favour of the wife in the latter part of the twentieth century; but even so, the rule of thumb that moneyed men will always find it easy to replace a wife with another – or with a stream of girlfriends – still applies. It keeps wives on their toes and gives them a tolerance towards infidelity that the wives of poorer men seldom have.

Like most of his relations and friends, Michael never saw any reason to deny himself the pleasures of the flesh. To all of them, morality had nothing to do with sex. Indeed, Michael went further than many of his sexually-liberated peers and lived by the rule of *droit de seigneur* in a way that would be totally unacceptable in today's world. 'As soon as Mrs Ziadie was out of the house,' our butler Edward told Joyce, his last nurse, 'Mr Ziadie used to go to the servants' quarters and demand to be let in by whichever maid had taken his fancy. He would never take no for an answer. They had to give him what he wanted. Once one of the girls said no and locked the door with the key. Mr Ziadie kicked down the door.'

Of course, we children knew nothing of our father's antics, so what the final straw for Gloria was, I will never know. What I do know is that by the 1970s, she was refusing to employ any maids at all. All servants, household and outdoor, were usually male, with the sole exception of the laundress, Eldred, whom she shared with Michael's sister Hilda, and who was definitely off the sensor of her husband's penile vane. 'Mummy has become a fag hag,' we children used to joke, even to her, especially when she employed a chef who was more queenly than Elizabeth I and II rolled into one. So the household staff remained resolutely male, if not always masculine, until Michael's body started to fall to bits under the progression of Parkinson's Disease. Then, and only then, did Gloria start to employ females again, first as housekeepers and then as nurses for him.

Towards, the end of his life, she even replaced one of the nurses when he complained that he didn't like her. 'She's too ugly,' he said. 'Get rid of her and get me someone who's easier on the eye.'

If Gloria had a measure of control over her husband's sexual conduct at home, she had absolutely none at the office. He and his brother Solomon regarded it as their right to sleep with any member of staff they wished. Doubtless the majority of their contacts were casual, but both also formed enduring relationships with members of their staff. In their scheme of things, it was perfectly all right to have a mistress who remained out of sight of their family and friends. There was evidently no problem and no conflict, so long as there was no overlap between the two worlds.

Inevitably, of course, circumstances arose which created a degree of interchange. One such incident occurred in 1979 when Michael was shot at point-blank range by a gunman who held him up at the store. As he collapsed on the floor, blood streaming out of wounds to his chest and back, the gunman took aim and would have doubtless finished him off if Mrs Powell, his senior floor walker, hadn't thrown herself between them and said that he would have to kill her before she would allow him to kill 'Mas' Mike'.

As soon as I heard how my father's life had come to be spared, I observed to my brother that Mrs Powell was his mistress.

'I don't believe that,' Mickey replied, always the last to believe that Spartacus was anything but a freedman. 'She's just a loyal employee.'

'Don't be so naïve,' I said. 'Only someone who genuinely loves someone else would do something like that. She's his mistress. And more to the point, she really loves him.'

'Daddy has never had a mistress. All of that is just Mummy's overactive imagination.'

'Why don't you ask Aunt Hilda and Aunt Doris if you think that?'

'What would they know?'

'Aunt Hilda has only worked with him for over thirty years. If she doesn't know, who does?'

The following year, Mickey and I were in Jamaica for Easter when I witnessed for myself the delicacy with which my parents avoided the true nature of his relationship with Mrs Powell. Aunt Doris's daughter Doreen, who had chronic high blood pressure and refused to take her tablets, saying they made her dizzy, was visiting Gloria when she keeled over, mid-sentence, on the back veranda. Gloria called one of the nephews who was a doctor and he sent an ambulance to take her to Nuttall Hospital. While she was in surgery, we were all alerted to the fact that Doreen was going to die and Aunt Doris would need our support, so all of us who were close to her headed for the hospital. I was sitting on the inevitable veranda of Doreen's hospital room – a room she would never use, as it turned out – trying to comfort Aunt Doris when Daddy walked in with Mrs Powell in tow. You could tell just by the easiness between them that Michael and Mrs Powell were intimate.

To say I was surprised by her presence would be an understatement. There seemed no good reason to justify her attendance – if he needed her emotional support, he should be doing without it until a more appropriate time – and I was somewhat offended on my mother's behalf that he was trotting his mistress out in a place where decorum precluded her admittance. This, after all, was a purely private family occasion, and interlopers of any kind were simply unacceptable. Of course, I was also intrigued to meet the woman who had saved my father's life, though I would have preferred to do so somewhere else than in a hospital while my cousin was dying.

My curiosity got the better of my rectitude, however, and as Michael introduced Mrs Powell to me, I eyed her up and down, assessing her with genuine interest. I noted that she was an attractive, personable, civil and civilized woman whose goodness of heart shone through her countenance. She was also a good thirty-something years younger than he was. Then she demonstrated how lucky my father was to have a mistress like her by greeting me with just the right amount of respect. She did not make the mistake of fawning, as so many other people did when meeting people like us. Then she walked over to Gloria and, while ostensibly sympathizing with her for the horror of having seen her niece by marriage collapse in front of her, treated her with the reverence royalists reserve for regnant empresses. 'She has the tact and decorousness of a true courtier,' I thought. 'She's also sensible. She sees that the way to maintain her relationship with Daddy is to be as respectful and non-threatening to Mummy as possible. And she has natural dignity.' I liked her immediately.

Later that afternoon, after Doreen had died and Michael and Mrs Powell had left, Gloria and I were waiting with Aunt Doris until the undertakers came.

'Is that Mrs Powell the same Mrs Powell who saved Daddy's life?' I asked, intent upon finding out my mother's true attitude to the woman who was clearly my father's mistress.

'Yes,' she said. 'She's a good girl.'

At that moment, I knew that the reason why Michael had been able to bring Mrs Powell into the hospital was that he already knew Gloria accepted the relationship and was completely indifferent to it.

Towards the end of her life, I discovered, while speaking about another member of our family whose husband has always had mistresses, Gloria's true attitude towards marital infidelity. 'She makes a fool of herself carrying on the way she does. As long as a wife's position isn't threatened, or he doesn't bring home unwelcome presents in the form of sexual diseases, it doesn't really matter what a man does. And men, let's face facts, will always be men. They can't help it. All men are unfaithful. A wife who even acknowledges that her husband is being unfaithful simply lowers herself in his eyes. If I had created a scene every time your father had another woman, I would have spent my whole life ripping my hair out. Where would that have got me? I had far too much self-respect for that.'

'So you really didn't mind?'

'When you're young and impressionable, you mind those sort of things, but, as you get older and learn the ways of the world, you realize there's little point in letting things like that bother you. As long as it wasn't done under my nose and I could ignore it with grace, it wasn't an issue. Women nowadays make far too much fuss about infidelity, but seem quite happy to tolerate things that my generation would never have done.'

'Like what?'

'Men who don't know, and don't want to know, how to take care of their wives. Whatever your father's faults, he always took good care of me. Man was made to protect woman and your father was a real man, not one of those namby-pamby freeloaders whom one meets so often nowadays. Believe me, it's better to be a man's darling –even an old man's darling – than any man's slave. I can truthfully say that I've never been any man's slave. Whether they've been my slave or not is something else,' she laughed.

'I suppose you might well have had another attitude if the outside *interests* had been social equals?'

'Whoa,' she growled, wagging her finger in a warning gesture. 'That would *certainly* have been another matter altogether. But your father, thank God, never did a Fatty-Boum-Boum on me.'

Fatty Boum-Boum was Michael's elder brother Elias. He had had a longstanding relationship with a lady of good background which caused a scandal within the family and led to a lifelong estrangement between him and the rest of them. They were all incensed on behalf of his wife, Lydia, that he could conduct an established relationship with one woman, and a lady at that. It was okay to screw ten or a hundred or even a thousand women, but to limit oneself to one lady was regarded as a huge solecism, even though Uncle Elias could hardly have been accused of flouting his relationship with her. Indeed, because she worked with him, they had the perfect cover for the time they spent together. This, however, made no difference to his disapproving siblings and cousins, who roundly criticized him until he withdrew from virtually all contact with the family.

It is always futile to judge people by the rules of another time, and the values of that age certainly seem breathtakingly hypocritical and unreasonable from a contemporary viewpoint, until one examines what motivated them and realizes that their objective was preservation of the family unit and conservation of the social fabric. Divorce was still something to be avoided at all costs, not only because of the disruption to family and social life, but also because it usually undermined the financial foundations of a divorced couple. As few marriages were conducted across class and colour lines, choice was also restricted, and there seemed little merit in 'swapping a black dog for a monkey', as Jamaicans used to say. Therefore a mistress like Miss Khouri, being wife material, was a living, breathing, throbbing threat to the social order, while a girlfriend like Mrs Powell was not.

If the values of that time seem bizarre to us, they did not appear so to those who lived with and by them. Michael, being a deeply conventional man, certainly did not think them odd. Indeed, he used them to insulate himself and his wife against his sexual adventures. 'I've never looked at another woman since I got married,' he would endlessly repeat to one and all, in front of his wife and children. I used to wonder why he felt compelled to comment so gratuitously upon such a personal subject, especially as his remarks always fell flat with Gloria, who pointedly ignored them. It was only after I had grown up and discovered through my aunts something of my father's peregrinations around the sexual terrain, that I came to understand why Gloria had always been so impervious to his protestations of fidelity. At first, I thought he was an utter hypocrite. Why, I asked myself, did he consider it necessary to lie so brazenly and openly in front of a host of friends and relations who all had to know that his fidelity mantra was so much rubbish? I also felt that he was cruel because, on the odd occasion that Gloria accused him of straying, he used to bark that she was 'mad'. The fact that she was, if not actually mad, pretty close to it, made it all the more inexcusable in my eyes.

When I was younger, I used to question whether his lies and denials hadn't helped to push her towards the precipice. Only later did I come to appreciate that he was giving her the message that all was well in their marital garden. Denial was honour; lies, respect; and the truth to be avoided at all costs unless you wanted to destroy the family unit. And the family unit meant a great deal to him, far more than it did to her.

Despite his commitment to his family, Michael had another flaw which made being married to him difficult. He had the most awful temper you have ever seen. Although he seldom lost it at home – Gloria simply would not tolerate such behaviour – he was notorious for his tantrums at work. On a daily basis, he would rant and rave, shouting at the top of his voice, completely out of control, his rage overcoming his stammer. As this was the only state in which he could freely communicate without impediment, his eruptions must have been quite a source of release to him; at all other times, he was a prisoner of his tongue and the frustration his inability to communicate consequently engendered.

Anything – and nothing – would set him off. On a good day, he might have only two episodes lasting twenty or so minutes. On a truly exceptional day, he might have only one; but on a typical day, his tirades would last an hour or two. Bad days were the worst. He would vent for hours on end without interruption. As bad days far exceeded good ones, no one could rely upon getting through an encounter with him at work without being subjected to the most extraordinary eruptions of rage.

Michael was lucky to live in a place like Jamaica at the time he did. People then were actually more attuned to the heart behind the voice than to the tone of voice itself. As long as they accepted that this was just your way, they displayed a degree of tolerance that was truly remarkable. As Jamaicans of all complexions and classes were inclined to passion even at the best of times, clerks, customers and business colleagues were prepared to accept that 'Killer', as his nephews drolly nicknamed him, had a 'bad temper' but that he didn't mean anything by it. This viewpoint was not without foundation, for all the evidence pointed to the fact that there was nothing personal, snobbish or racist in his tirades. He would as readily abuse a poor black man as a rich white man, a peasant as a prime minister, a pretty girl as an ugly woman, alluding to whatever about them struck him. He was utterly indiscriminate in his targets, and once the eruption had started, it would only end when he had spilled every bit of bile that was pressing upon him at that moment.

Although there was nothing funny about a scenerade while it was in full flow, sometimes he would be so over-the-top that you couldn't help laughing about it afterwards. Once he ordered an English salesman, who had come all the way from Yorkshire in England to sell him worsted – and with whom he had previously enjoyed cordial relations – out of the store for no reason at all, observing that the English were 'good for nothing except having sucked the financial blood of the world's population over whom you used to rule. Bad, worse, worst and worsted is what you all are.' Once he had calmed down, he did receive this Englishman, but whether the salesman ever returned thereafter is something I do not know, for one did not ask such questions in our family. However, when he died, the family did receive a plethora of warm condolence letters, including some from Yorkshire.

On another occasion, one of the clerks was late for work. Michael, having quite rightly observed that he would have to dismiss her if she continued to be habitually unpunctual – his underlying humanity made him loathe firing people who needed work – he then tipped over the edge. 'Don't think I don't know why you're always late,' he said. 'You can't leave your bed when you should in the morning because *nayger* is good for only two things – screwing and stealing.'

'Your father is out of order,' one of the clerks, taking umbrage, said to me under her breath. 'Not all *nayger* is a thief,'

'I notice you haven't taken exception to his remark about screwing,' I replied equally quietly.

'That me could never do,' she whispered. 'Everybody know all Jamaicans love nothing more than *cockie* and *pum-pum*. But him is still out of order to lump stealing with screwing.'

'Your father always had a bad temper,' Michael's sister Doris once told me.

'Even as a little boy, he would scream and shout when he got angry. He can't help himself.' Gloria's sister Marjorie also used to take a similarly tolerant view. 'Your father doesn't mean a thing when he blows a fuse. He's simply volatile. He's like a volcano that has to erupt. Then, once he's erupted, he's back to normal.'

It was easy for them to talk, for they didn't have to live on the slopes of Mount Vesuvius as the lava poured down the mountainside onto their heads. For his wife, children and staff, however, it was a different matter. 'He tried it out on me shortly after we were married,' Gloria recalled. 'Until then, I had never seen anyone behave like that. I made him know in no uncertain terms that I would not tolerate such conduct in my home. If I hadn't put my foot down, he would have made our home life the trauma his working life has been.'

Trauma it was. My first experience of it was when I was five years old. Eager to help Daddy, I had asked to be taken down to the store to 'work'. Although Michael had acceded, George, our chauffeur, must have been on standby in case he couldn't get through the morning without a tantrum. I can still remember Pretty da Mesa, one of his clerks, scooping me up in her arms when he started to rant out of nowhere about God knows what. She ushered the crying child out of the store for George to bring back home.

Thereafter, I got all too frequent glimpses of 'Killer' in action, for Michael believed that we children had to know where our money came from, and that meant that Mickey, Libby, Kitty and I had to work during the holidays. In the run-up to Christmas, Easter and, once Jamaica was independent, Independence Day as well, we could be found on our feet, from early in the morning until closing time (which at Christmas was late at night, pushed back from seven to eleven o'clock as Christmas Eve approached), signing bills, collecting money or wrapping parcels. If we so much as dared lean on a counter, run a joke with a clerk or be two minutes late in arriving back from lunch, 'the Tyrant', as I called him, would scream at us. Mickey and Libby were usually exempt from unfounded attacks, but I was not, for it was an accepted feature of our family life that I was Michael's anointed scapegoat.

Despite being an alpha male by inclination as well as a spoiled brat who was used to getting his own way, Michael had married an alpha female who was even more dominating, unrelenting, determined and spoiled than he was. He also regarded her as the oracle of all worldly wisdom, and, being aware of her social superiority, deferred to her in vast swathes of their life. This, of course, freed him from responsibility for those areas of their life over which she reigned supreme, which must have been a welcome relief for a man with little social interest but great pride and an exaggerated fear of failure.

Gloria's ascendancy over Michael was reinforced by the fact that he was more emotionally involved with her than she was with him. While she couldn't have cared less about displeasing him, he would get truly upset if he had perturbed her. This gave her considerable power over him, something she did not shy away from using as and when the urge took her. In the vernacular, he was 'pussy-whipped': a fact which was recognized within the family and even laughed about. Michael's niece Cissy remembers how her father Solomon used to mock his brother when he would refuse an invitation to go down to his house to play the games of chance which so dominated Ziadie family life, when Gloria wanted him to stay home with her. This despite the fact that he would then be in one part of the house reading while she was in another watching television or speaking to friends. 'I'm going to send you a box of Kotex,' Uncle Solomon would say, implying that he was a bleeding woman.

Unfortunately, nature earmarked me for my position of scapegoat by endowing me from an early age with an uncanny resemblance to my mother. This resemblance was so pronounced when I was young that everyone used to remark upon it quite spontaneously from the time when I was about three years old. Not only did I look like Gloria, I had also inherited her mannerisms, her way of speaking and even the unexpected way she had of phrasing things so that what I said, while in itself not extraordinary, was frequently construed as funny and would cause people to laugh. Till his dying day, Michael could not tell us apart over the telephone.

It was only when I went into therapy as an adult, and my therapist showed me how my relationship with my father had been influenced by psychological features of which even he was indubitably unconscious, that I began to appreciate the impact my superficial similarities with Gloria had had. There were, in effect, two versions of Gloria in the house. 'Maxi-Gloria' was Michael's wife and the person for whom he possessed a measure of consideration and a quantity of fear, while 'Mini-Gloria' was Georgie: the child who not only reminded him of Maxi-Gloria but was also an ideal target for all the bottled-up emotion he could not safely direct at his domineering wife without running the risk of damaging his marriage. So what did he do? He directed his antipathy at the version of Gloria who was vulnerable, and in so doing, not only scapegoated me but also gave himself the perfect marital safety valve. Who but a psychiatrist or psychologist would have recognized what he was doing?

There was one area of my life of which one might have reasonably expected him to be tolerant: the academic. Having been the brightest boy in his school, he revered academic accomplishment, and I was an academic highflyer. Libby was also academically brilliant, with the marks to prove it as well, but it was a precept of family life that she was the beauty, I the brains, and Mickey the fool. Kitty didn't even enter into the picture where categorization was concerned.

Michael expected me to come first at all times; and on the two occasions that I did not, he nearly tore down the house screaming abuse at me for being a lazy so-and-so when I was 'genius'. This was a word I had been hearing my parents use in connection with me since before I could remember. I thought this was just another instance of their chronic exaggeration, even though I knew I was bright. Indeed, I did not consider myself anything like a genius and gave it not another thought until, at the age of eighteen, I was given IQ tests during psychological examinations and discovered, to my surprise, that I actually did have a genius IQ. Not that this knowledge made any real difference as, by that time, I was totally fed up with the academic pressure which my father had heaped upon me, and couldn't have cared less whether I was first or fifth – so long as I was learning what I wanted to.

Michael had done some things to me over the years which had completely destroyed any desire I had to shine academically. One act of particular cruelty which I have never forgotten took place when I was twelve. I had come first, with an average, then virtually unheard of, of 92.8%. Libby had also come first, while Mickey, who had come about fourth or fifth, was actually studying for his 'O' Levels at the also unheard-of youthful age of fourteen. Our father had promised each of us a present if we came first that term, and over dinner that evening, we were calling in the promise. 'I'll give you what I promised you,' Michael told Libby. 'But you, Georgie, are getting nothing.'

The injustice of his remark burned even deeper then than it does now; and, believe me, even after forty-seven years, I am glowing with involuntary incandescence as I write this. 'Why not?' I asked. 'I came first too.'

'You didn't do well enough,' Michael said brutally, glowering at me, his gaze a beam of loathing.

'How can I not have done well enough when I did better than Libby and have an average of 92.8?'

'You coul…could…could've done be…been…better if you'd worked ha….har…harder,' he stuttered, his distaste displaced by the effort of getting out the words.

I could hardly believe my ears. There he was, someone who was always going on and on about honour and principle, right and wrong, fair play and decency, being as blatantly unfair and cruel as it was possible to be. He was using my academic accomplishment as yet another weapon with which to batter me figuratively

Life has decisive moments, and this was one. From that moment onwards, I no longer cared what my father thought of me. Until then, I had been pleased that he took delight in my academic accomplishments, that I was the fount for his pride in my supposed 'genius' which had, until then, been the one area of life where he showed me any approval. By snatching away my reward without good reason, he showed me that he was unfair and untrustworthy. I vowed I would never give him the opportunity to hurt me the same way again, and I never did. From then until he died, I never put my trust in him, not even after we had healed our breach.

If Michael destroyed something between us on that occasion, Gloria's response to his conduct showed why I still loved her. The emotion at the table was so palpable you could almost touch it. Libby and Mickey – who were not blind to the injustice that had just occurred – were looking at me, saying with their eyes how sorry they were for me. Gloria took a slow sip of wine out of her silver goblet and put it down with eloquent force, catching Michael's attention in the process. He looked at her as if to say: 'What now? You can't condemn me for trying to prevent slouching in school work?'

She looked straight at him, her face a mask free of all expression. 'You have to understand, Georgie,' she said lightly, her gaze locked with his, 'that the reason why your father scorns your academic accomplishment is that he always had an average of 115% when he was at school.'

Michael turned away, chastened by his wife – though not to the extent of reversing the unjust decision he had made – and I looked at Mummy, who cast me a look as if to say: 'Don't worry, darling. I'll make it better somehow.' Not, of course, that she actually ever did anything concrete about it. As I would come to realize, it was always the gesture with Gloria, never the deed. In this instance, however, that was a whole lot better than what I was getting from my father, and I loved her for her support.

Some weeks later, I was down at the store working in the run-up to Independence Day. Michael came up behind me.

'What did that woman want?' he snarled.

'We don't have what she wanted,' I said.

No sooner were the words out of my mouth than his hand flew in front of my face, missing it but knocking off my glasses.

'What did you do that for?' I shouted, raising my hand to the side of my nose, checking if there was any blood there. 'What did I do? I want to know. What did I do to deserve that?'

Mrs Satchell, one of the senior clerks, handed me my glasses, without which I was virtually blind. Although Michael could not see Gloria from where he was standing, and he clearly did not know she was nearby, I knew she was, so I simply edged close enough for her to overhear the kerfuffle, all the while shrieking: 'Why did you hit me?' As soon as Gloria heard me, she came over and demanded to know what had happened.

'Daddy boxed me for no reason at all.'

She opened up her eyes wide, indicating that one couldn't have divisions within the family in front of the staff.

'I assume you want the child to go home,' she said.

'Yes. Go to your precious home. Luxuriate in the lap of luxury, you goddamned useless waste of goddamned space,' Michael screamed at me, throwing two pound notes onto the floor so that I could get home by taxi. That one gesture showed me that he recognized he was in the wrong and felt guilty, otherwise he would have thrown down coins for me to take the bus.

That evening, Muriel Facey, a friend of my parents, was at the house for dinner. In all innocence, she hurtled headfirst into the minefield by asking me how work had been that day.

'Daddy was like a beast today,' I said before Mickey or Libby could reply.

Michael glowered at me.

'Beast? Beast? Is that what you think of your father?' he said without stammering, which I knew meant that he was in a rage.

Before I had a chance to backtrack, Michael threw back his chair, picked up his plate, which was laden with food, and hurled it at me. Aunt Muriel, who was sitting beside me, ducked to avoid being hit. Michael then moved into the second phase of his display, and, with an almighty bellow, like Samson tearing down the pillars of the temple or a wild beast growling before a kill, tipped the dining table over into the laps of Aunt Muriel, Libby and me. He then stormed off up the passage, repeating over and over: 'A beast. A beast.' Even after he'd reached his bedroom, a fact which we could not miss as he slammed the door with such force that it almost shook the house to its foundations, he kept on repeating 'beast...beast...beast' until finally we heard no more, and the latest eruption of Vesuvius had come to an end.

Chapter Eight

There was something else, something truly exceptional, which fuelled my father's distaste for me and further complicated our already disturbed relationship. I was being raised in the male gender, despite the fact that the more appropriate one would have been the female. While this was no fault of my parents, who cannot be criticized for the fact that I was simply born at a time when medical science knew far less about birth defects than it does now, the truth is that this circumstance caused my father grave embarrassment. Although I have no doubt that he wished me well in an abstract way, because I had not been born 'normal' meant that I was a visible offence to him; and the truth is that he often used to say that he wished I had 'never been born'.

Disability, of course, is always trying for any family, but as my brother Mickey observed shortly before dying, 'For a family as prominent as ours, it was especially difficult. And it was everyone's misfortune that it had to happen with a father like Daddy. Never was anyone less equipped for coping with something like that than he was.'

Mickey's assessment was right. Daddy made a bad thing much worse by his inability to cope with it at all.

The problem came to a head when I was thirteen. For some time I had been becoming increasingly aware that I had a monumental problem; but, as no one ever spoke about it, I assumed everyone else regarded it as no problem. This, I would learn in my twenties, thirties and forties, was definitely not so. Several relations had not only recognized the problem but questioned Gloria about it while I was still a very young child. The first time I was informed of this was when my cousin Enrique, whose parents Millard and Helen Ziadie were respectively my father's first cousin and Gloria's childhood best friend whose twenty-first birthday party had necessitated delaying her wedding, said to me, 'Mummy told me that she asked Aunt Gloria why you were being brought up as a boy when you were three.Your mother said the matter was in hand and she wasn't to worry.' Next up was my cousin Toni, who had much the same tale to tell. Then in 1993, Gloria's first cousin Jean told me much the same thing in London while visiting Mickey and me with her husband.'No one could understand what was going on,' Jean said, 'but since Gloria had said that she and your father had everything under control and they were getting the best medical advice, we respected the delicacy of the situation and didn't interfere.'

Gender is not as important to a prepubescent child as it becomes after puberty. It is, of course, important even in childhood, but you can navigate your way around misidentification with only slight misery. With the onset of puberty, however, gender becomes absolutely fundamental. One's every thought, feeling, action, ambition, goal, hope, fear, desire and, indeed, reason for living forks at the road of gender. In a very real sense, those who are misidentified are living a lie, and life becomes intolerable.

The enormity of my situation began to hit me when I was twelve, thanks to a remark of my brother Mickey's. He had a school friend called David Boxer coming for tea after school. 'Do try and appear less girlish,' he said to me. 'While you were cute when you were younger, you're now nothing but an embarrassment.'

Once Mickey's words had given form to the unspoken reality of my situation, there was no looking back. Painful, indeed cruel, though his observation was, it was also the truth, and I recognized that. The difficulty was: how to solve the problem? As I saw it, I could turn to no one about it except my brother Mickey and my sister Libby, who were only fourteen and ten and therefore of limited help and absolutely no influence with the only powers who could rectify this error: namely, Daddy and Mummy.

As the days turned into weeks and the weeks into months, I looked from one member of the family to another, turning over in my mind whether he or she could assist me. The fact that I never felt able to raise the subject with my mother says a lot about the nature of our relationship and about the way she conducted our family life. Favourite or no, I was expected to toe the line, follow the rules and abide by the regulations. Home life was her province. None of us was allowed ever to contradict her, even about the smallest thing. If I could not even question her interpretation of harmless and trivial events even when we were home alone and she was in a good mood, how could I possibly question something as enormous as the fact that I was being raised in the wrong gender?

There never was any question of my bringing the subject up with my father. All my life I had been the butt of his scorn and his rage. Nothing I had ever done ever earned anything but a curled lip or an irritated glance from him, save when he alluded to my brains. His dislike of me was so palpable that you could almost touch it, and it always had been. Instinctively I knew that going to him for help would be like a Jew asking Heinrich Himmler the way to the nearest synagogue.

Gloria's mother and sister were out. They had irretrievably damaged themselves as intercessors by having taken Mickey's side throughout the years when he had sought refuge with them against her various acts of cruelty. Nor did Gloria's various aunts and uncles and cousins seem suitable candidates either. They did not have the requisite level of influence with Gloria and Michael, or the relationships with them were not close enough. On Michael's side of the family, I could see no one who would qualify. Also, Gloria would have gone ballistic if I had turned to them instead of to her side of the family.

That left only Gloria's father Lucius. He seemed to be the only possible candidate. He was kindly, had influence with both Gloria and Michael, and he loved me. So I gingerly beat around the bush for one or two conversations, the last being the night before his murder. He had taken Mickey, my best friend Suzy Surridge and me to the movies and, after dropping Mickey at a party and Suzy home, patiently sat in his car while I tried to raise the subject. Whether he knew or guessed what I was trying to speak about, I will never know. Certainly he knew that something was bothering me, and that I was trying to get it out to him. Certainly he was patient, but if he knew, he definitely did not indicate. Then, the following night, he was murdered.

It would take me another three months before I worked up the courage to speak to anyone. The person I chose was Gloria's gynaecologist, Jimmy Burrowes. I think it says a lot about the nature of the relationships within my family that I felt safer going to a complete stranger, albeit one of whom my mother spoke warmly, than to my parents or relations.

My choice, as it turned out, was wise. Jimmy Burrowes was in favour of me being allotted the gender role towards which I was naturally inclined rather than forcing me to live in one I found antipathetic. Once my father discovered what his thinking was, however, he removed me from his care and put me under the charge of a husband-and-wife team of German doctors called Stamm. The leader of the team was the wife, who was a supposedly eminent psychiatrist. Her husband, an internist, was responsible for what would now be regarded as forcible chemical sex-change. Even before meeting me, the female half of this team had recommended forcing me to accept the gender role I had been allotted. I will never know for sure whether Michael told her that this was what he wanted, or whether she told him that this was what was best for me. The subject would remain such a hot potato between us that my father and I only ever danced our way around it.

Shortly before his death, when seeking to make amends, Michael indicated that it was Dr Stamm the psychiatrist who made the decision, but I suspect she did so after gleaning his preference, and that he had been at least as responsible as her. Not, frankly, that it made any difference to me by 1992, for I had long since forgiven my father for the part he had played in the wreckage of my early life. Indeed, by then I had a measure of compassion for the guilt he felt, though I have to admit in all honesty that this compassion was intermingled with less noble feelings such as just deserts. For Dr Stamm, I felt neither compassion nor forgiveness; and when Gloria told me on one of my visits home that the woman had died in a horribly painful way, my response was: 'So God really wasn't sleeping after all.'

'You shouldn't speak ill of the dead,' said Gloria, the arch-corrector who was ever willing to point out to others what their failings were.

'The woman was a sadist who enjoyed inflicting pain and suffering,' I said with rather more passion than I had hitherto realized I felt.

'That she was, but you don't have to be vengeful,' Gloria replied.

'I'm not the one who's been vengeful. God is. Did I make her die suffering so terribly? It seems to me if ever there was a case of "'Vengeance is mine,' sayeth the Lord" it is this one. And if you think I should feel guilty for taking ghoulish delight in her sufferings, think again. I don't and never will. If she suffered so terribly, it can only be a portion of what she caused for many of her patients over the years.'

Time has not lessened the intense loathing I have for that psychiatrist. Nor, I can now see, was there any prospect of it doing so. My feelings were too accurate a yardstick of the injury she caused me.

This started the day before my fourteenth birthday, when I was hospitalized and shot up with male hormones in an attempt to chemically alter my sexual characteristics. I was also subjected to repeated instances of intensive insulin shock therapy to force me to accept this violation of my body and my identity.

And where was Gloria in all of this? Playing, it has to be said, a very clever game: one whose motives and ramifications would take me years to unravel. At the time I thought she was on my side, even though her initial response, when Cookie had told her that I had left the grounds of the house without permission (to see Jimmy Burrowes for the second of my appointments with him), should have alerted me to what she was really about. She beat the living daylights out of me with Michael's leather belt, then consigned me to my bedroom for the remainder of the day until he came home. I was banned from speaking to the other children, and while she tried to pass it off as punishment for having broken the rule of leaving the premises without permission, I suspected that it was to prevent me from communicating with my siblings, lest they discover the true reason for my departure from home.

Later, when Michael came home and ordered me not to say anything about my real reason for having gone to Jimmy Burrowes, I knew I was right about the true reason for my quarantine.

Even at that tender age, I could see how unrealistic both my parents were if they thought that my siblings didn't already know all about why I had been to see the gynaecologist. Could they seriously believe that my siblings and I kept our gravest concerns from each other?

The following day, I was taken down to Tony Feanny's surgery by Michael. Quite why they even bothered to have me there has always been a mystery, as I was left outside in the waiting room while 'Uncle' Tony and my father dispensed with my fate. It was my mother's former love who came up with the Stamms.

A few days later, Gloria took me to see the female half of the husband-and-wife team. She was the psychiatrist who had overall charge of my case, and I had to meet her prior to being hospitalized. I would not meet her other and more humane (albeit still cruel) half, the internist who would violate my body with male hormones, until I was in the hospital. The mere fact that my mother was the one who was taking me to see this psychiatrist from hell should have put me on my guard, but because I did not yet know what was in store for me, or that my mother was utterly untrustworthy and would betray anyone's trust if it suited her, I did not appreciate that my parents were acting as a unit and were manipulating me so that I would accept treatment that was contrary to every one of my rights and inclinations. They knew only too well that, while I did not trust Daddy to respect my rights, I believed that Mummy would do so.

Even so, I was no fool, and after no more than three minutes with Dr Stamm, who was doing a mean impersonation of Rosa Klebb, the East German spy in *From Russia with Love*, I could see that she was an authoritarian personality who was enamoured of power and control. As our meeting progressed – and she displayed her contempt for my thoughts, feelings, wishes and inclinations by pointedly refusing to either ask me what my perspective was, or to listen when I said what it was – despite her lack of interest, I realized I was being consigned to the 'care' of someone who would most likely do everything but provide me with the care I needed. When she announced at the end of the encounter – it could hardly be called an appointment – that I would have to be checked into the hospital the day before my fourteenth birthday, I protested. 'Why can't I go the day after my birthday? I'm having a birthday party.' Her response was to turn that natural adolescent response into an issue of obedience and respect for authority, providing me with insight into her capacity for twisting innocent and innocuous facts into something they were not.

I can distinctly remember the journey back home from Nuttall Hospital, where Dr Stamm had seen me. I was filled with foreboding and tried to get an answer out of my mother as to why she was allowing this psychiatrist to turn my perfectly reasonable response to being deprived of my birthday party into an issue of obedience when no reasonable person could place such an unreasonable interpretation upon it. When she remained silent, I pressed home my advantage, pointing out that a far more reasonable interpretation was that Dr Stamm's insistence on depriving me of my birthday party had overtones of punishment.

Although I did not know it then, I had come perilously close to the truth. Prior to meeting me or having one test result, Dr Stamm had devised a course of treatment which involved treating my desire for the gender nature intended for me as an act of rebellion. This, according to her plan, would involve years of psychiatric treatment from her and (lifelong) hormonal treatment from her husband. It was her opinion that gender was a matter of nurture, not nature, and that, until such time as I accepted the gender assigned to me at birth, she would address my opposition to it with psychiatric treatment.

In tandem with this, her husband would artificially masculinise me with hormones. In her opinion, one of the reasons why I had never taken to the male role was that I was too naturally female; but she had every confidence that, after I was artificially masculinised by her husband and treated psychiatrically by her, I would eventually become resigned to the male gender. Tellingly, she never expected me to either like, or feel at ease in, that role, and envisaged me requiring lifelong psychiatric treatment. In other words, she and her husband were setting themselves up with a nice little money-spinner which would last for the rest of their natural lives.

There were other incentives for all the four adults playing the lead roles in this bizarre scenario. As far as the Stamms were concerned, there were medical as well as financial benefits. At that time, Gender Identity was a hot, indeed an exotic, topic. There were two schools of thought: one that gender identity was fixed somewhere between conception and birth; the other, that gender identity was not an absolute and that it could be adjusted, amended or shifted. Dr John Money at the Johns Hopkins Gender Identity Clinic was propounding the latter theory, using as his guinea pigs the John-Joanna twins. These were identical twins, one of whom had lost his penis when it was amputated after a circumcision went wrong. Dr Money's recommendation to the parents had been that the amputee be made a female surgically, which was duly done in early childhood, and that the child, renowned throughout the medical profession as Joanna, be provided with medical assistance as she grew up so that she would accept her new gender. In other words, at the same time that Dr Money was propounding his theory and trying it out on Joanna, Dr Stamm was effectively propounding the same in reverse with me.

There were substantial differences in the two cases, however. Firstly, Joanna was an infant when her amputation took place. She therefore never knew any other gender role than that of the female. I, however, was by this time a teenager. I had known all my life what it was to be raised as a boy. The role, however, had never taken, and now I wanted the farce to come to an end.

What I did not know, but the doctors concerned must have known, was that Joanna, though still a child, seemed no more eager than me to adopt the role assigned for her. As my teenage and her childhood trundled on, it would be with increasingly traumatic consequences for us both, and painful ones for our siblings. My brother Mickey and sister Libby were undoubtedly affected by my case, as was Joanna's brother John. However, while we would ultimately emerge with our lives intact, neither John nor Joanna did. Indeed, theirs was the most tragic outcome possible. Both of them committed suicide.

In 1963, however, while both medical experiments were underway, none of the doctors or parents knew what the outcomes would be. Doubtless both Stamms hoped for the kudos that John Money was achieving in America; and, had they not lost me as a patient sooner than they planned, there is little doubt they would have contributed papers on my case to the various medical publications, thereby enhancing their reputations and earning international prestige at my expense.

The Stamms were not the only adults who stood to gain in terms of reputation, had their treatment of me been successful. My father was also in line to be a primary beneficiary. Although I was not aware of it then, he had already decided that one of the main reasons why my gender must, on no account, be amended was that it would cause a scandal once I was openly acknowledged as a girl. There was every possibility that the scandal might not be contained within upper-class drawing rooms but might end up in the newspapers.

Michael's dread of scandal was not unique. It is quite extraordinary how the very prospect of scandal has always terrified a certain sort of upper-class person. There are few sacrifices they would not make to avoid that dreaded state. The terror of the prospect, of course, is invariably worse than the reality but all the more potent for it.

In Michael's eyes, he wasn't being unreasonable in requiring me to live a life in limbo just so he could avoid a scandal. As far as he was concerned, it was a small price to pay, despite the fact that there was already considerable chatter about my identity. As long as he and my mother continued to ignore the anomaly as assiduously as they had been doing all my life, it would remain only drawing-room chatter with no likelihood of developing into the full-blown scandal a role reversal might cause.

Although it would take me several decades to realize it, my mother was in cahoots with my father to the extent that neither of them wanted the anomalies of my gender resolved, though for different reasons. It is a testament to her manipulative skills that Gloria was able to persuade me for several decades that my father bore sole responsibility for the state of limbo in which I was forced to live throughout my teenage years.

In fact, I doubt that I would ever have come to realize how completely she had double-dealt if it hadn't been for my father, who indicated to me in 1993 that Gloria had backed him up all those years ago. This was a profound surprise to me, but when I turned it over in my mind, I realized that she had pandered to both him and me so that he accepted that she was on his side and I believed she was on mine, while she was actually pursuing her own agenda.

But what was that? At first, I thought it was to keep each of us sweet, but later on a doctor who knew us both provided me with a more convincing answer: Gloria wanted to keep me in limbo so that I would forever remain her obliging companion. What future did I have, without an identity, save to stay at home and remain her foil?

As soon as the doctor made this suggestion, I heard the truth bells ringing. I also knew it was not that rare an occurrence. Earlier in the century, Queen Alexandra had refused to allow her daughter Victoria to marry, forcing her to remain her lifelong and increasingly embittered companion. In the previous century, Queen Victoria had tried the same thing with her youngest daughter, but Princess Beatrice had outmanoeuvred her mother, without overtly rebelling, when she fell in love with Prince Henry of Battenberg. Even though she remained her mother's devoted companion once she was allowed to marry, she had dug in her heels and refused to give up the man she loved until the Queen relented and allowed the marriage. But I could not marry unless I was given my correct gender, so I was being set up to be the perfect perpetual companion.

As things would turn out, I did gain my gender. Not knowing the way Gloria had deceived me, I might well have gone on to fulfil willingly the Princess Beatrice role to Gloria's Queen Victoria, if she hadn't shattered our relationship as utterly as she would later do.

During my stay in St Joseph's Hospital, Gloria made it easy for me to believe that she was on my side when she and Dr Stamm crossed swords, and Dr Stamm banned her from the hospital for the remainder of my three-week stay. For years I was under the impression that the cause of their disagreement had been over my treatment, and that Gloria was upset over the way I was being masculinised chemically against my will and to my tremendous distress. Only later would I see that the source of their conflict was more fundamental: Gloria did not care whether I appeared to be masculine or feminine as long as I remained her adoring companion. The best way to ensure that was to keep me in limbo. As far as she was concerned, the issue wasn't whether a more masculine version of me would more readily 'pass' as normal. It was whether an altered version would remain as ideal a companion for her as I had hitherto been. Up to then, I had been developing in a way that suited her perfectly. Even those traits which Dr Stamm regarded as negatives, such as my love of clothes and my skill as a seamstress, she regarded as positives, for she – like her sister – was preoccupied with fashion, and this was therefore an interest which made my company all the more desirable as a result. As far as she was concerned, this was a case of 'if it ain't broke, don't fix it.' Both she and the psychiatrist were intent on keeping me in limbo, each for her own self-aggrandizing reasons and each with her own conflicting idea of what that limbo should resemble.

If my mother's self-interest is hardly laudable, neither was Dr Stamm's. Being a bright child, I could see right through the doctor even if I was blind to my mother. Although I was careful not to oppose Dr Stamm overtly, especially once I was isolated in the hospital, she had perfect recourse to the true level of my opposition to her insane determination to masculinise me: sodium pentathol – otherwise known as the 'truth serum' – with which she periodically shot me up so that she could get behind my diplomatic exterior to discover the way I really felt.

Having ascertained the truth, Dr Stamm then sought to use it to convince me to surrender all opposition by telling me time and again that there was little point in resisting my fate as it was only a matter of time before she wore down my defences with the drugs she and her husband were administering. This had the effect of instilling real terror in me, for I could tell that it would be an absolute disaster. More in touch with reality than she was, I could see that you cannot turn a sow's ear into a silk purse any more than you can turn a girl into a man unless she wants to become one, and as I did not, the consequences, both short- and long-term, would be catastrophic for me if she and her husband masculinised my appearance.

Things quickly reached a point where the mere sight of Dr Stamm, coming into my hospital room with an injection in the white pan in which she used to carry it, was enough to make me feel as if I were about to die. She certainly knew just how terrified I was, for once the drug took effect I would spill the beans, so to speak. While one would expect a doctor to have some compassion, especially for a terrified teenager, she had none.

Indeed, she went on to prove that my original instincts about her being a cold, inhumane caricature of the German concentration-camp guard type were accurate, when she graduated from psychological cruelty to the physical variety. The injections she administered became far more than just injections. Despite the fact that I had pronounced veins, and there had never been any trouble before with any competent doctor or nurse finding a viable entry-point for an intravenous injection – and despite the fact that she had had no trouble with my veins at first – once she appreciated how terrified I was of her, she developed ever-increasing 'difficulty' in inserting the needle. The first time she did it, she reduced me to tears, and I asked her to get the nurse to administer the injection. The look she shot me told me all I needed to know. She was tormenting me – and enjoying it at the same time. I was therefore not surprised when she had even more 'difficulty' in finding the vein that was popping out at her the next time she arrived with the injection and white pan. As I quivered with fear and pain, and she poked with pleasure, I derived some – albeit slight, but nevertheless real – pleasure from suggesting that she get my private nurse to give me the injection, since her eyesight was clearly not up to scratch. Her response was to jab the needle into my hand pointedly, hitting the bone and – no surprise here – missing the vein but inducing even greater pain and distress.

Finally, when Dr Stamm informed me that my father was in agreement with my staying in the hospital until such time as I began cooperating, I saw my predicament with unprecedented clarity. I was in the same position as Aunt 'Flower', my father's sister Ethel, who, family legend had it, had 'gone off her head when Hylton was hanged'. Hylton was a policeman who had been convicted of murder. Aunt Flower had struck up a friendship with him while prison-visiting. They became such good friends that he left her his slim worldly goods in his will. Naturally, she was upset by his execution, but I would later learn that this was not what had 'sent her off her head'. She was plain and plump and, by the time she became of marriageable age, her father was dead and therefore not in a position to arrange a suitable match for her.

This reduced her marital prospects significantly for, without her father to assist in finding her someone desirable, she was thrown back on her rather slender resources, if one can characterize being plain and plump in such terms. Although she was very sweet and loving, and indeed a capable businesswoman who would eventually have her own store, no 'suitable' man came along who was willing to take her off the shelf. Then a 'brown man' came along who fell in love with her and wanted to marry her. Solomon and Michael refused to countenance the marriage, and poor Aunt Flower was made to give up the one prospect she had for personal fulfilment, her so-called '*nayger* man'. Thereafter, she was condemned to a life of loneliness without any prospect of gratification.

As time passed, and Aunt Flower got older and plainer and fatter and no one of the right background came along to rescue her, she took to having affairs with men of colour which her brothers invariably broke up. One can imagine the frustration of a woman who is prevented from having gratification from the same sphere as the brothers who availed themselves of an endless stream of black and brown women, but that is not where the awfulness of Aunt Flower's story lies. It is in the fact that every time she began a new affair, the brothers would call in the men in white coats, who would literally cart their sister off to the hospital for shock treatment until she was docile and depressed enough to be beyond sexual urges.

Although at the age of fourteen I did not know all the details of Aunt Flower's 'illness', I was sufficiently aware of them to know that she now lived in horror of being hospitalized and had the real fear that, if she was not very careful, she would end up being permanently committed, despite the fact that she was definitely not mad, even if she was decidedly eccentric. To my mother's credit, she was the only member of the family with whom Aunt Flower would voluntarily go for out-patient treatment. 'I am the only person in the family who doesn't treat Flower like she's a dog,' Gloria, who never missed an opportunity to let the world know how wonderful she was, would proudly announce, grandstanding even when she was being kind.

Once I appreciated the parallels between my predicament and Aunt Flower's, I too began to worry about being incarcerated indefinitely, if not forever. I also saw that the longer I refused to cooperate with Dr Stamm, the worse things would be for me, both psychologically and physically. While I was unafraid of the psychological effects, the physical ones frightened me. By this time the male hormones with which her husband was shooting me up were producing visible effects. I was developing down above my upper lip, and my voice was lowering, though it is interesting to note that it would never become lower than the voices of other women in my immediate family and would always remain significantly higher than that of my grandmother Maisie, who had the most wonderful aristocratic *basso profundo*.

These changes nevertheless left me horrified, for I did not know if they would be lasting. Determined not to take the chance of having my body further changed by chemical means, and understanding that the longer I stayed in the hospital under the care of Stamm and Stamm, the worse the effects would be, I resolved to get the hell out of there as soon as possible. So I decided that I would cooperate with her, and started to agree to give living as a boy a shot, even though I knew only too well I had no genuine desire to do so.

This was the turning point. Although Dr Stamm must have known that my cooperation was more expedient than willing, she regarded it as significant progress. Michael, always careful about opening his wallet except for Gloria, Kitty and social purposes, was also thrilled. It meant that I could be released from the hospital for out-patient treatment, saving him a large proportion of the medical costs that were ratcheting up. As these included a private room, a private nurse, the cost of the drugs, food and incidentals, he would only have to pay for the fees of the Doctors Stamm and the cost of the male hormones I was being prescribed once I left the hospital.

Tellingly, when my autobiography was published in England in 1997, I received a letter from an eminent lady of Jamaican background named Margaret Tucker. Even though I had not mentioned the Stamms by name, and even though we did not then know each other, she felt compelled to write me. My description of the sadistic, concentration-camp style psychiatrist had been so evocative that she was able to identify her as Dr Stamm. It was reassuring for me to learn that others saw through the woman – though it has to be said that there was never a shred of doubt in my mind that I might have misjudged her. When evil stares you in the eye and pokes you in the hand, you know it.

But Dr Stamm's well-laid plan of using me as a guinea pig, while earning fat fees and medical kudos for herself and her husband, was doomed to failure. For all her arrogance and supposed medical knowledge, she was such a poor judge of character that she had made the fundamental error of assessing

Michael as the greater power in the Ziadie marriage. This mistake would cost her dear for, once I was released from the hospital and refused point-blank to go back to Dr Stamm or to take the male hormones which she had told me I must swallow every day, Gloria – who had developed an antipathy towards Dr Stamm after she banned her from the hospital on the grounds that her presence was undermining my progress – backed me up. The task was therefore left to Michael to inform Dr Stamm that I would not be returning to her for any more of her or her husband's 'treatment'.

Chapter Nine

When you've been to the bowels of hell, purgatory is a pretty good place to which to return. On September 6 1963, when Gloria collected me from St Joseph's Hospital and drove me back to that fraught and turbulent but physically comfortable place which I called home, I was never happier to see it, even though I was severely out of sorts and was actually returning to a way of life I had found intolerable only three short weeks before.

Hung-over from all the drugs I had been given, it would take months before the residual effects of the male hormones and insulin-shock treatments worked themselves out of my system, and I regained my natural equilibrium. I won't say it was exactly good to be back home for – my own problems aside – this was the period when Gloria would take up her nightly position on the front veranda, sipping port and sobbing histrionically while brandishing Michael's revolver and challenging 'any old *nagyer* out there' to come onto the grounds and see if he could get away with trying to do to her what Clifton Eccleston had done to her father. While she relished the idea of blowing this unknown trespasser to smithereens, I always sat with her, for it was a precept of family life that Gloria needed companionship at all times and, in the absence of friends or relations, it had to be me. Meanwhile, Mickey remained in his bedroom studying or listening to music when he wasn't boarding, while Michael, always eager to duck out of being alone with Gloria for anything more than ten minutes, was enjoying himself down at Solomon's, Doris's, one of the Seagas' or any another of their myriad friends' houses.

Libby and Kitty, who had returned to their convent within days of my release from the hospital, would never have been sitting with Mummy even if they had been at home. At that time, Libby's company was as antipathetic to Gloria as Mickey's had been, while she completely ignored Kitty and would continue to do so for another three decades. Despite the dramatics at home, it was nevertheless comforting to be back in an environment where the boundaries were more clearly delineated and the level of madness less threatening than at St Joseph's Hospital. Also, I had real compassion for Gloria's distress, not yet appreciating that it was less love for her father than self-indulgent wallowing that was making her tick. While sympathizing with her, I was also grateful that, though I was still condemned to limbo, at least it was no longer a limbo which would force a chemical sex-change on me. You cannot imagine the relief that was.

The following months were the calm before the storm. Michael had given Gloria a swimming pool and pool house to cheer her up following Lucius's murder, and this was the period when they were being completed. Once they were, in November 1963, they didn't seem to make such a discernible difference to either Michael or Gloria's lives; while she sometimes entertained around the pool, he only ever used it on Sundays and usually only on Sunday mornings at that, the afternoons being dedicated to dominoes with the men.

On the other hand, the pool and pool house changed the lives of us children beyond measure. We now had a meeting place well away from the eyes and control of our parents, who in any event allowed us unrestricted use of it during the holidays. We took full advantage of this, and so did our friends, the kernel of which were Mickey's school friends Bindley Sangster, son of the Prime Minister, and Andrew and Danny Melville, whose father John was a school friend of our father as well as the Bostich staple heir. As the 1964 summer holidays progressed, so did our popularity, word having spread amongst our contemporaries that the fun place to be was the Ziadie's pool. On a daily basis, between five and twenty friends would drop in for swimming. Our butler Edward would be up and down between the pool house and the main house, fetching soft drinks and ice and the occasional trays of fruit, which, of course, it never occurred to us to get or prepare ourselves, having been brought up never to do anything for ourselves lest we 'spoil the servants'. Then, of course, when lunchtime came, we couldn't very well eat without offering something to our friends; and before you knew it, Cookie was obliged to make sandwiches for everyone. Gloria never once complained or sought to discourage us from developing our burgeoning social lives. Indeed, she seemed to derive pleasure from seeing us blossom in a way that she approved of and deployed her considerable charm to seduce our friends into liking her.

What also helped to make Gloria the princess of cool amongst our friends was the fact that they were all allowed to smoke in front of her and Michael. Those were the days when it was the height of glamour to smoke, and just about every teenager smoked, though it was virtually unheard-of for parents to tolerate teenagers doing so in their presence until they were at least seventeen or eighteen years of age. However, I was allowed to smoke in front of my parents from June 1964. This was one of the few perks that living in limbo allowed me; it came about when Michael called in Dr Cooke, the psychiatrist at Belleview Hospital, the insane asylum, to keep me on the straight and narrow after I complained to Gloria that I really did not see how I could continue living without a gender.

My sessions with Dr Cooke were due to take place every Saturday morning on the veranda of the pool house. By this time, I was smoking twenty cigarettes a day and, finding it difficult to get through the first session without lighting up, asked him if I could. He said go right ahead, which I did. At the end of the second session, which he conducted in clouds of smoke emanating from me, he said: 'You do not have a psychiatric problem and I cannot continue to treat you when there is no psychiatric solution to your problem. I'm going to have to tell your parents that you need gynaecological treatment, not psychiatric.'

'Can you do me a big favour?' I asked. He nodded his assent. 'Can you tell my father that he must allow me to smoke in front of him? Smoking is the only outlet I have, and at the moment I can't do so in front of him.'

Dr Cooke, bless him, agreed and recommended to Michael that I be allowed to smoke openly. Of course, once I was permitted to do so in front of my parents, all the no-smoking restrictions were suspended not only for me but for my friends as well. It ought to be said that Michael, who had never smoked, did not approve of the habit, and would gladly have put his foot down and prevented all of us teenagers from smoking, but Gloria herself was seldom without a cigarette stuck into her carved ivory holder. Once Dr Cooke had made his recommendation, however, he was railroaded into tolerating something he would otherwise never have accepted.

During this period, it looked as if Gloria was also acquiring a more lenient streak. Although we were still expected to be perfectly behaved around her and her friends, we were further lulled into thinking that the leopard was becoming an antelope when Libby met Charles Matalon, who was much taken with her, and Gloria reacted in a way that seemed to be out of character. Her behaviour would, with hindsight, be entirely in character. Although Charles was about five years Libby's senior, Gloria judged him to be an eminently suitable beau for her barely pubescent daughter. This, I can now see, was not only because the Matalons were the richest family in Jamaica but because they were also old friends of hers and Michael's, and in her romantic scheme of things, the perfect outcome would have been for Libby to become Mrs Charles Matalon a few years down the line and make Charles a member of our family.

Michael, on the other hand, was the least romantic of men and had a very Middle Eastern view on dating. Left up to him, no girl would ever go out with a man until she had been safely propelled up the aisle as a virgin. He baulked at the idea of Libby going out with Charles, but Gloria – normally so strict that Libby wasn't allowed to wear even lipstick – not only allowed her to go out with him but to colour her lips and backcomb her hair as well.

'It's all perfectly innocent,' Gloria reassured the doubtful Michael, who nevertheless made sure he stayed up past his bedtime to let in Libby. He would then do what he always did with her, Kitty and myself whenever we went out on dates: open the front door and run his eyes over us from the top of our head to the tip of our toes, making it clear in his glance that he was checking to see that we had returned in the same condition in which we had left.

Mickey had not yet reached the age to obtain a driver's licence, but that did not curtail our activities, for Bindley Sangster had both a licence and his own car. Mickey, Libby, Suzy Surridge (Libby's and my best friend) and I would all pile into his Morris Minor station wagon and head off to nightclubs or to the cinema several times a week. At clubs, we were even allowed to drink the odd glass of rum punch or Red Stripe beer, for Gloria was a staunch advocate of the principle that all civilized people know how to hold their liquor and saw nothing wrong with us consuming alcohol. Michael, on the other hand, was like many other Lebanese of his generation. He practically never touched alcohol, not because he disapproved of it, but simply because he did not like its taste or effect.

The debate over teenage drinking has always been particularly fierce in the Anglo-Saxon world. I cannot help but feel that one thing my parents got right was the way they conditioned us into drinking moderately. Between Michael's abstemiousness and Gloria's alcoholism, they could well have tipped us into one extreme or the other. They did not, partly because Gloria herself demystified drinking for us by encouraging us at too early an age to consume alcohol as a discipline. I vividly remember her sitting me down at the age of twelve and teaching me to drink whisky and brandy. 'The Smedmores all drink a whisky in the afternoon and brandy after dinner,' she informed me, 'and the younger you are when you acquire a taste for them, the better off you'll be.' Although I was delighted to be treated in so grown-up a fashion, the pleasure palled when the first drop of whisky passed my lips. I disliked it intensely. Hoping that I'd like brandy better, I sipped it, only to discover I disliked it even more. To this day, I loathe the taste of both drinks, which just goes to show that premature introduction can result in more of a turn-off than a turn-on.

When summer ended in 1964 and school started again, the fun was over for everyone except our parents, who continued to pursue active social lives. I noticed, however, that Gloria was now opting out of many of the activities she had previously shared with Michael. No longer did she and I go to the race track every Saturday. She also stopped going to most of the poker games to which they were invited. Even when they were held at our house, she would stay in her bedroom, pointedly ignoring the fun taking place on the front or back verandas. She would still go to parties, however, and they still entertained constantly. She also struck up a close friendship with Victor Grant's latest wife, an exotic American called Gwen with whom she frequently hit the town, but something was clearly afoot, even if it was hard to discern precisely what. Gloria always played her cards close to her chest and never revealed her master plan to anyone, even though that did not stop her from dumping trivia openly and with relish on all and sundry, especially me.

'I'm an open package,' she would declare to whatever audience there was. As she came out with apparently indiscreet and deliberately shocking remarks about virtually every topic under the sun, some people might have been inclined to buy that statement. I knew better and was grateful when she developed a liking for Scrabble. Instead of listening to her moan and groan about everyone and everything, I could utilize more constructively the love of words we both shared as we played that most enjoyable word game.

Being articulate, with a wide vocabulary, she was a worthy adversary. I was no schlump either, being the only student at my school to ever have a 100% average in English Language, which I had now maintained for two years. I too had a fairly extensive vocabulary, so our Scrabble sessions were fun, made all the more so by the fact that it was always an open question which of us would win.

Then, one afternoon in November 1964, I went to the bathroom and came back to see Gloria rifling through the Scrabble pieces. I was so taken aback I questioned whether I was hallucinating. Surely Mummy wouldn't dislike losing so much that she'd actually cheat? Although on one level I immediately knew that answer to that question was yes, on another I was not yet able to face that fact.

There was also the question of what I could do about her cheating. If I humiliated her by making her aware that I had rumbled her, it would cause an adverse reaction whose effects could rebound detrimentally upon me. So I quietly backtracked and reappeared making enough noise to alert her to my impending arrival.

The next time Gloria suggested that we play Scrabble, I made sure I had an empty bladder. And the time after that. And after that as well.

Lo and behold, I suddenly found that I was on more of a winning streak. That had the curious effect of making Gloria more eager than ever to pit her wits against mine. Soon, she was encroaching on most of the free time I had, going so far as to send Owen to fetch me when I was visiting my best friend Suzy across the street.

Much as I enjoyed Scrabble, this latest development really cheesed me off. But saying no to Gloria was not an option. Not for the first or last time in my life, I was only too aware that my privileged status as favourite came at rather higher a price than I was willing to pay. Also not for the first or last time in my life, I would find myself torn in opposite directions by my mother: I loved her and wanted to be a good companion to her, but not to the exclusion of my own needs and desires. Yet here she was, setting things up so that I was being forced to put aside acceptable adolescent needs to satisfy her selfish ones.

But Gloria still had another trick up her sleeve. She started sending me inside at least twice during a game to fetch something for her. Sometimes it would be a pack of cigarettes. Sometimes it would be matches. Sometimes it would be ice for her gin and tonic. Sometimes it would be Kleenex. Or a fresh napkin. But it would always be something requiring me to leave the front veranda, where we invariably played, to go into the house for a few minutes.

I did not want to have unworthy thoughts, and I certainly took no pleasure in thinking that my own mother might be orchestrating things in such a way that she would obtain an unfair advantage, but as my winning streak receded into the background along with our uninterrupted games, my suspicions grew until I had to listen to them.

These suspicions presented me with a whole new dilemma. How was I going to deal with it? I could not very well accuse her. Aside from the fact that she was always standing on her dignity, her avowed stance in life was that she was never wrong about anything, not even the most trivial or accidental of things. To accuse her of cheating would be to state that she had not only been wrong but, worse, that she had done wrong, purposely and immorally. If I had been stupid enough to take that course of action, I would have been dead meat – and dead meat, moreover, that hadn't even had the satisfaction of getting an admission out of her, for I knew, even then, that Gloria did not do admission any more than the Pope did prostitution.

Since accusation was not open to me, what other options did I have? As I saw it, there were only four. Firstly, I could continue playing in the hope that she would desist from cheating, or secondly, I could continue playing with her and let her get away with her dishonesty. Although only fifteen, I wasn't naïve enough to think that she would stop cheating, nor did the role of dupe appeal sufficiently for me to collude in her taking advantage of me. I did consider laying a trap for her and catching her red-handed by doubling back unexpectedly early while she was still rifling through the pieces. However, I ruled that out on both expedient and moral grounds, the expedient being that if I mismanaged her exposure, I might find myself shoved out of the hallowed role of favourite into something akin to the victimhood of Mickey and Libby; and the moral being that it was wrong to lay traps for people. That left only the fourth and last option, which was to wait until the Scrabble set was packed away. Then, when no one was looking, I would send it hurtling to the floor, making sure that I threw away sufficient pieces while picking them up so that it couldn't be used again. I had no doubt that Gloria would conclude that one of the servants had been careless and that, in the absence of knowing which one to blame, she could blame none, so that plan seemed the best way forward.

I was aware that this last option had an obvious disadvantage, in that Gloria could replace the Scrabble set. But I felt it was my best bet as long as I played my cards properly and neither displayed relief at the loss of our Scrabble sessions nor suggested acquiring a new Scrabble set.

Knowing Gloria as I did, I anticipated that once the cycle was broken, she would most likely move onto something and hopefully someone else. Scrabble would then be a past interest, which is precisely what happened. Her niece by marriage and good friend Cissy was spending several months in Jamaica, and Gloria started to fill the gaps in her schedule by substituting Scrabble sessions with visits to Cissy down at Uncle Solomon's house.

Then came the addendum, and with it the realization that I had done the right thing in bringing not only her cheating to an end, but also her ruthless consumption of my free time. This came about when I found myself at a loose end one afternoon after school. Suzy was out and I wasn't allowed during term time to go beyond Suzy's or our other neighbour Tony's houses without parental permission. The servants said Gloria was down at Cissy's, so I telephoned to ask my mother if I could go and visit another friend. Cissy suggested instead that I get a Yellow Cab down to her house and join them there. I can still hear her saying, 'Your mother's here. It will be fun.'

Being my godmother as well as a close friend of both her uncle Michael and Gloria, Cissy had far more licence where I was concerned than most other people. But she was miscalculating, erroneously supposing that, because I was supposed to be Gloria's favourite, this would mean that she was desirous of my presence. It had never occurred to her that Gloria might not want to see me except as and when it suited her. Certainly it had never occurred to me for, like Cissy, I believed that being Gloria's favourite meant that she loved me and enjoyed my company. After all, mothers love their children, don't they? And their favourites more than their other children, which is why they are the favourites? I was about to learn a lesson to the contrary.

When I arrived at Uncle Solomon's house, Cissy met me outside and paid the taxi. While doing so, she greeted me as affectionately as ever then led me inside to her bedroom, where Gloria was lying on the bed drinking gin and tonic and speaking to Cissy's friend Anne, who was sipping a Red Stripe beer.

'What are you doing here?' my mother snapped. 'Can't I ever be rid of you? Are you my shadow? It's bad enough that I have to spend afternoon after afternoon playing Scrabble with you when I could be out enjoying myself, but now you're even tracking me down when I manage to give you the slip, as if you're a private detective and I'm your quarry.'

Even though I would often forget to live up to the wisdom I gained that afternoon, the scales fell off my eyes there and then. I saw exactly how little my much-vaunted companionship meant to my mother. I was not a companion whose company she valued. I was a time filler and, as such, of no real consequence. Any doubts I had about the way I had brought our Scrabble sessions to an end evaporated in that instant.

I had even wondered whether I had been unfair to my mother. Had I misjudged her? Had I been too harsh? Had I been too hasty in accepting my suspicions as well-founded, instead of giving her the benefit of the doubt until an external circumstance provided incontrovertible proof that she really was a cheat?

I had been waging a war between my intellect and my intuition, with my conscience as referee, and I had felt guilty that I might be doing her an injustice. What sort of a person would I be if I had been mean enough to deprive my mother, my one and only mother, of my companionship when she needed it? Just because a set of coincidences was sufficient to lead me to question how fairly she had been playing on the one and only occasion I had caught her rifling through the Scrabble pieces. Surely there had to be other explanations which might point to an innocent interpretation. Maybe a gust of wind had blown her cigarette ash over the pieces and she had been cleaning them off. Yes. If you thought long enough, you could come up with many alternative scenarios, some of which would point to her innocence.

Torn by such conflicting thoughts, I had even begun to regret being so precipitate and decisive, until I walked up into Cissy's bedroom, and Gloria shone the light of truth upon the callous and unfeeling way she had been using me.

Of course I was hurt. No daughter wants to think that her mother is using her. Of course I wished it were otherwise. Aside from anything else, it was pretty insulting and dispiriting to realize that what I'd always thought of as valued companionship was nothing of the kind. But I knew, as surely as I breathed air, that my mother had given me a real insight into what made her tick. Hurtful though it was, and much as I regretted having to accept it as a fact, I was also aware that I must not ignore the lesson I was being taught.

Although I was too young to understand all the ramifications, and although it would take me years to figure out that I, as well as my companionship, were of no real importance to my mother, and that I was there to be used and discarded as and when it suited her, I was thereafter intermittently aware that she had far less genuine appreciation of our relationship than she had led me – and everyone who knew us – to believe.

Any temptation I might have had to gloss over the type of person my mother was disappeared during the summer of 1965. Gloria proved then that she had definitely not changed species; and last summer's hiatus had been the exception rather than the rule. Although she still gave us great latitude in entertaining our friends during the school holidays, her ferocious and catty streaks were more to the fore than ever, and they played increasing havoc with the even tenor of family life behind the scenes.

Mickey was once again her target. He had recently passed his driver's test, and our father had given him Scrammy, having taken possession of Gloria's American 'hearse' which had reached the grand old age of four years.

Since she was far too important to drive an 'old' car, Michael had bought her a sexy new American model, which she preferred because it was newer and smaller than the 'hearse'. But it was still large enough to be comfortable and moreover was a powerhouse on wheels with a souped-up V8 engine beneath its sporty body, and she used to tear around town when the urge to put her foot down took her.

Once she saw how much Mickey loved Scrammy Gloria decided, for reasons which will only ever be known to her, that she was going to deprive him of it. She therefore instituted a malevolent albeit clever campaign with that objective in mind. First she prepared the ground, threatening to make Michael take away Scrammy every time Mickey said or did something she did not like. As these were always nonsense things, however, none of us perceived the real threat, especially not Michael, whose facial expression conveyed the message that he was not going to take away Scrammy for 'such nonsense'.

Gloria, however, was nothing if not relentless. To execute her plan, she had to shove Mickey out of the house, so she continued to lace into him for everything and nothing until he could stand it no longer. He discussed with Michael seeking refuge at Marjorie's house yet again, and our father, whose natural tendency was for a peaceful and happy family life, agreed with his set-upon son that it would be better if he left home for a while. So Mickey started sleeping at Marjorie's house.

However, he usually came home if he knew that any of his friends were going to be there. And they decidedly were there, the summer of 1965 being an even busier time around our pool than the summer of 1964 had been. Few days went by when we did not have anything from five to thirty visitors. While more peripheral members of the circle did not stay for lunch, our close friends usually did. Edward and Cookie were so rushed off their feet that they felt compelled to go to Gloria and ask her to intercede. She, reasonably enough, banned us from having any more guests for the next few days, 'to give the servants a chance to recover'.

That hiatus aside, our chums were at our house on a daily basis. Mickey had a new best friend, Michael Silvera, who also attended Jamaica College with him, as indeed did most of the other boys. Michael had a motor-bike and it was he who usually went up to York Castle – Marjorie's new house after Lucius's murder forced her to sell her old house – to inform Mickey to come down to join his friends, for communication between the houses of the two Smedmore sisters wasn't straightforward. Marjorie did not have a telephone, having recently moved into her house and the Jamaica Telephone Company having not yet run telephone lines up to it.

It was this communication problem which Gloria exploited to create the mischief she had in store for Mickey. Whenever she saw that none of his friends was there, she would send Owen, our head gardener, up to her sister's house with the message that Mickey had to come down immediately to play host to his friends. He would arrive, find nobody there and leave, perplexed that his mother could lie so brazenly and seemingly stupidly, for she was being caught out each and every time.

However, Gloria's game plan was cleverer than we gave her credit for. She then started to send Owen up to Marjorie's with the message that Michael had telephoned and said that he needed Mickey to come down to the store to help. Mickey would dress, drive downtown and arrive at the store only for Daddy to say that he had not rung for him.

The apparent pointlessness of Gloria's behaviour might have been lost on us, but it wasn't on her. She knew it was only a matter of time before Mickey, who was more assertive than the rest of us, ignored the summons Owen was bringing in the belief that it was false. Sure enough, the next time she sent Owen up, Mickey told him to tell Gloria that he wasn't going anywhere, as he knew Michael didn't want him at the store.

About two hours later, Mickey showed up at the house and came up to the pool, where Libby, Kitty and I were ensconced with Suzy Surridge and Bobby de Mercado: a friend whose family had been the original partners in Lascelles de Mercado, the basis of the family fortune of the late Princess Royal's husband. He told us how Gloria had tried to send him on yet another wild-goose chase and we, naturally enough, sympathized with him. Unfortunately, unbeknownst to us, this was the one occasion upon which Michael genuinely had asked Gloria to send Owen for Mickey to go to work.

Gloria had laid the trap well, and Mickey had walked right into it. Now all she needed to do was lie in wait until her notoriously hot-tempered husband came home and did her dirty work for her.

We all noticed how uncharacteristically quiet Gloria was that day. Since she had not complained of having one of her migraine headaches or sinusitis attacks, her conduct was a puzzle, especially as she kept to herself in her room the whole time. The mystery, however, didn't last more than a minute past Michael's return home from work.

As usual, he announced his arrival not only to us and the servants but to the whole neighbourhood by sitting on his horn from the moment he turned into the driveway until he stopped the car. He didn't do 'waiting', and there would be all hell to pay if they were not dutifully lined up waiting to open the car doors and start to unload whatever it was he had brought home as soon as he stopped the vehicle. They were, however, so well trained in dropping whatever it was they were doing and running to greet his arrival that he never had to issue reprimands.

Usually, when he arrived home, Michael would head straight for the front veranda, where Gloria would be sitting awaiting him unless she was out. He would bend down, kiss her on the cheek, go into his bedroom and change into something more comfortable while Cookie prepared his tea. Within minutes he would return to the front veranda, flop onto the chaise longue opposite her favourite chair and spend the next twenty minutes or so listening to her while she jabbered on as he consumed the cake and sandwiches laid before him with his cup of tea. Then, as soon as Edward came to clear the tea, he would get up, say he was 'off to r…r…rest' and head back to his bedroom, where he would bathe, read and rest until guests arrived for the evening or the dinner bell rang. Sometimes, Michael might break his routine by coming up to the pool and saying a brief hello to us, but by and large, he didn't. This afternoon, however, we all knew trouble was brewing when, within seconds of arriving home, Michael was booming out without a trace of a stutter: 'Mickey. Where are you? Get down here right now.'

In that instant we all knew that Mickey was in deep trouble. He started to blink overtime, always a sure sign that he was nervous. He got up from the chair he was sitting in on the veranda of the pool house to head into the main house. We tried to be reassuring, knowing that Michael was angry, but none of us had any idea just how deep the trouble would be because none of us knew how adeptly Gloria had laid the ground. Nevertheless, we knew it was going to be dramatic enough to be required viewing, so the rest of us headed towards the front of the house by walking down the driveway while Mickey went into the house through the back.

We took up our positions outside the dining-room windows. Gloria, we saw, was in the adjoining breakfast porch, while Michael was pacing up and down the back veranda which adjoined the breakfast porch, thereby giving us a perfect view of the whole drama as it unfolded.

'Why didn't you come down to help me when your mother sent Owen for you?' Michael bellowed as soon as Mickey reached him on the back veranda.

'I thought this was another one of Mummy's stunts,' Mickey explained.

'Are you going to stand there and let this ne'er-do-well that you spawned abuse me?' Gloria demanded of her husband, her voice ringing out from the portals of the breakfast porch. Fortunately for us, her back was to us, so there was scant chance of her realizing that we were witnesses, for then she would have sent us back up to the pool.

'She's always sending Owen up to Auntie's to tell me you want me at the store when you don't,' Mickey said in a reasonable tone of voice.

'So now it's a failing on my part to ask my son to help his father when he needs his help, but it's not a failing on his part when he shirks his duty in preference for a day of pleasure around the pool with his friends,' Gloria said, intent on stoking Michael's fires until they flamed uncontrollably.

'Is it some crime for your mother to want you to assist me?'

'That's not what I said, nor what I meant,' Mickey said, his voice as calm and modulated as possible in such a heated atmosphere.

'What did you mean, then?' Michael asked, still angry but plainly on the verge of letting light in upon the situation.

'Are you going to stand there, like a big *mumu* and let this good-for-nothing talk you out of the consequences of his actions – inactions, actually? Are you a man or a mouse, a doormat or a fool?' Gloria demanded.

'What a push-fire your mother is,' Suzy whispered to Libby and me.

Taking his cue from his wife and proving that he really was more mouse than man, Michael chose anger over reason.

'I told you to come and work,' he shrieked. 'You didn't come. You didn't even phone. You are a good-for-nothing so-and-so.'

Mickey stood his ground splendidly. He remained as calm and reasonable as ever, doubtless the only indication of nervousness being his eyes, which by then would be blinking sixty to the dozen. 'Daddy, if I'd thought that you'd really sent for me, I'd gladly have gone.'

Michael, ever predictable and as easily read as a baby book, started to issue a warning. 'If ever this…' he started. But before he could finish saying what punishment he would decree if ever this happened again Gloria, intent upon having blood spilled, interrupted and thereby kept Michael from wavering off the course she had predetermined.

'You must be the biggest idiot God put on this earth if you fall for such a brazen disclaimer. It's also an outrageous insult to me. I will not stand here and allow Mr Consequential to twist and turn things to his advantage. He may have my sister and mother fooled, but he doesn't have me, and he'd better not have you, if you know what's good for you.' Then, directing her next words to Mickey, she said, 'You're no good. Absolutely no good. I should have crushed you between my legs when I was giving birth to you. That's what I should have done to you.'

It was obvious even before Michael moved towards Mickey that Gloria was pulling his strings. Nor would she stop until he delivered up what she pleased. And that was to beat Mickey.

Mickey knew it too, and stepped back as Daddy advanced towards him. 'I could blow my brains out,' Michael said, reluctance battling for ascendancy with frustration and rage. 'How much can one man stand?'

'You'll have to stand a lot more if you don't nip this in the bud,' Gloria observed.

'God, what a push-fire,' Suzy repeated under her breath. 'She's not going to stop until your father beats Mickey up.'

Surrendering to the greatest power present, Michael let out the most almighty howl of anguish. It was a sound more akin to a suffering animal than a human being. With that he unbuckled his belt, whipped it out of his trousers and, grabbing the buckle, shortened it to a more manageable length by wrapping the first few inches around his hand. As he was doing this, Mickey, who had been standing still, suddenly mobilized himself and bolted for the door leading to the back garden. Fired with fury, Michael ran after him and, blocking his escape, started to flail at him. As the lashes rained down on Mickey, Gloria stood behind Michael, goading him.

'Let this be a lesson to you,' she said to Mickey. 'You're no damned good. You never were. You never will be.'

At first, Mickey took the blows without trying to protect or defend himself. But, as the beating persisted and it became apparent that Michael was actually out of control, Mickey then tried to head for the sofa, presumably to use it as a shield. Michael, however, was having none of it. Every movement Mickey made, he shadowed; and, as often happens in real life, all the onlookers realized at more or less the same time that there was a real danger that he could kill Mickey.

As if be prearrangement, Libby, Suzy, Bobby and I looked from one to the other, each of us seeing our fear reflected in the eyes of the other. 'You'd better go and break this up, Bobby,' the three of us suggested in more or less the same words at the same time, while he uttered the same thought with the pronoun 'I' substituted for 'you'.

Bobby was over six feet tall and well built, so there was no doubt he would be able to handle Michael, who, though a six-footer himself, was slender rather than brawny.

The realization that her son's life might be in danger hit Gloria more or less at the same time as us. 'Enough, Michael, enough,' she ordered. 'Stop now. Do you hear me? Stop right this instant. Stop, I tell you. Stop,' she said, her words having absolutely no effect.

Help, however, was on the way. It took Bobby no more than two or three minutes to run around from the front to the back of the house. In the intervening period, Mickey had curled up into a standing approximation of the foetal position, protecting his face and the front of his body, even the back of his head, which he was covering with one arm, while Michael lashed away as if he were a Roman solider and Mickey Jesus of Nazareth being scourged before the crucifixion.

'Stop, Daddy, stop,' Libby and I were wailing, but if Michael heard us, he never let on.

Bobby sensibly announced his arrival before grabbing Michael from behind. 'Mr Ziadie, it's Bobby, sir. I'm going to grab you now. Okay, sir,' he said and seized him from behind. Michael struggled only momentarily, allowing Bobby to pull him off Mickey and take control of the situation. I suspect he must have been grateful for the intervention. Gloria certainly was.

'Thank God you're here. Mr Ziadie's got a little carried away, I fear,' she said, as if she were an innocent bystander who had been witnessing something that was odious to her, rather than something which she had engineered and enjoyed until it looked as if there would be unforeseen repercussions.

Michael seemed to come out of a trance, visibly returning to normal as he beheld his battered son.

'See what you've made your father do?' said Gloria, as unconscionable and normal as ever.

Michael, always the more conscionable of the two, acknowledged the reality of what had happened by saying, 'Just go outside.' He wasn't ordering; rather, he implored. He must have been frightened of a recurrence of the uncontrollable rage which might well have ended in his son's death.

Mickey stepped towards the door leading up to the pool then stopped dead in his tracks as Gloria said to her husband: 'Are you insane? You're sending him to the very place he was so eager to go to that he couldn't help you at work. Well, you may be an old *mumu*, but I'm not. Mickey,' she declaimed, 'your father and I are taking Scrammy away from you. Let's see how consequential and independent you are without wheels.'

Mickey shot Gloria a look of such dignified inscrutability that I had to take off my hat to him. I would not have been able to contain how I was feeling, but he did.

'Go. Just go, before I do something I regret,' Michael pleaded with Mickey.

Mickey left the back veranda and headed towards the pool, where we rejoined him. We all sat down, commiserating with him and reflecting on what had happened. None of us could quite believe what we had witnessed. Libby and I – and, to a lesser extent, Suzy – had all seen Michael in action before, but Bobby had not. Yet he was no more shocked than we were. 'Killer' really had almost killed; and it was a sobering, indeed frightening thought, to realize that we had come so close to witnessing the murder of a brother and a friend. Yet none of us blamed Michael so much as we did Gloria. Having seen the whole thing unfold, it was apparent to all of us that she had been the main proponent. Even though Daddy had been the person who had actually delivered the blows, ultimate responsibility lay with her, for she had knowingly goaded him, a man with scant control of his temper, into delivering the first blows, by making out that he was a weakling who lacked the resolve to discipline his son, even though he had clearly been trying to shy away from the physical abuse she was intent upon provoking. Furthermore she had then encouraged him to continue when it looked as if he might stop.

Mickey, Libby, Suzy and I agreed that Gloria was a real bitch. Bobby, who did not have as much knowledge of her usual conduct as we did, remained silent while we decried her demeanour and motives, discussing how she had manoeuvred and manipulated throughout the summer, sending Owen up to Auntie's house with false messages, so that she could lay the ground for this scenario. While Mickey, Libby, Suzy and I talked, Bobby listened; and I could tell, he was half wondering if we were not being unfair to Gloria. It was hard, very hard, for anyone who did not know her well to appreciate what a Machiavellian witch she really was. Like all intriguers, she was careful to conceal most of what she was up to behind a misleading façade; but those of us who knew her well had some of her measure – though I wouldn't say any of us ever really had it all. It is extremely difficult for people who are not devious and destructive to put themselves into the shoes of those who are. It is even more difficult for people with a conscience to actually reconfigure themselves as someone without one, so it was always difficult to tell quite what her objective was until her latest scheme had come to fruition, or to predict how she would actually execute it.

However, her children were not clueless as to what sort of person she was. Indeed, Gloria herself used to boast, 'I'm the biggest bitch you'll ever meet, and no one had better forget it.' This she was always saying to us children, to Michael, to the servants and to her sister and mother. While we queried the necessity of her trying to instil fear in us, Mickey, Libby and I did not query the basic veracity and accuracy of her statement. It was one with which we concurred wholeheartedly.

'Mummy really is the biggest bitch you'll ever meet,' I now said.

'If she takes away Scrammy, I'll never speak to her again,' Mickey said.

'She's determined to ruin our lives,' Libby said.

'She's not going to ruin mine anymore,' Mickey said. 'I'm moving out. I'm going to speak to Grandma about living with her. Bobby, can you take me down to my grandmother? She lives on Fairway Avenue.'

When Bobby agreed, Mickey, who had precious little stuff at Auntie's house, went into the house to pack a few of the possessions which would see him through until he was able to come back up to our house to get the remainder.

While Mickey was inside, a pall of doom descended on Libby, Kitty and me – and, to a lesser extent, Suzy, who was so close to us that she was almost an additional sibling.

Mickey was due to get his 'A' Level results in a week or two, and if he had passed all his examinations, he would have to decide what he wanted to do with his future: whether he would go to university and what he would study. Although he didn't have a hope in hell of becoming the musician he wanted to be, both Michael and Gloria having made it plain that that option was not open to him, they did expect him to enter one of the professions. So he had to come up with a decision of one kind or another soon.

Up to this point, Michael and Gloria had been able to keep from the world at large the true level of cruelty which passed as care and discipline at home because no one outside the inhabitants of the household had witnessed one of those scenes. Not even Maisie and Marjorie had ever been present during one of the fully-fledged dramas that had resulted in Mickey leaving home so often, though Suzy had been present for enough of the build-ups to have gained an accurate picture of what went down once she was sent home.

This time, however, the curtain of discretion had been torn aside. Bobby was a good friend of Michael's sister Doris's sons, and was often at her house. There was not a prospect in hell of a lid being kept on this incident; and, sure enough, within days Michael's nieces and nephews and brother and sisters were singing from the same page as Gloria's mother and sister.

Despite the misfortune of having been born to a woman as cruel and calculating as our mother, we children had been lucky otherwise. Our paternal relations were as systematically kind and thoughtful as our maternal ones. Within days, we had discernible proof of this. Maisie and Marjorie took up for Mickey, our grandmother going so far as to say that she would support Mickey and pay for his education if Michael did not. Daddy, however, refused that offer, saying that of course he would pay for Mickey's education even if he had left home, and moreover he would continue to give him pocket money, but no one was to tell Gloria.

We children were all upset at the loss of Scrammy, not only because she represented independence but also because she was something of an institution in the family. Michael was a hopeless driver, so she had been badly broken in and had a top speed of fifty, a starter that was as unreliable as his temper and an inability to climb steep hills without a helping push from all of us. This, however, only made her an object of affection and amusement amongst us; and it was a sad day indeed when Michael's mechanic Victor Rose came up, the day after the incident, to collect her for resale or scrapping, whichever proved to be more feasible.

Then Michael's niece Audrey stepped into the breech and gave Mickey the black Volkswagen Beetle which she had been using as a run-around until she got her new car.

The first we knew of this was when Mickey drove up to the house to show Libby, Kitty and me how our cousin, as beautiful inside as out, had rectified our mother's atrocity. Not only did Audrey's compassionate generosity reaffirm our basic belief in the goodness of humanity – a belief our mother's aberrant behaviour might well have undermined, had we lacked such humane and supportive relations as Audrey, Maisie and Marjorie – but the black Beetle was actually a better car than Scrammy.

Now 'we' had new wheels, and if the Beetle did not have the virtue of Scrammy's failings, it nevertheless had another appeal entirely: it drove well. Doubtless with the passage of time we would grow to love her too. We were busy talking in the study about the Beetle and Scrammy when Gloria, who must have been eavesdropping, appeared out of nowhere.

'Where did you get that car?' she demanded of Mickey.

'I'm no longer living here so I don't think you need concern yourself with how I came by it,' he said calmly and reasonably.

'Whether you live here of not, you are my child. I gave you life. Now I will ask you again,' she said, her voice as cold and hard as steel. 'Where did you get that car?'

'And I said, since I am not living here anymore, it's none of your concern.'

'You think you're so consequential,' Gloria sneered, 'but you're not. I know that your cousin Audrey gave it to you. Well, you'll have to give it back.'

'I'll do no such thing,' said Mickey, still calm, his tone of voice still pleasant.

'You will.' Gloria trilled. 'I have decreed what you will do, and *my will shall prevail*.'

Mickey said no more, which was sensible, for Gloria, unable to spark off his replies and not in the mood to engage in one of the fully-fledged scenes which were her speciality and which required no response at all from her victim, stood still for a moment, seemingly assessing the damage she had done, and having accounted it worthy of her talents, harrumphed haughtily and departed.

In truth, none of us thought that Gloria could impose her will in the circumstances. The car, after all, wasn't hers to give, so it could not have been hers to take away. Mickey left with every confidence that Gloria could not force him to return the car. When Michael came home from work that day, however, she started in on him as soon as he was walking up the back passage towards the back door. For once, she was so impatient to see him that she wasn't waiting for him to come to her but was sitting on the back veranda, ready to intercept him.

Before he even had a chance to reach the house proper, she launched her attack. 'Your niece Audrey has made a mockery of my punishment of Mickey's selfish disregard of you. She has given him a replacement for Scrammy. That undermines my authority, and I will not stand for it. I demand that you make that consequential little worm give Audrey back the car.'

'Gloria, for God's sake,' pleaded Michael, bending down to kiss her on the cheek, desperate to avoid a row. 'The child isn't even living here anymore.'

'You *mumu*, it doesn't matter whether he's living here or not. He's still our child, and we still have a duty to discipline him. I will not have my authority undermined. You will order him to give that car back to your niece. It is too much that I'm always having to cope with the interference of family: first

Mama and Marjorie and now Audrey.'

'Please Gloria, he's young...'

'Are you a man or a mouse?' she sneered. 'Where's your backbone? You'd better find it if you know what's good for you. I will not tolerate this situation, nor will I allow you to expose me to it by taking the easy way out. That sorry excuse for a human being whom you call your son might be able to make a fool of you, but I won't be allowing him to make one of me. Nor will I be allowing you to have him hold me up to ridicule. You let those damned children lead you around by the nose, as if you're a racehorse and they're your groom. But this time you will behave as a proper father, a protective husband and a *man* should. You will see that Mickey gives Audrey back the car. You will order him to take it back to her. And you'd better make sure she takes it back, if you want peace in your family. Mark my words. I said *your* family. Audrey is *your* family, not *mine*, and any disruption will affect you a hell of a lot more than it will affect me. And you can bank on it: there will be a severe rupture in my relations with the Ziadie family if you allow them to interfere the way you've allowed my mother and sister over the years. And don't console yourself with the thought that because I've let Mama and Marjorie get away with their interference, I'll let the Ziadies. Mama and Marjorie are my family, and what I will put up with from them I will not be putting up from the Ziadies. I hope I've made myself clear?'

'I'll have a word with Mickey,' said Michael, looking sheepish.

'You do that,' Gloria said, sailing out of the house into the back garden.

If Gloria thought she had found an easy way to torment Mickey, she reckoned without the ingenuity of her son and his first cousin. Since her objection lay in the car being a gift, Audrey then sold it to him for the princely sum of £25, £20 of which she gave him, though Gloria and Michael never knew that detail. If, however, we hoped that such finesse would be enough to deflect Gloria from her objective, we were wrong.

A few days later, Michael came home after stopping off at Maisie's house to see his mother-in-law and son. Having learned of the new arrangement, and considering it to be a win-win situation for all concerned, he came home and told Gloria about it. I was in my bedroom when I heard her raised voice, always a sure sign that she was even more serious than when her voice was at its normal pitch – not, it must be said, that anyone who heard her threats uttered at her usual pitch ever thought that she wasn't serious. Malevolence of such potency didn't need volume to reach the recipient's ears or heart. 'I don't give a continental damn whether he has bought the car or Audrey has given it to him. He cannot have it. You will telephone him at Mama's right now and inform him to take it up to Audrey immediately and drop it off. Then he is to find his way down here and report to me so that I can see for myself that my instructions have been obeyed.'

'Don't yo…yoo…oou th…th…think yo…yo…you're blow…blowing this th…th…thing out of a…a…all proportion?' Michael stammered.

'If you'd prefer, I'll telephone both Mickey and Audrey,' Gloria said, her voice laden with menace. Michael knew, as well as I did, that what she was telling him was that he had better do it, for if she did, she would create so much havoc that he'd always regret that he hadn't been the henchman. Quite what she would do, one didn't know. But one knew that she was capable of doing pretty much anything, and in so vicious a way that the damage would be far greater than if he did her dirty work for her. So he duly telephoned both Mickey and Audrey, and within an hour Mickey was standing in front of Gloria, confirming that he had executed her wishes.

This incident, more than any other, showed me how ruthless and cruel my mother was. This really was a step too far. Although I had spent my whole life seeing her torment Mickey and Libby, I don't think I had ever faced the fact before that she was really a very calculating and Machiavellian sadist who not only enjoyed inflicting pain but was also someone who would go to extreme lengths to set up situations that caused it. There was something chilling about her conduct, and it froze out a lot of the affection and regard I had hitherto had for her. Of course, I was not stupid enough to let on to her or anyone else – indeed, not even fully to myself – how I felt, but I had started along the long route to seeing my mother for what she was.

For a long time I had wondered how life would be if Daddy should die. Now, for the first time, I started to imagine what it would be like if Mummy died too. Though I did not wish harm to befall them, the prospect of being an orphan, I can assure you, had its appeal.

Chapter Ten

Within weeks of the loss of Scrammy, Mickey got his 'A' Level results. He had passed and, at the age of nearly seventeen, had to choose what he wanted to do with the rest of his life. He had no interest in joining the family business. While it might have surprised others to hear that Michael did not want his son following in his footsteps, we all knew that Daddy hated what he did and felt that the rewards, though great, were not really worth what one had to endure on a daily basis. 'Mo…money isn't everything,' he used to say.

'You co…ould become a doc…doc…doctor or dentist,' he said when the subject of Mickey's career came up, 'but you don't have the br….brains to do medicine, so do den…dentistry instead. It will give you a good living without having all the pro…problems bu…business has.'

The idea of shoving his hand down the mouths of strangers had no appeal for my fastidious brother, who not only washed his hands several times a day, as if he were competing with Lady Macbeth in the cleanliness stakes, but went further and was always smelling them as well as anything he picked up, whether it was a book, a record, an ornament, even car keys, to assure himself that they were perfectly clean and smelled accordingly. 'I'll do law,' he decided. 'Not that I wanted to,' he would later say. 'It was simply something to do and seemed preferable to Daddy's suggestions.' Michael arranged for the family solicitor George Desnoes to take him into his firm as a pupil, and within weeks Mickey was on his way to a career in law that would turn out to be distinguished.

While Mickey settled into his new life, our father kept a close eye on him, often stopping off at Maisie's house to see him on the way home. This was more than can be said for Gloria. She had cast herself firmly in the role of martyr to an ungrateful son and not only acted as if she had been the wronged party but refused to speak to Mickey until he apologized to her. As he quite rightly felt there was nothing for which he should apologize, he declined to do so. In that, he had the support of each and every member of the family, with the occasional exception of our father, who would beg him to apologize from time to time 'for the sake of peace'.

If anything, Mickey was even more determined not to speak to Gloria than she was not to speak to him. He had not forgiven her; and, as often happened in our family, the situation quickly degenerated into farce. Mickey still came up to our house to see his sisters, and Gloria did not dare to put a halt to those visits, for she knew that to do so would make her position untenable with the wider audience, which was the only entity she cared about. Had she kicked Mickey out in the first place, she might have been able to object to his presence in her house, but because she had not, she was forced to endure it as and when he wanted to be there. This showed how preposterous was her supposedly moral stance of boycotting her mother's house on the grounds that Grandma was 'harbouring the viper there', for Maisie too continued to come up to the house to see us. This added yet another ridiculous dimension, for Gloria pointedly refused to speak to her mother, calling her 'a treacherous whore' behind her back, which I took to be a sign that she was aware of the insecurity of her own position, otherwise she would have been making the abusive comment to her unfortunate mother's face. Grandma, well used by now to her daughter's behaviour, simply ignored Gloria's ignoring her.

On one or two occasions, Mickey and Maisie were present while there was a houseful of guests, none of whom realized that mother and son and mother and daughter were not speaking. It is small wonder that people who knew us well said that we lived in a 'madhouse'.

I was now the only one of my parents' children living at home. Libby and Kitty were away at boarding school for most of the year, and with Mickey at Grandma's house, I still had to sit with Mummy when she wanted me to. I cannot say I derived any real pleasure from these sessions. I could no longer look at her without seeing behind the mask to Machiavelli. This reinforced the sense of being used by her that I had sometimes felt ever since that cutting remark she had made in Cissy's bedroom about there being no escape from me when I had been the one who had wanted the escape from her.

I was now beginning to see more clearly than ever that Gloria had no scruples about turning the tables on others as and when it suited her, and that she did so without justification, compunction or regard for the feelings of the person she was targeting. This sometimes made it extremely difficult for me to present as uncritical a façade as she required, for there were times when I was practically bursting with the desire to puncture her flow and tell her a few home truths. However, I only needed to think of Mickey or Libby to see where assertiveness had got them. No. Gloria required uncritical adoration, or the appearance of it, at all times; and, unless I wanted to join the ranks of the abused, I had better play the game the way she determined it should be played. So I kept my counsel and retained my position of favourite, trying not to think about what was happening whenever my affection for her was overridden by these thoughts.

Human relations are complicated, none more so than when one party has all the power and the other none. But character is destiny, and I could no more escape from myself than I could from my abusive mother. I now found myself embroiled in an ever-increasingly layered relationship with her. The underlying affection I had entertained for her from early childhood was still there, albeit diminished and receding progressively into the background, but it nevertheless popped out with the slightest encouragement. So, as time marched on and I relaxed into this newly complex set of emotions, there were times when I would feel love, pleasure, mistrust, discomfort, pressure, pain, hatred and the urge to flee all in the space of a half hour. The internal turmoil this induced needs little elaboration; and there were times when I felt as if I would explode from the strain of it all.

Fortunately for my ultimate well-being, I never questioned my right to feel what I did. Nor did I have the urge to rationalize my feelings and dress them up as something they were not. This acceptance of reality, above all, made it possible for me to get through such a conflicting phase with minimal emotional damage. Indeed, by accepting the contradictory feelings I was experiencing, I was actually doing something healthy, for the greatest problems that the victims of contradictory personalities such as Gloria experience, result from them denying what they have been through or how conflicted they feel about their experiences.

Ironically, the one emotion I now seldom felt for Gloria was one which I had possessed in spades while a child: sympathy. I could see that she used emotion rather than felt it; and I arrived quite naturally and without any conscious desire at the emotional detachment my brother and sisters had always had where she was concerned. It was as if she were a character in a play of her own devising rather than a sensitized being to whom one could or should relate. She never seemed to have a natural or an expected emotion and certainly none to the degree that anyone else did. Everything was either at over-the-top fever-pitch or unnaturally tepid and, more to the point, seemed predicated on her immediate needs, whether for attention, admiration, excitement, to alleviate boredom or whatever. Inevitably, her every response was about what suited Gloria, Gloria, Gloria, to the exclusion of everyone and everything else – unless, of course, she wanted to impress some poor sucker who didn't know her well. Then she would turn on the charm, trot out the emotions she only displayed when in the company of those she wished to seduce, after which she would revert to type.

It was not only her coldness and self-centredness that was pointing one in the direction of the monstrousness of her reality but also her lack of empathy, genuine emotion or consistency. Her 'nerves' were a case in point. From ever since I could remember, she had gone on and on about her 'nerves'. It was an accepted fact of life that 'Gloria suffers from her nerves' and 'Gloria is so highly strung that she must do exactly as she wants without restraint or resistance'. Later on, I would come to the conclusion that she was actually an emotionless sensationalist who used sensation as a substitute for the lack of emotion she felt, whipping herself up into frenzies to conceal from herself as much as anyone else that she occupied an emotional desert.

Although I had been too young to analyze her motive for playing the 'nerves' card with the relish she did, even at that age I could sense that there were sound reasons why someone like her would play that game. In the 1960s, 'nerves' were regarded as a mark of refined sensibility rather than an indication of an emotional disorder, and nervous breakdowns were much in vogue with a certain type of lady who had nothing wrong with her except pretensions to sensibility or a desire to manipulate people into letting her have her way. Medical confirmation of 'nervousness' provided the ladies concerned with proof that they were far more delicate constitutionally than normal women, thus innately superior. Nervous breakdowns were not something suffered by lower- or middle-class women, or indeed by your average upper-class female, but only by socially superior women of superior sensibility. Of course, once they had the diagnosis and a track record of 'nervous trouble', everyone would have to relinquish his or her will to them and give them their way, lest the frustration of unrealized desire push them over the edge into another 'nervous breakdown'.

It was a neat game, one which many an emotional terrorist had been playing for centuries. There was nothing new about 'nervousness', and indeed history and literature are littered with a variety of women who held their families hostage to their 'nerves', including another Jamaican, the poet Elizabeth Barrett Browning, who was too ill to even walk downstairs for much of her life, yet subsequently managed to elope through an open window with fellow poet Robert Browning, once she found a man to love, and even produced a child in middle age despite having been bedridden for most of her adult life. Yes, there was nothing new about Gloria's game, though I doubt that the reasons for it were apparent to her friends or relations.

Gloria had been claiming to have nervous breakdowns since we were children, but none of her progeny could see any discernible difference between our mother having a nervous breakdown and our mother being her normal self. Of course, none of us yet knew the tale of how Dr Mosley had told her parents that she was too 'highly strung' to hear the word 'no', ever since which she had been relentlessly playing the 'nerves' card. Because none of us appreciated that she needed to produce the occasional 'nervous breakdown' to retain credibility, we actually saw through the game in a way that the adults surrounding her, who had been primed over the years with Dr Mosley's diagnosis, did not. Indeed, none of us children could see that she had genuine 'nervous' trouble at all. If anything, she had nerves of steel, or in the alternative, lacked ordinary nerves. Much that upset others left her untouched. With the exception of her histrionic outpouring of grief in the months succeeding her father's murder – and one had to remember that these scenes always took place following her daily consumption of a bottle of gin and while she was working her way through her nightly bottle of port – nothing save admiration seemed to move her, except when she did not get her own way, at which point you could depend upon a release of bile.

Gloria's 'breakdowns' struck me as more of an expedient concoction of her own imagination than anything else. She did not go into the hospital when she had them. She never had medical treatment. She might take to her bed for a day or so, but there were several breakdowns to which she alluded which seemed to have occurred in the middle of what passed as normal family life with us. Not yet knowing of Dr Mosley's diagnosis, or how Gloria had exploited it over the years to get her own way, my siblings and I nevertheless knew that we were pawns in a game where fact and fancy were interchangeable and seldom recognized as such by the adults surrounding us.

The Scrammy episode, however, had caused such waves within the family and gained Gloria such universal disapproval that it was only a matter of time before our ever-resourceful mother set about regaining the ground she had lost. This she now did by seeking refuge in her 'nerves' but only after she had tried, and failed, to brazen her way out of her predicament. The one thing she could not stand was disapproval from everyone surrounding her, but this is what she was getting from one and all. When she tried to justify herself to her Smedmore Aunt Maud, she was met with – as Aunt Maud recounted it to me – 'stony silence'. She fared no better with her Smedmore Uncle Rodney, who told her what a fine young man Mickey was. When she turned to her closest Burke aunt, she got an even worse response. Aunt V told us how she demanded that Mummy change the subject when she brought it up; and when Gloria persisted, she informed her that she had been cruel and malicious to Mickey, who was a nice young man of whom any parent should be proud. She would have encountered similar responses from the Ziadies had she been stupid enough to raise the subject with them, especially as Audrey was involved, but she was no fool and wisely went to ground instead.

After a few weeks without her support system of sympathetic relations, Gloria came up with what she thought was the perfect plan to shift the blame. She made an appointment to go and see a psychiatrist, and recounted the encounter to everyone who came to the house for the next few weeks. 'My dear,' she would say dramatically, 'I went to see Dr Whatever [I've forgotten his name] because Michael has been telling me for so long that I'm mad that I'd thought I'd better check it out. "So, Mrs Ziadie, why are you here?" he said as soon as I sat down. "Because I'm mad." "Did you say you've come to see me because you're mad?" "Yes." "You can't be mad, Mrs Ziadie. Mad people always think they're sane. So if you think you're mad, you can't be. Has anyone been telling you you're mad?" "My husband tells me all the time. He's always saying

You're mad, Gloria. So I've decided to come and check for myself whether I am mad. Because I think he's mad." "Does he say he's mad?" "Michael admitting he's mad?"' she would recount, injecting her voice with an unmistakeable dose of incredulity. '"Never. He'd sooner die rather than admit that he might be mad." "Maybe he is the one who should be coming to see me," he said, which tells me that he thinks Michael is the one who's mad, not me.'

If Gloria hoped to swing opinion behind her by such means, she failed. Everyone in the family circle, as well as among her close friends, was of the opinion that she was indeed half-cracked, if not wholly so; and while many of those same people also thought that Michael too had a screw or two loose, the consensus was that he was the saner of the two. Moreover, he was generally acknowledged to be kinder.

Whether it was the failure of her psychiatric ploy to regain lost ground from the Mickey episode; whether she was embarking upon a distraction exercise; whether she was now bored and decided that she could do with another drama, and one moreover in which she would remain the centre of attention rather than have that attention diverted to third parties such as her injured son; or whether her motives were an amalgam of all three, I will never know. But close on the heels of that visit to the psychiatrist came another of her rather dubious nervous breakdowns.

One Sunday morning she got up and announced, right after she had taken her orange juice with the requisite number of sachets of gelatine to strengthen her hair and fingernails and before she took the first sip of the inevitable gin and tonic, that she was having a nervous breakdown. I could see no discernible difference between this breakdown victim and the normal Mummy, still suspiciously in evidence, especially when she told me, as calmly and regally as ever, to telephone Jimmy Burrowes and arrange for him to have her checked into Medical Associates. Why, I asked myself, was she having a gynaecologist check her into the hospital where she had had her hysterectomy two years before, and which she often said was 'just like a five star hotel', rather than consulting a psychiatrist who might – or might not – then decide whether she needed hospital treatment? It seemed to me that she was doing nothing but setting up an attention- and sympathy-seeking diversion, and one moreover, which would be as luxurious as her daily life. Sure enough, when she proceeded to pack an assortment of silk and lace negligee sets, full make-up and decorative jewels and then ordered Owen to put the luggage in the car boot, together with a twelve-bottle case of Louis Roederer champagne, I had all the confirmation I needed. This nervous breakdown was nothing more than a ploy to regain centre-stage and garner sympathy.

Although I did not, at the tender age of nearly sixteen, realize that there were elements to her motives beyond attention-seeking and sympathy, over forty years later I can see how accurate my assessment was, even if I was not yet mature enough to figure out that the other elements included such tawdry motives as reasserting her ascendancy and enhancing her glamour.

To those who might query the glamorous element, I ask them to ask themselves: what is more poignant than a beautiful woman bejewelled and fully made-up, lying in a magnificent negligee of the finest silk and lace, drinking champagne and bravely fighting a nervous breakdown while she remains as entertaining and cheerful as ever? The fact that she had her hairdresser go to Medical Associates to style her hair should have provided me with a clue, but I fear at that age much eluded me that makes sense now that I am older.

If I saw at least some of what was happening, the adults around me saw none.

One afternoon Michael took me to see Gloria. 'How do you th...think you're mo...mother's doing?' he asked me afterwards.

'She seems her normal self to me,' I said.

'To me too,' he replied.

We drove along in silence, as we always did. Just before we reached home, he said, 'Your mother's be...being very brave.'

'How do you mean?' I asked.

'It mu...must be very difficult to present a br...bright face to the wo... world when you...you're having a bre...breakdown,' he said.

'I suppose,' I said, finding it difficult to believe that an intelligent man could be so easily duped. 'But at least she's brought Grandma and Auntie to heel,' I said, introducing some reality into the conversation. They were both speaking to her again now that she was 'ill'.

Michael shot me a quizzical look.

'Well, she's got them talking to her again,' I said.

'I don't know what's wr...wrong with your brother. If it was my mo... mother in the ho...hospital, I'd wa...want to see her.'

'But your mother wouldn't have whipped your father up into a frenzy so she could have an excuse to take your car away from you,' I observed.

'Huh,' Michael grunted noncommittally, reverting to our accustomed state of silence before I presented him with too much truth.

If one of the benefits Gloria obtained from her 'breakdown' was having her sister and mother visit and speak to her again, and if it also got her a lot of the attention she sought, in that friends and relations visited her in vast numbers, her son proved to be a much harder nut to crack. He stayed firmly away.

After nearly a week's stay in the hotel-hospital, Gloria returned home. Everyone had visited her except Mickey, Libby and Kitty, the last two of whom were at boarding school.

I suspect that Gloria timed her departure to coincide with her consumption of the final bottle of Louis Roederer, but maybe I am doing her a disservice and maybe she returned when boredom set in and she needed something new with which to entertain herself. Whatever the reality, she duly returned and whatever passed as normal at home came back with her. She was such a dynamo, such a powerhouse of energy, such a force of nature that, whenever she was absent, the house seemed peculiarly still, almost deadly in its calm, and it has to be said, a lot duller than when she was in residence. Then the place would throb, often unpleasantly, but always vibrantly.

With Mickey staying at our grandmother's house, and with no indication that he would ever return home, Gloria needed to cast another of her children in the role of her primary victim. To no one's surprise, she alighted upon Libby, who, up to this point, had been her secondary victim.

I have no doubt that I would have been thrown into the cauldron if I had been injudicious enough to let on how much regard I had lost for her, but since I did not, and since Kitty was off-limits as Michael's favourite, Gloria promoted Libby to the hot seat and started to roast her at every opportunity.

In many ways, Libby was the ideal victim for a mother as competitive and compulsively self-centred as ours. Aged fourteen, she had realized her early promise and grown into a beauty: one, moreover, who looked somewhat like her mother. Although Gloria looked much younger than her thirty-eight years and was always thrilled when people said that she looked more like our sister than our mother, she was nevertheless acutely aware that she was no longer as young as she had once been. Even if she still managed to attract as many admirers as she had when she was younger, forty was then held up as the cut-off point for beautiful women to retain their desirability, and even though she was hoping to extend that deadline beyond its established limit, she was not stupid. She knew that nature must inevitably take its toll. At that point, she would then be forced to share centre-stage, and maybe she would even be relegated to the wings – prospects that were both anathema to her.

With such an attitude, the passage of time and the diminution of her attractiveness must have filled Gloria with a foreboding that only someone as vain and self-centred as she was can truly understand. I don't pretend to get even near to comprehending the emotions that she must have been experiencing, but I do know that fury, bitterness and envy manifested themselves, for these were what she directed towards Libby. It is almost as if she felt that, by targeting Libby, she could somehow freeze time and preserve herself as the captivating beauty before whose altar all men and gullible women fell.

Although Libby had a break from our mother's malice once she returned to boarding school, when she came home that Christmas for the holidays, Gloria was ready and waiting for her. No matter what she wanted to do, she could not. No matter what she said, Gloria found a way of twisting its meaning. She was constantly accused of rudeness and impertinence when she had only been politely responding to whatever it was her mother had asked her. She found herself being sent to her room so often that she started to stay there out of choice to avoid the scenes that she knew would be inevitable if Gloria caught sight of her anywhere else in the house.

Gloria, however, wasn't Gloria for nothing. Once she twigged as to Libby's tactics, she started to demand that she come outside, criticizing her for being a recluse etc, etc, etc. Libby would then be forced to leave her bedroom, only to find that she was being banished back to it within the hour, as Gloria had trumped up yet another reason to abuse and punish her.

Not content with tormenting Libby directly, Gloria came up with another way of causing her grief. She had a new beau since earlier that year, her relationship with Charles having failed to progress because of the age difference. Bruce was someone whom Gloria actually liked and approved of. He was a lovely person: warm, kind and decent. His background was impeccable. Indeed, as so often happens within old families, there was a connection: something along the lines of his great-uncle having married the sister of Gloria's Aunt Estelle's husband St Elmer Brooks. But it was Bruce's ready laugh, allied to his superb manners, which were the secret of his success with Gloria. He would laugh uproariously at her comments, which were genuinely witty but required an appreciation of true drollery, which not everyone had. As he always treated her with the respect that she felt was her due, she melted under the appreciation and deference. Till her dying day, she never had an ill word to say about 'Brucie-Baby', as she called him.

Despite liking Bruce, Gloria felt no compunction in doing everything in her power to keep him and Libby apart. Sometimes he would be banned from coming to the house because Libby had done something which required that she be put in punishment, even though these infractions were always covered in mystery and known to no one but Gloria herself. Otherwise, when Libby wanted to go out – say, to the cinema – she would often require Libby's presence at home to babysit her, even though she and Libby never spoke except when necessary and would therefore not spend one minute in each other's presence, Libby staying in her bedroom reading while Gloria remained on the back veranda watching television. But Gloria's objective would be satisfied, for it wasn't to have Libby's companionship but to frustrate her and punish her for being young and beautiful.

One of the more distressing features of Gloria's personality was her ability to explore the dark side of every scenario. She could come up with nuances for additional torment which would never have occurred to anyone else. She now utilized this talent by finding yet another club with which to batter Libby. 'That child is a born bitch,' she started to complain to Michael. 'She stayed in her bedroom the whole time you were out. She wouldn't even sit with me.'

'Do...don't you know yo...you're supposed to pro...provide company for yo...your mo...mother?' Michael would then angrily reprimand Libby, who of course was not about to sit with Gloria when every time she did, she found herself dragged into a row entirely of her mother's making.

But Gloria had another motivation for behaving as she did. She wanted to drive as deep a wedge as she could between father and daughter, one of her favourite games being to use Libby's presence in much the same way that she had used Mickey's, turning them into whipping posts in her crazed version of persecutor as victim.

Michael, always determined never to put Gloria in the wrong, would arrive home to find his wife pressing his protective buttons. Sometimes he would dismiss her complaints. Sometimes he would be irritated by them, telling her to 'get off my back. I'm sick of your nagging.' Sometimes he would reprimand Libby. With each incident, however, you could see that he was torn more and more, and struggling to retain whatever composure he had. He did not want to explode, to lose control, to have a repetition of the Mickey episode. Yet each time he returned home to Gloria's diatribe, he was being driven closer and closer to breaking point. I suspect he feared what might happen if he reached it. If I am correct, he was right to do so, for when he did reach it, he did something that was so awful that it was truly unbelievable.

That, however, was in the future.

In the meantime, Gloria set about sowing seeds of discord between Libby and myself with the same facility she utilized when doing so between father and daughter. She knew that Libby and I were close; so, to instil envy and resentment, after she had prevented Libby from going out with Bruce, she would then give me permission to go, even though neither he nor I wanted me to be there. Of course, neither Libby nor I realized how she was trying to divide and rule, using my status as favoured child as yet another club with which to beat my beloved sister over the head, while at the same time hopefully triggering not only yet more pain but also enough sibling rivalry that Libby would resent me.

In my ignorance of Gloria's true objective, I would leap right into the cauldron and try to utilize my favoured status to get her to allow Libby out. These appeals of mine were nothing new, for I had been using them for years to rescue Mickey from the boiling water he frequently found himself in. But I was no more successful than I had ever been, though that did not stop me from trying to help my siblings each time something new occurred.

It was only decades later, when Mickey was dying and his and Libby's resentment about my favoured status cropped up in conversation, that I began to understand what a clever game Gloria had played. Her Machiavellianism had seeped into every aspect of our lives, and in the process, she had made even our love for each other into weapons which she could use to wound us.

By the time Libby returned to school in January 1966, she had endured such a dose of her mother's malevolence that she was smoking like a chimney, and her hands shook like leaves. My heart went out to her, and I tried as best as I could to commiserate; but there really was very little I could do to improve her situation beyond the efforts I had made.

Our father, the only person with the power to make a difference, did even less. 'Whether your mo…mother is wrong or ri…right, she's right,' he would rumble every time she appealed to him directly. That was the only contribution he was prepared to make. .

I, however, had problems of my own, and they were arguably worse than Libby's. I could no longer face living in limbo and had been thrashing about trying to find a way to resolve my situation. Then an unexpected event occurred which provided me with the cover to act.

The priest who took our English Language classes had informed us that we could write anything on any topic we pleased for our end-of-term examination paper. Sick of the hypocrisy that surrounded one everywhere and unable to call my parents' bluffs, I decided to call his. So the topic I chose was 'Sexual Freedom'. In the essay, I stated that the law should be changed to make prostitution and homosexuality legal and that all true Christians should support such a move, for Christ himself cautioned against casting the first stone. Although I expected the essay to raise a few eyebrows, I did not anticipate the reaction it generated. Father Quinlan, the headmaster, expelled me, informing my parents of his decision in a letter enclosed with the end-of-term school report.

For some years, I had been intercepting my reports. I make no apologies for having done so, as Michael's unreasonable criticism of my academic performance made such conduct necessary. There would always be an ungodly scene when he saw my report. If my marks were particularly high, he would limit himself to verbal abuse about how I had not worked hard enough and what a lazy good-for-nothing I was. But if they were not, he would punish me. The outcome I always hoped for was the one where he shrieked that I wasn't 'going out for a year', because he couldn't maintain such a patently extreme punishment and I'd be out and about after a few days. However, if he screamed that I wouldn't be 'going anywhere for a week', you could depend upon it that I'd have to cool my heels for every one of those seven days.

Rather than have him ruin the holidays, I took to withholding the report until after the new term had begun, when my freedom of movement was curtailed in any way as a natural consequence of the resumption of school.

I had been planning to run away for some months – ever since Dr Cooke had withdrawn from my treatment, in fact – but money was a problem. I got the princely sum of two pounds a week pocket money, so saving wasn't possible. I usually got money for Christmas from certain relations, however, and once I saw that I had been expelled, it mobilized me. My parents would blame the expulsion rather than my need to obtain my correct gender as the motive for running away. That would remove the sting of implied criticism of their actions which would be an inevitable link with the gender issue. So I hoarded every penny of the money I had been given for Christmas and bought a one-way ticket to Miami. I packed shoes, brassieres, panties and dresses which I had been smuggling home from the store for months, and caught a flight to freedom and an integrated identity the day the new term began. I left the report and a letter informing my parents of my expulsion on my bed, where the servants would find it and take it to Michael or Gloria.

I was acutely aware that earning money in my new life would be difficult. I had been brought up to do nothing for myself. I could not even boil water. Nevertheless, I reasoned that if maids could do it, so could I, and set about getting a job as the one thing that needed no qualifications except love of children: a nanny. I hoped to earn enough to seek competent medical help, for up to that point I had been kept in the dark by my parents, with refrains that I was 'too young' every time I sought an explanation for what was going on. I was pathetically ignorant of the real medical issues. Not only did I have no in-depth information, but I also had absolutely none as to how much it would cost to resolve. The limbo in which I was living was therefore not only a matter of living without a gender but also without any information concerning it.

Both my parents were secretive by nature and both loved the power and freedom mystery gave them. This was an ingrained aspect of both their characters, and allowed them to function with a degree of liberty that openness would not have afforded them. If people don't know where you stand, or where they stand with you, that gives you the advantage of acting and reacting in any way you please. Since you don't need to explain how or why you have behaved in any given circumstance, you can pretty much do whatever suits you: which is precisely how my parents conducted their lives, not only with people close to and distant from them, but also with each other. The fact that they were brushing me off like a fly that didn't deserve acknowledgement or information was therefore nothing unique to me. It was simply their way of doing things, even if it had for me the inevitable effect of heightening rather than lessening the uncertainty surrounding my problems.

Once I was in Miami, I was finally free to face the world as the person I really was. However, no sooner did I check into the Hotel Leamington than I could see how utterly unprepared I was for functioning in the world at large. Although I managed to land a job as a nanny within a day, I did not deceive myself about how difficult it would be to cope with learning how to do things that most other people had been doing all their lives and expected anyone working for them to do as a matter of course.

Not for the first time I would see how double-edged a sword privilege was. My father's horror of scandal would not have been so great had we been from a lesser-known family. Privilege was still making it difficult for me to escape from the insufficiencies of my background, the gender issue being only the most glaring of them. I intended, however, to give the job my best shot, for with success would come an integrated identity as well as liberation from a background that was more a prison than anything else.

On the first day of my job, however, I realized it was only a matter of time before my complete inexperience betrayed me. When that happened, I would find myself in an even more invidious position with my parents than I would have been had I voluntarily turned myself in.

I now saw that the inadequacies of my over-privileged status prevented me from escaping from the limbo-like aspects of that same background. This was one of the most depressing and frightening consequences of running away, made worse by being wholly unexpected. There and then I understood how much harder a road I had ahead of me than children who were born with similar birth defects but without the handicap of supposed 'privilege'.

Nor did I deceive myself that many people would spare me the compassion they would have given to anyone else who had similar handicaps but a less lavish lifestyle. I had already come to discern in the last year how compassion was a commodity which few considered the privileged deserved. This came about as a result of a passing comment from a third-tier friend from a happy but not particularly rich family who, having overheard Michael lambasting Mickey down in the house, ended up saying how lucky we still were because we had so much more of all of this world's goods than practically everyone else.

Perplexed how any human being could make such a statement, I spoke to Libby's boyfriend Bruce about it. He then pointed out to me that many of our peripheral friends ignored all the personal anguish which Mickey, Libby and I had to live through, not only considering us luckier than most of our peers but also envying us our privileges.

That, it has to be said, was a lesson that life has never allowed me to forget, if only because I have over the years had so many different people in so many different countries make it clear to me that no one from a privileged background has a right to feel pain, much less to be deserving of compassion for the pain which they do feel. It is as if they think that privilege inures the human being from the ordinary feelings that all human beings possess in some degree.

Faced with the invidiousness of my predicament, I decided I had better be sensible. So I telephoned Gloria's cousin Dolly, who lived nearby, and told her I was in Miami. She said yes she knew, Gloria had telephoned to tell her, and she would come and pick me up.

Dolly's response to my telephone call surprised me. It alerted me to the fact that if my parents knew where I had run away to and how I had got there, they were already 'on to me'. Knowing how punitive they could be, I was mightily relieved that I had not tried to brazen it out, and that I had left the school report on my bed. Bad as things would be for me when I got back home, they would have been immeasurably worse if Michael and Gloria knew my real reason for running away.

It's just as well I behaved as I had. Within an hour of Dolly picking me up and taking me to her house, Marjorie, Mickey and Suzy Surridge, who had flown up from Jamaica in pursuit of me, walked in through the front door. Seeing me safe and sound, they immediately lost all anxiety and started to tell me excitedly what had been happening at home in the two days since my departure. They recounted how Michael had telephoned the American ambassador, who had agreed to get the FBI to search for me if I did not show up soon. As they were retelling these events, I was glad to see that they were doing so with levity.

'I don't think you'd have liked your picture plastered all over the place on "wanted" posters,' Auntie scolded with a glint in her eye and a smile on her lips.

'Or being on the Ten Most Wanted List,' Mickey riposted.

The vision these comments induced caused Dolly, her husband Walston,

Auntie, Mickey and Suzy to start to laugh so hard, Marjorie ended up with tears in her eyes. Although I joined in the laughter, the very visions which they found so funny actually chilled my blood when I saw how close I had come to causing an international incident.

'I think you won't even be punished,' Marjorie added, making it clear that I had most likely escaped all disagreeable consequences. 'Your mother hasn't been at all perturbed by what you did, though your poor father has been beside himself with worry. You know how his stomach acts up when he becomes nervous. He took to his bed, sick as a dog, throwing up constantly. Dr Sleem had to come to the house and give him something to settle him down.'

It was the first time in my life my father had ever displayed any positive concern for me, and I cannot deny being secretly delighted at the discovery that maybe, just maybe, intermingled with all of that loathing and embarrassment might just be the tiniest bit of love. That was an even better payoff than the discovery that Auntie was going to treat my escapade as an enormous jape which had the unexpected benefit of giving the four of us an all-expenses-paid holiday in Miami. We moved into the MacAllister Hotel, hit the shops and tourist sights, and I hugged the knowledge to my skinny bosom that maybe my father didn't hate me totally. It had not yet dawned on me that maybe Gloria's essential indifference was something with which to concern myself, possibly because she had always been careful to dress it up in pleasantries which had me as deceived as everyone else.

After four glorious days in Miami, Marjorie, Mickey, Suzy and I headed back to Jamaica. It had been such fun. 'Next time you run away, can you go to New York?' Suzy ended up saying to laughter all around. 'I've never been there.'

When I returned home, it was to a chastened Michael. He had been so worried that he was just glad to have me back home, so did not punish me. However, Father Quinlan did, thinking that by reversing the expulsion he was doing me a favour. While I appreciated his gesture and compassion, I did not like being at the school any more than I had before running away. I saw that there would nevertheless be no escape from it unless I could get into an American university on the strength of my 'O' Levels. With that in mind, I set about making applications to various American institutions.

My escapade also heightened Michael's latent paternal instincts with regard to Mickey. He begged and begged and begged him to return home until he did so – but on certain conditions. These included not being required to apologize to Gloria and being given the unrestricted use of Michael's car when he wanted to go out. If he and Michael both chose to go out at the same time, our father would have to use Gloria's car, otherwise Mickey, who had been having unrestricted use of Maisie's and Perez's cars, would be placing himself at a disadvantage. We all knew what Gloria was capable of. Had Mickey not protected himself with that agreement, every time Michael went out, she would keep her car in the garage and Mickey a prisoner at home rather than lend it to him. Because Mickey knew that our father was an honourable man who would keep to his word once he had given it, he returned home.

One consequence of that agreement was that Gloria tried to use it to her advantage, suggesting to Michael, after he had lent his car to Mickey, that they go somewhere together rather than he go out on his own. Then, when the time came for them to depart, she would change her mind and in so doing, have caused him to stay at home, because by then it would be too late for him to join whatever poker or domino games he had been planning to attend. Michael was very slow on the uptake where his wife's machinations were concerned, but after she'd pulled that stunt a few times, even he began to see through her. Things came to a head one night after he'd turned down an invitation to poker at Albert and Madge Seaga's house to accompany her on a visit to Victor Grant's house. Then, when she declared that she couldn't be bothered to go, he shrieked at her: 'I will not have you turn me into a goddamned prisoner in my own house. You can't keep me dangling at your whim. Georgie, come and sit with your mother. I'm going to poker.'

'You'll simply make a fool of yourself, turning up to a game when they already have a full complement of players,' Gloria observed acidly.

'Then I'll sit and watch,' he bellowed, no hint of a stammer confirming his fury. He stormed out of the house, slamming the back door with such force that the wood would have split had it not been so thick.

Meanwhile Mickey and Gloria were still barely speaking. Neither one would budge: she from demanding an apology, he from refusing to give it. Gradually, however, as they coexisted on a daily basis, the barriers fell away and they began talking directly to each other. Things appeared to be back to normal, except that what was now normal in our house was anything but.

At this juncture, we – meaning Mickey, Suzy and I – had become friendly with an American seminarian called Andy Charbonneau, who used to teach me at St George's, the Jesuit Seminary I attended as a day student. Being a believing Roman Catholic, my father was pleased. Little did any of us envisage how such an innocent friendship would end in the distressing consequences that now ensued. One evening we asked Andy to go to a midnight movie with us at the State Theatre. Midnight movies actually began at eleven o'clock, which nevertheless made us perilously close to the edge where our curfew was concerned. Mickey, however, was sure we wouldn't have a problem driving Andy back downtown to the seminary before heading up to the foothills of the Blue Mountains, where we lived. So he didn't tell Daddy what sort of movie we were going to see. For no particular reason I decided to cry off, so wasn't a part of the drama that unfolded.

The first hint of trouble was when Mickey was dropping Andy back at St George's after the cinema. The back tyre developed a puncture. Opening the boot to take out the spare, Mickey discovered that this was flat too. He left the car there and got a lift home. The following morning, Daddy arose to see his car missing. Mickey and I were sitting on his bed talking about what had happened the evening before when Michael came into Mickey's bedroom to ask him where the car was. Mickey started to explain when Gloria, overhearing what was being said, loomed into view. 'The child is making a damned fool of you yet again,' she said, stoking the embers in the hope of causing a conflagration.

Michael, seldom in effective control of his temper, ordered Mickey to continue in a tone of voice that betrayed a loosening grip. 'But why were you at S…St. George's?'

'Andy came with us,' he said.

'You don't expect your father to believe that nonsense,' Gloria said. 'He's not a fool, you know. Even he knows that priests and seminarians can't go out on the town at night. What were you doing there? Whore-mongering?'

Only in Gloria's scheme of things would anyone take a whore to the grounds of a seminary, but it did give a clue to her way of thinking. Bluff and double-bluff were so much a part of her way of doing things that, had she been a man seeking to screw a prostitute in safety, she would have taken her to a seminary in the confidence that neither the police – who patrolled the lover's lanes and New Kingston for 'action' – nor the priests – who were safely tucked up in bed with thoughts of God and Hellfire but not visiting prostitutes – would think to look there. Undeniably, she was clever, but not so clever as to realize that few other people functioned in her world of elaborate ruse and counter-ruse, and certainly not her son. Had she cared to employ a little more reason and a little less suspicion, she would also have seen that such fantastical reasoning was beyond the character and possibly the intellect of the young man she had labelled 'the Fool'. But then, while Gloria was consistently abusive, she was not consistently reasonable. Indeed, reason usually had very little to do with her behaviour or motives.

Mickey looked astonished when Gloria accused him of whore-mongering. He was a devout Anglican who went to church every chance he had and lived by Christian precepts. He purposely did not look at her but at Michael instead, to whom he addressed his reply. 'I told you what happened,' he said solemnly and calmly, clearly offended by the suggestion.

'Are you going to stand there and let that little whippersnapper make a complete ass of you?' Gloria said to her husband before turning to her son and saying: 'If you don't start spilling the beans this instant, I'm going to box the truth out of you.'

'Don't you dare touch me,' Mickey said. 'I've done nothing and I will not have you strike me.'

'You are stinkingly impertinent. I gave you life, and I can do any damned thing I please with you. Remember that, and your life will be a lot easier,' she said, trotting out a few of her favourite phrases as she fired a slap across his face.

'How dare you?' Mickey said, raising his voice for one of the few times in his life.

'Don't shout at your mother like that,' Michael said.

'I didn't come back home for this,' Mickey said and started to walk out of the bedroom. We all knew where he was going: back down to Grandma's, even if he had to do so on foot.

'Your father and I are not through with you yet,' Gloria said in her most imperious tone.

Mickey ignored her.

'You'd better stop him if you know what's good for you,' she said to Michael.

'Mickey, stop now,' he said. 'You heard your mother.' No hint of a stammer, which meant that anger had loosened his tongue.

Mickey continued walking.

Michael, rooted to the spot, glowered as Mickey passed through the doorway.

Gloria sprang into action and shot after Mickey, grabbing his shirt by the scruff of the neck. He tried to shake himself free, but she was hanging on for dear life.

'Are you going to let your son break my wrist?' she said, appealing to Michael's protective instincts.

I knew what she really feared was a broken fingernail, for those were the days before repair kits when long manicured fingernails were the mark of a lady, and she took pride in hers. Indeed, whenever she hitched or, God forbid, broke a nail, the way she carried on, you would have thought a new drought was wiping out a whole continent.

'You're hurting your mother,' Michael said, stepping towards Mickey.

'I don't see how I can be hurting her when she's the one who has got hold of my shirt and is strangling me,' Mickey observed, putting his hand between his shirt and his neck in an effort to loosen her stranglehold.

'Michael, Mickey's hurting me. Stop him,' Gloria said in as pathetic and whimpering a tone as she could come up with.

She's clearly intent on getting Daddy's sympathy, I thought.

'You're hurting your mother,' he repeated, stepping in closer to mother and son.

'Let go of me. I can barely breathe,' Mickey said. I was amazed by how calm he was. He had barely raised his voice.

'Michael, please make him stop,' Gloria said in her most pathetic, innocent, please-help-and-protect-me voice. 'Please make him stop.'

My stomach churned. I could tell that she was as sincere as an actress on a stage. No wonder people were always saying she should have been an actress. At that juncture, however, I concurred with Annabel Surridge, who once said: 'Your mother isn't dramatic. She's much more than that. She's operatic.'

That was the point at which all hell broke loose.

'I told you to stop,' Michael screamed, seemingly unconscious of the fact that someone cannot stop something he has never started doing. He tore into Mickey, dragging him away from Gloria, whose eyes shone with gratification and excitement as he started flailing at him with blow after blow. Mickey did not fight back but tried to protect himself.

'Stop. You're hurting me,' he said over and over again.

Michael, however, was beyond the voice of reason. Now totally out of control, he soon had Mickey down on the bed. He then jumped on top of it, breaking the mahogany frame in the process. Rather that continue to witness what was happening, I decided it was time to flee, so I ran out of the room. Nevertheless, I stood outside in the passage in case Mickey called out for me to help him, though what I could have done escaped me then and escapes me now. If Mickey and Daddy were unevenly matched, the former being five foot eight and about one hundred and forty pounds, the latter being a six footer who carried an additional fifty or so pounds of weight, I was five foot six and weighed a mere ninety-six pounds, so Daddy could have flicked me across the room with his fingers.

Weight, however, was not the decisive factor, as Gloria soon proved. Within minutes she used her voice and the power she had over her husband to bring this latest episode to an end. Calmly at first and thereafter in an ever more urgent tone, she said to her husband, 'Are you going to kill yourself? I don't mind if you kill that pathetic little shit, but I do mind you killing yourself. Stop before you get a heart attack or a stroke. Do you hear me? Stop right now. Stop, I say. Michael, come to your senses, for God's sake. Michael, listen to me. Stop now. God damn you, you blasted lunatic, stop when I tell you to. You'll kill the little shit if you don't stop, so stop right now.'

Afterwards, Michael was full of apologies, but Mickey had had enough.

'Mummy is an evil stinker,' he said. 'And Daddy a wild beast. I will never live with them again. They are nothing but monsters: she a calculating and malicious bitch, he a semi-lunatic who isn't in possession of his faculties half the time. Sometimes I don't know which one is worse.'

He moved down to Maisie's house yet again, though this time with the declaration that no amount of begging from Daddy could induce him ever again to live under his parents' roof.

Within months, he had left for England, to read law at the Bar. He sat his dinners at Gray's Inn and took rooms in the house of Miss Birtwhistle, the venerable old lady who had taught Queen Elizabeth the Queen Mother when she was a little girl. His childhood, together with the torment and vulnerability that his cruel mother and out-of-control father had inflicted, was over. But that merely left a breach which Libby, and later on I, would fill.

Chapter Eleven

Some months before Mickey left to pursue his studies in England in September 1966, I had been accepted by the Fashion Institute of Technology. Because of the credits system in the United States and FIT being a college of the State University of New York, those who wanted to major in apparel design had not only to take all their artistic courses but also a full Liberal Arts load in order to graduate. I had always been of academic bent and loved nothing better than to curl up reading about history or world affairs, so I was as delighted as my father when we discovered the full extent of the academic courses I would have to take. I wanted to become a dress designer, a choice of career which both my parents accepted and approved of, but I also planned to continue feeding my mind, for the one thing over which I was in accord with my father was the pleasure learning brought. He too was a voracious reader, as indeed were several others members of his family, including Libby and his niece Audrey.

What my father would not accept, however, was my leaving home before the age of eighteen, so even though I could have gone to New York that September of 1966, I had to remain at home because I had only just turned seventeen. 'You're too young to fend for yourself in a strange city,' he decreed. When I pointed out that I would be under the watchful eye of Frances Bacal, the greater consideration came out. 'You can't leave your mother alone with no one for company, and we can't interrupt Libby's education to bring her home until next year, after she has sat her 'O' Levels.'

I was not best pleased, I can tell you, to have to stay in Jamaica, especially as Michael insisted that I still had to attend St George's, a school that I loathed because of the anomalies my genderless identity caused. My true status was an open secret among my friends, but this did not extend to school, where the student body was a more mixed and unsophisticated bag. I consequently came in for a fair amount of daily ribbing, to put it mildly, and I set about bringing that to an end by skipping school as much as I could. No sooner would Daddy drop me off outside the school gates in the morning than I would turn tail, hop on the bus and seek refuge at a friend's house – usually Patsy Taylor's. Her mother was one of the few mothers in our set who worked; and her father, who was even stricter than Michael, approved of me, partly on the grounds that he and Gloria had been friends while growing up. So I could hole up at the Taylors' house for hours on end in the knowledge that, if I were discovered, Patsy and I could come up with some tale that would explain away my presence without raising too many red flags with her parents and mine. Fortunately though, we were never caught.

Home life that year settled down into something approximating peacefulness. Gloria seemed more content than in a long time. She and Michael argued less frequently, and even though she did not resume going to the races, she did occasionally relent and play poker, as long as it was with people she regarded as fun. She also had Michael attending what he viewed as a bewildering number of nightclubs. She loved dancing, and both she and he were excellent dancers, so practically every week she would make sure that a large group of friends went out to the most fashionable nightclub for dinner and dancing. Otherwise, she would organize evenings out with friends at fashionable restaurants, and, whenever there was a party, she made sure he went whether he felt like it or not.

'You may be an old man, but I am young and want to enjoy myself,' she would say.

His response was always the same: 'I'm a bore and proud of it.'

'That's fine, as long as you bore yourself in public and not me in private,' she would respond, making it clear that she would brook no opposition from him.

With my siblings away and my friends banned from the house during term time, I would have been awfully lonely but for two factors. The first was that I was seeing some, if not all, of my friends during the day while I was supposed to be at school, and the second was that I still had Suzy, my best friend and neighbour, who lived opposite us. Every afternoon I would go to her house, or she would come to mine, and we would shoot the breeze until we heard Michael's car horn. It wasn't only the servants, I can assure you, who ran like the seven devils out of hell when they heard it blare. I did too, flying across the road and rushing to the pool house, where I would sit, my nose buried in a schoolbook, pretending to be studying, on the off-chance that Daddy came up to see what I was doing. Although he never greeted me socially, not even in company, he was assiduous in checking whether I was doing my schoolwork. This was in marked contrast to Gloria, who never once, throughout the scholastic lives of any of her four children, ever checked up on us or indeed enquired whether we were doing any work at all. She had absolutely no interest in our scholastic activities, which with hindsight was negligence of the highest order but was, at the time, a welcome counterbalance to her exacting husband. He frequently came up to the pool, looked to see that I was doing my homework, grunted when he saw the schoolbook I was holding up, turned tail without speaking to me and returned into the house. Sometimes, when he was in a bad mood, he would berate me, informing me – and the neighbours, for his voice carried like no one else's – what a disappointment I was. 'God gave you such a brilliant mind. You've done nothing with it, and all the signs are that you never will. You will amount to nothing. Nothing. You will always be a big zero. What am I going to do with you?'

I bitterly resented these uninvited attacks, but they were nothing compared with the ones he started to mount on me once I resumed my agitation for a resolution to the genderless existence I was still enduring.

If he came home in a bad mood and Gloria was out, he would start in on me, the absence of a stutter telling me all I needed to know. 'You are a nothing. A nothing. You will always be a nothing. Do you seriously think any man will ever want you? What man would want a freak like you? Men want a woman they can be proud of, not one they'll have to explain away. Give up your ridiculous quest.' Other times, he would say, 'I will not let you besmirch my good name with scandal. You will never, never – you hear me, never – wear a dress as long as I draw breath. I am not going to have you ruin my good name.'

He was not above threatening me with committal either. 'I can have you locked up and the key thrown away,' he would sometimes warn. 'Don't delude yourself into thinking I won't do it. Push me far enough, and you'll be pushing yourself right into confinement.' By far the most extreme mantra, however, was when he recommended that I solve my problem by taking 'a dose of rat poison'. I could tell that he meant it too. He would have preferred to see me dead rather than having to endure the scandal that rectifying my situation might bring in its wake.

Another tactic which Michael used to loosen my grip on the desire for my correct gender was threatening to prevent Mickey, Libby and Kitty from seeing me 'if you bring scandal down on our heads'.

'Think about how you will ruin their lives,' he would counsel. 'No one will want to marry them when the whole world knows they're related to an acknowledged freak.'

Not knowing what Michael really would and would not do when the time came that I was openly declared to be a girl, I had to face the prospect of living without the brother and sisters whom I loved. Not even that, however, could override my need for an integrated identity.

It now occurred to me that there would inevitably come a time when we children would all be grown up enough to be beyond his control. I therefore made that point to him, after which I heard no more about my siblings being banned from seeing me when the time came for this limbo-like farce to be brought to an end.

None of that was anything as demeaning, however, as the ploy Michael came up with when he saw that his invective wasn't wearing me down. If I was near my bedroom, or in it, he would start by dragging me fully clothed in front of the full-length mirror. 'Don't think I can't see right through you. I can tell that nothing I say will ever move you. You are determined to ruin my life and everyone else's in the family.' Then he would order me to remove my clothes, and, when I refused to, he would tear them off.

'Look at yourself,' he would say. 'Look at yourself. You are a freak. A big nothing. Nothing. Nothing but a freak. No man will ever want you. God knows what I've done to be cursed with a child like you.'

The first time he did this, I felt so defiled that words alone cannot convey the full extent of the violation. Repetition, however, brought liberation of a sort; and by the fourth or fifth time, although still feeling defiled and violated, I was also sufficiently outraged to fight back when he started hurling his invective at me.

'I may be a freak, but at least I'm not a bully or a coward,' I screamed right back at him, functioning on the principle that however loudly he had shouted,

I would top him by shouting louder and that in itself would be a victory of sorts. 'And, lest you forget it, God in His wisdom created me a freak. I don't recall Him creating you a bully or a coward, simply a baby. So leave me alone and take your complaints to God. But while doing so, reflect upon the fact that my freakiness hasn't debased me as a person, while your bullying and cowardice have debased you. Take that and chew on it. And while you're doing so, reflect upon the fact that you're quite right in saying that nothing you do say or do moves me. And, do you know why? Because, unlike you, I'm not a gutless wonder. I have character and self-respect, and any insult from you is like a compliment from anyone else. So, go on, give this your best shot, but do so in the certain knowledge that it will never be good enough to reach me, you despicable bully.'

After that tirade, Michael never dragged me into the bedroom to humiliate me like that again. Whether it was because I had humiliated him more than he had humiliated me, or because I had reached that part of his soul where fair play and decency or maybe even just self-recognition resided, I do not know. Either way, he limited himself to verbal abuse instead of physical degradation thereafter.

Frankly, I was glad when Libby and Mickey came back home for the summer holidays, not only because I was happy to have their companionship but also because misery loves company and I had discovered that, with them away, Michael was as monstrous towards me as Gloria had been towards them. I was relieved to spread the misery between the three of us rather than having to carry the whole load on my back alone.

That summer, however, so much else was going on that neither of our parents was bored enough to need to amuse him or herself with tormenting any one of us exclusively. Firstly, there was the issue of my gender, about which I was now in open rebellion, demanding that I be taken to the Johns Hopkins Gender Identification Clinic at John Hopkins Hospital in Baltimore, where I knew time would be called on the diabolic delays that had characterized my father's way of dealing with the problem. My demands had an urgency born of desperation. I was due to start a new life as an apparel design major in New York that September, and I did not want it being destroyed by a limbo-like identity the way my teenage years in Jamaica had been. For the first time, I therefore started to be overtly assertive to my parents about my right to have my sex. Although Gloria never ignored me and always responded with a show of understanding, Michael either ignored me or then opposed me, so I became more and more vociferous until I was in open opposition to him.

While formerly I had masked my loathing and contempt for my father except on the few occasions when he privately pushed me into revealing how I felt, I now made no bones about my attitude. I had always been articulate, an advantage he did not have, and I started using that facility to run rings around him. This was the age of the Sexual Revolution, and I delighted in making him look like an old-fashioned stuffed shirt. If he objected to Libby's attire or make-up, I would pass some withering comment along the lines of 'This is Jamaica 1967. Get out of the Middle Ages and the Middle East' in the expectation that I would be pressing his buttons. Over the years, I had heard Gloria disparage his nationality so much that I figured he must be vulnerable there – otherwise she wouldn't belabour the point the way she did.

Seeing no merit in keeping the fight in the hinterlands when I could take it to the heartlands, I also now threw down a general challenge to his authority every chance I had. Michael had always lain down the law about morality and principle, fulminating about how 'the world has gone to the dogs. No one has morals or manners or respect for authority anymore.' The fact that his complaint was one shared by many of his generation all over the Western world, as the sexual and class revolutions took hold, and Baby Boomers like me threw over the traces of the old order in favour of love, peace and liberty, gave my actions a spurious sort of validation, with me linking myself to the progressive movement within society generally, thereby casting my father onto the scrapheap of reaction. 'Why should youth respect age if age has no sense and is out of step with a better way of doing things?' I would ask, launching into a reasoned and articulate attack that undermined even further the authority he was trying to shore up. Sometimes the intellectual in him got the better of the bully, and he would say, 'You ought to become a barrister, you know.' Other times, however, he would storm off into his bedroom, humiliated and feeling even more ineffectual than before he had opened up his mouth.

Where I led, my two siblings followed. Mickey, who was visiting for the summer from England, had always been politically liberal, which was anathema to his extremely right-wing parents. But he had hitherto been careful to keep the full extent of this liberalism to himself, even though the hints he used to give always earned him rebukes for being a 'communist'. Now, every time

Michael opened his mouth about politics – something of a nightly exercise when there was company present – Mickey would assail him with an alternative point of view.

Michael invariably retorted with a heartfelt 'The *Manchester Guardian*,' spat out so pejoratively that all listeners had no doubt that he regarded the newspaper his son read as an insult as well as an epithet.

Mickey would invariably persist in developing his theme with all the confidence and balance of the barrister he was studying to become. This of course only resulted in Michael accusing him of being a communist. At this point, Gloria would hop into the fray, pointing out 'you can see the use your hard-earned money is being put to.' As the summer wore on, however, and Gloria did not plot and scheme against her son the way she used to do before he went to school in England, and Michael's accusations of communism never escalated into rage, I began to see that both Michael and Gloria were changing their attitudes towards Mickey.

This was bad news for Libby. Whether anyone else was aware of it or not, she was being prepared for the role as the new number one victim, and she was only too aware of her painfully primary status. But Libby's way of coping was not like Mickey's. Where he had stood his ground, she tried to sidestep all arguments with both parents by avoiding being in their company as much as possible. If we were going out, however, she would have no choice but to pass them as we were leaving the house. Gloria always jumped on her at that point and turned Libby's clothes and make-up into the battleground, doubtless because she hated seeing a younger, equally glamorous version of herself who was garnering praise and attention she regarded as exclusively hers.

Gloria was actually playing a clever game, undercutting Libby at the same time that she was playing upon Michael's Near Eastern sexual attitudes. She only needed to raise her eyebrow, harrumph disapprovingly, ensure that a gentle 'uh' escaped from her lips or mock Libby by passing a catty comment about her clothes, hair or make-up, to convince the prudish Michael that any teenage girl who dressed so captivatingly must be up to no good. This usually had the desired effect of setting off an eruption of the volcano known as Michael Ziadie. As he fulminated about Libby's motives for looking like a 'trollop' (which she most decidedly did not), I knew what lay in store for her unless I nipped things in the bud. He would whip himself into such a frenzy that she would be sent back into her bedroom to change or to stay there in punishment, sometimes for days on end. So I would wait until Michael paused for breath before leaping in.

'Don't be so ridiculous,' I would sneer. 'This is not Lebanon under the Ottoman Sultan. What she has on is the height of fashion. You ought to know that, considering you're a merchant. That's how everyone dresses nowadays.'

'I don't care what everyone does. I only care about what my children do,' Michael, always predictable, would reply whenever I started on about what everyone else did.

His very predictability made it easy for me, because I would then silence him with the same rational argument every time. 'So we're supposed to function in splendid isolation,' I would conclude, 'inside some bubble that bears no relation to the outside world or the values and mores of civilization. How are we supposed to function in or adjust to the world at large, if you so despise modes of behaviour which everyone except dyed-in-the-wool prudes like you find acceptable?'

Gloria, sitting in wait for the right moment to press Michael's buttons and get Libby into more trouble than she was already in, started to leap in with comments suggestive of the possibility that Libby was dressing like that to 'advertise her wares'. She knew as well as us that the one thing that was guaranteed to send Michael – and indeed all fathers of his generation and background – into an apoplectic frenzy was the prospect of his wife or daughters being 'untidy' sexually.

Always taking care never to interfere with or interrupt or contradict Gloria, I now used my newly-found brass to take the fight right to the heart of the matter as soon as Michael started to accuse Libby of dubious conduct. 'Libby is not sleeping with anyone, nor does she want to, but so what if she did?' I would challenge, asserting her innocence at the same time that I was forcing him to defend his moral posturing.

The first time I posed the question, Michael practically frothed at the mouth. Immediately, his decibel level rose to its loudest; and he boomed with such force that Gloria had to interject and ask him if he wanted the neighbours to hear every word he was saying. 'You are disgusting,' he boomed at me, ignoring her. 'You are condoning immorality. Repeat what you said if you dare, and I will box you so hard your head will swivel 180 degrees.'

Having introduced the unthinkable, I now waited until the next time before elucidating upon my argument.'There's nothing wrong with sex before marriage,' I pointed out when the subject next arose.'All that stuff about walking up the aisle a virgin is simply old-fashioned rubbish, totally irrelevant nowadays.'

'You are not only a freak, but morally corrupt,' Michael spat out, storming into the house and seeking refuge in his bedroom, where he slammed the door with such force that it was a wonder the hinges didn't spring out of the wood.

As the summer wore on, Gloria, I noticed, was the odd one out.While she was an active contributor to the political discussions, taking pot shots at 'the communist' whenever he aired his liberal views or cattily referring to Libby as 'the Jezebel' and pointing out how she was 'painted like a harlot', once the subject of sex outside of marriage was under discussion, she limited her comments to reminding everyone that she had gone up the aisle a virgin and had only ever known one man. It struck me as odd that someone, who was always so expansive on just about every other topic, would be so quiet on this one. I cannot, to this day, figure out whether it was because she did not want to attack me or whether the real reason was that her beliefs dovetailed too closely with mine and she didn't want Michael to know this, as that knowledge would undermine her position as the 'pure' wife which, by this time, we children all suspected she was not.

In the middle of the tumult, Gloria's brother-in-law Ric, who had never really recovered from Lucius's murder in his house, died of a heart attack aged forty-two in front of our Aunt Marjorie. We children all loved Auntie passionately, far more so than our own mother, and Uncle Ric had always been such a loving part of our lives that we felt the loss not only for her but also for ourselves. Gloria had always got along well with her brother-in-law, and we fully expected her to be really distressed. Maisie, who loved her son-in-law, certainly was: taking to her bed for over a week, as was her wont whenever anything terrible happened. Gloria's reaction was so muted, however, that it was apparent that, despite her professed fondness for Ric, her true feelings did not cut deeply.Where she was concerned, his death seemed to be more a case of casual regret than real loss; and her complete absence of positive grief was one of the pointers I would employ, as I navigated around the shoals of her personality, to conclude that she really had few, if any, profound feelings for others.

Indeed, Gloria's opportunism came to the fore when she used Uncle Ric's death as the excuse for ducking out of taking me to Baltimore so that I could be openly declared a girl. 'Your aunt needs me,' she said, informing me that I would have to wait for a more convenient time to receive the medical treatment I needed.

Rather than challenge her, which would have done my cause no good, I got into Michael's car and drove up to York Castle. 'Auntie, Mummy says she can't take me to Johns Hopkins because you need her here with you,' I said.

Auntie, always loving towards us, shot me a look. 'How many times has she come up here since Ric died?' she asked. 'Two, maybe three, counting the day of his death and the funeral. Your mother really is too much. Just get right back in that car and tell her I say she's to get her backside onto that plane and get you your sex.'

Armed with Auntie's riposte, I did exactly as she suggested. I went straight back down to our house, confronted my mother charmingly and respectfully but determinedly, my diplomatic skills excising the word 'backside' in the retelling, and thereby threw the bundle right back in her lap. Cool as an Alpine stream in March, Gloria then informed me that I was nevertheless not going to Baltimore, that the reasons were medical and that she had tried to spare my feelings by pretending otherwise. When I enquired what they were, she said she was not at liberty to tell me, and I knew she was lying, hoping to con me into thinking that there was some profound reason beyond my comprehension that she could not impart. Does she really think I'm that stupid? I had to ask myself, or does she think that I am obliged to believe any lie she tells just because she is the one who has told it? I would dearly have loved to be in a position to call her bluff directly, but since I wasn't, I did the next best thing. I did it indirectly, taking an overdose of Valium, but only after I made sure I informed Mickey and our good friend Michael Silvera first, so there was no chance of me dying. I did not intend to leave this earth before I had first had a fair shot at living as myself.

My cry for help captured my self-absorbed parents' attention for all of a day or two. Although Gloria seemed slightly chastened by my actions, I would hardly say that Michael was. His initial response was to delay calling the doctor, thereby giving the pills time enough to take effect and kill me. 'Are you mad?' Gloria said and rang Dr Sleem, our family GP after Tony Feanny was replaced following his marriage. Dr Sleem was another scion of another 'good family', for my parents would have no more had someone outside of their circle attending to us than have a servant sit at the dinner table with them. He arrived and recommended calling an ambulance to take me up to the University College Hospital, so that my stomach could be pumped. My parents vetoed that suggestion, because they wanted to hush up what had happened and there would be no way of doing so if I were hospitalized. So Dr. Sleem somehow got me to regurgitate the contents of my stomach, and he and Gloria spent the rest of the night pouring coffee down my throat, walking me up and down the drawing room, until he judged it safe for all of us to go to bed.

Within a day or two I was fully recovered, but my actions had had the desired effect. Dr Sleem pointed out to my parents that in cases like mine suicide was a real prospect unless the patient was given meaningful treatment. What he meant was that my treatment should proceed in accordance with the recommendations of Dr Cooke and Jimmy Burrowes, namely that I be openly declared to be of the female gender. Michael still had a few more rolls of the dice, however, doubtless in the hope that I would kill myself before I sullied his precious name, preferably in such a way that he could blame it on something else.

I believe that Gloria was fully aware of what was happening and was indeed assisting him by preparing the ground in case I did commit suicide, so that they could be able to pass it off as something unrelated to my birth defect. 'Genius is very close to insanity' was a comment she started uttering with chilling repetitiveness – invariably with a little chuckle – almost always shortly but seldom immediately after asserting that 'Georgie is a genius.' This was to give people the chance to make the link for themselves between my supposed genius and the attendant mental instability which they would then blame when I killed myself, thereby ridding them of a scandal while providing their vanity with the kudos of having been the parents of a genius, albeit an ill-fated one.

I was not then aware how much covert assistance Gloria was providing for Michael or how involved she was in batting for his team. I did receive the odd indication, such as when she fobbed me off then lied about taking me to Baltimore, but by and large she led me to believe that she was on my side. 'We have to wear down your father gradually,' she used to say to me.

With hindsight, I can now see that Gloria never had any intention of helping me, nor of jeopardizing her relationship with Michael by sticking up for me when he was so terrified of scandal. Her real reason for behaving as she did towards me was to maintain my goodwill and the companionship which she assumed flowed from it. I was still her number one companion within the family, and as such, her actual number-one companion in life, because she let few people see behind her socially captivating mask or – in the case of my father – her aggressively feminine role-playing. Had she known that my companionability was motivated more by fear and expediency than by love, she would have been surprised.

If I was deceiving her, she was also deceiving me. She would always mouth gentle but ultimately meaningless platitudes when the subject of my gender came up. 'God never gives us more than we can bear,' she would say. 'The Lord tries those He loves.' She would then tell me how I must have courage as 'nothing lasts forever' and 'everything comes to an end, not only problems but also life'. This meaningless show of sympathy convinced me that she was on my side in the 'War of Georgie's Gender', when the sad fact is she was on her own side, keeping in with both Lenin and the Romanovs so that both sides would think how loyal and wonderful she was.

It would take me decades before I would unravel the Junoesque game she was playing. The proof that she was more heavily involved than I realized was always right under my nose, however, for she was the conduit between Michael and me. It was she who told me, in the summer of 1967, that, rather than going to the Johns Hopkins Gender Identification Clinic in Baltimore, Michael had decided that my mental state following my overdose would be assessed by a psychiatrist at the Columbia-Presbyterian Hospital in New York. This should have alerted me to the fact that she was a lot more involved in the decision-making process than she led me to believe, but at seventeen one does miss many a trick, especially if one is not suspicious by nature.

'Why do I need to see a psychiatrist when Dr Cooke himself said that I don't have a psychiatric problem and that psychiatry cannot provide a solution for what I'm suffering from?' I asked her, knowing that my father was jerking me around yet again but unaware of her covert complicity with him.

'It's because you took an overdose. The doctors need to see that there's nothing wrong with you before they can deal with the "other matter",' she said. The 'other matter', needless to say, was the euphemism she used to address my birth defect.

'But the only reason why I did so was because it was the only way to get medical treatment. I can't believe that doctors are so stupid as to think that a human being can live without a sex forever or that I am the only human being on earth who has no feelings. How would they like to live without their sex for even an hour, much less a day or a week or a year? I've been having to do so for seventeen years. It's unreasonable and unconscionable.'

'They need to satisfy themselves that your overdose isn't indicative of an underlying psychological problem.'

'For four years I've been battered from pillar to post medically, and not one doctor has been able to come up with anything psychologically wrong with me. Don't think I don't know that Daddy's had them searching in the hope that he can then rule me out of having my sex. It seems to me someone is hoping that if I'm deprived of my sex long enough, I will develop mental problems, which will then be used as the excuse to prevent me from having in adulthood the one thing everyone else has had since birth. The total lack of logic of it all, not to mention the rank injustice, is an insult to my intelligence, and should be to yours as well,' I said.

Gloria, as ever, nodded sympathetically. Looking back on it, she really was a superb actress, for she never overplayed her hand. She would do the minimum and let your imagination and expectations do the rest.

However, I must have been more aware unconsciously of what was really going on; though still believing that she was on my side, I did not take Gloria's word. Indeed, I could smell a rat, so unbeknownst to my parents, I took the precaution of driving up to Dr Sleem's house and asking him if he thought that I needed psychiatric treatment. He was surprisingly candid, stating that he was rather horrified by the inhumane way in which I had been treated. 'I've told your parents that my concern is that any further delay in getting you the treatment you need will damage you psychologically. I've made it plain to them that there is nothing wrong with you that sorting out your gender won't solve. I am definitely not in favour of any further delays and will be including my observations in the medical notes I send to New York,' he said.

Thanking him for talking to me, I asked him if he would refrain from informing my parents that I had been to see him. His response was such that I could tell that he didn't want them knowing about my visit any more than I did.

In New York, Gloria and I would have a second conversation about the pain the delay was causing me. This was after my first visit to the psychiatrist in New York that September of 1967. It was on this occasion that she came out with her 'confession' of how she had hated Mickey from before his birth because Michael had had a 'woman' while she was pregnant with him, but that she had loved me from the first time she saw me.

'If you really love me,' I then said, 'you'll help me. I cannot continue living like this. If I can't have my sex, I will kill myself. I mean it.'

I did mean it. And I knew that she knew that I meant it.

'You won't need to do that,' Gloria said in her most sympathetic tones. 'I promise you, after the doctor has confirmed that you have no psychological problems, I'll see that you get your sex.'

Like the gullible fool that I was, I believed her. It did not occur to me that the mother who claimed to love me – and who I believed did love me despite the hateful aspects to her character – would actually be shallow and vain enough to want to gain brownie points by reassuring me about a life-and-death matter without ever having the slightest intention of carrying through on her promise. Yet that, I would learn only too soon, was the case.

Chapter Twelve

With me out of the way in New York, Libby was brought in from the Servite Convent to be the child at home. She was enrolled to sit her 'A' Levels at The Priory School: the most fashionable day school in the country run by Henry and Greta Fowler, patricians who had a touch of Hollywood glamour about them, Greta's daughter Jennifer being married to the movie star Robert Shaw. Situated about three miles from our house and a few hundred yards from King's House, the official residence of the governor-general, and Jamaica House, the official residence of the prime minister, Libby now got a taste of what it was like to be an urban schoolchild in our family.

Jamaica was becoming increasingly violent. It was generally agreed that it was unsafe for a Have to walk the streets. White Haves were deemed to be even more vulnerable than coloured or black 'Haves', who were not identified by the colour of their skin but by their clothes and demeanour. Female Haves were obviously more at risk than male Haves, but even the latter were reluctant to take their lives in their hands and walk more than a few yards, every other journey being negotiated by car.

Despite the dangers and despite the fact that these very problems had been used by Michael to curtail our freedom when his children wanted to go out socially, neither he nor Gloria saw anything hypocritical about, or contradictory in, letting us fend for ourselves on the streets of Kingston on the way home from school. So Libby found herself sharing the fate I had been subjected to at St George's College. Michael dropped her off in the morning as he had dropped me off, but at the end of the school day, she had to make her way home on her own by bus and by foot, notwithstanding the fact that Gloria had absolutely nothing to do and could easily have picked her up. 'Had I not made arrangements to get lifts with people whom I barely knew, she would have exposed me to the daily danger of being mugged, raped or kidnapped in preference to inconveniencing herself to make a ten-minute car journey,' Libby once observed to me.

I suppose a mother who is as indifferent to the fate of her favourite child, as Gloria was with me, can hardly be expected to care about a child with whom she has never had an affinity and has moreover selected as her supreme victim. If she had loathed Mickey because of the attention he used to get from her sister and mother, her fury was nothing compared with what she now directed towards Libby. Where Mickey had been the prince within the family, Libby was the beauty queen before the world. The breadth, scope and degree of the attention she received was a daily reminder to her egocentric but aging mother of how her time was passing and the spotlight was shifting away from her. Of course, most beautiful women find the aging process more difficult to come to terms with than women who have never had the advantage of overwhelming physical attractiveness. Beauty is undoubtedly a marvellous source of pleasure and praise, and used wisely, it can enhance one's life; but, like many of life's other blessings, it is a double-edged sword, and unless you wield it carefully it cuts both ways, lacerating not only what you want it to but also what you don't intend it to.

In our family, there were many beautiful women who had used their looks productively and lost, or were losing, them sensibly. Maisie, though never a great beauty, had been a very attractive woman as well as a man-eating *femme fatale*. She had come to terms with getting older without bitterness. One of her sisters was a raving beauty who had managed to circumvent the rocks of the aging process without rancour – albeit with the help of the surgeon's knife – and Gloria had various first cousins who were her contemporaries and were more or less successfully facing up to the loss of their universal appeal without turning into venom-spewing shrews. Even her sister Marjorie, handsome rather than beautiful but every bit as stylish and vain, was aging magnificently both physically and mentally. There was also a plethora of Ziadie cousins renowned for their beauty who were facing the loss of their youthful looks in a manner worth emulating, none more so than Sir Peter Jonas's mother May and her sister Toni de Acevedo. But then none of them was an out-and-out narcissist with histrionic tendencies the way Gloria was. It was the fundamental flaws in her character that had been playing havoc with her life and ours while she was in the full flower of her beauty, and now that this was fading, her egocentricity would feed her bitterness and envy until she had wreaked as much damage as she could.

Of course, beautiful women who possess narcissistic and histrionic personalities find aging a far more traumatic process and react far more adversely than normal beauties, largely because they have relied too much upon their looks to gain the attention they require. Faced with the loss of both looks and attention, they go into a tailspin. Many commit suicide or withdraw from life, such as the famous Countess of Castiglione in the Second Napoleonic Empire, while others turn their fury outwards and try to damage others the way they perceive a cruel life is damaging them.

Gloria was too intelligent, with too great a sense of her own dignity, to blind herself to the realities of what was happening to her. 'I don't intend to make a complete ass of myself the way Violetta Riel does,' she would say, 'acting as if she's still thirty-five when she won't even see seventy again, except on a mile post. Nor will I allow my vanity to get the better of me the way Mama does, hoping that men will still find her alluring even though she's nothing but an old goat.'

The problem was that Gloria had no personal resources to fill the void. Like all egocentrics, the world began and ended with her. She had no interests except for the admiration and adulation others provided her with. Although she was superficially interested in gardening, she had not developed this hobby beyond learning enough to stock her own garden with rare and exotic plants from all over the world. These were tended by the gardeners. She would occasionally walk through the garden admiring it, or take people on tours and soak up their praise for handiwork which really wasn't her own, even if the overall concept was. Even this was hardly enough of an interest to sustain her into middle and old age. The challenge for her would be to develop sufficient interests to replace her beauty and the attention it had brought her before her looks went the way of all flesh.

Even though Gloria was aware that time would sooner or later erode her looks and the catholicity of appeal which they had brought her, she now failed to rise to the challenge of developing alternative sources of gratification. Indeed, her initial response to the aging process was to ignore the problem, doubtless in the hope that, if she ignored it long enough, she would have been proven to be wrong about its existence and then the problem would solve itself by disappearing. Such self-delusion is not uncommon amongst narcissists, but it usually coexists alongside the awareness of the problem that one can't quite wish away. So it proved to be with Gloria.

As she thrashed around, wavering between recognition of – and the need for a solution to - her problem, Gloria's lack of responsibility exacerbated it in a way that would prove fatal to her ultimate self-interest. She was a dedicated lover of pleasure who felt that her one obligation in life was to enjoy herself, something Michael had allowed her to get away with. Unlike most other ladies of her background, who had the good grace to do minimal chores such as going to the supermarket or ordering in groceries from the shops, she had long since refused to do any such thing. Until I was old enough to drive and took over the chore of grocery shopping, Michael had to get the staff at his business to organize all the food in the house.

Gloria's inaction in this regard was symptomatic of a larger problem of which irresponsibility was only a part. I would say that the real flaw lay at the very root of her character. She was not only self-centred but also self-regarding to the point of self-idolatry. Nothing was ever her fault. How could it be? She was perfect. Never wrong. When people and events did not measure up to her exacting demand that they serve her and only her, she reacted with a fury she felt was justified. As far as she was concerned, because everyone and everything existed for her exclusive benefit, if anyone or anything fell short of her expectations, they had failed her and were therefore deserving of her rage. Being the only person around whom the world revolved – and the only perfect one at that – she had also never had an ignoble motive, never committed a dubious deed, never been anything less than a wonderful, noble, marvellous human being who was always deserving of adulation and admiration. This attitude is what made it so easy for her to turn her every vicious act around and convert it into the fault of her victims.

All of this would have been destructive enough, even if she had not exacerbated the problem with laziness. But she did. 'It's as if she thinks it's beneath her dignity to do anything,' Libby said in adulthood and tried to solve the problem by pointing out to her mother how pleasurable activity could be. I knew what Gloria's response was even before Libby told me how scornful and contemptuous it had been. As far as Gloria was concerned, she was far too important a personage to have to do anything for herself, much less for anyone or anything else. The result was that she died without getting herself even a glass of water. Till her dying day, she never once boiled water, made a cup of coffee or did any of the other things that even people with staff sometimes do.

With that fatal combination of arrogance, irresponsibility, anger, self-importance, laziness and helplessness, Gloria was hardly likely to help herself in coping with the problems of aging. So she did what she had always done. She blamed others for what was really her own fault. As she looked at the young, beautiful daughter who was on the threshold of her life and envied what lay ahead for Libby and mourned what was fast coming to an end for herself, Gloria turned her fury outwards to the daily reminder of the youthfulness and beauty which were slipping out of her hands.

Things had been bad enough when Bruce was courting Libby, but once Michael's great-nephew Ben Lazanne came on the scene as a suitor, and Libby started taking him seriously, Gloria lost all inhibitions and gave full vent to her sadistic, Machiavellian streak.

A contributory factor was the way she felt about Ben's father, whom she despised as well as 'scorned' (her word, not mine). This made her indifferent to how her behaviour was viewed by Ben's family, for while Bruce's family were people for whom she had enough regard to care about what they said about her, with the result that she would have exercised a measure of self-restraint even if she had not liked Bruce as much as she did, this was not so with the Lazannes.

In fact, Gloria's attitude towards Ben's father was the recognition one shark has of another. 'Nasser' – as she accurately nicknamed him after the Egyptian dictator – was as disagreeable a piece of work as she was. A contemporary of Michael's and the younger brother of his eldest sister Mathilde's husband George, Nasser had also married Michael's niece, with whom Gloria had been to school, at the tender age of fourteen. This of course became a handy tool for Gloria to use against them, even though two of her first cousins had eloped at fourteen and sixteen respectively. 'But their parents didn't give their consent,' Gloria crowed when I tried to subtly point out that kettles should not call pots black. 'It's disgusting that your aunt could have unleashed that monster on her young daughter,' she said with finality, and I kept my counsel, realizing the futility of pointing out that she was trying to make into a savage practice what had until recently been the done thing in aristocratic and royal circles, as the marriage of Princess Ira von Furstenburg to Prince Alfonso von Hohenlohe-Langenburg a few short years ago proved.

Although our two families were not pitched together frequently, Gloria's path crossed Nasser's enough for a natural antipathy to have developed into mutual loathing over the two decades of her marriage.

As luck would have it, Michael wasn't too keen on Nasser either. Although he was fond of his niece, he was happy to give her husband a wide berth. This had been easy enough to do while we children were growing up, for the Lazannes lived in some comfort in a converted hotel in the country while we lived in town. Once a decade or so, we went to visit them, usually for a funeral or some such family event, at which time Nasser would come into his own. He was the most gracious and welcoming of hosts, the complete opposite of what he was outside his own house.

Then the elder Lazanne children came to town to go to university and started living with their grandmother. As so often happens in upper-class circles where families intermarry with bewildering frequency, Aunt Hilda also bore the surname Lazanne, having married one of Nasser's cousins. Thereafter, we saw an uncomfortable amount of Nasser, who frequently visited his children, for my siblings and I were fond of our aunt and often visited her. As a result, we got to know our Lazanne cousins and their father very well. He, unfortunately, could always be relied upon to pass the one comment that would wound and generally made a pain of himself, but everyone put up with him because they liked his wife and children.

If the father was a pill, however, his children were genuinely nice. I struck up a particularly close friendship with his daughter Lorraine, another of the beauties for which our family was known. She often came up to our house to see me, and sometimes she would be accompanied by her eldest brother Ben, but only after he had met Libby at another cousin's wedding when she was sixteen. Then his eyes had been on stalks; and before long Lorraine was telling us how beautiful he thought she was. But Libby seemed to have no real interest in him, still having eyes only for Bruce. Then Bruce went to university in Canada and everything changed.

This I discovered when Libby was visiting me in New York over Easter 1969. Ben had been paying her serious court in Bruce's absence, and she was now torn between him and Bruce. To say that I was gob-smacked would be to put it mildly.

It should be emphasized at this point that neither Michael nor Gloria had anything against Ben himself. Indeed, they both liked him. From my father's point of view, he was perfect son-in-law material if one could forget about his father. He was almost as avid a follower of the turf as Michael, who spent hours talking about horses with him. He enjoyed playing poker, dominoes and backgammon. He was charming, intelligent and well-mannered, which had appeal for both Michael and Gloria, who also found his personable approach appealing.

So far as Michael was concerned, Ben had another quality which put him streets ahead of Bruce in the beau stakes: he was about to qualify as a doctor and would be specializing in cardiology. That meant that his wife would be assured of a comfortable lifestyle, even if one discounted his father's considerable material assets. Bruce, meanwhile, had just started university in Canada, so would not be in a position to marry Libby for years. Moreover, Bruce's father was not as well off as Nasser. As I would discover to my cost in a few years, Michael was dead keen to see his daughters suitably married at the earliest opportunity, in keeping with the more traditional approach to life which was then still prevalent in the upper reaches of society.

It might surprise people from more modern or pedestrian backgrounds to learn that there was nothing unusual or untoward about Michael's wishes. All well-bred girls were nothing but marital fodder. No matter how brilliant or talented a daughter was, a responsible father and mother had no higher aspiration than that she marry suitably. That meant marrying a kind, decent, preferably physically attractive young man from a good family, who should have enough money to support his wife in the lifestyle to which she had been born. If he had lots of money, so much the better. A grand name, meaning household or titled, wasn't an absolute must, but if as a consequence of hitting other targets, you got that as well, so much the better. The pressure to marry suitably was intense. All well-bred girls felt it. Indeed, there was so much spoken – as well as unspoken – pressure upon young girls to marry before their twenty-fifth birthday that you felt your life wasn't worth living if you hadn't gained the marital stamp of approval by then. There is no doubt in my mind that Michael would have influenced Libby by overt and covert means to come to the 'right' decision, without realizing that when she did, Gloria was getting the perfect weapon to use against her.

Once Libby made her choice, Gloria went to work with a vengeance. This woman who could never find the time to pick up a child from school and only once every few years bothered to write to any of her children when they were away at school or university, now turned her attention to tormenting Libby, using her relationship with Ben as licence to cast self-restraint to the winds. She would sit down in her favourite chair on the back veranda plotting and scheming, picking at Libby for nothing, then moaning to Michael about what a 'little bitch' Libby was. This went on day in, day out, month in, month out, until Libby wrote to me in New York to say she didn't think she could stand much more of it. Things were building to a crescendo, and what a crescendo it would prove to be.

The drama started one Sunday afternoon at the beginning of summer 1969. Michael had gone to play dominoes, and Libby was at home in her bedroom reading, while Gloria was in hers resting. Ben, who was on call at the University College Hospital where he was a resident, popped down to the house to see Libby. Deciding that it made more sense if he took her to the hospital, where he had the use of the residents' quarters in case his services were needed, he played right into Gloria's conniving hands by being considerate enough not to wake her up and tell her what he was doing.

A couple of hours later, when he dropped Libby back home, he did not realize that Gloria had so pumped up Michael that Libby's life was in danger.

No sooner did Libby get inside, however, than Michael started to rant and rave. Gloria had been filling up his head with pictures of his daughter and great-nephew indulging in carnality in those residents' quarters.

After several more hours of his wife's goading, Michael, who had resisted losing his temper with all the slender resources he had at his disposal, finally snapped under the pressure. 'I'm sick of you and your nagging. You always find something to taunt a man with and drive him to distraction,' he screamed at Gloria before going to the cupboard where he kept his gun, taking it out, and screaming, 'I could blow my brains out.' Gloria, never one to back down or to miss the chance of escalating a drama up to hysterical proportions, suggested that he turn the gun on his errant daughter instead. Michael then stormed into

Libby's bedroom, where she was reading, and put the barrel of the loaded revolver to her head. 'I feel like blowing out your brains and mine,' he shrieked in anguish.

'I cannot tell you the terror I felt,' Libby said a few weeks later, when I returned to Jamaica from New York for the summer holidays and went down to Maisie's house, whence she had fled after that scene. 'I didn't know whether he'd pull the trigger or not. I could tell *he* didn't know whether he'd pull the trigger or not. He was totally out of control. You cannot imagine how I felt as I wondered if these were going to be the last few moments of my life. Was this how I was going to die? No one who has not been through something like that can ever really understand how you feel. After what seemed an eternity but must have been a matter of minutes, sanity reasserted itself, and he took the gun away from my head and apologized. I said nothing, absolutely nothing, in case anything I said set him off again. I just looked at him. After he left my bedroom, I turned off the light and tried to get some sleep, but of course, I got none. I could still hear that bitch next door trying to wind him up. I didn't know if she'd succeed and he'd come back into my room and maybe finish off the job. To say that I was terrified doesn't begin to describe how I felt. Finally she shut up, and everything went quiet. I don't think I'll ever get over the sheer terror of that night. Ever. The following day I telephoned Grandma. She came for me, and here I am.'

The pattern established by Mickey's presence at his grandmother's house now repeated itself with Libby. Every afternoon, Michael would stop off at Maisie's and apologize to Libby and beg her to come back home. Gloria, needless to say, kept a wide berth. She knew her mother was furious with her, and that other close relations, such as her sister and sisters-in-law, had been made aware of this latest incident, but she didn't care. Her attitude was that, as long as the world at large thought that she was marvellous, what did the disapproval of a few piddling relations matter? Moreover, she was able to convince herself that she was blameless, for she had not held the loaded gun to Libby's head or threatened to pull the trigger, so she could not be blamed for what had happened. Accepting no blame for the part she had played in pumping up her volatile, moralistic husband, she even managed to put a positive spin on her actions, maintaining that she was only trying to preserve Libby's reputation lest Ben ruin her chances for matrimony by carelessness that could be misconstrued as immorality. Yet again Gloria was demonstrating her remarkable ability for attributing noble motives to dirty deeds.

When I got back home for that summer of 1969, I still had my own problems to contend with and could therefore be of no help to Libby. Aside from commiserating, there was little else I could do. I had to protect my own position, and with a father as deeply hostile towards me as our mother was towards Libby, I was hardly able to fight battles on her behalf. Furthermore, I now had a new worry. Suppose Michael turned the gun on me? I had little doubt he would pull the trigger and that he and the police would cobble together some story that let him off the hook. I had heard them recommend to him on too many occasions, while chatting to my parents – usually while waiting for the latest dismissed servant to gather together their belongings prior to removal in the back of the paddy wagon – that the way to deal with thieves was to shoot them dead, put a piece of pipe, a hammer, a toy gun or a cutlass into their hand, then call the police. I had little doubt that the rule that allowed patricians and the police to form a mutual protection club would apply to my murder, if my father should repeat with me what he had nearly done to Libby.

Worried about the possibility of being shot by Michael, I did not have the option of turning to my mother for protection. She had eroded any residue of trust I had once had in her when she had dishonoured her promise to help me achieve my gender, once the New York psychiatrist confirmed that there was nothing psychologically wrong with me. This he had done in May 1968, bringing the period of psychiatric assessment to an end and in so doing, triggering an adverse reaction from the father who would have rather seen me dead than declared a girl.

Desperate to bring what I now called 'this cruel farce' to an end, I reminded Gloria of the promise she had made in that New York hotel bedroom in September 1967 to help me. I asked her to take my side and convince Daddy to either consent or then step aside and let my treatment take place without his assistance or opposition. Her reaction took my breath away. 'I have no recollection of making any such promise to you,' she said in that cold, harsh way she had when she wanted you to know that she meant business.

'But you must remember, Mummy. It was in your hotel room when you said...' I started, unusually tenacious and insistent.

She cut me off icily. 'Look here child, let me make one thing clear. I knew your father long before I knew any of you. Long after you've all flown the coop, he'll still be there. I have to think about my relationship with him. I'm not going to take a stand that's diametrically opposed to one he takes *on any issue*, and certainly not on one that's as emotive as your "matter". So you may as well get it out of your head that I ever promised you anything. I never did and I never will and that's all there is to that.'

'So I'm supposed to live in limbo,' I said, close to collapse but insistent nevertheless, for I could tell she remembered only too well the promise she had made.

'You will just have to cope until you're twenty-one. The law says you can't do anything without parental consent between now and then, and you can bank on it, your father won't be helping you, nor will I be going against him.'

As I write this, the reaction I had, of disbelief and horror that any human being, much less a mother, would be so heartless and brutal, comes back with discomfiting intensity. I also remember only too clearly that, at the very moment I was experiencing those unwelcome emotions, I was also only too cognisant that Gloria was simply being as ruthless and selfish towards me as I had seen her be towards Mickey, Libby and a myriad of other people. Although one part of me was shocked, another part was prepared. I had never been the sort of person who believed that I was in any way so special that what A did to B, A wouldn't ultimately do to me, and having seen so many instances of Gloria's cruelty and heartlessness over the years, I accepted that my turn had come.

A part of me was grateful that I had been emotionally distancing myself from her in recent years, and that I had possessed sufficient faith in my own powers of observation and intuition to have prepared myself for this moment. Make no mistake about it, though, this was a very frightening time. It was a real turning point. Not only did it show me how utterly unfeeling and unscrupulous my mother truly was, but it also removed the last vestiges of hope I had for a relatively painless resolution to my problem. Thereafter, I could not kid myself that she would help me. I had hoped, until then, that she would pay for the corrective surgery which she had said I would need prior to my papers being amended so that I could be officially declared a female and live in the female gender without fear of arrest. Until then I was liable to prosecution unless dressed as a male because my papers stated that my gender was male and it was against the law in the United States and British territories to dress in any but your legally assigned gender.

I did not then know that I did not need any surgery to have my papers altered. Worse still, I also did not know that I had been in the position legally to sign the surgical consent forms ever since I had turned eighteen. All that nonsense about me needing to be twenty-one was just another delaying tactic. Gloria duped me with a barefaced lie, actively assisting Michael in perpetuating my misery in the hope that I would be worn down before time ran out. I still find it almost beyond belief that my own mother was prepared to deceive me on such an important matter as the age of consent. Thanks to her, my agony was prolonged for another two and a half torturous years.

Of course, one must also acknowledge that I should have known by this time that someone as unscrupulous and self-centred as Gloria should not be relied upon, especially about important matters, but at eighteen I could not conceive of any person being so monstrous as to deliberately mislead another upon a point of such importance. You can imagine how utterly betrayed I felt when I eventually found out.

I thought then, and think now, that there was no excuse for her deception; and though I ultimately forgave her for what she had done, the futility of wasting my time so flagrantly has never left me.

Those who do not remember the past, George Santayana observed, are condemned to repeat it. Throughout history, mankind's reluctance to face facts and learn the lessons of bitter experiences has meant that time and again we are compelled to dig ourselves out of holes into which we would never have fallen if only we had learned our lessons the first time around. So it would prove with me nearly forty years later when, in another sleight of hand, Gloria would cheat me out of hundreds of thousands of dollars instead of time.

Where Gloria was not misleading me in 1968, however, was in the degree of cooperation I would need from her and my father to have my legal status regularized. Under the British system, birth certificates could only be amended if a genuine mistake had been made at birth, as had happened in my case. My parents would have to confirm that error in a Statutory Declaration, as it was called, which would be the basis upon which my gender changed legally from male to female. Without that process, I would be consigned to perpetual legal limbo, with no possibility of a normal life, normal employment or even matrimony. I was not prepared to accept a perpetuation of the anomalies with which I had been saddled all my life, for those were much worse than any of the nonsense I had to put up with to stay in Gloria's good books. I opted for the lesser of two evils– wisely as it turned out. I kept in with Gloria.

No matter how sceptical I was growing of my mother, I could not let her know that I was seeing through her. She was such a punitive and vengeful personality that she would never have cooperated with regularizing my legal status if I had fallen foul of her. I knew only too well she would gladly, indeed righteously, have consigned me to a perpetual limbo-like scrapheap and taken pleasure in the discomfiture her lack of cooperation was causing me. I had seen her sadism in action too often to doubt that I would be spared from it unless I played ball with her, and having lived the first part of my life in one sort of limbo, I would have ignored just about anything she threw at me or anyone else, rather than run the risk of living out the rest of my life without a defined legal status. So the devoted, uncritical, obliging Georgie of the past remained ostensibly devoted, uncritical and obliging; and whenever Gloria wanted me to become the pair of ears she chewed off, I cooperated with all the willingness of the truly desperate and tried as best I could not to deviate from my martinet mother's manifesto.

Gloria's abandoning of my cause, however, forced me to rethink my future. In the two and a half years since I had run away to Miami, I had grown up a lot. My earning capacity had improved, and eager to obtain the funds for the corrective surgery I still thought was necessary to regularize my position legally, I started to supply fashionable boutiques such as She and Abracadabra in New York with designer outfits. I was now well and truly a fully-fledged dress designer, even though I was still at college. My outfits retailed for between \$60 and \$250, and I sold them to the boutiques for between \$30 and \$125, making okay money for those days, though the target figure of \$5,000 which I had set myself was proving difficult to accumulate quite as quickly as I had hoped.

If progress was slower than I wished, I was now definitely on the road to resolution. As soon as I returned to New York in September 1968, I found out, with surprising ease, the name of a gynaecologist who specialized in cases like mine. This confirmed the suspicion I had developed over the years that my parents were using doctors to hinder rather than assist me. If, in a lay capacity,

I had access to specialists so readily, why didn't their high-fee doctors? I went to see this gynaecologist; he took me on as a patient; and thereafter the only hitch to solving my problem was when I could afford the surgery. Life, I was discovering, was really simple if you wished it to be. Maybe not easy – but simple.

Armed with the knowledge of how my parents had mucked me about, pretending to seek medical help when they were intent on medical hindrance, I gained an invaluable insight into the sort of people they were. However, I tried not to think about it, or indeed to see too clearly what it was that experience was shining a light upon. Too much knowledge can be a poisoned chalice when you have to keep drinking from the well of callous and selfish people, so I suppressed as much conscious recognition of the knowledge I was acquiring as I could.

This was a phase of my life when the last thing I wanted to do was return home for any of the holidays. However, my presence was required at Christmas and in the summer, not only to help at the store but also so that my father could make sure that I had not contrived to succeed in my goal for an integrated identity, and to keep my mother company.

In the summer of 1969, I delayed my departure from New York for as long as I could. When I could delay no longer, I flew into the maelstrom whose fallout was still taking place after Michael had put the loaded revolver to Libby's head. Determined to preserve my position as best as I could, I took a leaf out of my father's book and played Pontius Pilate impersonating an ostrich, and when Libby returned home from Maisie's house and Gloria tore into her on a daily basis, I pretended nothing untoward was happening. Beneath a bland exterior, however, I was so upset that I could not wait to 'escape from this prison' as I put it.

Libby had been due to go abroad to university that September. She and Ben, however, were aware that their relationship would end in marriage; and since he was due to stay in Jamaica for another year before joining the staff of a Canadian hospital, she decided to stay home and attend the University of the West Indies instead.

In the seven years since Independence, Jamaica had changed significantly. It was well on the way to redefining its identity as a black country with diverse but racial minorities of diminishing importance, rather than as the multiracial country where each race was equally important. There were practical reasons for this change. Some were indigenous, such as the fact that a hefty majority of Jamaicans were of African descent, but others were due to the ethos of the age. This was the period when Black Power in neighbouring America was a nascent movement. Black Jamaicans identified with their American brothers and sisters and adopted many of their ideas and slogans. Having discovered a pride in being black, they embraced an anger of what whites had been doing to them for centuries and started asserting themselves and their rights in a way they had never done before.

Student unrest spread throughout the Western world in 1968. Whether in France, England, America, Germany or Jamaica, students had taken to the streets, organized sit-ins on campuses and loudly demanded that governments rectify the errors of the past. One of those errors, of course, was what the whites had done to the blacks before, during and after slavery.

In some ways, Libby could not have chosen a worse time to attend the University of the West Indies. The student body, mostly black, was largely left-wing with Black Power sympathies. It takes no imagination to see the sort of reception a white girl who bore a household name synonymous with wealth, mercantilism and old-fashioned privilege was going to receive. It says much for her powers of endurance and diplomacy that she was able to function for a year, rising above the racist taunts the more radical students threw her way. It must be said in defence of many less radical black students, however, that they had nothing against white Jamaicans and would not have condoned the treatment meted out to her. Like me, they were in the invidious position of having to shut their mouths and defer to the powers of hatred.

Reluctant silence, I fear, is also what my situation was forcing me to adopt at home. I was only too aware of how vulnerable I was where Gloria was concerned. I was, as she herself would have put it, 'on thin ice'. I made sure I neither skated nor fell into the water but stayed absolutely still and silent as I watched her abuse Libby. However, Libby's torment was coming to an end, not only up at the University of the West Indies but also at home. She and Ben decided to get married prior to his departure for Canada in June 1970.

Gloria was not about to let an opportunity escape her to poke an adversary in the eye, and she now turned the announcement of the engagement into the perfect stick with which to beat Nasser.

Ben revered his father. Although Nasser knew of his son's unofficial intentions, when Ben asked Michael for Libby's hand in marriage and made the enterprise official Ben quite rightly wanted to tell his parents face-to-face, before his great- uncle and great-aunt officially announced the engagement in the newspapers. So he asked Daddy and Mummy to delay the announcement until he had had a chance to go home that Sunday and tell his father. They agreed, and that Sunday morning Libby, Ben, his younger brother Babe and I set off for the country anticipating the joy the news would bring his parents. No sooner did Ben's car pull up to the house than we knew something was wrong. Nasser was standing by the front door, awaiting Ben's arrival, his face a testament to anger, the newspaper in his hand beating time on his leg. 'What is the meaning of this? Why am I the last person in the country to know that you're engaged? What sort of a son are you, letting me read about your engagement in the newspaper? Where is your respect for your mother and myself? Are we no better than every stranger in the land?' he demanded, seeking an explanation for the lead story in Violetta de Barovier-Riel's Social Column.

'Uncle Mike and Aunt Gloria said they'd delay the announcement,' poor Ben tried to explain. 'It hasn't been announced yet. Look, Dada. See. There's no announcement in the Engagements Section. Aunt Gloria must have confided in Violetta. It's not our fault. We all tried to keep the news secret until after telling you.'

I had my doubts. Knowing the way my mother functioned, and knowing Violetta, who was very correct, I could not see that venerable lady breaking an embargo. On the other hand, I could easily envisage Gloria being alert to the mischief she would cause if she kept her word to Ben by not announcing the engagement officially in the Engagements Section of the newspaper but nevertheless leaking it through the Social Column.

The following Sunday, Violetta dropped in to see Gloria after Mass, as she often did. I pulled her up to the swimming pool to show her some orchids, which were in full bloom, and taking advantage of the moment, asked her if Mummy had told her to hold off on publishing the story until after Ben's parents had been informed of the engagement. She said no, she hadn't, and asked if it had caused a problem. I said only a slight and temporary one, which had already been rectified; and she asked if she should say something to my mother. I said better not to, and having received confirmation of how Gloria had 'laid the trap' (one of her favourite expressions), that was the end of the matter.

Despite her character flaws, this self-regarding daughter of Narcissus was an able organizer who had done many successful charity events in her time. With Libby's wedding, she now had a personal event to sink her teeth into, and there was never any doubt in the mind of anyone who knew her that she would pull it off splendidly. It would, of course, be Gloria's show with Libby the obligatory central figure only as and how she had to be.

Although Libby found none of it a laughing matter, Gloria was so outrageous it was almost funny. Weddings in those days were customarily held before sundown, because British law prevented marriages from taking place at night. The mother of the bride, however, was never going to shine as brightly during the day, when she would have to wear the required hat and dress, as she would in the evening, when she could be resplendent in an evening gown and diamonds. So Gloria got special permission to have the wedding ceremony conducted as late as possible. Next, she went to see Cardinal-Archbishop McEleny, the Roman Catholic Primate, who was about to depart for a new posting in the US. She called in the favours he owed her from the time she had been chairman of the Alpha Old Girls' Association and got him to postpone his departure so that he could officiate at the wedding. As she recounted it, he was almost honoured to oblige her, which may not have been too far from the truth, for Gloria had the uncanny ability to get people to feel honoured to do favours for her when the honour really was all hers.

As she set about planning the wedding with the precision of a military campaign, you could see her deliberately crushing every one of Libby's ideas or suggestions. Her attitude could not have been plainer: if she could have eliminated Libby from the show altogether, she would have done so.

Libby was frequently in tears or so upset that her hands would shake as if she had Parkinson's disease. I swore that, if I was fortunate enough to get married one day, I would never make the mistake of letting my mother loose on the arrangements. When my time actually came, I eloped rather than let her reduce me to a nervous wreck and a resented central figure of the Gloria Ziadie show the way she reduced my sister.

However, even Gloria could not prevent Libby from being the star of the show, so she set about making sure that her daughter was the perfect foil for her. Libby had to wear a dress and have a hairstyle of which she approved, and there were endless rows surrounding both. Libby wasn't allowed to wear make-up which Gloria didn't approve of either. In those, pre-wedding planner days, the mother of the bride was the producer of the show, and our mother wasn't only a megalomaniac but one with a heightened sense of grandeur and an eye for beauty. Demonstrating what energy and ability she had when she could be bothered to put them to use, she was busy from morning till night for nearly two months, ensuring the wedding would be one the guests never forgot. No detail was too small for her to overlook. She even telephoned members of the family whose formal attire she did not like and instructed them to order new suits. When Michael remonstrated with her, saying she would cause offence, she said she didn't care how much offence she caused as long as they showed up as she required. Her knowledge of, and love for, flowers now came into their own, as she ordered just about every florist on the island to buy in and refrigerate a variety of blooms. Then, in the last two days before the wedding, she set about decorating the church and Caymanas Country Club, where the reception was being held, turning them into settings reminiscent of a Hollywood film.

In the days immediately after the announcement of the engagement, while Gloria had been whirling around town like a dervish executing her plans, Libby was making arrangements to enrol in university in Canada. One afternoon she, Michael and I were on the front veranda talking when Gloria arrived home. Mother asked daughter some question about visas; daughter answered; mother accused daughter of not answering properly; daughter denied saying what mother was accusing her of having said, and before you knew it, they were in the midst of a monumental row with Gloria threatening to cancel the wedding. Libby warmed my heart when she called her bluff, saying: 'So go ahead and cancel it. As things stand, it's more for your greater glory than my marriage.'

Gloria, appreciating the veracity of that statement and never being one to deny herself an opportunity for sparkling brightly in social settings, quickly diverted the argument into more opaque waters.

'You are an ingrate. An ingrate. You have no gratitude, after all I've been doing for you.'

'I am not an ingrate, and I don't see what gratitude has to do with a visa. We were talking about visas. How does a visa connect with gratitude? You haven't helped me with my visa so how can I be grateful to you?'

Libby, hoping to bring the row to an end before it escalated further, started to depart for her bedroom. Gloria, however, was going to do her darnedest to keep her in the line of fire for as long as she could.

'That child is nothing but an ingrate and a parasite,' she said to Michael. 'It's always take, take, take. She doesn't give a damn how I'm knocking myself out on her behalf. All she cares about is herself. She'll suck, suck, suck till we have no marrow left.'

I can still see Libby, in the drawing room, sneering scornfully before taking a few more steps towards her bedroom. Her message, non-verbal though it was, could not have been more graphically conveyed: You are a pathetic termagant, but I won't be lowering myself to respond further to your preposterous accusations.

Gloria, however, was not about to give up without another push or two. 'Can't you see that she's using us, you self-deluding old fool?' she said to Michael, quick as a flash. 'She's a parasite, using me for my labour so she can show herself off in front of her friends with a lavish wedding, and you to put her through university after she's a married woman. What I want to know is: if she's such a hot-shot big woman that she can be rude to her mother, why does she need our money to educate herself?'

Libby, enticed back into the argument, returned to the front veranda from the drawing room. 'What are you saying?' she asked, a look of such shock intermingled with horror on her face that I was seriously tempted to tell her to go back inside. But I knew if I did, I would also be implying that Gloria was trying to deprive her of the opportunity to go to university and that would blow my future along with Libby's. So I kept my trap shut and listened.

'I am very sure you understand what I'm saying only too well,' Gloria said haughtily, springing her trap. 'You're intelligent and always have done well in English, which is your native tongue, so there should be no doubt in your mind what I'm saying. But in case you need to hear it again, I will repeat it. You are an ingrate and a parasite who will suck your father and myself dry if we let you. Ben will soon be your husband. If you want to go to university, let him pay for you to go. Why should your father and I pay?'

'You pay?' Libby asked in disbelief. Gloria never paid for anything – not for herself and definitely not for her children. Michael was the walking, talking cheque-book.

'Are you going to sit there like a lump and let her talk to me like this?'

Gloria demanded of Michael.

'Apologize to your mother,' he said meekly.

'For what?' Libby said.

'The problem with these children is that they've been spoiled rotten. We've indulged them at every turn, and they think they're entitled to everything when they're entitled to nothing. They're nothing but parasites and leeches, and this one here,' Gloria spat dismissively, looking at Libby, 'is the biggest parasite of all. I say, if she's so independent that she can be rude to her mother, let that nephew of yours whom she's marrying pay for her to go to university.'

'Gloria,' Michael said, trying to be conciliatory, 'he's ju…just starting out in li…life. Things will be a str…struggle enough for him to su…support himself and a wife without the add…additional expense of un…un… university. I'm ha…happy to pay for all my ch…children's education. You know my mo…motto: Governments can take your la…land, your investments, your mo…money, but they can't take what's in your he…head.'

'You may have your father deceived, but you don't have me,' Gloria, determined to prevail, hurled hatefully at Libby.

'Once that wedding ring is on my finger, I won't condescend to take a penny of your precious money,' Libby said and with that walked off into her bedroom.

I waited for a decent interval, so that Gloria wouldn't think that I was offering support to my sibling, then went inside too. As soon as I reached my bedroom and had closed the door loudly enough so that my mother would know which room I had gone to, I exited by the other door and headed for Libby's room. 'Don't let her do this to you,' I said. 'She'll count your refusal to go to university as a victory. I say, defeat the bitch. Take Daddy's money and go.'

'I'm sorry,' Libby said. 'I will not allow anyone to make such preposterous accusations to me and think that she can get away with them without me showing her that I need my dignity more than I need her or her wretched money – money, incidentally, which we've all helped to earn, if you consider the amount of free labour they've got out of us over the years during the holidays.'

'All the more reason to take the money and run,' I said.

'I will not give that bitch the satisfaction of seeing me take any money from them once I'm married,' Libby said.

'Personally speaking, I'd take the money and not give her the satisfaction of winning, but I can see why you feel as you do,' I said.

Thereafter, Libby and Gloria were not really on speaking terms. It was peculiar to see the arrangements for a wedding continue with the bride being sidelined so totally, but all of us had long since been used to the most bizarre scenarios being treated in our house as if they were ordinary situations. I suspect that Gloria might even have been secretly pleased to have rid herself of the necessity of referring occasionally to Libby out of good manners.

As the big day loomed ever closer, she was so busy she no longer had the time for daughter-bating, so the combination of non-speaking and ignoring worked in Libby's favour.

On the day itself, Libby and Gloria went to the hairdresser in the morning. Afterwards, they headed for the bank, where Gloria's jewellery was stored. Then Libby went to Maisie's house, where she and the bridesmaids were dressing. Gloria came back home to dedicate herself to the all-day beautification process which was an integral ritual of her social life. Before going out, she always had her hair done, then manicured her nails herself. 'No manicurist can do them as well as I,' she always maintained, bestirring herself for a process that invariably took several hours. Only when she was satisfied with how her hair, fingers and toes looked would she then glide into her bathroom for her bath. Having cleansed herself, she would then powder herself, scent herself, put on her underwear and hose, sit in front of her dressing table, to apply her make-up, which took about an hour. When that was finished, she would put on her jewels and last but not least, her dress.

Gloria had treated the dress she was wearing to Libby's wedding as if it were a state secret. This, it would turn out, was not so surprising. When she started down the aisle, her hair piled high, her body encased in an empire-line gown of shimmering silver silk georgette, escorted by her great-nephew by marriage, 'Oh Toothless One', in formal evening wear, there was a decided rustle as people turned around, followed by audible gasps – first of admiration, then a hum of barely audible chatter which coursed through the church, like a wave ebbing towards the shore – as people realized that the vision of loveliness walking down the aisle wasn't Libby dressed in white but Gloria in silvery almost-white.

Gloria did indeed look magnificent, but as her Aunt Maud later said to me at the reception: 'I thought: Why is Libby proceeding to a Bach toccata, and where is her father? It was only when she got closer to the family pews that I realized it was Gloria and not Libby.'

Aunt Maud, a great favourite of us children, owing to her tolerance, sweetness of nature, understanding, and plain good fun, was the relation Gloria called 'The Scold' even though I never once heard our great-aunt disapprove of anyone but Gloria. And never did I see her disapprove of her niece more than on this occasion. She shook her head and said, 'I don't know how she could do something like that on a day like this.'

Nor was Libby blind to why Gloria had chosen to wear the dress she did. 'Mummy deliberately tried to steal my thunder by wearing a dress that would look white in the distance so that everyone would think she was me,' she quite rightly said. Gloria herself gave the game away when she proudly crowed, to one and all over the next few weeks: 'You cannot believe the number of people who told me that they thought I was the bride when I started up the aisle.' Although she didn't say so in as many words, there was no doubt that she had intended everyone to think precisely that.

Despite Gloria's scene-stealing competitiveness, she nevertheless organized a wedding that was sumptuous, elegant and a jolly good show; and Libby still has an album full of photographs to prove it. At the time, all the sentiments associated with Gloria might have been negative; but she had never cared about any of our reactions, and you could tell she counted the event a roaring success, solely because for ninety seconds everyone thought the forty-two-year-old Gloria was the eighteen-year-old bride Libby.

What struck me about her attitude wasn't even how pathetic such vanity was but how shameless she was about basking in limelight that any conscionable person would have done her utmost to avoid.

Chapter Thirteen

With Libby a married woman living in Canada, I once more became the only child at home. Mickey was still in England studying to become a barrister. Kitty was sitting her 'O' Levels at her boarding school in the country, after which she would come home for the summer and stay. It was now generally accepted that I would go to New York right after my twenty-first birthday in August to get myself sorted out. As no one, myself included, knew what my plans would be following the surgery which would allow me to become whole not only physically but also legally, Kitty was being brought home to replace Libby as the resident child of the house and chief babysitter to our infantile mother.

How I came to be at home at that time says much about the way Gloria operated. I had graduated from FIT in January 1970. I fully intended to remain in New York until I was old enough to sign the release forms for the surgery. In mid-February, however, Gloria telephoned me. She and Michael were in Florida for the races at Hialeah, and she initially suggested that I fly down to Miami for a few days, as my presence was required to sign some trust papers. After I had bought the ticket, she called again to tell me they had changed their minds and I wouldn't need to sign any trust documents after all. 'Exchange the ticket and come to Jamaica for a few days instead. Your father and I miss you.'

Well, telling me that my father missed me was like saying that Hermann Goering had decided to convert to Judaism. 'Come on, Mummy, you know as well as I do that Daddy doesn't miss me,' I said, knowing that this was one of the few times in her life when I could contradict her without fear of rousing the beast that lurked within.

'Yes, he does, and so do *I*, ' she said in that artificially light tone of voice that I knew meant she was conceding the point without acknowledging the concession. 'Come for a few days. The break will do you good. You'll get away from the cold weather, and we'll have the pleasure of seeing you.'

I should have smelled a rat. Never once, in the whole of my life, had Gloria ever before said that she missed me. I had not yet learned my lessons so well that I remembered them, and like a fool, I agreed to return home for a few days.

A week or so later, I boarded a Pan American flight for Jamaica with hope in my heart for a speedy return to New York and a total lack of the scepticism I needed to offer me protection against my manipulative mother's machinations.

From the day of my arrival, Gloria turned her fusillade of charm on me to convince me to stay in Jamaica until after my twenty-first birthday on August 17. By now it was accepted by my parents that I intended to sign the release forms for the surgery, as soon as I could officially do so, and she used this fact skilfully.

'Stay and help me to make your father see the light. You're my favourite child, and I don't want any friction between you and the man I love.'

Asking me to stay in Jamaica was asking a lot. Although I had only a half-life in New York, I had no life at all in Jamaica, unless you could call the freaky nothingness I was forced to endure, together with its relentless embarrassments and perpetual abuse, a life. I explained this to my mother, whose response was: 'You've got to stay and help me with your father.'

Gloria could see that I did not want to stay, but once I hesitated, I was lost. She wheedled and wheedled and wheedled, making me feel like a complete heel if I didn't assist her in assisting me to assist my father to accept the inevitable. Finally she wore down my resistance, and against my better judgement, I agreed to stay.

No sooner had I done so than she telephoned Frances Bacal in New York and instructed her to close out my apartment on East 81st between First and Second Avenues. 'But it took ages to find that apartment. It's not easy to find good and cheap apartments in New York,' I protested, seeing my life slipping out of my hands. 'You'll find another,' she retorted airily, instructing Frances to store my clothes and possessions in her basement until I had another apartment.

'But you don't understand,' I said. 'Frances doesn't have the time to pack up all my clothes and books and records and things. She's up before seven in the morning and doesn't return home from work until six-thirty, if she's lucky. And she doesn't have servants who can help her lift the boxes that she packs the things into, much less lug them.'

'She can hire packers or give everything to charity,' Gloria said, again airily, which I can now see covered her determination if not her lack of empathy.

'She will not be giving away any of my things, thank you very much,' I heard myself say with naked forcefulness, so outraged at my mother's lack of regard for my possessions that I could gladly have throttled her at that moment.

'So it's the packers, then,' Gloria said lightly, as if the matter were of no importance at all.

'But you didn't tell her that she could hire packers,' I said, feeling that she was taking advantage of Frances's kindness.

'Child, you're being extra *pazevie*,' Gloria rasped, using a word of her own invention which meant much ado about nothing. 'She's a big woman and can cope perfectly well with a tiny favour like this.'

If I had any doubts I was doing the wrong thing, within days of that conversation, I began to see what a big mistake I had made. Gloria and Michael had not once brought up either the subject of my future or of my father's attitude towards the scandal he feared surrounding it, and I began to get the picture: I was there to babysit my mother. The nonsense she had spewed about my assisting her in assisting Daddy had been only so much flannel with which to obtain my approval. Now that she thought I was stuck, the 'real reason' I was in Jamaica would be forgotten, just as she had 'forgotten' her promise in September 1967 to help me 'get my sex'.

If my mother thought she could roll me over so easily, she had underestimated me. 'I'm going to telephone Frances and tell her to pay next month's rent on East 81st Street,' I said one afternoon, while we were sitting on the patio under the macca tree on the front lawn. 'I can tell my presence here isn't going to help you with Daddy.'

'But it is helping,' said Gloria, bold as brass, in her sweetest, most confidential tone of voice. 'Just because you aren't privy to all that's going on behind the scenes doesn't mean that nothing's happening.'

I fear I'd been down that route one time too many to let her slippery assurances stand. 'What is happening, then?' I asked in as level and pleasant a voice as I could muster.

'It isn't in your interest for me to say too much, but you can take my word for it, I'm making good progress with your father. Much better than I'd be able to make if you weren't here.'

Although I wasn't convinced by what I then felt were barefaced lies – something that was subsequently confirmed by my father – I didn't dare call her bluff in case I alienated her. So I stayed, trapped by my deceitful, self-centred mother into being her ostensibly obliging companion.

As the weeks turned into months, and the tension in the family became unbearable, what with Gloria's relentless abuse of Libby and Michael's hostility towards me, I did not even notice that I had lost my appetite until Ben pointed it out.

'You've developed something called "anorexia". No doctor will ever operate on you if you lose any more weight,' he informed me when I hit the scales at ninety-four pounds.

He prescribed Peryactin, a drug which was supposed to increase the appetite but had the side-effect of inducing sleep. Once, while speaking to his brother Richard, I fell asleep in the middle of a sentence.

As I went into a real slump, the Peryactin made me sleep almost around the clock and increased my appetite so that I was ravenously hungry. However, I was so tense because of all that was going on at home that my throat would seal every time I tried to eat. Sometimes, I would be so eager to get the food down that I would try to override the tightness in my throat by determinedly swallowing nevertheless. I cannot convey the dreadful feeling as my body rebelled against my desire to feed it, and I would have to flee from the dinner table for the lavatory, where I would end up draped over the seat retching nothing but air and whatever gastric juices were in my stomach.

Even after such episodes, I was so highly motivated to lose no more weight that I would return to the table and try to swallow more food. On good occasions, I would manage to get down something, but often the whole process would begin again and I would end up going to bed disheartened, hungry and terrified about what was happening to me. There were times when I felt like the proverbial kitten inadvertently stuck against its will in a washer-dryer which is being whirred round and round, in danger of asphyxiation when the water doesn't threaten to drown it. Ben finally came to my rescue with the best advice anyone could have given in the circumstances.

'If swallowing is a problem, eat ice cream,' he suggested. 'Don't worry about a balanced diet or nutritional content. All that matters is that you consume a minimum of 2,000 calories a day, preferably more. Ice cream is the easiest way to do it.' Thereafter, and for the next several months, I literally lived on ice cream, and while my throat continued to constrict at the sight of food, I was mightily relieved to know that come August 17 my struggle for a life worth living would be at an end. I had no doubt that once my basic problem was cleared up, everything else would fall into place and it would only be a matter of time before my ability to eat normally returned.

Throughout all of this, the only people who displayed no concern were my two parents. Not once did either of them even acknowledge that there was anything untoward about this child of theirs who was visibly disappearing before their eyes, struggling so obviously but unsuccessfully to eat.

Once Ben and Libby left for Canada following their marriage, his brothers and sisters took me under their wing. They were kindness and compassion itself. I often went on crab hunts, to the cinema, to nightclubs, to the country or just visiting with them. Ben's younger brother Babe in particular was wonderfully supportive, partnering me at the races, which was a development Michael had not foreseen and which rendered him speechless. Babe was one of his favourite nephews, and when he showed even greater solidarity with me by taking me onto the dance floor at Aunt Doris's party, I half expected Michael to throw a fit. However, he decided to act as if nothing out of the ordinary was happening, not because his attitude towards me was softening, but because he did not want to jeopardize his relationship with Babe. Neither Babe nor I realized that his overt support of me was not lessening Michael's fear of the consequences the resolution of my problem might bring. All of us youngsters were hopeful that come September, their uncle and my father would see sense.

If my father failed to rally, my grandmother did. One afternoon, I was resting when one of the servants called me to the telephone to speak to her.

'Georgie, I need you to come down and see me as soon as you can. Your Aunt Marjorie has just told me something that I had no idea about and I need to speak to you.' Auntie was staying with her, having recently separated from her second husband Alex Stanton, with whom she had been living in Grand Cayman since their marriage two years previously.

Curious to know what the grandmother with whom I had always got along well wanted to speak to me about, I waited until Michael came home, borrowed his car and headed down to her house.

I hadn't put my foot through the front door properly before Maisie pointed to a chair. 'Would you like some cake and tea?' she asked.

I grimaced, the thought of food enough to make me sick, and asked for ice cream instead, which she and I went into the kitchen to fix.

'You have to believe me,' she said while dishing out the ice cream, 'I have never known anything about your problems. If your aunt hadn't made a stray comment about the difficulties you're having at the moment, thinking that I was in on the secret, I'd never have been any the wiser. I cannot understand how your mother could have kept something as important as that from her own mother – and for so many years. I cannot tell you how distressed I am to hear about your situation,' said Maisie, a pillar of honesty and rectitude – except where marital infidelity was concerned. 'I am so sorry I didn't know.' You could tell she felt deeply ashamed of her lack of support on this issue over the years.

I must have looked as shocked as I felt. Could I really be hearing correctly? All these years, Grandma had known nothing about my birth defect. Auntie, presumably, had assumed that Grandma knew, while Mummy had deliberately made sure she didn't. I could well see how the non-communication had happened. We lived in a world where good manners dictated that people did not ask awkward or penetrating questions, not even within family circles. This was the well-bred way, and my mother's family, whatever their failings, were well bred and conducted themselves accordingly. I could also see that, when one factored in the turmoil that Auntie and Grandma had endured over the years because of Gloria's mistreatment of Mickey and Libby, it made it almost inevitable that 'The Favourite's Matter' had been shunted to one side.

But no more. Maisie, who was as indomitable as she was loving and responsible, now solved all my problems in a few short sentences. 'What your parents have put you through is inhumane. You will have your sex, and I will pay for the operation. Your aunt has said she'd like to show solidarity and make a contribution, but we both want you to know you are not even to consider the expense. Whatever it is, I will gladly pay twice over, and so will your aunt.'

I could hardly believe what I was hearing.

'I don't think I'll ever be able to thank you enough for this, Grandma.'

'Go back home and find the very best doctor. You can't afford a botched job. You don't have to say anything to your mother or father. I'll handle them.'

Handle them Maisie did. I never found out what she said, but within days, Gloria was calling me outside to sit with her under the macca tree, a favourite seat because none of the servants could eavesdrop there.

'Mama, Marjorie and I have decided we're going to pay for your operation,' she said. 'Why don't you make an appointment with Sydney Williams [Jamaica's leading plastic surgeon] and see whether he can do it? If you have it done in America those greedy bastards are going to try to empty our pockets. And your father and I would be much happier if we can have you nearby us so we can take care of you afterwards.'

'My gynaecologist in New York is making arrangements with one of the top men in the field there,' I said. 'I don't want to put myself under the care of anyone who isn't an expert. I can't afford to have anything go wrong.'

'How much will this cost?'

'I don't know exactly, but all in, surgeon, anaesthetist, operating theatre, hospital room, nurses, it should be about $5,000.'

'I've spoken to Sydney Williams already. He says he can do the operation. Go and see him. Remember, your grandmother, aunt and I aren't made of money, and without your father's help, it's going to be a struggle.' Gloria was the very voice of reason as she played with a diamond ring that was worth at least twice what all my medical treatment would cost. 'You really are a piece of work,' I thought but preferred having her along for the ride than in the opposing camp. I played along with the farce, though I did not tell her that Grandma had already told me that I should go to the best, that money was no problem and that I knew that the sums involved, while huge for me, were very manageable for each of them individually, and collectively a doddle.

I suspected the only reason Gloria had offered to pitch in her two cents' worth was because she was aware of what a callous cow she would have looked in the eyes of the world if word got out that her mother and sister had helped me out while she had not. As for her claim that she and Daddy wanted me close to them after the surgery to take care of me, the hypocrisy of it was so awesome that I would have wanted to puke even if the two of them hadn't already reduced me to feeling as if I could do so constantly. Did she seriously think that I was so blind that I had not seen how many times throughout my own life, as well as the lives of my siblings, she had done everything in her power not to care for us? She was simply hopping on the bandwagon to protect her precious name, and I knew it as surely as I knew she was my mother. No matter the provocation, however, I was not going to fall out with her or give her an inkling how onto her I was. I needed her goodwill to change my papers, even though I did not need her financially anymore. Also, I hoped that once this sorry business was over and done with, I could put it all behind me and maybe rekindle something of the old relationship we had once had.

To humour Gloria, I did indeed go to see Sydney Williams. I asked him if he had ever performed a vaginal reconstruction and a clitoral reduction before. He said he had not. He assured me he could do them and even explained what he would in theory do if I had been reckless enough to allow him to use me as a guinea pig. I politely thanked him for his time, paid him for the consultation and went back home, where I informed my mother, hovering and salivating like a ghoul greedy for information, that I was definitely going to New York. My tone of voice was so adamant that she did not, for once, try to wheedle me out of what I wanted to do. In fact, if she had tried, I had already decided how I would handle her. 'Grandma has said she'll gladly pay the New York expenses twice over,' I would say. This would undoubtedly have silenced her, for she was always mocking her mother for being 'cheap', meaning tight-fisted, because Grandma liked living simply though comfortably, preferring to spend spare money on land rather than clothes and jewels or entertaining.

Intent on bringing my protracted limbo to an end as soon as I could, I now turned my attention not only to the medical arrangements but also to the financial ones. Organizing the doctors was relatively easy. I had been through so many by this time that there was almost a glut to choose from, and I got all the cooperation I needed from some of the previous medicos. The money, however, was something else altogether. In 1970, most governments, including the British and Jamaican, had foreign exchange controls which restricted the flow of funds from one country to another. Businesses and families with international dimensions like ours worked their way around these with a contemporaneous version of the old-fashioned letter of credit. Tens and hundreds of thousands of dollars were pledged on the shake of a hand or the nod of a head, with delivery of goods taking place in one country and delivery of funds in another. Indeed, I had been running money from Jamaica to New

York for my parents' friends ever since I had been attending school there. Sometimes it would be $15,000, sometimes much more, always in cash in US dollars, always to pay for goods purchased in New York which were essential for their businesses in Jamaica but for which the Jamaican Government, in its wisdom, would have denied them permits, to 'keep the wealth of the country in the country'. The friends rightly supposed that the Jamaica customs, who were obsessed with catching currency smugglers, would not bother with a child, and indeed they never did.

As I remember it, Gloria took over the financial arrangements and led me to believe that she would be giving Frances's brother in Jamaica the $5,000 Maisie and Marjorie had pledged, together with her contribution. Of course, she was as secretive as ever about what sum she was donating, and I never did manage to winkle that information out of her. She did mention in passing something about Frances being provided with a few dollars more for extras, which I took to mean hundreds, not thousands, but this did not ring any alarm bells. As and when I needed to call upon the funds, Frances would dispense them to me in New York.

Once everything was in place, I booked my ticket and prepared to leave Jamaica. 'Isn't your mother going with you?' Maisie asked.

'No. She says Daddy needs her.'

Grandma said nothing, but she didn't need to: the slight pursing of her lips said it all.

I too felt that my mother should have been coming with me. After seven years of dramatics and histrionics, in which my father's stance had been a refusal to precipitate a scandal and my mother's had been that my birth defect was such a monumental problem filled with hidden pitfalls about which I was much too young to be informed, it seemed somewhat anticlimactic, not to mention breathtakingly hypocritical, to adopt the diametrically opposite position and act as if Everest were now an anthill which I could easily step over on my own. Why, I asked myself, if it had never been anything but an anthill, had it been made into such a steep peak? And why, if I was too young at twenty years and three hundred and sixty four days for my parents to sign the surgical consent forms, was it suddenly such a bagatelle that I could not only sign the consents myself but also attend to myself post-operatively at twenty-one years and two weeks?

Something didn't add up, that was for sure, but I was more focused on having the identity I had so far been denied than trying to square my parents' circles. I simply continued making arrangements to leave home, possibly forever. The prospect of scandal was looming large in my father's consciousness and, it has to be admitted, in mine as well. The popular press was then obsessed with sex changes, the April Ashley case in particular having provided fantastical fodder throughout her divorce from Lord Rowallan's heir, the Honourable Arthur Corbett, and though I was not changing sex but merely obtaining the gender I should have had from birth, there was every possibility that the distinctions between the two cases might be lost and I might be billed as the first of the born patricians to have changed sex – April Ashley having come from a working-class background. Although I had a great deal of sympathy for people like April Ashley, who, in my view, hadn't had any more choice than I did, or indeed brown-eyed diabetics or perfectly healthy blue-eyed babies do in being born the way they are, I dreaded almost as much as Michael did the prospect of being turned into a newspaper sensation. Unlike him, however, I was not prepared to sacrifice my life to avoid it.

When children have unrealistic and egocentric parents, they either become like them and surrender to the lack of perspective which blows everything out of proportion as priorities get scrambled, or they develop level-headedness. This sense of proportion provides a touchstone with reality in compensation for what is lacking in their background. Although I still had some way to go to before becoming as level-headed as I now am, I was already well on the way without even realizing it. Therefore, I made no plans to return home or to deal with newspaper publicity if it should come my way or indeed to do anything but get myself on that plane to New York so that I could be united with my gender.

So what if Gloria didn't want to come with me? I didn't really want her to, if I were honest, for I could well do without her self-obsessed antics, even though I did think it was her maternal duty to come.

God and the surgeon, however, weren't sleeping; and the day after the operation, when the nursing staff discovered the trouble I had eating anything at all – it would take me an hour or two to get down a quarter of a small cup of jelly – the doctor refused to release me from the hospital except into the care of one of my parents. He emphasized to Frances that I was perilously close to the point of irreversible weight loss, which would result in death. He said that he would never have operated on me if he had known about my eating difficulties. Like everyone who has an operation, I had lost weight after it, and he had to protect himself against being held liable in the event that I now died.

Frances telephoned Gloria and Michael to give them the doctor's verdict. Michael told Gloria she had no choice but to fly to New York the following day. Ironically enough, the doctor then released me from the hospital prior to her arrival on the strength of the fact that she was coming. So Frances and I could well have pretended that she was coming when she was not. Neither of us would have done something so underhand, however.

I was watching television in the sitting room of the apartment Frances shared with her sister Belle when Gloria arrived from the airport. Once she saw that I was the only person at home, she dropped the mask of agreeable charm which she had had in place and let rip. She was royally cheesed off that Frances, who was not yet home from work, had not taken time off to pick her up from the airport, so she had been faced with the bother of taking a taxi from JFK to the Bacal apartment. Having got that off her chest, she turned the fusillade in my direction, moaning about what a 'nuisance' I was, how she was 'sick and tired of all the problems' associated with me and how 'inconvenient' it was that that 'blasted doctor had dragged' her 'from the comfort of home' to New York.

I cannot deny I was cut to the quick. Hurt fought with a sense of injustice jostling with indignation, but nevertheless I started to apologize, explaining that it hadn't been my choice or Frances's but the doctor's. I explained that he was simply trying to protect himself against a possible lawsuit in the event of my death from anorexia. 'No one ever died of starvation in the midst of plenty,' she sneered, jumping on her authoritative soapbox and dismissing his concerns as so much rubbish. 'Just you make sure that you don't get in my way while I'm here. Since I've been dragged up here quite unnecessarily, I intend to enjoy myself. Make sure you keep out of my way. Do you understand me, child?' she rasped.

'Yes, Mummy,' I said with more compliance than I felt.

'Now go and fix a gin and tonic the way I like it. I'm dying of thirst,' she ordered. So I trotted into the kitchen, the farcicality of the situation firmly tugging me between laughter and outrage. Fortunately for the sake of peace, I chose to 'rise above' my mother's inconsideration. Frances came home, and Gloria – 'in her element' (her words, not mine) – turned her attention to the serious business of enjoying herself. She pumped Frances for information about what were the latest plays worth seeing and which restaurants they ought to go to.

'Do you think Georgie's up to all of this?' Frances naïvely enquired.

'Well, if she's not, we leave her here,' she replied as if the alternative of staying in with me were beyond contemplation.

'Do you feel you're up to coming?' Frances asked me, knowing something of what sort of person Gloria was.

'I'm sure I can manage going to dinner, though I don't know about sitting for a length of time in the theatre.' I replied.

'Let's go to dinner tomorrow evening,' Frances suggested. 'Maybe Georgie will be able to get down some of that chicken cacciatore she used to like so much.'

Gloria shot her and me an irritated look, as if to say: 'Don't bore me with this'.

'Book us some tickets for a few shows,' she said. 'Georgie can stay here and rest.' With that, she steered the conversation away from me back to her social diary and the activities with which she wished to fill it.

Having exhausted that subject, she turned her attention to something even nearer to her heart.

'Can you arrange to take me to that wholesale diamond house we went to when I was up here to enrol Georgie at school? I'd like to see if they have anything I can tempt myself with.'

Frances duly made the arrangements the following day; and the day after that Belle and Gloria left to visit the Belensky Brothers in the Diamond District. They came back several hours later, Gloria's excited chatter telling me how well things had gone even before she had properly set foot in the apartment. I of course was then obliged to fetch her the inevitable glassful of gin splashed with a *soupçon* of tonic. In a ploy typical of the way she controlled her children and close relations, she declined to provide me with any information of what she had bought, and when Belle started to tell me she cut her off and changed the subject. Yet, when Frances came home from work, she regaled her with the tale of her purchases, which she then spread out for her to see: a large pear-shaped diamond engagement ring with baguettes on the side set in platinum; a dinner ring consisting of clusters of diamonds set in white gold; a diamond watch bracelet, with the watch-face concealed beneath a cover of diamonds so that it looked like a bracelet while performing as a timepiece, set in platinum; and a parure of rubies and diamonds set in yellow gold.

'Michael is going to kill me,' she said, her statement more a boast than a complaint. 'I simply couldn't say no, even though I didn't have nearly enough money to pay for everything.'

Belle laughed. 'They know Michael's good for the money.'

'He's not going to be thrilled that I bought so many things,' she said truthfully. Michael was always complaining that Gloria's love of jewels was excessive and that 'she'll drive me into the poor house'.

'But he'll have no choice but to pay once I go back and tell him what he owes them,' she said.

'Didn't you bring any money?' I asked naïvely.

'Of course I did. That's what I bought the two rings with,' volunteered Gloria, unusually for her.

'You paid for the watch bracelet as well,' Belle reminded her. 'It's only the ruby and diamond suite that hasn't been paid for. Remember, Gloria?'

I saw a flicker of something behind Gloria's inscrutably bright expression. Here we go again, I thought, wondering what my mother was now up to. No sooner was Belle out of the room than I found out.

'Come into the bedroom with me,' she whispered. 'I have something I want to say to you.'

Once safely inside the bedroom she was using, she shut the door behind us and motioned towards the bed, indicating that I should sit on it. She stood over me.

'This is going to be our little secret,' she said gently, conspiratorially. 'I used the money that was left over from the operation to buy the diamond watch bracelet.'

I knew that something was left over. The surgery had turned out to be much easier, once the doctor had opened me up, than he had anticipated, with the result that I had been in the operating theatre for half the allotted length of time. That saved on theatre costs. Furthermore, because nature had been kinder to me than he had envisaged, my stay in the hospital had been cut from a week to three days.

It now turned out that Gloria had got her mother and sister to make contributions well in excess of the $5,000 I thought the three of them had made, with the result that there were several thousand dollars left over.

'But Mummy, that money should rightly be returned to Grandma and Auntie or then turned over to me. It was given to me, so it's my money,' I said.

'Look here, child, you need my goodwill if you're going to have anything approaching a normal life. I've been mightily inconvenienced by your goddamned problems for many a year, and it's time I got something for my trouble. If you know what's good for you, you'll keep your trap shut. If I ever hear you've broken faith with me and let your grandmother, aunt or father know about our little secret, you'll wish I'd shut my legs and crushed your skull when you were coming out of the birth canal. Now go and get me a gin and tonic,' she said in an evocation of her oft-stated boast that she was 'as cold and impersonal as the grave'.

The worst, however, was not yet over. A day or two later, Gloria accompanied me to the doctor for my post-surgical check-up. After the examination, he showed us into his office, where he had a typewriter.

'You'll need to have your papers changed,' he said. 'I'm going to give you a letter that reflects the medical facts.'

He then sat down, typed the salient facts concisely and handed this document to me. I took it, read it and passed it to my mother for her to see it while he took out an envelope. Gloria extended her hand to receive it.

'I'll keep this,' she announced, playing the concerned mother. 'It's far too important for a child to have. She might lose it.'

With that, she folded the letter and placed it in the envelope he had handed to her, then slipped it into her handbag. Meanwhile, I was thanking him and he was saying that he would like to see me again in two weeks, after which Gloria and I departed.

'Can I please have the letter, Mummy?' I asked, once we were outside. 'I'll need it to get through Customs and Immigration and ultimately to change my birth certificate.'

'Absolutely not. You don't think I'd be mad enough to let a child have responsibility for such an important document? Frances can get photocopies of it, and I'll keep the original safe and sound. You never know when you might need the original. Learn one thing, child: one never lets an original go unless one has to.'

Little did I know it, but Gloria had seized this important document, not to protect me but to prevent me from using it. The fact I did not cotton on to her was partly due to her subtlety. 'I am so subtle I have gone beyond subtlety to *subtility*,' she used to declaim, using a word she knew did not exist to convey the thought none of us wished to face.

I know that I share some of the blame for not seeing through Gloria.

Although she was careful to conceal her game plans, over the years she had provided enough clues to her intrinsic Machiavellianism for someone as astute as I to arrive at an accurate assessment of her venality. I like to believe, however, that my failure to do so was actually born of a virtue and not a vice, and that my inability to see how and why she was using that doctor's original document as a blocking instrument was because people with a heart find it almost impossible to contemplate how people without one can function so heartlessly. That is the advantage the antisocial personality has over the social one.

In 1970, however, much of what was to follow had not yet taken place. Nevertheless, Gloria was laying the ground carefully and cleverly, having realized, as I did, how important that medical document was. She surrendered possession of it only long enough for Frances to take it into her office and photocopy it, after which she handed me two of the photocopies and told me to use them to get through Immigration.

A few days later, Gloria and I flew out of New York to Toronto. Libby and Ben were living in nearby London, Ontario, and she had decided to 'park' me with them and give herself, ever the inveterate traveller, a chance to see a place she had never been to before prior to returning home to Michael.

I am not sure exactly when Gloria noticed that she had got rid of one daughter who was competition only to find herself saddled with another. Possibly it was while we were in New York and several of her friends were commenting on how beautiful they thought I was. Or possibly it was after we had flown up to Canada, and the stewardess, not knowing why I was leaving the aircraft in a wheelchair, asked with obvious concern and some curiosity how I was. Upon being told by Gloria that I was simply recovering from relatively minor surgery but couldn't stand for the length of time it would ordinarily take to clear Customs and Immigration, she replied how glad she was that I wasn't seriously ill for she thought I was 'one of the most beautiful sights I've ever seen and I'd wondered if maybe she was gravely ill'.

Until Gloria had seen me in New York and Canada, she had never actually witnessed me fully dressed and made-up, because I had been banned in Jamaica from being properly togged up by my parents. So she had really had no idea of the impact my looks had on others.

Now, however, she did. We hadn't been at Ben and Libby's apartment for more than an hour when, out of thin air, she launched into me, sneering that

I was a 'freak' and she was 'sick to death' of me. She had never before referred to me in such terms, and I was profoundly shocked and far more upset than I had been when my father had spoken of me in a like manner. I started to protest tearfully, and she cut me off in much the same way she had dismissed Mickey and Libby over the years. So I retired to my bedroom for the night, furious, perplexed, hurt and mystified as to the reason for her attack.

The following day, however, everything was back to normal and, not connecting up the dots, I failed to see that the attention my looks were receiving meant that I had triggered her 'seek and destroy' mechanism the way Libby's looks had. I mistakenly marked her conduct down to having been in a bad mood, dismissed it as an aberration and gratefully dropped the thought, with all its attendant odiousness.

Little did I know that this was the harbinger of what was to come. Gloria had found herself another enemy, another competitor to see off: another daughter to destroy. This time she wouldn't stop until she had tried to ruin my looks – literally ruin them.

Chapter Fourteen

The 1970s were a period of momentous change not only in my life but also in Jamaica's. There had been pockets of civil unrest since the student riots of 1968, and as the date of the next general election approached in 1972, the island, always intensely political, erupted into sectarian violence, with supporters of the ruling Jamaica Labour Party and the opposition People's National Party embarking on furious gun battles on their 'patches' in downtown Kingston. These areas, such as Trench Town, became bywords for violence all over the world and through the songs of Bob Marley and Jimmy Cliff spread the gospel that only political conflict could result in political empowerment. Large areas of downtown Kingston became no-go areas, even – indeed especially – for the police. Uptown, where the élite lived, life went on in much the same way as before.

Beneath the graciousness and lavishness which typified upper-class Jamaican life, however, there was anxiety reminiscent of the pre-Independence days. Once more people started talking about the possibility of a coming 'revolution', except that this time it was ominously linked to the intentions of Michael Manley, the leader of the PNP. 'He's a communist,' many people said and cast their eyes ninety miles to the north towards Cuba, where Fidel Castro ruled, as an awful warning of what would happen to us if Jamaica went the way of our neighbour.

In the years since Castro had come to power, too much had happened in the West Indies for sophisticated Jamaicans to repeat the pre-Independence error of thinking we would be rescued from our fate by the benevolence of a greater power. If Britain had been Pontius Pilate when the time to protect our interests had come in the early 1960s, America was viewed as worse: inept and insular. One only needed to look at the pig's ear they had made of the Bay of Pigs to see that they couldn't even launch an effective invasion on an island where they already had a military base. 'If they can't dislodge Castro when they already have Guantanamo Bay,' people started saying, 'what hope will there be for them to overthrow Michael Manley if he too turns Jamaica communist, when they don't have a foothold here?' Wisely, the Jamaican Haves understood that they would have to fend for themselves and started to make plans accordingly. That translated into liquidating sufficient assets to give themselves a nest-egg abroad – usually in the United States or Canada and occasionally in Britain – in case they had to flee.

While the Haves were uptown facing the prospect of ruin, and the Have-nots were downtown fighting their turf wars, I had to consider whether to return to the land of my birth. If I did, I opened myself up to the very real threat of newspaper publicity. This would damage my ability to lead a normal life in the future. The world in which I was born and raised had an abiding horror of any publicity which went beyond glowing mentions in social columns or birth, death, engagement and marriage announcements. I would, in all likelihood, find it difficult to live down the 'scandal' that newspaper publicity would be regarded as, for the prevailing ethos in upper-class circles was that anything is acceptable as long as it doesn't spill out into the public domain. On the other hand, if I returned home and there was no newspaper publicity, I stood a good chance of living down my upbringing as a boy. I had no ambition to do anything but lead the life into which I had been born, namely that of a socially acceptable young lady whom the magic of matrimony would convert into a socialite matron the way my mother and aunt had been.

If there was one virtue my difficulties had given me, it was a level-headed comprehension of reality. When people said I was courageous, as they had taken to doing by this time, I always explained: 'It's not so much that I'm courageous as that I know from bitter experience that everyone pays the price for any decision, for any action and inaction that they and others take. The price of courage is seldom higher than the price of cowardice. In fact, life has taught me that it is usually lower. So one may as well be courageous, not out of bravery, but because it's the most sensible way to lead one's life.'

Although Jamaica might be experiencing problems, it was still my country and the life of an exile did not appeal to me. Therefore, when I returned to New York from Canada for my check-up with the doctor, I had to decide whether I wished to spend the rest of my life avoiding Jamaica just because I ran the risk of triggering a scandal. To my way of thinking, I had done nothing wrong, so why should I avoid a place I had more right to than most? The prospect of leading the rest of my life skulking around in foreign parts, as if I had done something shameful when I had not, had no appeal. Indeed, it offended my sense of justice and dignity. I decided that the best way to face my future was to do so head-on. If there was going to be a scandal, let's get it over with so I could then know what I was dealing with. And if there was not one, so much the better. Thereafter, I would be able to live in the light, without fear of the shadow-land that living with a 'secret' brings in its wake. As far as I was concerned, I had had quite enough of living in limbo to last me a lifetime, and I was not going to be relegated to another version of it so soon after I had managed to work myself free of the last form.

All I now needed to do was ask my parents whether they wanted me to return home, for such a course of action might well have consequences for them as well, and I very well couldn't return without their assent. Before I even had a chance to bring up the subject, my father telephoned me in New York to tell me he wanted me to return home before Christmas because, as he put it, 'Your mother is lonely.' There were no children at home, Mickey, Libby and I being respectively in England, Canada and the United States, and Kitty being at her convent boarding school. I knew that he was as terrified of a public scandal as I was, though Gloria was blithely indifferent to whether there was one or not. This, together with the need for me to return and be Gloria's companion, thereby releasing him from babysitting duties and giving him the freedom to do as he pleased, provided a calming effect upon Michael and, I must admit, upon me as well. So I agreed to return, filled though I was with misgivings.

Unlike her husband and daughter, Gloria seemed to be looking forward to the dramatics associated with my return to Jamaica after such a profound transformation. Whether there was a scandal or not, this was just too good a drama for her to miss out on. She was doubtless relishing the attention being the mother of the talked-about Georgie Ziadie was bringing in its wake, for I was the hot topic in smart circles. So much so that friends would subsequently regale me with stories about strangers making the most bizarre assertions of close acquaintanceship with me, just so that they too could lay claim to knowing me. For the first, though by no means last, time in my life, I was discovering that when one is the flavour of the month, truth and accuracy fly out of the window, to be replaced by false claims and untrue stories, some of which are so weird that you really cannot help laughing at them.

If I was disinclined to condemn strangers for their pretensions, that was only because my own mother was cannily milking the interest in me for its dramatic worth. Before my plane had even touched down at Palisadoes Airport, various people had let me know that Gloria's response to the chatter was to cast herself as a stalwart martyr to a cruel life, telling all and sundry how *she* had suffered over the years as a result of having had a child with a 'matter' like mine. My own suffering, of course, was ignored. Once when I called her on it later on, she actually had the gall to tell me: 'A mother always feels the pain of her children more acutely than they themselves do. Just because I'm not vulgar enough to parade my heart on my sleeve doesn't mean that I don't feel things deeply.' I refrained from responding, but I knew that she had felt my suffering about as acutely as Tiberius felt Mary's after Jesus was crucified.

As Gloria prepared for the starring role she had allotted herself in this for-once-genuine drama in a life filled with histrionics in which the most mundane and ordinary events were blown into extraordinary extravaganzas, I swallowed long and hard and headed for home.

When I returned, I immediately saw how Gloria intended to cope with a situation that cried out for explanation. She acted as if it's an everyday occurrence for a girl to be assigned the male gender for twenty-one years of life, then, as if the world is a magician's stage and the cloak is flamboyantly pulled aside to reveal the treasure of feminine pulchritude that was always lurking underneath it. 'The doctor who performed the operation said it was a sin that it hadn't been done years before,' she casually told all and sundry, paraphrasing what he had actually said, which was that it was a 'pity' it had not been done years ago. I could also see that she was implicitly criticizing Michael by making out that he alone had been responsible for the unconscionable delay. If she wanted to poke him in the eye while standing up for me, I reasoned that it was only what he deserved, though with time, I have come to see that what she was really doing was garnering sympathy for herself for being married to such an insensitive man while at the same time misleading me and others into believing that she had provided me with support when she actually provided none. It was a clever rewriting of history and is one of the many instances of the disloyal self-aggrandizement which would ultimately lead me to conclude that she was conscienceless as well as a classical narcissist to behave as she did.

Whatever Gloria's motives, I was grateful to her for her show of support at this most vulnerable time of my life. That is, until her sensationalistic streak got the better of her, and I caught her exaggerating what I had been through to enthralled visitors. 'With due respect,' I said to her, right in front of her audience, 'since no one else here would consider it appropriate for us to be discussing their private parts, I must insist that the same courtesy be extended to me too.'

'What a way you're touchy,' she said airily, laughing off my reprimand.

'No I'm not,' I said furiously. 'I am merely a human being with human feelings and even though that fact was ignored for the first twenty-one years of my life, it doesn't mean that you or anyone else should ignore it ever again.'

It's interesting how people react when you speak a palpable truth. You would have thought I had slapped the face of each and every one whom she was regaling. The air was suffused with embarrassment, not only because I had justly reprimanded my sensationalistic mother but also because I had unmasked their prurient appreciation of her violation of my right to dignity and privacy.

In fact, the only person present who did not display any embarrassment whatsoever was Gloria. Nevertheless, my scolding had the desired effect. Like many sensationalists, she was acutely attuned to the sensory temperature of her audience, and she changed the subject immediately, much to the relief of everyone present. For the remainder of her life, she never brought it up again when I was present, unless she was using it as a tool of blackmail or control, though I have reason to believe she dined out on it as and when it suited her purposes.

By January 1971, I had been back in Jamaica for nearly two months. To my immense relief, there had been no newspaper publicity, and though I did not yet know in which country I wanted to live, as long as I was at home, I would, of course, reside with my parents. That was the practice with young ladies of my generation. Only 'sluts' or spinsters long past the age of eligibility – which meant their thirties – moved away from home. All others stayed until they walked down the aisle. I was not about to buck that custom, for I saw only too clearly that doing so would add a question mark about my marital desirability, conveying the message that my family and I believed that my past had rendered me unmarriageable.

In fact, within weeks of returning home, the reception I had been accorded by one and all was so positive that it quickly became apparent that I was regarded as marriageable. That was a huge relief to my father because he soon made it clear he wanted me off his hands as quickly as possible, and to me because, like every other girl of my age and station, I had only one ambition in life: to be married.

As normality sprinkled its golden dust on my life, I took the necessary steps to regularize my legal status. After all, I could hardly travel without incident on a passport that said male, nor walk up the aisle with a man unless my birth certificate were corrected to provide my true gender. I made enquiries and discovered that the procedure was relatively simple. My parents had to swear a Statutory Declaration confirming that I had been mistakenly registered at the time of my birth owing to a physical defect. This they now did in front of Metry Seaga, their good friend who was also a justice of the peace and uncle of Eddie Seaga, Jamaica's finance minister at the time and subsequently its prime minister. The following day, I made an appointment with the Registrar of Births, Deaths and Marriages, and the day after that I drove to Spanish Town, the ancient capital of Jamaica where the Registry was located. I met with her, and after I had handed over the photocopy of the doctor's letter together with the Statutory Declaration, she said, whether through compassion or because it was true: 'There must be something in the water that causes cases like yours. We've had several over the years so we're now practised at dealing with them.' She then informed me that my papers would thereafter be kept under lock and key to preserve my privacy. She asked if I had ten minutes to spare or whether I wanted her to post me my new documents, and when I said I'd take them, walked across the room and pulled out a blank document.

'This is a Short Form Birth Certificate,' she explained. 'We use it mostly for adopted children but also for corrections like yours. You see, by law we can't change a birth certificate, only amend it, and since the Long Form will have all your previous and present details, you should use this instead. There's no embarrassing information on it.' As she was explaining, she wrote out my name, Georgia Arianna Ziadie, my sex, female, my date of birth, August 17 1949, and handed it to me. I was home and dry. Legally and indisputably I was finally being acknowledged for what I truly was.

Once this process was over, I was filled with gratitude for having been born in the country I was. No matter how awful Jamaica's reputation was becoming worldwide, the fact remained that Jamaicans were by and large warm, compassionate and humane.

By the time I left her office, I could see that, important though the procedure had been, it had also been straightforward and not the big deal my parents had for so long represented it as being. I tried to suppress the thought that something as simple as this could and should have been done years before it had been, and, to an extent, I succeeded, for it would not have been possible to have a relationship with my parents if I held things against them. And I wanted to have a normal relationship with both of them. Little did I know that I was bashing my head against a brick wall, not because of Michael, who settled down to being a fairly okay father once the deed was done, but because of Gloria.

If there was something anticlimactic about the regularization of my legal position, there was nothing ordinary about the way society reacted to my presence once word got out that I had returned to Jamaica and was supposedly a ravishing beauty. Overnight, everyone who didn't know me wanted to meet me. One such person was Nell Bourke, an American telephone heiress who had married Pat Bourke, brother of Jennifer who was married to Robert Shaw the movie star and the son of Greta Fowler, who owned Priory School, where Kitty was due to follow Libby to do her 'A' Levels later that year. Nell asked Libby, with whom she was friendly, to arrange a meeting between us. I did not mind, for I had heard a lot of positive things about her from my sister, but Libby was furious. 'Don't go. How dare she turn you into an object of curiosity?'

While I could sympathize with Libby's point of view, the fact was, people were curious about what had happened to me, and, had I been in their shoes, I would have been as well. Without pandering directly to their curiosity, I had nothing against them seeing that I was as normal as anyone else – and if they also wanted to rave about my looks, as they had now started to do, so much the better.

When you're twenty-one and living at the centre of a social event that has the possibility of blowing up in your face and ruining the rest of your life, you don't stop to think how you developed the tools to get through the attention that is, at best, a mixed blessing. Although I did not analyze or indeed recognize it at that time, I was using my egotistical mother's stylish – if self-centred – sweep through life as a coping device. All my life I had seen Gloria accept the attention she managed to orchestrate and generate as if it were her due. This she had done not only with an attitude of entitlement but also with dignity and grace, and while I disliked the intense attention I got for the first few months after I returned home, and rose above it as best I could, it was simply a variation on the negative attention living in limbo had generated throughout my teenage years. So I continued to accommodate it exactly as I had in the past. Subsequently, friends and relations would say I displayed a remarkable level of grace; and if I did, I can only say that I owe a partial debt of gratitude to my mother, for it was she who provided me with the role model for gracious acceptance of attention.

Another leaf I had taken out of her book, without then being aware of it, was the technique of deflecting unwanted subjects of conversation. All my life I had seen her ignore what she did not deign to acknowledge, and to do so with such grace that people could not even accuse her of disdain. I had adopted a similar attitude while living in limbo to avoid anyone embarrassing me by raising the matter of my upbringing. As far as I was concerned, it was a no-go area, akin to that of a friend of the Bacals who had been in Auschwitz. Although everyone knew what had happened to her, she never discussed the subject, not because she was ashamed of it, but because it was so painful and emotive that the only way to keep it in its proper place was to relegate it to the past and leave it there, where it belonged. I felt exactly the same way about what I had been through. Though I never denied it, speaking about it was too distressing. Indeed, anything but the most delicate allusion was so upsetting I was determined not to be sucked into reliving and revealing my pain just so I could gratify people's curiosity, no matter how valid it was.

There were times, of course, when it became necessary to allude to what had happened to me. I was not my mother, and I had no desire to cut a swathe through life dominating all proceedings and acting as if I was the only person on earth whose concerns should be considered. So I developed a few stock sentences to explain the situation in as non-violating a manner as possible: a policy I have adhered to throughout my life with the result that the only time my 'history' is ever raised is when the subject of birth defects or handicaps are under discussion, or in press interviews, when journalists bring it up, little realizing how they stomp over ground that others recognize as too tender to tread upon. At all other times, my birth defect simply isn't an issue, and as I get older, I can see how sensible I was to refuse to let it become one by giving it more attention than it deserved.

Coping well with scandal requires a refusal to acknowledge the unsavoury possibilities that lurk beneath the surface, and by this time I was more adept at that task than most of my elders and just about all of my contemporaries. This was partly because such skills had been perfected in my mother's family over the centuries. Not only had she had to ignore talk about her 'boyfriends', and her mother had had to present a serene face to the world as her adultery was discussed in drawing rooms for twenty-five years before it was splashed over the pages of the gutter press, but Gloria's maternal great-grandmother had also been involved in a society scandal in the nineteenth century, so I really was fortunate in having been born into a family with a track record of 'rising above it'.

Nevertheless, I was acutely aware of how uncomfortable one felt every time one showed one's face in public: how every time one entered a room, one had to compose oneself to act as if one was just another person, even though one knew people were gossiping about one. Towards the end of Gloria's life, when I was curious to discover what had made her tick, I tried to find out if her *sang froid* concealed as many emotions as my display of that trait had done. The terms in which she replied made it clear that what lurked beneath was every bit as cool as the face she showed to the public. This I found chilling and rather sad, and I could well understand why she had been so miserable, for people who feel very little can't be fulfilled.

Just as Michael and I were beginning to relax about the threat of publicity, his niece Doreen arrived at the house one evening with a story which brought an end to our fear. She worked at the *Gleaner*, the nation's leading newspaper, as the editor Theodore Sealey's secretary. 'You will never believe what happened today,' she said after dinner. 'Someone rang up Ted Sealey and asked him why he wasn't writing about Georgie. People are too much, don't you think? But he was ready and waiting for them. He said, "I could never do that to Gloria Ziadie's daughter. Not after all she's done for charity." Afterwards, he said to me: "Isn't Mr Ziadie your mother's brother?" I said yes. He said: "Go and tell them no newspaper in Jamaica will ever write about their daughter.

I'll make sure of that."You can relax about Georgie, Uncle Mike. She's safe.'

We were all delighted. Michael and I because of our lucky escape, Gloria because she was being given credit for it and for many years afterwards never missed an opportunity to let me know how her charity work had spared us all from the ignominy of a public scandal.

Finally, I could afford to let the sunshine in. So I set about leading my life with a confidence I had lacked as long as the cloud of scandal hung over me.

At first, it looked as if the future that all girls of my background were supposed to have might fall into my lap with extraordinary ease. Within two months of my return to Jamaica, two of the country's most eligible bachelors declared an interest in me. Although I would sooner have died a virgin than contemplate anything but escape from the first, the second was another matter altogether. His name was Maurice Shoucair. He was the scion of a well-known family and was in fact a distant cousin of my father's. I had met him once or twice years before but knew him so slightly I wouldn't even have recognized him had he not been introduced to me at a party given by my old friends Andrew Melville and his then wife, Pam Seaga.

Like all well-bred men of good family, Maurice knew that the way to a parent's heart was by impeccable behaviour, so he asked for my father's permission to take me out. Michael said yes. 'You could do a lot worse than marry him,' added Gloria, always central to every issue. 'He's from a good family, and everyone says he's a very nice person. Unusually for a Shoucair, he's also good looking.'

Then she went to the hairdresser and, doubtless while gossiping about me, was informed by one of the ladies there that Maurice's father SN had left the bulk of his considerable fortune to the elder brother, Eddie. This was unusual in Mediterranean families, who functioned under the principle of the *Code Napoléon* whereby all children are left a proportionate share of the estate. That was all Gloria needed to hear to put her foot down. She came home full of mystery, hinting that she had a secret which she was hugging to her bosom. Then Michael returned home from work, and she launched into an account of what she had been told. When I said that I already knew that SN had left Eddie the lion's share and didn't care whether Maurice had money or not, she said: 'Don't you think you've caused enough scandal already? You cannot and will not go out with a married man.'

'He's not married,' I said.

'Have you seen his divorce absolute? No. I thought you hadn't. You cannot go out with a married man. That's all I have to say.'

'Oh, for God's sake, Mummy, do stop being such a hypocrite,' I said impatiently. 'We all know you don't give a fig about whether he's divorced yet or not. The money – or lack of it – is all you care about.'

Gloria shot me a look of absolute hatred. I had dared to challenge her and worse, to speak the unvarnished truth while doing so.

'It's your reputation I care about,' she said, denying the undeniable.

'Oh, come on,' I said, getting annoyed. 'Yesterday you were full of how suitable Maurice was and today, after going to Veronica's and hearing about SN's will, you object on the grounds that he's not divorced yet. If you're going to object, why don't you come clean and do so on the real grounds?'

'Your mother is right,' Michael said. 'If Maurice has no money and he has children to support, what sort of a husband will he make? You can't go out with him, and that's all there is to that.'

To say that I was furious is an understatement. Because there was a dearth of suitable bachelors who were my contemporaries, I now faced the prospect of either settling for someone I did not want, in the form of the first of the bachelors who had shown interest in me, or of playing a waiting game. Why, I reasoned, should I do so just because my mother was obsessed with money? Indeed, my siblings and I were all convinced that this was the reason she had married our father and had stayed with him.

Libby wrote to me from Canada and suggested that I sneak out and meet Maurice behind our parents' backs, but I would not do so. Partly this was because I did not want to alienate them but partly also because I had discovered that Maurice had a bad heart and 'with my luck, he'll die on top of me' as I wrote to Libby. So I hit the social scene, my objective according with what my parents wanted for me, and within a few weeks I had met the first of the series of suitable beaus I would have.

In life, one can't legislate for the spark that makes something special. Unless it happens of its own accord, there is nothing you can do to create it. At this point in time, my parents were not applying pressure on me to settle down, and I wanted someone I loved and who loved me. Marrying for advantage was anathema to me, and I have to admit I used my mother as an example of all I should avoid. Sure, Gloria had an attractive husband who loved her and sure, she had money and position, but really, she had nothing. I felt that a large part of her problem lay in the fact that she had chosen to live with a man she didn't really love while selling herself out for money and the means to support a gracious secular existence. Of course she hated the negative effects of such a dreadful bargain. But the choice had been hers, and I really didn't see how anyone – myself included – could escape from the negative consequences of what I regarded as marital prostitution.

By this time, I had scant sympathy for Gloria's choice, so I was hardly likely to make the same mistake. In fact, I was of the firm opinion that she would have been better off taking the alternative route the way some of her friends had done. Charles Matalon's stepmother Barbara, for instance, had left Charlie Fox with two young children and gone out and got a job rather than stay in a marriage she was not happy in. Gloria, I felt, could have done the same thing. She could have left Daddy, reduced her standard of living, moved to a smaller house, got a job and tried to make a life for herself and her children until she met someone else, just as Barbara had done. Even if she didn't, she could have become a 'gay divorcee' in the old-fashioned meaning of the word. But I knew that the thought had either never occurred to her, or then she had considered it and rejected it out of hand, because there was no way she was going to reduce her standard of living.

Later I would come to realize that Gloria had been wise, not because her choice had made her happy, but because the alternative would have made her no happier. Sadly, she lacked the ability to love a man. What she did possess, instead, was the ability to use a man as a marital meal-ticket. Any man, no matter how wonderful or obliging, would have been nothing more to her than that. The sad truth was that like all narcissists, she only wanted to use 'loved ones' for what she could get out of them, while at the same time despising them.

This proclivity carried over into Gloria's concept of 'romance'. Although Michael would have divorced her instantly if he had caught her cheating, he did not mind her having a lovelorn 'swain' in the tradition of the Renaissance 'lover'. Her lust for admiration certainly demanded that she not only have an adoring husband supporting her financially but also a worshipful beau professing undying love for her right in front of her husband. During her late twenties and early thirties, Tony Feanny and Frank Watson had fulfilled these roles. Although Vida MacMillan stated that Gloria admitted to being genuinely in love with Tony Feanny, it is arguable that she would have ultimately been any happier with him than she was with Michael, irrespective of the outcome of their relationship. Some people lack the capacity for real happiness, and I believe my mother was one of them. She had the emotional depth of a teaspoon, and I think her love for 'Uncle' Tony was more about romance and attention than the depth of feeling one needs if one is to have a fulfilling and successful long-term relationship.

If one considers that Tony was feeding Gloria's ego by being the lovelorn suitor who would never get to first base – a role which Michael must have fulfilled in the early days of their relationship before he tired of it, hence his toleration of some other schlump filling his shoes – it is entirely possible that she was speaking the truth when she denied ever being in love or sleeping with him.

Whatever the true nature of her relationship with 'Uncle' Tony, there is no doubt she was never in love with 'Uncle' Frank, as we children called the multimillionaire owner of a chain of betting shops which, ironically enough, Michael had refused to partner him in on the grounds that money from gambling would take the bread out of the mouths of poor people, so it was morally tainted.

For about four or five years after the reign of 'Uncle' Tony, 'Uncle' Frank was more than a prominent member of my parents' circle, He was ever-present, and there was no doubt he was sweet on Gloria. 'Frank Watson, you are too old and ugly for any woman to love,' she used to say to him, as she would dance and flirt with him, instructing him to 'come and give me a kiss' as she presented her cheek. She frequently regaled everyone with the story of how he had wanted to marry her when she was seventeen; how he had offered her £40,000 cash and a house in her own name (equivalent to several million dollars at today's rate) if she said yes; and how she had responded: 'What, marry an ugly old man like you? You're the same age as my father, you vain old goat.'

According to Uncle Frank's daughter Anne, he told her that he definitely had an affair with Gloria immediately after ending an affair with her friend Carmen McNaught. But his son Anthony says, 'Who knows? What I do know is that Daddy thought your father had the best manners of anyone he'd ever met. He used to say, "Michael Ziadie is the ultimate gentleman."'

Whether her relationships with both men were sexual or not, Gloria was always intensely self-interested, and I suspect that, even if she had been in love with Tony Feanny, there is no doubt that she never regarded Frank Watson as a feasible marital prospect. Even though he was richer than her husband, he was not good-looking – in our family good looks were a prerequisite along with social position and enough money not to ever have to think about it. 'Frank had been divorced for so long that he was too difficult to control,' she once told me. This meant that she couldn't wrap him around her little finger the way she wrapped Michael, and as Gloria herself used to admit: 'I don't tolerate people standing in my way.' 'Uncle' Frank finally was downgraded and married someone else. He and his wife remained on friendly terms socially with my parents, but you could tell that Gloria had lost any interest in him and was only going through the motions of civility on the odd occasions they got together. Afterwards, she would always pass some disparaging comment about him which called her sincerity into question.

Whether my mother had tried to swap husbands or not, I believed that she had destroyed her life – and to a large extent her family's happiness – with false values, and I was determined I would not follow in her footsteps. So, as I settled down to the serious business of husband hunting, I did not appreciate that I was simultaneously setting myself up as a target for someone who possessed all the competitiveness, envy, resentment of youth and loathing of aging, which are such pronounced aspects of the narcissistic personality.

Indeed, at first, I naïvely thought Gloria was enjoying having me at home with her. I did not realize that, while that may have been the head of the coin, the tail was developing in an altogether more negative tandem beneath the surface.

'Come and sit with me,' had always been one of her favourite refrains, and it was one I now heard yet again on a daily basis. Though there were pressures building beneath the surface which would pop up soon enough, I took at face value the easy companionability that seemed to have been restored to our relations.

This being an unusual period of relative calm and pleasantness, I let my guard down and dared to hope that the turbulence of the past was now behind us. Indeed, as I surveyed the scene, there were sufficient positive signs to hope that life was on an upswing not only for me personally but for the family as a whole. Although Gloria and Kitty were no closer than ever, when my little sister came home from boarding school for the holidays, Gloria did not interfere with the fun she had going to the Yacht Club; being up at the pool with her boyfriend; going out with her friends; or being ensconced in her bedroom nursing her ulcer (something she had endured since the age of twelve), the way she had with Libby. Whether our mother abided by a hands-off policy because Kitty was Michael's favourite and she knew he would not have tolerated the abuse the way he had with Mickey and Libby; or whether Gloria did not consider her an adversary because Kitty, though cute-looking, was not feted as a 'beauty' and therefore was not competition, the fact is, she let Kitty enjoy the life of a privileged young girl about town without trying to ruin her good time

During this period, Gloria's relationship with Libby even improved now that she was married and living abroad. Although one could not have called it cosy – if only because Libby could not forget that the woman who now presented herself as benign had previously been so malign – the mother-driven animosity was a thing of the past, and their relationship was superficially pleasant and respectful whenever Libby visited from Canada, which she did most winters.

This newfound harmony appeared to extend across the board when, early in 1971, Mickey returned home from England, having 'eaten his dinners at Grey's Inn', the vernacular for qualifying as a barrister. In a total *volte face*, Gloria treated him with respect and even got her friend Victor Grant, the Attorney General, to employ him as one of his two assistants.

Gloria even declined to use that old bugbear, transportation, as a stick with which to beat her son when it reared its head. Mickey's job required a measure of travelling to the country for rotating Magistrates' Courts. Otherwise, he was at the Attorney General's Department in Kingston. How he would get around became a problem; he did not have a car and it would have been unthinkable for him to take the bus or taxis. 'I don't believe in buying children cars,' said Michael, in a display of frugality which he would also apply to me as well. 'But what I'll do is give you the proceeds from an insurance policy which I took out when you were born to buy one for yourself.' Gloria nodded her head in benign acquiescence, her manoeuvrings regarding Scrammy and Audrey's Beetle a thing of the past.

So Mickey finally got himself a set of wheels that Gloria did not covet, and he settled down to a pleasant life in his native land for the first time since he had been born.

However, he made sure that he did not live with his parents.

'I'd never live there again,' he said, alluding to all that had happened before his sojourn in England. Instead, he lived with Maisie, who was quite determined that her treasured grandson would never be put in the line of fire again. So, once Mickey made it clear that he was back in Jamaica for good, she actually bought adjoining townhouses that were under construction – one in her name for her and Uncle Perez, the other in Mickey's name as a gift to him – and announced that she would sell her big house.

In the meantime, Grandma was absolutely thrilled to have 'Grandson' living with her. Gloria, meanwhile, acted as if she and Mickey had always been great friends. It chuffed her no end to say 'My son is the Assistant Attorney General and he's only twenty-three.' 'The Fool' had well and truly transmogrified into the Legal Beacon, and I looked on in fascination as my brother utilized the freedom men had in circles like ours to come and go as he pleased.

My movements, on the other hand, were as restricted as ever. The Sexual Revolution may have taken hold in the world at large, but as far as my father was concerned, his daughters' virtue was still something to 'protect'. Whenever I went out on a date, Michael would always let me into the house, looking me over from head to toe with ill-disguised intent to establish that I had not been 'tampered with'. It was so silly one couldn't take it seriously. Rather than feeling that my rights were being violated, I used to laugh about it and sometimes even hammed it up with him. To his credit, he used to smile sheepishly, not of course, that it stopped the inspection that or the next time.

With Mickey back on cordial terms with both parents; Libby safely married abroad and thereby deserving of respect; Kitty visiting home without any conflict; and with my problems sorted out, life seemed to have changed for the better. Not only did I let my guard down, but I was actually naïve enough to believe that the interest Gloria started to show in my activities was sincere. I suppose at twenty-one no one is so mature as to consider that another human being, especially a mother, is simply lying low and biding her time, watching to see how the land lies before she converts yet another child into her target.

Knowing that Gloria was an incorrigible romantic who loved to involve herself in the love affairs of others when she was not watching celluloid versions at the movies or on television, or casting herself as the central heroine over whom some lovesick swain was mooning, and believing that she was genuinely interested in my future, I surrendered to long girlie chats with her while she pumped me for information about this guy and that. These, I must confess, I thoroughly enjoyed. I noticed that she never gave advice or even passed an opinion beyond the most anodyne and noncommittal remarks, usually 'that's nice' or 'um' uttered with a slight smile. But that didn't strike me as ominous.

Had I known then what I know now about narcissism, I would have been able to see that the reason why she hid behind a mask of benign neutrality was that she was essentially indifferent to my fate and was simply using the conversations as time-filling entertainment, while gathering information which she could use against me as and when it suited her purposes. Libby did try warning me. 'Stop telling Mummy everything,' she'd say. 'No matter what you tell her today, she'll twist and turn tomorrow. You're making a big mistake. She can't be trusted.'

Although I did not tell Libby that I thought she was mistaken, I actually did think her bitter experience at Gloria's hands had so jaundiced her against our mother that she was misapplying it to my situation. As I saw it, our situations could not have been more dissimilar: I had always been Gloria's favourite child and she had been the dartboard. I therefore refused to allow her to influence me negatively and continued confiding in our mother, little understanding that my relationship with her was in a state of transition and it was only a matter of time before my new role as her latest target was revealed.

Ignorant of that fact, I had no idea that every time I filled Gloria in on a new event in my life, I was stoking the fires of her envy and competitiveness while also giving her information she could potentially use to my disadvantage in the future. Even when she did not use it, her display of interest was less about Georgie the person than about obtaining information. She loved being well-informed, not only about me but about anyone else whose life was of interest in the social orbit. 'Everyone confides in me,' had always been her proud boast. 'I know more secrets than anyone else.' There was more than a smidgen of truth to that statement, for she was a great friend whenever there was a drama – as long as those involved were socially desirable – and even after she died several people commented on how wonderful she had been while they were going through their divorces, affairs and scandals or whatever the peak points in their lives had been, death excepted. Gloria didn't 'do' death, except if she was immediately involved, such as with the deaths of her father and son. Otherwise death was too unglamorous for dramatic possibilities, and Gloria wasn't about to get herself bogged down in anything she couldn't convert into a drama or a pleasure.

Later on in life, I would run across other sensationalists and would then see the parallels between their conduct and my mother's. At this period in my life, however, I really did think that Gloria had turned over a new leaf, not only with me but with her other children and that our companionable relationship was as sincerely treasured on her side as it was on mine. I was truly delighted that we were back to a loving relationship into which I could relax, free of the watchfulness and caution I had been obliged to develop during my teenage years. I marked the difficulties of the past down to an extraordinary set of circumstances which would never be repeated and felt it was unfair to apply the standards required for ordinary life to such an unusual situation. Excusing her as I now excused my father, with whom I was already building a more cordial relationship free of the animosity of the past, I looked forward to a future in which my mother would indeed become one of my better friends.

As I examined the past, I even felt guilty about having had such a negative attitude towards Gloria over the previous five or six years. I came to the erroneous conclusion that I had misjudged her. Ignoring the evidence of her past conduct, I neglected to apply the lessons I should have learned by this time. I therefore discounted the fact that her vanity required her to be an integral part of all important happenings in her social circle; that her charm is what sucked people in; that when she was through with them she would spit them out and move on to the next novelty with no more interest in their ultimate well-being than she had in a block of cement; and that of course she would be interested in my activities, for I was one of the hottest tickets socially at that moment and she was definitely not going to deprive herself of being an integral part of that show. Mother-love might have had something to do with it, but no more than two or three percent, if that.

Lulled into a sense of false security, I even deliberated with Gloria over where I should live. Masculine pickings in Jamaica were so slim I really could not see how staying there would result in matrimony unless I was incredibly lucky and someone fell out of the sky like manna. There simply were no men of the right age and background available, whom I found attractive. As life had taught me not to trust to luck, and settling for some rich but boring older man did not appeal to me after the rush of desirable beaus I had encountered in New York, including top athletes and socialites, I could not see how remaining in Jamaica would lead to anything but protracted spinsterhood. Time, moreover, was of the essence not only because the clock was ticking and I had arrived at the ancient age of twenty-one without that magical wedding certificate to provide me with the stamp of approval that all girls of my generation regarded as the most important thing in life but also because the safe harbour matrimony was supposed to be had great appeal for me after the stormy seas of my past.

Of course, I could have jumped on the bandwagon that many of my generation were on and expanded my options to include coloured or black men, but this had little appeal for two major reasons. Firstly, such a union would have been anathema to my parents; and secondly, the only men I found attractive were a particular type of Caucasian. There was no way I was going to kiss, much less marry, a man I didn't fancy.

Faced with that matrimonial dilemma, I settled into my new life in Jamaica with the view that it was more a holiday than anything permanent. Only too soon, however, I was bored rigid. Living in the lap of luxury with nothing to do except chat with your mother and visit friends and go to parties, restaurants or nightclubs night after night might seem desirable, but I can assure you, those attractions quickly pall unless one is unnaturally lazy or unintelligent. It induces *ennui*, and with that, life loses its otherwise natural sparkle. So I looked around for something to do. Although Gloria made it obvious that she was happy for me to stay at home keeping her company, Michael was providing an inadvertent incentive to further activity by being anything but Mr Generosity in terms of an allowance. He was providing me with the princely sum of five pounds a week, which went no further than buying the cigarettes I chain-smoked. Even if I didn't have to pay for rent, food, petrol, clothes, shoes or any of the everyday things other girls had to, I couldn't even go for lunch with a girlfriend without asking Gloria to subsidize the activity.

Turning to my newest confidante, I discussed with her what I should do. Should I get a job or should I go into business as a freelance dress designer? Gloria advised me to go into business. 'You can have a boutique. I'll get your father to back you. We'll have only the most exclusive clientele and I'll drop in as and when I can and help you out. We'll serve champagne and canapés to the customers, all of whom we must vet carefully.' Ye Gods, I screamed to myself, she's planning to take over my business before it's even in existence.

Had I planned to stay in Jamaica, I would have scratched Gloria's idea on the grounds that it would become a ball and chain. Instead, I quietly went about my original idea of being a freelance dress designer and spread the word amongst friends that I would be available for one-off commissions. I also freelanced designs to the fashionable boutiques, just as I had done in New York, and modelled: something I had also done in New York. As the orders poured in, Gloria kept me company while I sewed. Whether I wanted her to or not, she sat with me; and only too soon the past was reasserting itself and the total focus of her monologue was her own preoccupations. At no time was she ever speaking to all my father's sisters, and whichever one was the enemy of the moment would be the target for her bile. It didn't take long for me to get the message. She was as oppressive as ever and too reliant on my companionship for comfort or good health.

It had never taken me long to get the picture, and the one I was now getting was that I had better find a way to move out of my mother's orbit unless I wanted to be stifled by her. Out of nowhere I received the catalyst I needed. His name was Bill and he was six foot three inches tall, well-built, athletic, blond, with green eyes and more sex appeal than anyone should be allowed to have. Even before I discovered that he was from a socially acceptable American family, I knew from his demeanour that he was a gentleman. Even if he had not been, I would not have cared less, for he was the most sexually appealing man I had ever met – or indeed have ever met.

Luck must have been on my side, because I met Bill by accident. I had gone out with various cousins to the Jonkanoo Lounge, then a fashionable watering hole, to kill time, as one did rather more of than was good for one in those days. One of my cousins knew one of his group, though this was almost unnecessary. As soon as I walked into the Jonkanoo Lounge, our eyes locked, and even before Elaine and Billy started talking, Bill and I were edging towards each other in what were the opening steps of a torrid ritual.

Although Bill was returning to New York the following day, he was due back in Jamaica in a few weeks. He was helping to set up a carpet factory for Monsanto, the conglomerate for which he worked. So began a relationship which I soon saw would please my parents as much as me if it should lead to marriage. I decided to move back to New York to give it whatever chance it had to develop.

My parents responded to my decision to return to New York in different ways. 'How do you propose getting from here to there?' Gloria asked acidly, betraying her irritation at losing her companion. 'Your father and I are sick and tired of paying for you to travel the world as if you are a millionairess.' I needed to hear no more to know that she would not be helping me to jump ship.

In the seven months since I had come back to Jamaica, I had made quite a name for myself as a dress designer and model. This I now used to advantage. Air Jamaica had the distinction of being the only airline with an in-flight fashion show. One of my friends did their public relations, so I asked her if they would be interested in swapping designs for tickets. Maxine said 'yes'. All I needed to do was make the twelve garments they required for my first-class return ticket to New York.

My father's response was also telling. 'I'm not go…going to stand in your wa…way if you want to go. Kitty will soon be here per…permanently, to keep your mother company.' So there we had the unvarnished truth in two sentences. My financially-flush father, who had tried to handicap me with penury so that I would remain a captive audience for the wife whose company he found too burdensome to share except in the most limited way, was not prepared to offer me any financial assistance while I was abroad, not even the paltry five pounds a week he gave me as pocket money. I could go if I wished, not because he cared whether I was here or there, but because my presence in Jamaica was no longer necessary. Kitty would be leaving boarding school in a matter of weeks to live at home for the first time since she was five years old. She would be attending The Priory School in September to study for her 'A' Levels. The role of babysitter would therefore be filled. I had become redundant – at least as far as Michael was concerned.

The cold draught of my parents' selfishness had once more blown my way, but I still wasn't ready to get the message. Instead of seeing them for the insensitive, self-centred people they were, I dismissed their meanness, in the face of all that money, as a desire on their part to encourage me to become financially independent. Where I got that noble motive from is a testament to the hoops I was jumping through to avoid facing painful truths, when the reason why they were not giving me money or assistance was the same as in the past, and as it would remain in the future. You give to those you care about. If you don't care, you don't give. They didn't give because they didn't care, at least not about what I wanted, only what they wanted, which was for me to remain trapped as Gloria's companion. It was as simple as that.

And yet this episode was not without its merits. Although I did not yet know it, I had taken the first tentative step to a new, foreign life which would liberate me from my mother. However, it would also destroy the positive remnants of our relationship, and that, paradoxically, would save me in a way no amount of excuses ever could.

Chapter Fifteen

While I was in New York enjoying the myriad matrimonial prospects, including Bill, Gloria remained in Jamaica. She was now dealing with aging in an interesting way. Previously she had always had an overtly heterosexual admirer whom she called a 'boyfriend' and who was in nightly attendance. 'Uncle' Frank had been succeeded by Morton, whom we children nicknamed 'Pop'. But he had recently jumped ship, after years of visits, to get married.

Rather than replace him with yet another heterosexual swain, she abandoned sexual allure in favour of political influence, while making sure that she received the steady diet of admiration and entertainment she needed by adding to her circle what was then called 'perennial bachelors'.

Her two closest male friends, however, were not any of the artists or musicians who could now be found at the house on a nightly basis. They were two of the country's heaviest hitters: the Chief of Staff of the Army and the Attorney General. It is a testament to Gloria's gift for steering relationships in the direction she wished them to go that, though both Brigadier Rudolph Greene and Victor Grant married, during the peak years of their friendships with her, she managed to retain the hold she had over both men while also befriending their wives. Indeed, she was so adept at seducing the wives as well as the husbands that she became best friends with Rudolph's wife Margaret and Anna, who had replaced her former 'close' friend Gwen to become Victor's fourth and final wife.

Rudolph and Margaret, Victor and Anna – and before her, Gwen – were constantly at our house; and every bit of concern Gloria could never give to her children or immediate family she lavished upon these men and their wives. Her seductiveness remained asexual and as self-interested as always, for what she was achieving in these relationships was influence or, at the very least, a show of it.

So far, the common thread in everything Gloria had done was power and its exercise. In her teens, she had used her sexual allure to conquer a rich man, whom she married and then led on a merry chase. In her twenties, she had used that allure to become a star of the social world as well as the star of one romantic show after another. Whether, as she maintained, these relationships were devoid of sexual intercourse is beside the point. They were intense romances; and, as anyone who has been in love or lust knows, you don't actually have to have sex to be hoisted on the petard of sexual desire. There is actually a strong case for the fact that by withholding her sexual favours – if that is indeed what she did – she opened up a void that allowed her to manipulate the relationships so that her cravings for attention were satisfied while those of the men with whom she was involved were not. Thus she exploited her personality as well, using it to become a popular and envied hostess.

In her thirties, Gloria seemed to become bored with so much popularity; and she graduated, at least within the immediate family, to the naked exercise of raw power. Gradually, the mask of charm started to slip before an ever-widening circle of people, and the monster beneath became more and more visible, even though, I noted time and again, people would discount the evidence before their eyes and seek to explain it away in some anodyne fashion.

Although Gloria had retained her youthful looks and continued to capitalize upon them to bewitch man after man and to cut a glamorous swathe through Society, she seemed to have decided that the time had come to feather another nest before the feathers in her old one blew away. Being no fool, she would have been aware that no woman in her mid-forties, no matter how beautiful or captivating, can escape from the fact that her sexual allure is diminishing. The reality of life is that virtually all men are attracted to nubile young things, and once a woman approaches middle age, she loses the universality of her appeal. That is not to say that she ceases to be attractive to men from a wide age group, simply that the proportion of men who are now attracted is reduced. And with each passing year, the reduction increases.

If Gloria was learning how transient sexual power is, it was not the only source of power whose transience she was about to discover. The year 1971 was the last one in which 'old' Jamaica existed. The way of life that families like hers had known for four and a half centuries was coming to a rapid close with the ousting of the ruling political party. Michael Manley, the handsome, *café au lait*, five-times married lothario who had been Gloria's first boyfriend, much to the annoyance of her colour-prejudiced parents, was elected prime minister in early 1972. A renowned but vain orator who, like Tony Blair, was in love with the sound of his own voice, he began his term of office as he intended to continue. Rousing the rabble and terrifying the Establishment, he announced in parliament shortly after his accession to power that he intended to break the backs of the oligarchs who controlled the wealth of the country because the people had 'suffered' and 'been oppressed' long enough. If these oligarchs didn't like the changes that he was going to institute, he declared, there were 'five flights a day to Miami' (his words, not mine) and they could leave the country.

The problem with politicians who are enchanted by their own rhetoric is that they seldom allow the facts to interfere with what they are saying. The proof of this is that ten short years before Michael Manley was blaming the Jamaican oligarchy for having oppressed the 'people' for centuries, his father, Norman Washington Manley, the former premier of pre-Independence Jamaica, had lain the blame for their oppression firmly at the door of successive British governments.

The British Empire was a thing of the past by 1972, however, and there was no political advantage to be gained from continuing to hold the former colonial power responsible. So Michael Manley, whose avowed ambition was to become a leader of the Third World alongside Kenneth Kaunda and Julius Nyrere (a feat he would achieve with ridiculous ease), came up with a new set of oppressors. According to him, there were twenty-two families – generic, not nuclear – who controlled the wealth of the country. Although he did not name them officially, he allowed his henchmen to circulate unofficially what became known as the 'List of the Twenty-Two Families'. The word on the street was that all the members of these Twenty-Two Families should either get out of the country, leaving their assets behind, or run the risk of being forcibly shorn of their wealth and possibly suffer an even worse fate.

Needless to say, this intimidation spread panic amongst the people on the list, who, contrary to the catchy and politically astute sound bite, did not number a mere twenty-two families, or even a few hundred, but many thousands of people. By using generic families and counting all their relations, the prime minister had cast a very wide net that included just about everyone in the country with any connection to anyone with assets.

As Michael Manley strode and strutted upon the world stage, garnering praise from all left-wing sources for his 'love of the people', he showed those of us in the know why his relationship with Gloria could never have succeeded. They were both irresponsible dramatists who would say anything to achieve their objective, which was always ultimately to push themselves forward, irrespective of the cost, to obtain the admiration and approbation they felt was their due. Fairness never even entered into the equation. So what if he was intermingling racism with anti-materialism, whipping up the impecunious who would then embark upon the senseless and self-destructive slaughter of a multitude of innocents? The ruling PNP felt justified in arming their supporters with guns and turning a blind eye as these thugs rampaged throughout the country, shooting and stealing without fear of punishment in the Jamaican version of ethnic cleansing. What did the lives of the several thousand murdered as a direct result of the prime minister's political irresponsibility matter? He was playing to the gallery, and his audience was not the thousands of decent black, brown and white Jamaicans who worked hard for a living and were entitled to every penny they had earned but the uneducated poor as well as 'democratic socialists' all over the world, especially in England, where he became, within months of his election, the darling of the *Guardian* newspaper set. As the British people would later learn with Tony Blair, few in a nation can afford the luxury of a prime minister whose priority is earning international approbation at the expense of the well-being of his citizenry.

Joshua, as Michael Manley immodestly called himself in a Biblical allusion to another saviour, went everywhere with his rod of correction, giving anyone who wished to see the message that he had megalomaniacal tendencies and that he would brook no opposition to his dream of a 'free' Jamaica where all men were equal: which is to say, equally impoverished. Those who questioned whether he meant what he said needed look no further than to his closest political ally, Fidel Castro. The Cuban leader had also implemented a policy of equal poverty for all except the government and ruling party, and when he sent over 'political advisors' to assist in the 'democratic socialization' of Jamaica, Jamaicans had all the proof they needed that their country would follow where Cuba had led.

At first, the political advisors were only a handful, but by the end of the 1970s, they numbered several thousand. They were in every town, village, hamlet, city and suburb. They were ever-present, watching with an avidity peculiar to totalitarians, whose avowed 'love' of the people always rules out such 'counterrevolutionary' conduct as trust or governmental non-interference in its citizens' everyday lives.

Jamaicans discovered that Michael Manley was more Castro than Joshua, however, when he built beside the army headquarters in Kingston, with Cuban assistance, a concentration camp which the government, in typical totalitarian nonsense-speak, named the 'Gun Court', despite the fact that it was neither a court nor truly gun-related. The only discernible link to weapons seemed to be the guns which the government planted on their political opponents so that they could detain them in the Gun Court.

To onlookers, it was obvious the camp had been built with intimidation in mind. Had you not known better, you would have thought it was a film-set for a Nazi concentration camp. It had high fences topped with barbed wire and twisted metal. There were barbed-wire no-man's land gaps between inner and outer perimeter fencing, and gun towers manned by guards wielding machine guns, who operated a shoot-to-kill policy.

I was not unique among Jamaicans in being appalled by what Michael Manley was doing to the country. Unlike the average person, however, I was fortunate enough to have actual verification of how hypocritical Manley's posturing was because my family knew the Manley family personally. In fact, our family had known them over three generations, and it was this knowledge that gave one a sickening sense of the pointless unproductiveness of it all.

Though perfectly civil, the Manleys were hardly freedom fighters. In fact, they were more privileged and discriminating than most other families, coloured or white, Jamaican or foreign. Both Norman Washington Manley and his wife Edna were renowned in social circles for their pretensions. They did not mix socially with 'the people'. Indeed, they did not condescend to mix even with the merely bourgeois. They mixed only with the *crème de la crème*. So elitist were they that everyone in their circle had to be at the top of their category, whether social, artistic or professional. While most patricians, my parents included, would plump up their circle with some mediocrities, the Manleys made it plain that they were too sensible of their own greatness to make space for, or waste time on, anyone but those of the first rank. Elitism taken to such lengths goes beyond snobbishness to something even more odious; and, because the Manleys were arch-proponents of it, one would have laughed about the ludicrousness of their posturing as protectors of the people had their mockery of the facts not been so serious, indeed deadly, for the nation as a whole. Nor is that an exaggeration. Tens of thousands of Jamaicans lost their lives as a result of Michael Manley's policies, some through state-sponsored murder such as the Green Bay Massacre, others through more random violence, but an unacceptable number through poverty as well. Never before nor since have Jamaicans starved to death.

The 'matriarch' of the Manleys, as the family pretentiously referred to Edna, was an English sculptress of considerable talent. At the beginning of her career in the 1920s, when she was young and recently out of art school, she was regarded as one of England's finest artists, on a par with such greats as Duncan Grant. However, she married Norman Washington Manley and moved to Jamaica. Thereafter, she was out of the mainstream of the Modern British Movement, and while she would achieve recognition as one of Jamaica's finest sculptresses and painters, the fact remains that being at the pinnacle of a small country's artistic community is not commensurate with being at the pinnacle of one of the great Western nations' Modern Movement. Edna was acutely aware of having swapped a big pond in which she could have been a big fish for a small pond in which she was a whale.

Edna was actually a rather charming woman. Tall and imposing in the grand manner, I have actually heard her deplore some of the racist nonsense which her son was responsible for when he became prime minister. One such incident she recounted at the house of the eminent artist David Boxer, who was a great mutual friend. Edna was in high dudgeon because a black man had come up to her and asked her: 'Where you get Michael from?'

'I'm afraid I don't understand you,' Edna Manley said she said.

'Where you get Michael from? You must 'ave thief 'im. You don't expect black people to believe that a white woman could give birth to such a great black man?'

Although Edna deplored such consequences of her son's political policies, there is no doubt she enjoyed being cast in the role of Jamaica's Queen Mother, just as she had enjoyed being the wife of the premier when her husband had been the pre-Independence head of government. I thought this harmless stuff, though the family's pretensions to greatness, with all the disastrous consequences for the nation, were another matter altogether.

The 'patriarch', Norman Washington Manley, was a half-black, half-white barrister whose English cut-glass tones had long since eradicated all evidence of the Jamaica of his birth in favour of the Oxbridge persona he brought back home after qualifying in the Mother Country. He was what both white and black Jamaicans mocked as being a 'black Englishman'. Even at the height of summer, when the thermometer hit the nineties, and the humidity was so great that sweat poured off anyone who walked ten paces, irrespective of how many or how few articles of clothing they had on, he could not be separated from the woollen, three-piece suits, complemented by a fob watch and chain, which were the uniform of the professional classes in England. It was as if he feared being identified as just another Jamaican of colour if he got rid of the Anglo-Saxon attire which was then perceived as a badge of superiority by those not in the know. Had his politics not been so aggressively in favour of Independence, he would have been seen by the people as an 'Uncle Tom'. But because of his nationalism, he was elected premier of Jamaica under the British colonial masters, and his pretensions were accepted as civility

Cold, stiff and aloof, Norman Manley was a parody of naturalness. Renowned, except amongst his supporters, for his grandiose political ambitions, he didn't actually dislike the British, whom he aped in everything. No true Jamaican patrician would ever have done such a thing. He simply saw no reason why Jamaica should have any leader but one with the name 'Manley'. He didn't want to get rid of the British way of life or the British system. In fact, he was an advocate of both. All he wanted was to replace the British political leaders with the Manley family. His plan was that first he, then afterwards, his son Douglas, would become prime minister. This was as clear a refutation as exists of the principle of democratic self-determination, for no truly democratic country is governed by hereditary prime ministers.

Norman Manley's – and Jamaica's – tragedy was that Douglas, a more balanced creature than his younger brother Michael, ruined his father's dynastic plans by turning out to be a politically inept liability whose alcoholism was the worst kept secret in the country. So, in true Caesarean fashion, Norman Manley turned his gaze towards his vain, priapic, visionary second son Michael. Duly anointed head of the National Workers Union, the trade union affiliated with the PNP (yet another flagrant display of antidemocratic nepotism), Michael Manley cut his political teeth with rabble rousing on a par never seen in the country before.

As Adolf Hitler said in slightly different words, it is a sad but true fact that uneducated and disadvantaged people are more apt to believe a lie the bigger it is. The biggest lie of all was that Michael Manley loved the people. He really loved only himself, and those who do not believe it should read his daughter Rachel's excellent memoir *In My Father's Shade*. Whether she intended to or not, this former girlfriend of my brother Mickey paints a devastating picture of her father as a self-indulgent narcissist whose vanity was so insuperable that it was exceeded only by his well-concealed coldness – a coldness which she successfully describes as taking a variety of forms, some chilling and all destructive of his children's lives, even if she neglects to enumerate that they were also damaging to the country at large.

If Michael Manley proved to be a political disaster for Jamaica, he was also the perfect illustration of how easy it is to mislead the desperate with false promises comprising equal measures of hot air and silken words. Practise enough illusion and they'll love you until hunger hits them in the belly. One used to want to cry every time some poor person said that 'Joshua is going to lead the people into the Promised Land.' You dared not ask them how they thought the Manley Government could achieve the impossible of creating this 'Promised Land' where all poor people became rich, while they were impoverishing the rich, depriving money-makers of the means to make money and fighting off every source of future investment as if wealth and its creation were pariahs to be sacrificed on the altar of Fidel Castro-like demagoguery.

Knowing the Manleys, I was sure Michael Manley had to be aware, as he was nurturing his image as an anti-American, anti-Establishment, anti-materialistic leader of the Third World, that man cannot live by shit alone, nor can countries consume it just because their prime minister is full of it and shoots it out of his mouth with pathological frequency. I had no doubt that he knew only too well that he was deceiving the people. But he didn't care. As long as he, Michael Manley, played the role upon the world stage that his vanity dictated he ought to have, what did it matter if the people suffered and starved? So, for nearly a decade, the people swallowed the false promises whole, and as the Promised Land failed to materialize, and Joshua blamed everyone but himself and his government for his failure to deliver the prosperity which he had promised but which his policies prevented, their bitterness increased until Jamaica was labelled one of the most violent and lawless places on earth.

Only when Michael Manley's political diarrhoea resulted in the financial collapse of the country in 1980 did the deceived unfortunates vote Joshua and his rod of correction out of power in a landslide that ought to have buried him permanently. The electorate, however, gave him another chance some years later, when communism was no longer fashionable, and he had recanted his 'democratic socialist' ideals in favour of the newly fashionable western-style capitalism which Mrs Thatcher had done so much to make acceptable all over the world and which former 'democratic socialists' and communists from Russia to Angola embraced with an alacrity that was truly amazing, showing that the only thing rarer in politics than predictability is integrity.

The second time around, Michael Manley proved to be as inept as ever at everything but making speeches; and by the time he left office he was an embarrassment more than anything else.

I find it difficult to forgive Michael Manley for three things. Firstly, the destruction of the country's economy; secondly, the racism that made every white or light-skinned person in Jamaica a target for nearly a decade, and cost the lives of thousands, who were brutally murdered by the very people he had encouraged with his irresponsible rhetoric to 'take' what was 'rightfully theirs'; and thirdly, the destruction of a way of life that had evolved over nearly five centuries and was, for all its imperfections, as close to multiracial Nirvana as had existed anywhere on earth at that time. With more responsible government, he could have fostered instead of destroyed, and Jamaica would indeed have been even more of the island paradise people all over the world had thought of it as being prior to his election as prime minister.

My mother and her former boyfriend had more in common than I felt comfortable with: neither scrupled to consider their duties to others nor to respect the rights of others when they stood in the way of their ambitions. Michael Manley was as adept at demonizing vast swathes of humanity as she was. Yet the facts were more complicated than he pretended, and he knew this to be the case, because the very class of people whom he first demonized was the sector of the population from which he drew his friends, his wives – save one, Beverley Anderson, who was the 'face that fit' while he was on his Black Power, democratic socialism kick – and all his mistresses, several of whom were friends of mine or my mother's. To hear him talk, you would have thought everyone with a white or fair skin and two cents to their name spent every waking hour plotting how to do in black people when the fact is very few of our kind were socially irresponsible. Even people like my father, who had a terrible temper and could be verbally abusive to anybody and everybody, had such a highly developed social conscience that he paid his workers above the going rate. I witnessed him on many an occasion bending over backwards rather than dismiss someone who deserved it because he knew that jobs were scarce and if he fired them, they would experience real hardship. Nor was my father unique. Although there were – and always will be under any system – heartless people, he was representative of his class. The old concept of *noblesse oblige,* though about to become derided by the very people it had been designed to protect, as a result of prompting from politicians such as Michael Manley, meant that no one with a conscience was ever blind to his or her obligations to those less fortunate than they were.

The national decline was reflected in the decline in our family's prestige and influence. Though Gloria maintained a close relationship with the Chief of Staff of the Army throughout the eight years of the Manley regime, within two or three years of the PNP victory, our family name, once synonymous with worldly success and privilege, had been twisted to symbolize the oppression of black people.

I was not alone in being racially abused when I walked the streets of Kingston. No white or fair skinned person could avoid being called 'pork' – i.e. white pig – and while words cannot really hurt you, sticks and stones do break your bones, and guns do kill or maim you. Murders of the Haves by the Have-nots now became commonplace. In an ominous extension of previously unheard of racial prejudice, holdups involving white or fair skinned women, or black Haves – who were lumped with whites by the criminal element of the Have-nots – seldom took place without rape also being involved. The women lucky enough to tell the tale all recounted how their rapists set out to humiliate them, justifying their conduct on the grounds that they were settling scores going back centuries. Joshua had opened up a can of worms, and the Jamaican Haves' situation closely paralleled that of the French aristocracy's during the revolution.

I was surprised at how well Gloria adjusted to the changes taking place around her. Although she regretted the diminution of the political as well as general influence which she had enjoyed while the JLP was in power, she was dextrous enough to forge 'personal' friendships with such non-political appointees as the prime minister's private secretary. Fortunately for her, this lessening of influence was to an extent concealed from the world at large, partly because her first cousin, the Hon Danvers Williams, was a minister of government and member of the cabinet, and partly because Michael's cousin Delroy Ziadie was also involved with the government.

Those of us who knew how much Gloria loved possessing influence realized that its loss must have been acutely painful. Yet she showed an unexpected aptitude for flexibility which she intermingled with admirable dignity and integrity. Unlike many of the patricians who started to 'find' blackness where none had previously existed or who now admitted to a 'touch of the tar brush' which they had been denying for decades and in some cases for centuries in the hope that by joining the opposition they would redeem themselves, Gloria held her ground with neither unseemly display nor apology. She remained as plainly and proudly patrician as ever, and while she started using some of the vernacular which conveyed the message that one was *à la mode*, she never pretended to be common or black. Indeed, she used to mock those who did, and for once I was completely in sympathy with her, for it really was pathetic to see the lengths to which characterless people would go to deny an identity they had been happily inhabiting for a lifetime.

I freely admit that Gloria adjusted better to the new Jamaica than any of her children, with the exception of Mickey, who had always loved black people with a passion that only an unloved white boy with loving black nannies can summon up. Her feistiness, fearlessness and competitiveness gave her a freedom to respond to Black-Power situations in a way that our more traditional reserve did not. What we ignored, her dominating streak refused to; and sometimes you actually could see how her more maverick behaviour worked in her favour. One such incident, which was witnessed by friends and reported back to us, took place when she was cut up by an aggressive driver at Cross Roads, a part of the city near a no-go area. Refusing to give way, Gloria ended up blocking rush-hour traffic. The driver of the other car, hoping to bully her, actually dragged her out of her vehicle and started to abuse her verbally in front of a gathering mob which was initially baying for the blood of the 'white woman'. Now, the one thing Jamaicans of all backgrounds respect is pluck, and whatever her faults, Gloria had that quality to excess. As this five foot three, slender forty-something lady held her own against the hulking bully and the baying mob who were hurling invective at her and telling her to 'go back to 'merica', the mood changed when Gloria said: 'The one place none of us came from is 'merica, as you so charmingly call it. I tell you what. Let's agree that whichever one of us came here last has to go back to where they came from first.'

The man, transfixed by Gloria's feistiness, agreed.

'Well, here's the fact. You're black, so you either came here from Africa as a slave of the Spanish or the English. Which is it?'

The man evidently looked uncertain.

'Let me help you,' said Gloria, quick as a flash. 'Are you a Maroon?'

'No. Me don't come from Nanny Town.'

'If you're not a Maroon, you're not descended from Spanish slaves. That means that you're descended from English slaves. The English captured Jamaica in 1655 from the Spanish, so your ancestors came here after 1655.'

'Bwoy, what a way the white woman know she history,' one of the crowd said admiringly.

'Yes, I know my history, and I know where I come from. My maternal grandmother's family were amongst the first settlers of Jamaica. They were Spanish Jews who came here in the early 1500s when the Inquisition was at its height and the only place Spanish Jews could practice their religion free of persecution was in the New World. Jamaica has the oldest colony of Jews in the New World, and my ancestors were among the first of those families to come here. So, if anyone is going to clear out of Jamaica, it's going to have to be you, not me. But I tell you what, if you stop disputing my right to drive on the road free of your interference, I'll extend you the courtesy of allowing you to stay in *my* country with my blessing.'

The man stepped aside, someone in the crowd opened Gloria's car door for her, and, cheered on by the remainder of the crowd, she drove off, having turned hostility to admiration in a matter of minutes.

When the incident was reported back to me, I told Michael about it.

'One of these days your mother is going to get herself killed,' he said. But I had my doubts. In the new Jamaica, engagement in the form of argument entered into as an equal rather than as a superior earned the respect of the masses. It was patrician reserve, I suspected, which actually elicited antagonism.

Topping others in face-to-face arguments was not the only ploy Gloria adopted to deal with the new order. Now that luxury was suspect, and driving expensive cars was an invitation to every crime from car-jacking to simple verbal abuse, she traded in her fancy American car for a middle-of-the-road English model. Socially, she expanded her horizons to include representatives of the new elite. For instance, Mickey had been at Grey's Inn with Maurice Bishop, and they had remained friends as my brother became recognized as one of Jamaica's leading lawyers and Maurice achieved notoriety as the communist leader of Grenada. Maurice, who would ultimately be assassinated by the Americans during their invasion of that island nation, was always received by Gloria whenever he was in Jamaica and entertained both *en famille* and more formally. His reception by my parents surprised me, not because he wasn't a fit person to mix with socially – he was charming and civilized – but because his politics were anathema to them and only a few short years before, he would have been deemed unacceptable not only on social grounds but also political ones. Yet here he was, being treated like a member of the family by Gloria, who had the good grace, when he was killed, to condemn the American government's actions, and, until then, she always gave him a rousing welcome every time he came to Jamaica.

For all her flexibility, Gloria must have found adjusting to the new order difficult. Her husband, mother, sister and children remained so adamantly supportive of the previous ruling party that she was left no room for manoeuvre to switch allegiances. There was little doubt in all our minds that that is precisely what she would have done had we not made it impossible for her to do so by our vociferous condemnation of the government's policies. 'Mummy is a PIP,' we used to say, meaning 'Party In Power', refusing to condone silently the steady stream of racist, democratic socialists she might well have allowed to flow through the family home as they engineered to shove families like ours out of the country and she preserved her precious political influence. Our vociferous opposition meant that Gloria's days as a political hostess were over, at least for the foreseeable future, until the JLP were returned to power, if they were ever allowed to, or if the PNP changed its policies.

Nor were Gloria's days as a purely social hostess faring much better. As the Manley regime turned its screws on the moneyed classes, the Diaspora began. The Established Families left in droves, along with many members of the middle classes who might not have been socially desirable but were nevertheless fundamental to the smooth and civilized running of the country. This meant that she no longer had a ready pool of friends to call upon or entertain, and she would feel this loss acutely for the remainder of her life. Rather than expanding, Jamaica was contracting, and with it, the interest one could draw out of life there.

Worst of all, however, was the element of financial insecurity which now crept into everyone's life. Taking a leaf out of Adolf Hitler's book, Michael Manley set about divesting the Haves of their assets the way the German chancellor had done to the Jews. Law after law was drafted with the aim of stripping certain people or categories of the population of particular aspects of their property. One of the early targets of the government was the destruction of land values. Collective farming as practised by Lenin and Stalin was then being upheld as an ideal by the Manley Government, despite the disastrous effects that policy had had upon Russian agriculture, the Russian peasantry, the Russian landowning classes, the Russian economy generally and any other economy which had subsequently followed the disastrous Russian example. Michael Manley should certainly have known this to be a fact: he was a graduate of the London School of Economics. To force families such as ours to sell our farms and estates, Manley increased the land taxes by several thousand percent per annum. As farms and estates became an expensive luxury rather than a manageable foil to city living, families such as my mother's, which jointly owned a pimento farm called Windsor – named several centuries prior to the Saxe-Coburg-Gotha family's adoption of that moniker – had little choice but to sell their properties. Within eighteen months, farms and estates that had been selling for hundreds of thousands of US dollars, sometimes for millions, prior to the change in the law, now fetched forty and fifty thousand dollars apiece. This was at a time when a brownstone on the Upper East Side in New York fetched $225,000, which should give an idea of what the true scale of the losses was.

Next on the chopping block was urban property. To engineer his economic 'miracle', Manley had to pass no law beyond those he had already passed. The collapse in urban real-estate values became a natural extension of the collapse of rural ones, especially when it was combined with the circulation of the List of the Twenty-Two Families. People were so desperate to get out of the country before they lost everything or were arrested and imprisoned that they reasoned that salvaging something, no matter how little, was better than losing it all. Also, it suddenly became unsafe to live in those ambassadorial-style villas which the upper classes occupied in Kingston, for no amount of burglar bars or security guards could assure your physical safety. My father's cousin Victor Ziadie, whose Millsborough house occupied the most desirable position in the whole of Kingston, actually moved out of it, and it remained unoccupied for the next thirty-five years!

Reflecting the average Jamaican's appreciation of humour, many a car soon bore the wry commentary on the political situation in the form of a popular bumper sticker: *Would the last person in the island please turn out the lights?*

Having seen the bottom fall out of the property market, Michael Manley then turned his attention to acquiring the Haves' investments. Unlike Stalin and Lenin, who had simply nationalized any company or industry they coveted, Manley believed in doing things legally – like Hitler. He allotted farcical values to assets, for instance forcing my father to surrender shares worth millions of dollars US, for the arbitrary figure of $50,000. All perfectly legal, without any possibility of rectification in the future, for the assets had not been confiscated or seized but bought, albeit forcibly for a fraction of their true value, by the government.

As Gloria faced a future in which her husband's financial worth had a zero lopped off it, her response was interesting, to say the least. She couldn't bring herself to condemn the man whom she had once called a boyfriend and who she said 'gave kisses sweeter than wine', not because she had any residual affection for him but because he was in power and she respected political power even when it was appallingly misused or malign. Instead, she blamed the other Michael, her husband, for their reversal of fortune 'I told you to move your money out of the country,' she said, not without a certain amount of justice. 'But you wouldn't listen. Every time I told you what he would do you said: "He wouldn't dare." Well, he's dared, and we're one step away from the poorhouse.' This last assertion wasn't true, however, for they were still worth well into seven figures.

I cannot begin to imagine how Gloria must have felt as she reviewed the wreckage of her world. I try to put myself in her shoes and wondered how I would feel if I had married a man for his money. How it must have felt to have stayed with him for it, given up my liberty and peace of mind for it, then had woken up in my late forties to find that ninety percent of the fortune has disappeared, owing to the crazy policies of my ex-boyfriend. One could not fail to have a measure of sympathy for her. And once more, I used her example as an awful warning of where false values lead.

Chapter Sixteen

I was in Jamaica staying at home when Michael Manley was first elected prime minister. I vividly remember listening to his address to Parliament when he warned families like mine that there were 'five flights a day to Miami' if we didn't like the changes he proposed. However, when you are twenty-two, the antics of verbally incontinent prime ministers seem irrelevant compared with the more pressing problems of finding a suitable husband. So it was with me.

After my last stay in New York, I had decided I would prefer to base myself in Jamaica, where living at home afforded one every creature comfort, rather than remaining in a city where the standard of living was inferior. Admittedly, New York offered a richer array of people to meet, but that very wealth of choice meant that one had to be far more assertive than I was comfortable with being. Indeed, I loathed how New Yorkers spent half their time letting everyone know that they were worth knowing. Personally, I preferred having others blow my trumpet for me. I also objected to the sensation I frequently experienced, that everyone in New York was valued more for attributes such as their looks and family connections or money, than for their characters. Whatever the failings of the world of my birth, I was discovering it had one virtue: character was more important in established circles than it was in transient societies such as New York.

When all was said and done, I wanted a husband, but could never accept one unless I truly loved him and he truly loved me. Without being in the least romantic, I had developed an uncomfortably deep attachment to sterling virtues such as constancy and sincerity as a result of seeing how false values had ruined my mother's life. I could no sooner envisage myself with a man whom I did not respect than I could imagine myself emulating Gloria's example.

In a way, I was marking time throughout the early part of 1972. Although I did fulfil the occasional modelling assignment, I was reluctant to return to dress designing, slightly because I found it intellectually stultifying but largely because I could not stand being a captive audience for my garrulous mother. That seemed inevitable as long as I had to sew the garments I designed, for she would insist upon 'keeping me company' and chewing off my ears until I felt like screaming.

My cousin Babe came once more to my rescue and arranged a job for me in the Department of Obstetrics and Gynaecology at the University Hospital of the West Indies. Although I had no secretarial training, I could type like a demon, having been taught by my grandfather when I was ten years old. So now I put that skill to good use as a departmental secretary.

I also bought Mickey's Volkswagen Beetle from him, using money Michael provided from the proceeds of an insurance policy he had taken out for me at birth and which had now matured. That gave the message to one and all that I was in Jamaica to stay, which, without realizing it, was the worst message I could have sent to my mother, for it put me firmly in her sights as the target to seek and destroy.

Blissfully ignorant of the trouble that would inevitably brew behind the scenes when her narcissistic need to annihilate the competition kicked in, I set about leading the life of a young lady lying in wait for a husband. I was frequently out on the town with beaus, none of whom moved me. I also went out with friends and even with my parents sometimes, for there were several social events to which we were all invited.

It was around this time that I started to connect up some dots which had been jumping before my eyes for the last year. Every time Gloria and I were asked to the same party, she would call me to help her get dressed while I was dressing. This had started in February 1971, at a time when people had started to rave about me being a 'great beauty'.

'You're so much better at putting on make-up than I am. And my eyesight is going to the dogs. I can't see what I'm doing even when I do it with the magnifying mirror,' became her refrain.

Now, the one thing no one could do was refuse any request of Gloria's. So

I would help her, interrupting my own efforts to get myself together. In those days, all young girls wore false eyelashes and lots of eye liner, and it was fairly standard for me to have one eye done but the other undone or half done, as I was called away from my own mirror to hers.

When I had finished acting as her make-up artist, I would return to my bedroom to finish off my own preparations. Invariably, however, Gloria would throw open her bedroom door before I had a chance to finish and announce, 'We're ready. Let's go.' As she never waited for anyone, I would have to depart without the finishing touches that are so essential to good grooming, or then do them in the car. This meant appearing in public with sloppily applied make-up, for it isn't possible to put on make-up properly when a car is bouncing along Third-World roads.

I don't know whether it was the interruption of the months spent in New York, or the resumption of this practice, which did the trick; but one evening, after Gloria had done this for the umpteenth time, I began to ask myself if she could be doing this deliberately, to ensure that I was not as well groomed as she.

Although I knew deep down that the answer was yes, that my competitive, Machiavellian mother was up to her tricks, I nevertheless underwent a period of tussling with myself. How could I think such an unworthy thing of Mummy? Surely no mother would sink so low? Worse, was I following in her tradition of bitchy suspiciousness by thinking the worst of her when she was possibly innocent?

Giving her the benefit of the doubt, I pushed these negative thoughts to the back of my mind. Each time she interrupted my dressing schedule, however, I came closer and closer to acknowledging that my thoughts, no matter how negative, had been accurate all along.

Once I reluctantly faced the fact that something untoward was going on behind the scenes, I resolved to beat her at her own game. I therefore decided to get dressed so early that, when she called me to 'help' her, all I had to do, when I was finished with her beautification process, was put on my dress and shoes.

Sure enough, when the next time came, I was ready and waiting. She called me, as she had been doing for the last year, and I departed from my bedroom, fully made-up, every hair in place, ever jewel I would be wearing glittering from my earlobes, neck, hands and wrists. When I walked into her bedroom, to see her making a great show of 'struggling' with her mascara, she looked up and was so startled she did not have time to conceal her surprise.

'Ha, did you start to get dressed last night or yesterday morning?' she snapped, betraying annoyance.

'No. I simply decided to give you all the time you need,' I replied pleasantly.

The look of pure loathing she shot in my direction gave me all the confirmation I needed. Gloria was trying to sabotage me deliberately.

In situations as subterranean as this, it takes a while to get beneath the surface of what is apparently going on to the reality of what is actually taking place. Because I had not confronted her directly, Gloria couldn't be sure that I was either onto her or had bested her. She learned soon enough, however, for each time that she repeated her 'requests for help', I showed up in her bedroom groomed to bandbox standard. When she realized that she could not sabotage me, she stopped asking for my help. Her eyesight, so perilously in danger of failing her when she stood to knock me out of the beauty stakes, suddenly restored itself to its previously adept standard, and thereafter, every time we were going out together, she would give me a sour look as we were leaving the house.

Had I understood that Gloria was a narcissist and that narcissism was – as Dr Len Sperry observed in his *Handbook of Diagnosis and Treatment of the DSM-IV Personality Disorders* – a disorder in which arrogance, impatience, hypersensitivity and competitiveness result in destructive behaviour, I would have been very worried indeed. As it was, I thought Gloria's little game pathetic – stupid even. It didn't occur to me that she was building up to something truly malevolent. After all, people don't behave like that, do they?

I should have known, by this time, that my mother was not 'people' and that the way she behaved was so bizarre because she had a disordered personality. Certainly, she could say and do things that were so grotesque, so off-the-wall, so unexpected and out of the ordinary, that you couldn't really consider the ramifications dispassionately without also facing the fact that she was either evil, insane or both.

As Theodore Millon and Roger Davis put it, the narcissist's belief that he or she is superior is merely a facet of a generalized disdain for reality. According to these two authorities on Narcissistic Personality Disorder, the Glorias of this world do not feel constrained by rules, customs, limits or discipline. Plausible to a fault, they have no difficulty in justifying self-centred or inconsiderate conduct. They have powerful and uninhibited imaginations, never question the rightness of their belief and simply assume that others, and not they, are always in the wrong. Their self-deceptiveness often comes to their rescue so that facts are twisted to fulfil their fantasies. While devaluing others as a matter of course and inflating themselves and their accomplishments, their grasp of past memories is sufficiently elastic to allow them the luxury of changing the salient features of those facts so that they fulfil their contemporaneous requirements and needs. Even their past relationships are therefore illusory, the licence they give themselves to rewrite history in self-glorifying terms negating the actual relationships themselves. Their world is full of fiction. They dismiss conflicts and convert failures into successes with an alacrity that allows them to maintain their inflated sense of self. Their fundamental difficulties mostly lie in their lack of connection with reality. If that disconnection is allowed to flourish, as it was with Gloria, their thinking becomes increasingly deviant and peculiar, and their defensive manoeuvres become increasingly obvious to onlookers – as indeed Gloria's now started to become to me.

Of course, no one wants to think of their mother as insane or, worse, evil. So, instead, I personalized the message, making light of it. 'There Mummy goes again,' I would start telling myself and everyone else, 'being Mummy.' In so doing, I discounted the reality and thereby missed the significance of what her conduct meant.

A case in point is how she behaved when Max Langner, a German shipping magnate who was sweet on me, came to Jamaica. The subject of marriage came up, and while I was fond of Max, who was a truly lovely man, it was more in the way a niece is fond of an uncle than a girl is of a man. He was some forty years older than me, and I did not fancy him in the least. I had met him at the Vienna Opera Ball in 1970, and thereafter I used to go out with him whenever I was in New York. It was all very innocent and courtly, though he would have liked it to be more sensual. When he came to Jamaica and met my parents and the subject of marriage came up, my father tried to encourage me to marry him.

'Are you nuts?' I asked Michael. 'Why would I want old age creeping all over me?'

'He's a good man. He's ki...kind and decent and can ke...keep you in a way that means you'll never have to worry about mo...money for the rest of your life.'

'I am not a piece of meat in a butcher's shop, displayed in the window for the delectation of all and the purchase of one,' I retorted hotly. 'What you are suggesting strikes me as being too akin to prostitution for comfort.'

'Don't be so ch…childish.'

'Money isn't everything,' I said.

'Spoken like someone who…who's always had it,' Michael observed levelly.

'I want to marry someone I love.'

'You can't e…eat love.'

'I only want for myself what you wanted for yourself. You married someone you loved. I don't see why I can't.'

'And su…suppose this lo…love doesn't come along?' Michael said. 'Look at how many me…men you've been out with in the la…last year. It's my du…duty as your fa…father to steer you in the right di…direction. Max will make a go…good husband.'

'For someone of Mummy's age, not mine,' I said.

Michael left to go into his bedroom, leaving Gloria and me alone.

'You surely don't think that Max wants to marry you for yourself?' she said, once she heard the bedroom door shut. 'Why would a man of that sophistication want a silly young girl like you? It's me he really wants.'

I was so flabbergasted I could only say, 'Come again?'

'I could tell last night, when we were at Blue Mountain Inn, that it's not really you he's interested in. It's me. He wants me, not you.'

'How do you arrive at that?' I asked, dumbfounded.

'It's as plain as the nose on your face. It's me he's in love with. He's come here for me, not for you.'

'You will have to explain to me how it is possible for a man, who had never met you before he came here last week, to have come here for you. I'm obviously missing something, and I want to know what it is,' I said rather more calmly than I felt.

'He's heard all about me and come to pursue things with me,' she said, as if this were a self-evident truth seen by all intelligent people but missed by the imbecile that her supposed genius daughter was. 'He can't do it overtly, because I'm a married woman, so he's doing it through you.'

'Well, I've lived to hear everything,' I said, walking off inside to get my car keys and drive down to Mickey's new house, where he now was living after moving out of Grandma's big house. I recounted the conversation to my brother, who laughed along with me. We agreed that the one thing our mother had was a very high opinion of herself. Even after we had laughed ourselves silly about it, however, I still could not shake the feeling that there was something ominous about my mother's thinking, and this extended way beyond either humour or ego.

After Max left Jamaica, I continued enjoying myself both socially and at work. About two months into my secretarial stint at the O&G, UHWI, however, the (female) head of the department told one of the other consultants that I was a disruptive influence because I was such a magnet for the young doctors. They congregated in the department's office at the slightest excuse in a way they had never done before, and she felt the department would be better off without my presence. Hugh Wynter, the consultant to whom she voiced these concerns, and who subsequently replaced her as department head, opposed her plan to shove me out. Instead, he suggested that they use my family connections to raise much-needed funds to buy expensive equipment such as a foetal heart monitoring machine, instead of having me work as a secretary. So I was offered a new position: fundraiser for the Department of Obstetrics and Gynaecology, University Hospital of the West Indies.

The catch was that the new position paid nothing. While the departmental head might have thought this couldn't possibly be a problem for a member of the Ziadie family, it was for me. Without my salary, I had no money at all. All the money I had earned in New York over the years had been spent the year before while I was living there. My father, however, agreed to give me sufficient pocket money to enable me to fulfil this new position. He did not specify what the sum would be, and only after I had agreed to the changes did I discover that he considered the sum of ten dollars per week to be adequate. This, of course, would keep me in cigarettes and nothing else, but by this time I already given up the secretarial job along with the modest salary, and feeling thoroughly tricked, I asked Gloria to intercede. 'Don't you think you've caused enough problems between your father and me over the years? You'll have to find someone else to fight your corner for you. I've done as much as I intend to do,' she snapped, making out that she had been valiantly protecting my interests over the years in yet another false claim to glory, as Michael would later confirm to me.

As I set about creating a fund-raising committee of the nation's leading socialites, I turned over in my mind how best to solve the problem of my severe financial embarrassment. I surmised that my parents, who had no compunction about being as mean as they could engineer in private, would not want people whose opinions mattered to them to think ill of them, so I went to Michael's first cousin Joe Joe Ziadie. He was not only one of the nicest, kindest and most generous members of the family but, being one of the richest, had the respect of both my parents. His sister Toni was also a great friend of mine as well as of my mother, and I supposed that a word from him would embarrass Michael into stumping up more than the paltry sum he was offering. It did, for all of two weeks, when I was given twenty dollars a week. At the end of the third week, however, Michael handed me ten dollars again 'Business is bad,' he said. 'If it gets better, I'll in…increase your pocket money.' I knew I was being fobbed off and determined that I would not let him delude himself into thinking I was deceived. 'I wondered how long your *generosity* would last,' I replied sarcastically. 'Joe Joe gives Mark more than the twenty dollars you were straining with, and says you can easily afford to give me much more,' I continued, referring to Joe Joe's youngest child, who was several years my junior. 'How do you think I'm ever going to amount to anything if you don't give me the most basic assistance? You should be ashamed of yourself.'

'It's all right for Jo…Joe Jo…Joe to ta…talk. He doesn't kn…know my pressures,' pleaded Michael, who played the sympathy card with as much relish as Gloria whenever he too wanted to avoid anything.

So, virtually penniless, I set about raising hefty sums for charity.

I had never chaired or been solely responsible for the organization of a large charity event before, though I had sat on the odd charity committee in New York. However, I had a good role model in Gloria, whom I used to accompany when I was a child as she 'touched' half the business community and all the rich relations for donations to her causes. Through her example and my innate common sense, I knew exactly what was needed to make the event a success.

Gala charity events raise their funds from three primary sources: ticket sales, sponsorship and programme advertising. Ticket sales might appear, to the uninitiated, to be the primary source of revenue, but in fact they are usually the least profitable part of the enterprise. Sponsorship takes care of many or all of the expenses associated with an event, such as the cost of the venue; the cost of the artist if it is a concert and a band if it is a ball; even the printing costs, for tickets and programmes cost money – and a lot of it – to print. The lion's share of the revenue therefore usually comes from the advertising in the programme.

Should I organize a ball or a concert? I decide to go with a concert rather than a ball for several reasons. Two of my New York friends were the French pianist Andree Juliette Brun and her boyfriend, Jim Anderson, who had actually started out as a beau of mine before retiring into friendship. Andree was a fine musician who had given concerts everywhere from the sovereign's palace in Monaco to Carnegie Hall in New York. I loved music, as did my brother, and as indeed did Gloria; and I thought it would be easier to fill a concert hall than a ballroom, as balls rely solely on Society types while concerts do not.

'Bums on seats' is a phrase that all charity organizers use to describe the essential matter of attendance, and I saw that a concert with a pianist of the international calibre of Andree would assure success, for we would get 'bums on seats' not only from music lovers but also from the Society figures who appear at all socially desirable events. I therefore approached Andree and Jim about the possibility of donating her services in exchange for an all-expenses-paid, first-class holiday in Jamaica, which was still regarded as one of the most glamorous places on earth at that time.

Once they agreed, I went to see Dudley MacMillan, husband of Gloria's erstwhile best friend Vida, about booking the State Theatre, which he owned. He gave me a 'good date', which is crucial to the success of any venture; and I next went to British Overseas Airways Corporation, as British Airways was called in those days. David Creedy and Richard Pavitt, the head and number two respectively, gave me Andree's and Jim's first-class tickets, and I was on my way.

The Fund-Raising Committee of charity events of this kind serves an invaluable but unobvious function. The people on such committees usually do very little work, but their illustrious names act as a magnet for those snobbish or worldly enough to want to be a part of a prestigious 'do'. Although I had a stunning committee on paper (the only person who refused to sit on it, even in the capacity of joint-chairman, was Gloria), the hard graft of raising the funds nevertheless fell to me. Day after day, usually with a friend such as Suzanne Silvera but often on my own, I dropped in on one successful businessman after another. Those to whom I was related or connected through marriage or friendship all gave generously, and even though the event was well in the black some two months before the concert date at the end of June 1972, I nevertheless cast an ever-widening net, going to see businessmen I was neither related to nor knew, but all of whom would have known of my family.

To the credit of everyone, I only had one refusal. Suzanne and I had called upon a gentleman whose Christian name I have forgotten but whose surname was Henderickson. He owned the National Baking Company and was known to be very rich. When I made him my set pitch about the necessity of purchasing vital equipment to protect the lives of mother and child during delivery, he interrupted me and started to berate me for having chosen such a 'white, snobbish, old-fashioned thing as a classical piano recital when this is the new Jamaica and you should be appealing to the masses and putting on a ska recital.' I could hardly believe what I was hearing, but the one virtue of having had a mother as unpredictable and aggressive as Gloria was that I thought on my feet and responded to attacks immediately, instead of six hours later, like the uninitiated. I therefore gave him a piece of my mind, pointing out to him that it was he who was being snobbish and racist, for what made him think that none of the masses would attend a classical music concert? Patently, I pointed out to him, he had never been to a Jamaica School of Music recital, otherwise he'd have known that many of its supporters, and most of its students, were drawn from the masses. Having said my piece, I then stood up. 'Come, Suzanne,' I said before he had a chance to reply. 'Let's get out of here before this jerk makes me do something I'll regret.'

That one incident aside, the fund-raising process was astonishingly agreeable, with everyone being so supportive that it reaffirmed my faith in humanity.

Only too soon, the date of the recital loomed. Bums on seats now became a pressing issue, so I turned my attention to drumming up publicity. This was as easily done as said. Tino de Barovier, whose mother Violetta was Gloria's good friend la contessa, and Consie Walters, whose daughters were my good friends, were responsible for the television and radio stations; and they gave us plug after plug and agreed to interview Andree when she flew into the country. Aunt Violetta also plugged the event in her social column, building up anticipation with the paying public as we held reception after reception at such places as the French Embassy, helping, through her efforts, to turn it into a desirable social event.

The Governor-General Sir Clifford Campbell was attending in an official capacity as the Queen's representative, and Gloria's good friend Rudolph, Chief of Staff of the Army, could not have been more helpful as he liaised with King's House on my behalf. Everyone, in fact, could not have been kinder or more helpful, with the sole exception of Gloria. 'No. Keep me out of it,' she would say in that neutral, cards-close-to-the-chest way of hers, which meant that something was brewing beneath the surface, every time I tried to involve her. 'This is your show, not mine.'

Although I did not know it then, narcissists tend to become inaccessible and withdrawn when feeling threatened, as Lorna Benjamin confirms in the 1996 publication, *An Interpersonal Theory of Personality Disorders: Major Theories of Personality Disorder.* And Gloria was, unbeknownst to me, very threatened, for not only had I trespassed on her territory by emerging as a feted 'beauty' but I was now invading her other realm, the charity world. With hindsight, I can see she hoped that if she withheld assistance I would fall flat on my face.

Her lack of involvement was so glaring that I should have realized trouble was brewing. However, I was too busy, and frankly, I was no longer focused on my mother's moods or schemes. She was my mother. We lived in the same house. We sometimes went to the same parties or concerts. But really, we were different generations with different goals and ideals, and it would have been pretty pointless to bog myself down thinking about what that immature woman was cooking up when I had more important things to do. So I ignored what was happening, little realizing how momentous the trouble would be when it did come.

A few days before the concert, Andree and Jim arrived. The snobs went into paroxysms of delight when, in the process of her television and radio interviews, it emerged that Andree was a princess as well as a highly regarded pianist whose provenance included being a student of the great Marguerite Long and a teacher at Pepperdine College in California.

By the day of the recital, there was a real sense of excitement surrounding the gala. As long as there wasn't a tropical downpour, which always kept people at home even if they had bought tickets beforehand, and as long as Andree played well, the event was sure to be a howling success. I bounced out of bed filled with anticipation for the success that lay ahead. After eating breakfast, I asked Gloria, who was still in her dressing gown, if she wasn't planning to change and come to the hairdresser with me. She never went out without her hair being done.

'It's your show, not mine. I don't want to steal your thunder,' she said neutrally, always a dead giveaway that she was concealing something.

'You won't be stealing my thunder. Come on. Andree is a superb pianist. You'll enjoy her playing. And everyone is going to be there.'

'All the more reason to stay away,' she said, again neutrally.

'But Mummy, I want you to be there,' I said, hoping that by accepting her explanation at face value and ignoring the spoiled 'if-I-can't-be-the-centre-of-attention, I-want-no-part-of-it' sulk that was also taking place behind the veneer of neutrality, she would respond in kind and agree to attend.

'Well, you can't have everything you want. You'll just have to content yourself with my absence,' she said dryly, terminating all future discussion as she took another sip of her inevitable gin and tonic.

For the remainder of the day, I was perturbed by Gloria's determination to keep herself apart from the event. Although I suspected that her reason for doing so might be related to her self-centredness or her competitiveness, the Pollyanna in me hoped that I was wrong, and I struggled to reconcile how any mother could wilfully deprive herself of the opportunity to witness an occasion when her child flourished.

The evening turned out to be as successful as the harbingers had been. The one jarring note was when the governor-general, a venerable old man who was notorious for falling asleep in the evenings, started to snore. I looked to Rudolph, who was seated on my other side. He looked to Lady Campbell, the g-g's wife, who looked straight ahead, quite obviously used to having to tune out moments such as this. So, taking a leaf out of my mother's book, I 'inadvertently' jabbed him in the side with my elbow, and he awoke with a start. End of problem – at least till the next time he nodded off. Thereafter, every time his head started to droop like a weeping willow, I simply moved my arm close enough to put pressure on his, and fearful of another gutting, he snapped to attention for a few more minutes. Afterwards he endeared himself to me when he said that he had never had a 'prettier alarm clock'.

Sir Clifford's snoring aside, the gala could not have been more successful. The event raised a substantial sum, the O&G department got their foetal heart monitoring machine and whatever else, Andree and Jim fell in love with Jamaica and ended up having a wonderful stay both in town and the country, spending much time at Windsor. Jim even sealed my fate with my competitive mother by saying to Michael and her, 'Your daughter is an extraordinary girl. Most twenty two-year-olds couldn't organize their way out of a nightclub without help, yet she put on a gala that Sol Hurok would be proud to be associated with. When I first met her, I thought she was a pretty unusual nineteen-year-old, not only because she was so beautiful, but because she was so stylish. But after last night, I can see that her beauty and style are only the tip of the iceberg. You must be proud of her.'

As if that wasn't a red enough flag to waive before a bullish mother, within days Hugh Wynter, the consultant gynaecologist whose idea it was to turn me from secretary into fundraiser, appeared at the house with another compliment which was bound to goad my competitive mother into paroxysms of envy. 'Gloria, you should have seen your daughter as she escorted Sir Clifford down the aisle. She was truly magnificent. People were oohing and aahing. Zoe,' he continued, referring to his daughter, who presented the bouquet to Andree at the end of the recital, 'captured the mood when she said, "Daddy, is that beautiful lady a queen or a movie star?"'

Little realizing the impact his statement would have, Hugh chuckled delightedly. Gloria responded with a neutral 'My dear,' which could mean anything the person interpreted it as meaning. Doubtless, he thought she was being agreeable and benevolent, but I was only too aware that Gloria's neutral comments usually hid anything but neutrality, and I found myself wondering what was wrong with her and made her derive so little pleasure from compliments that would have thrilled most other mothers. I did not know, as Sperry observed in 1995, the success of others generates envy in the narcissist.

There was little doubt that Gloria was hardly pleased with me at this point. Although I suspected that her nose was out of joint because I was getting too much attention in the social world, I attributed some of the blame to her disapproval of a relationship I had started about a month before. I had been at Epiphany, then the most fashionable discotheque in the city, with friends when a tall, handsome stranger standing beside me asked me if he could buy me a drink. 'You can't just come up to Michael Ziadie's daughter and talk to her,' said Michael Silvera, a great friend of mine. I laughed, thanked Michael for his protectiveness and allowed the handsome stranger to order the proffered drink.

As we talked, I rather liked him and definitely found him attractive. He was just my physical type: well over six feet tall, burly, good-looking. It turned out he played rugby for Jamaica, despite being Welsh, and was in the country working as an accountant at Peat Marwick. After a few dances, Ron asked me if I would like to go to a party with him the following day. I agreed, Michael and his wife Suzanne dropped me home, and the following afternoon the handsome Welshman duly arrived at the appointed time to pick me up.

I was sitting on the back veranda talking to Gloria when he was shown in by one of the servants. You could see just by the way he was looking around that he was impressed by his surroundings. That, of course, was not a good sign. I had already realized that he was not 'one of us' as soon as he had opened his mouth the evening before. I couldn't have cared less that his accent was resolutely middle-class, and, now that he was making it so apparent that his family had as little money as background, I cared no more about that either. I liked him. That was all that mattered. So I ignored the awe and introduced him to my mother.

'How are you, my dear?' Ron said to Gloria by way of greeting, clearly making a misguided attempt to level the playing field, as if by being overly familiar he would eliminate whatever feelings of inadequacy the disparity in our worldly standing had triggered within him.

'Very well, thank you,' Gloria replied icily.

'Well, we're off. See you later,' I said airily, trying to act as if nothing untoward was happening.

'Is your mother always so cold?' Ron asked before I had barely put my foot in his car. 'The way she treated me, you'd have thought I'd crawled out from under a rock. What a snob she is.'

'She's used to being treated with rather more respect than you showed her. It's no big deal. I'm sure if you meet her again and leave off the "my dear", she'll be fine,' I assured him before changing the subject.

He changed it right back and gave me a lecture on how people like my mother thought they were better than everyone else because of their wealth and position, but they really weren't any better than anyone else. I agreed with his hypothesis and said so, but then pointed out to him that even though that was so, the fact remained that she was his elder and on those grounds alone she was deserving of being given a degree of deference. Even snobs, I said, are entitled to being treated with respect by their children's friends. He hotly disputed this, however, stating that such shows of respect were upper-class conventions calculated to keep others in an inferior position. I disagreed, pointing out that the average Jamaican peasant expected to give respect to his elders. Before we could conclude the conversation, we were at the party and Ron had shot up in my estimation not because of his opinions but because he 'thought about things'.

So began my romance with Ron and as well as the problem of him and Gloria. He nicknamed her 'the bitch' from that first encounter, and while I am the first to concede that she really could be an awful bitch, I have to say in her favour, he had a massive chip on his shoulder the way only a class-conscious Brit can have. If there was one instance when she had right on her side, it was this one. Gloria's loathing of Ron was excessive and indicative of what Aaron Beck and Arthur Freeman describe in *Cognitive Therapy of Personality Disorders* as the excessive anger of narcissists when they are not accorded the respect they demand.

From that first meeting, however, Ron was antagonistic in a way only a British petit-bourgeois professional, on the lookout for slights from people he fears regard him as inferior, can be. Every time he saw her, he made a point of calling her 'my dear', and no amount of pleading from me to desist got through to him. As far as Ron was concerned, everything, from the colour of one's eyes to the clouds in the sky, could be traced back to class, even when class was the one thing that had nothing whatsoever to do with anything. He simply could not see that courtesy does not demean those who employ it and that showing it to all classes of people is not infra dig.

Up to that point, I had never encountered anyone who was so rabidly class-conscious. But then, I had never lived in England and therefore did not know, as I would later discover when I lived there, that such class-awareness was neither unique nor unremarkable, no matter how undesirable it was. There were whole swathes of the British population who hampered themselves with self-defeating class misconceptions which might once have been understandable, in the days when Queen Victoria sat on the throne and class-stratification was the order of the day, but were now nothing but self-defeating and anachronistic irrelevancies.

In the eight months that Ron and I went out, I would be a very rich woman if I had a pound for every time he introduced class into something which had absolutely nothing to do with it. Although he was undoubtedly intelligent and could be both fun and charming, he spoke about class so much that my brother Mickey, left-wing by any interpretation, started to refer to Ron as a 'class bore'. Nor could Ron ever see that it was the chip he had on his shoulder that caused problems where none needed to exist. Admittedly, Gloria would never have regarded him as her equal, but she had no choice except to tolerate him if I wanted him in my life. The quality of our personal relationship rather than the disparity in our worldly stations should have been the focus of his attention, but he was having none of it. He was on a real class kick, fomenting issues where none arose, causing problem after problem until finally, when he tried to incite my cousin Joe Joe Ziadie's servants to walk out on Christmas Day, telling them that our family were oppressors of the poor and taking advantage of them (they reported Ron's comments right back to Joe Joe), not even the advantages of his six foot three frame or undeniable intelligence could compensate any longer for the hassle, and we came to a parting of the ways shortly after that.

'The peasant', as Gloria called him, became history, though not before his presence in my life had made her realize that I was past the point of deferring to her wishes the way I did when she had scuppered my relationship with Maurice Shoucair. By going out with Ron long after she had made her disapproval known, I was wordlessly telling her that I was putting my wishes before hers. This was not a message Gloria liked hearing. As Lorna Benjamin makes clear in *An Interpersonal Theory of Personality Disorders: Major Theories of Personality Disorder*, within their personal relationships, narcissists take presumptive control of others and behave with contempt towards them. They expect their wishes to be granted, and when they are not, they react with rage. Unbeknownst to me, this is what Gloria was building up against me, not only because I had dared to become a competitor in the beauty stakes, but also because I had committed another solecism that narcissists cannot tolerate: I was functioning as an independent person, when this daughter of Narcissus's attitude towards her children was that they are not separate individuals but sources of need gratification.

Marjorie now arrived in Jamaica from Cayman, where she was living, having reconciled with her second husband, and inadvertently added fuel to the fire that was consuming my relationship with my mother. Unusually for her, Marjorie was staying with us. Maisie had recently moved from the big house into the townhouse adjoining the one she had bought for Mickey. Marjorie had been to the hairdresser and returned with a tale which had given her much pleasure and which she confidently and naïvely hoped would give all of us equal pleasure when she recounted it. 'The funniest thing happened at the beauty parlour,' she confided. 'One of the ladies came with a cutting from an American paper. Knowing that you go there, Georgie, she thought Veronica would like to see it. It said that you'd been modelling in a fashion show for the Jamaica Tourist Board at the Stony Hill Hotel and that you're regarded as one of the most beautiful girls in the world. Isn't that a lovely compliment?'

'Ha. If she's one of the world's most beautiful girls in the world, I must be the most beautiful woman in the universe,' Gloria harrumphed dismissively.

'Don't you listen to your mother,' Marjorie said to me, rolling her eyes. 'No matter how beautiful she might consider herself as having once been, she's never been as good-looking as you. Take it from me. I've known her from the day she was born.'

'I can see you plan to pack this child's head up with as much rubbish as you packed Mickey's up with,' Gloria said caustically. 'As if I don't already have enough problems to contend with.'

'I never packed Mickey up with any rubbish, and I'm not packing this one's up with any either. There's no harm in her knowing the nice things people say about her. God knows she had to live through years of listening to people saying the most awful things about her while you ignored what was going on, and if that didn't warp her, you tell me how a compliment published in an American newspaper is going to harm her? Let me tell you something, Gloria, if you think I've come here to have you pick a row with me, think again. I'll pack my bags and move to a hotel right now if I hear another word out of you,' Marjorie said firmly.

'My goodness,' Gloria said jokingly, 'what a way you've become oversensitive since you married Alex. Can't anyone even joke with you now without you pouncing on them? Just because your birthday is in August doesn't mean that you have to attack like a lioness over every little joke.'

'Anyway, darling,' Marjorie said to me, cutting her sister out of the conversation, 'I thought you'd like to know what the American papers are saying.'

'Thanks, Auntie,' I said, no doubt making things even worse than they already were. 'It's nice to know, though I try to keep a sense of proportion about that sort of thing. One must always remember that age withers all beauty and therefore it behoves no one to put too much reliance upon one's looks. Even if I were truly as good-looking as my more enthusiastic admirers say, which, let's face it, I'm not. On any given day, there are countless better-looking girls than me walking down Fifth Avenue or Bond Street if not King Street.'

'You see,' Marjorie said triumphantly to Gloria, 'the child has more sense at her tender age than you've ever had, and by the looks of it, ever will have.'

Gloria's response to all the attention I was garnering was not immediate, but when it came, it was decisive and vicious and out of the blue. Kitty recounts what happened. 'You and I were sitting on the floor in your bedroom one afternoon listening to music. I remember it was a Wednesday because Daddy was at home resting. In those days, stores closed at midday on Wednesdays. All of a sudden, the door burst open and Mummy stormed into the bedroom and started to attack you. She rained down blows on you, punching and hitting you. You tried to defend yourself as best you could without responding in kind, and I ran to fetch Daddy, who I remember was fast asleep. He pulled her off you and said, "Are you mad? You must be mad. Leave the child alone. She's done nothing. You can't go around beating up someone who hasn't done anything to deserve it."'

Kitty says the memory of the incident is emblazoned on her mind for several reasons. 'I've never forgotten it because the attack was completely unprovoked. Daddy was so unnerved by it that he asked us if we felt it was safe for him to go and play poker that night at Uncle Wesley's house. We told him we thought it would be fine so he went.' Michael offering to forego a pleasure was as memorable as Gloria being benevolent to her children when there was no audience present to register her wonderfulness.

Tellingly, I have absolutely no recollection of that incident, possibly because it was followed by another shortly afterwards which was so dreadful that the subsequent one is fixed in my mind with all the immediacy of something that happened twenty seconds ago.

It was November of 1972. I had recently returned from spending two months in New York and Canada. While away, I had given careful thought to avoiding further conflict with my mother. It bothered me that in the last year our relationship had deteriorated to the point that practically every conversation seemed to end in a squabble. As I saw it, the problems between her and Ron were really an irrelevancy.

No matter how well-intentioned I was, Gloria somehow always managed to twist and turn everything I said or did so that I ended up having an exchange I had not wished for or expected. I knew from past observation of her *modus operandi* that it was virtually impossible to pinpoint the precise moment in any conversation when it derailed from pleasant to unpleasant, for she was a past-mistress at pushing exchanges in a direction people did not intend or desire. So I resolved to avoid all future conflict by ignoring any of her manipulations which would raise the temperature to a greater heat than I desired – and I wanted no heat at all.

Filled with those good intentions, I returned to Jamaica and, within days of my arrival, I had been presented ample opportunity to test my resolve. No two words out of my mouth failed to elicit a mocking or sarcastic response from my mother. Determined to avoid falling into the pit of further squabbling, every time she dribbled poison, I ignored it, acting as if she had said and done nothing untoward.

If I thought my tactic would successfully prevent further conflict, I was mistaken. A fortnight after my return home, I was lying on my bed drying my hair with one of those old-fashioned dryers which had a plastic cap that fitted over one's head and was connected by a hose to the machine. I was ignoring, as best I could, what was going on outside. Gloria had been in a mood for hours that was vitriolic even by her standards. There was a new and very ugly housemaid who replaced the last of a series of houseboys. This unfortunate woman had not polished the floor in the breakfast porch to Gloria's exacting standards, and she had made her clean it thirty-six times. I know it was that number of times because Gloria had been counting them. 'Ma'am, I beg you, show me what I'm not doing,' the poor woman had been pleading for well over an hour. But her sadistic mistress refused to point out the error of her ways. 'Figure it out for yourself, you lazy nigger,' Gloria would say. 'Do it again. You *will* do it until you get it right.'

Because my bedroom shared a window with the back veranda, where Gloria was sitting spitting out instructions and invective, I could hear with uncomfortable clarity what was transpiring.

Had I not come back from New York with the resolution to steer clear of any conflict with my mother, I would by this time have interceded on behalf of the poor maid. But, intent on avoiding falling into what Gloria called her 'wasp's nest', I kept my counsel.

'Thirty-six times you've cleaned the blasted floor,' Gloria finally said, 'and it is still as black as your damned heart. God must have created you to try white people's patience. You'd better pack your bags and go before you make me do something I'll live to regret.'

'You going fire me for this?' the incredulous maid asked.

'That's right, you lazy nigger. Anyone who can't clean a floor isn't fit to work for decent people. Now get out of my sight and pack your bundle of rags. I'll be out to deal with you when you're ready to leave.'

Although those of us who lived with Gloria knew the form, the maid did not. As she bemoaned her fate and made the truthful observation that her employer was being unnecessarily harsh, I could stand by silently no longer, so I went out to where Gloria was sitting and, to give myself justification for interceding without it appearing that I was interfering, I said to her, 'Would you like me to help you?'

'Go and tell that raucous *nayger* woman that she'd better shut her trap before she gives me a migraine – unless of course she wants me to go outside and beat her to a pulp with that selfsame mop with which she couldn't shine the floor,' Gloria said in grandiloquent, almost quaint, fashion.

Armed with the permission I needed to intercede, I went to the maid's room. I strongly counselled her to be quiet, to accept her dismissal without further protest, to pack her bags and to depart as quickly as she could. 'What about my two weeks' severance pay?' she asked, bringing up the bugbear that always resulted in the police being called.

'You won't get it from Mummy, but if you go quietly, and stand on Wiltshire Avenue until Daddy comes home, I'll get the money off him and bring it out to you or send it out with Owen, ' I said.

Having sorted that out with as much justice as one could reasonably hope for when dealing with Gloria, I returned to my bedroom via the back veranda, where she was sitting imperiously sipping her gin and tonic. 'I hope you made it clear to the monkey that she'd better be off the premises before I run out of patience?' she offered by way of a 'thank you'.

'Yes, Mummy,' I said gently and headed back inside to finish drying my hair.

No more than ten minutes could have elapsed before the room to my bedroom was pitched open ferociously and there stood Gloria, a cigarette in her hand and her face distorted with rage.

'You think you're so special just because people are packing up your head with all sorts of nonsense,' she spat as smoke poured out of her nostrils. I was transfixed, not only by the double-action of railing while smoking, but also by the non-sequitur of my being special, which had absolutely no connection with the dismissal of the maid or anything else that had transpired that day.

Having resolved in New York and Canada not to respond to any provocation, I decided the wisest course of action would be to do nothing. Nothing at all. Except continue drying my hair. As if nothing untoward were happening. So I looked at my crazed mother and neither said nor did a thing.

Gloria, however, was spoiling for a fight; and what Gloria wanted, Gloria intended to get. Menacingly, she stepped towards me, switching the cigarette from her index and middle fingers to her index finger and thumb, so that it now became like a weapon.

'You are nothing but a self-satisfied little stinker. But I gave you everything you have, and what I have given, I can take back. Do I make myself clear, Ravishing Beauty?' she spat, stopping by the foot of my bed.

I knew that at this point I was supposed to say, 'Yes, Mummy', which would have allowed her to twist the scenario any way she wished, whether it was accusing me of being impertinent or ungrateful, or disrespectful or argumentative or of being any of the myriad other accusations which she customarily hurled at me and had been hurling at Mickey, Libby and the servants from ever since I could remember. I had determined not to function according to her script, however, so I remained silent.

'Great beauty indeed! Well, I gave you your beauty, and I intend to take it back as you don't deserve it, you stinking little bitch,' she said, moving towards where I was sitting on the bed.

Sometimes things unfurl in slow motion. What takes a second seems to last a lifetime. This was one of those occasions. As Gloria bore down upon me, I remember wondering what she was on about. How could she take back my looks? They weren't hers. They were mine. What was she on about now?

Like all of her children, I was so used to her ravings that I regularly discounted what she was saying. I was about to discover to my horror that this was not the time to be discounting anything. She was now standing no more than a foot in front of me, and a second after I had discounted her threat to take back the beauty she had given me, she lurched forwards and jabbed her cigarette in the direction of my right cheek. Whether it was instinctive self-preservation or the detachment that had come from my earlier resolve, I will never know, but in that split second, I had somehow moved away. What happened next I do not know, for this was the one and only time in my life that I blacked out. When I came to again, I had Gloria pinned down on the floor in the passage outside my bedroom.

'What I gave, I can take back,' she was snarling, and I was straddling her, banging her head on the floor as if it were a ball. 'Shut up, you bitch,' I was saying to her 'I said shut up. If you don't shut up, I'll make you.'

'You can't make me do anything I don't want to do. No jack man can make me do anything I don't want to do, much less a nonentity like you,' Gloria sneered as I bounced her head back and forth on the tiles and warned her to shut up.

When she realized that I had no intention of stopping until she was silent, Gloria started to shout, 'Owen, come and get this lunatic off me! Come here right now! Owen! Owen!'

This scenario must have continued for a good few minutes – quite how many I have no idea, for time was immeasurable in such a situation. Like an endlessly-repeated cycle of action and reaction, I straddled her, bouncing her head and ordering her to shut up while she hurled invective at me between bellowing for Owen.

Finally, Owen arrived, the other servants having run outside into the garden to fetch him. Then a peculiar thing happened. Owen did not lift me off Gloria, or in any other way touch me. He hauled her from beneath me, as I continued battering her head on the floor. 'You notice, Miss G, I didn't touch you,' he said later to me by way of explanation. 'I figured if I drag Gin and Tonic out from under you, that way it hurt her more and give you the chance to get in a few more blows.'

Once Owen had us separated, Gloria and I squared off, like two snarling animals.

'Get out of my house,' she screamed. 'Get out of my house this instant.'

'It's not your house,' I screamed right back, determined to stand up to her no matter what she said or did. I could hardly believe that my own mother had tried to destroy my face, but I also knew that that was precisely what she had attempted, and moreover, that she had done so out of a perverted fit of envy. 'It's my father's house. I'm going nowhere until he tells me to leave.'

'This is my house and you will pack your little knapsack right now, otherwise I'll call the police to throw you out,' she said in the manner and phraseology she used with the servants.

'Why don't you do that?' I said sarcastically, walking towards the telephone in the passage and picking it up. 'Would you care to tell me the telephone number of Mathilda's Corner Police Station? God knows you should know it by heart by now. You use – or should I say *ab*use – it enough.'

Gloria looked at me, and realizing that I had called her bluff and she could hardly call the police on me without creating a monumental scandal once word got out, harrumphed, turned on her heels and walked back outside onto the back veranda. 'You wait until your father comes home,' she shrieked. 'He'll fix your wagon for you.'

'There is not one goddamned thing either he or you can do to me,' I said.

'Striking your own mother,' she said.

'Trying to burn your own daughter on the face, you vicious, demented bitch,' I said, following her outside. 'It's not enough that you tormented that poor woman. No. You had to try to ruin my face, just because people think I'm beautiful and you think the only person on earth who should ever get attention or a compliment is you. Well, get used to it. From hereon in you'll be getting fewer and fewer compliments and less and less attention until in the not-too-distant future you'll be getting *none*. *None*. Do you understand what I'm saying? *None at all*. Because in the natural order of things, you're past your glory days and from hereon in you're only ever going to be a fading – soon to be faded – pathetic creature who once was a beautiful woman but who is now nothing but a raddled, vicious, twisted, envious, jealous, vicious bag who didn't develop any soul and therefore is left with *nothing* – do you hear me? *Nothing!* – to replace the looks which you once relied upon to the exclusion of all else. You have to be pretty sick if you think that by destroying my looks it helps you with the loss of your own.'

With that, I walked back into my bedroom and located, under my bedside table, the butt, which was all that was left of the cigarette with which she had tried to burn my face, the rest having disintegrated and scattered all over the floor. 'What nature of beast seeks to destroy the face of her own child?' I thought, looking at it. Rather than answering the question, I picked up the butt and walked outside with it, to the back veranda where Gloria was sitting in her inevitable chair. Standing over her, I had it poised to drop it in her lap. 'Here is your handiwork,' I said. 'You might like to cogitate upon what you've just tried to do, you demented bitch.' Then, thinking better of getting rid of the evidence, I said, 'On second thoughts, I'll keep it. Knowing what a liar you are, I'll hang onto the proof of your efforts. Let's see you lie your way out of this one. You really are the biggest bitch anyone can meet,' alluding to her proud boast of being the biggest bitch anyone would ever encounter.

'You'd better believe it,' Gloria said proudly, as if evil were a worthy accomplishment.

After that response, there really was nothing more for me to say or hear. It had all been said and done. After telephoning my Aunt Hilda to ask her if I could stay at her house until I had decided what to do, I went back into my bedroom to await my father's arrival, knowing that he would most likely take the side of the woman who was always right 'whether she's wrong or right'. It would be intriguing, nevertheless, to see how he justified such a glaring violation of the rights and well-being of one of his children.

Of course, I hoped that he would take a moral stand and order his unscrupulous wife to apologize for an act that would have resulted in disastrous consequences for both of us had she succeeded in disfiguring me. What Gloria had tried to do was so beyond the pale, so inexcusable, so potentially destructive that she had, in the moment she had tried to disfigure me, destroyed whatever remained of the positive aspects of our relationship. Thereafter, we might have a formal relationship, but I would never again feel any degree of warmth or affection for her. She had well and truly finished off our relationship, and we both knew it.

When Michael came home, Gloria was waiting, like a praying mantis, to poison proceedings. She ordered him to dispense with the maid, who was waiting in her bedroom, informing him that she had a far more important matter for him to deal with as soon as he had got the 'impertinent, lazy nigger off the premises'. One benefit of what Gloria had tried to do to me was that the woman was actually one of the few members of staff she had ever dismissed who got her two weeks' severance pay without any question, for Gloria was

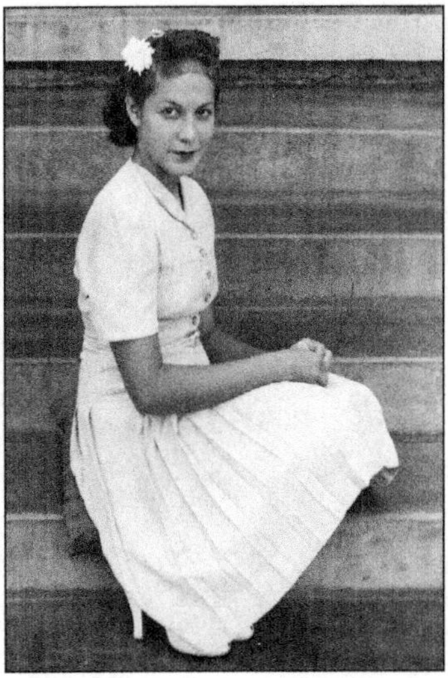

The fifteen-year old Gloria, already aware of the power of her wiles, around the time she captivated Michael

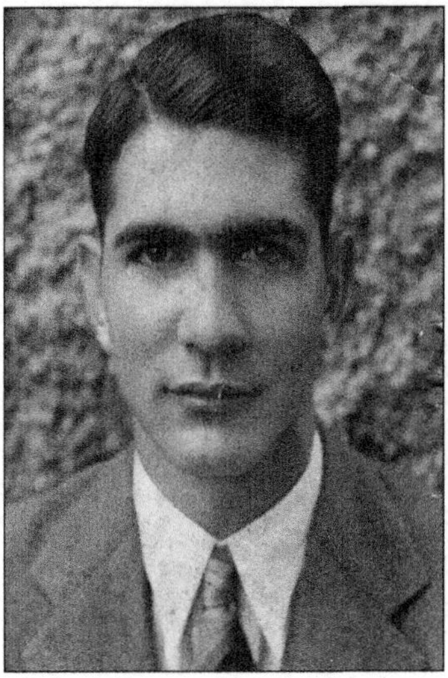

Michael just before marriage, aged 29

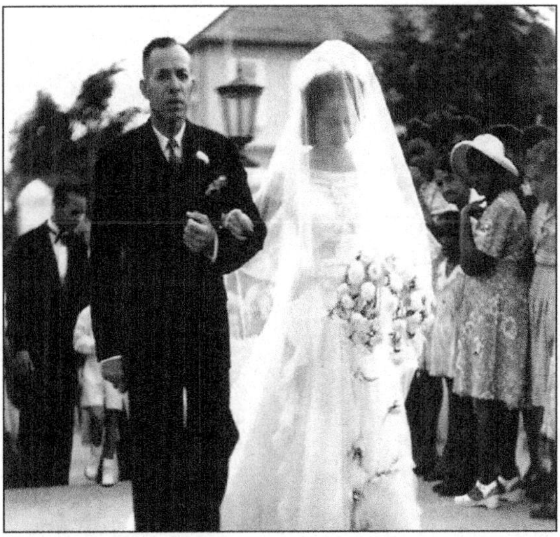

The diaspproving Lucius Smedmore escorts his daughter into the Cathedral for her marriage, observed by a gathering of respectful spectators in hats

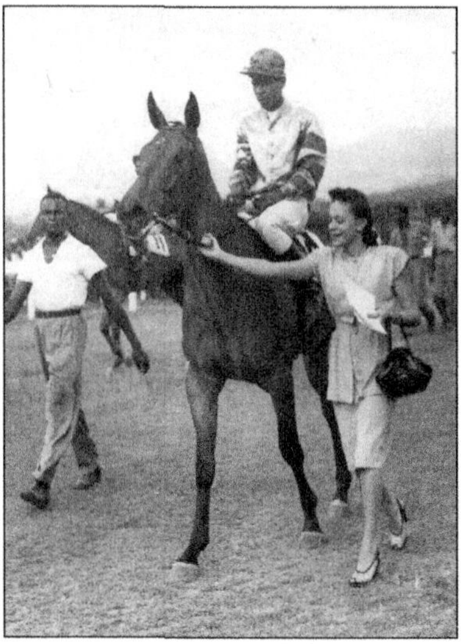

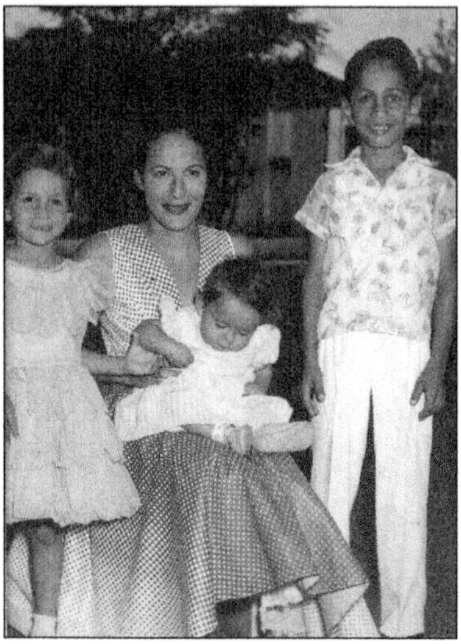

Marriage brought forseen riches and the glamorous lifestyle that included such tasks as leading in her husband's winners

Gloria at twenty eight knew how to project the socially-acceptable image of the devoted mother when in fact she was anything but to Libby, Kitty and Mickey, pictured with her

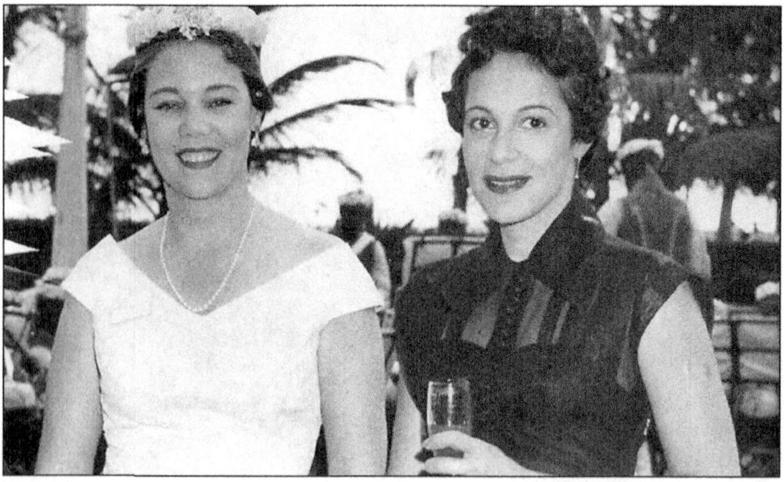

More to Gloria's taste was socialising with friends such as Vida MacMillan, by courtesy of the Jamaica Tourist Board

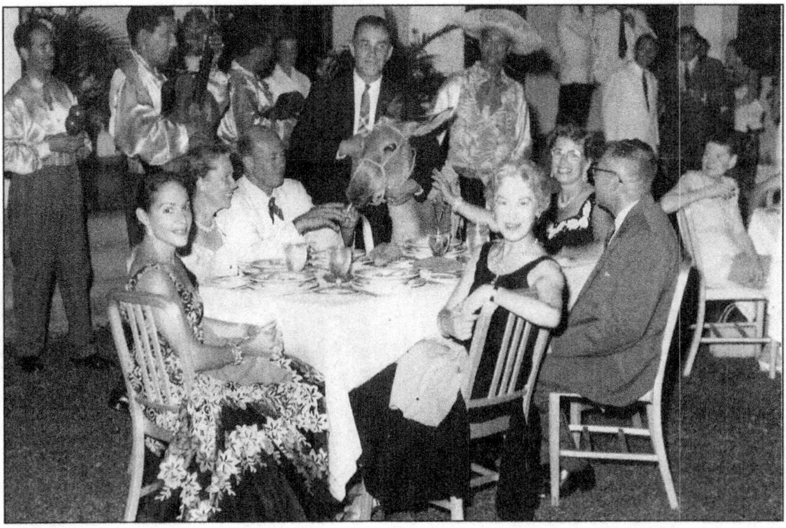

Gloria (far left) with Lucius (back to camera) at the Tropicana in Havana, Cuba, the year before the Revolution

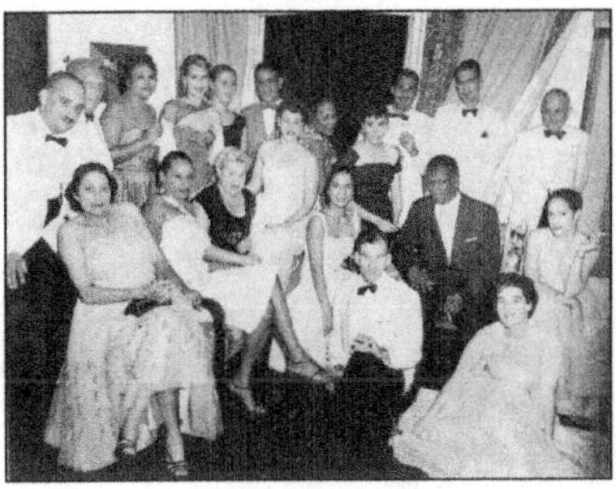

Dudley MacMillan (left) and Vida (standing in white) at their reception for Nat 'King' Cole with Michael standing behind and Gloria sitting to his left

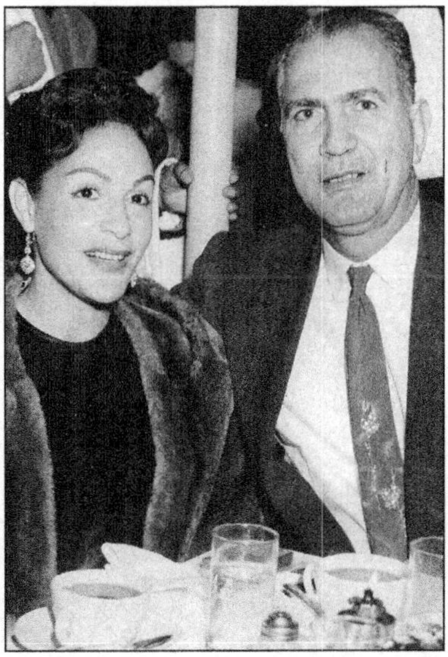

Michael and Gloria nightclubbing in Mexico in the mid-sixties

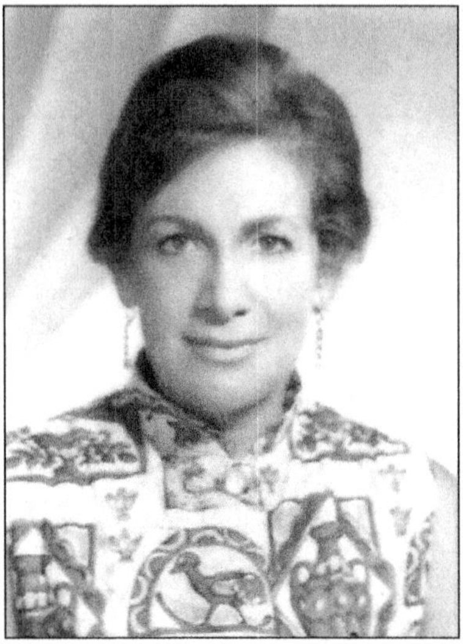

Marjorie, who was handsome rather than beautiful and a far better mother to her nieces and nephew than her sister Gloria

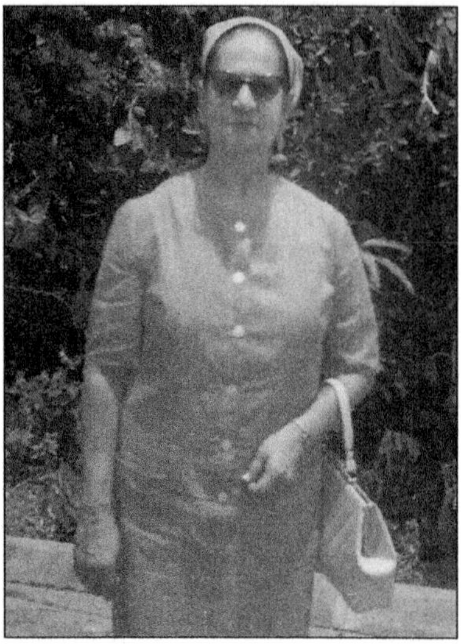

Maisie, the redoubtable and non-conformist matriarch of the family

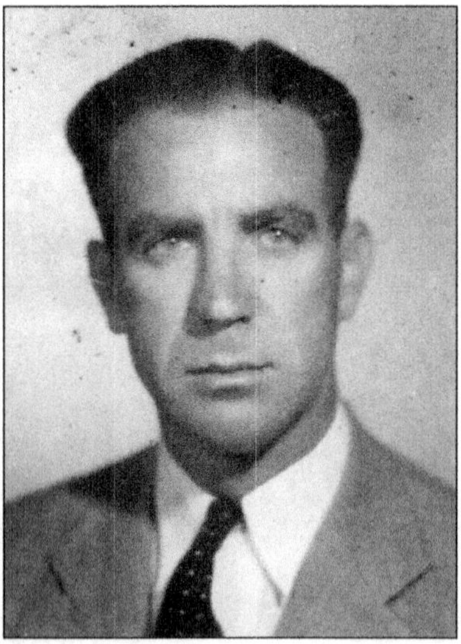

Rafael Perez Guerrero, the lover whose existence raised questions about Gloria's paternity

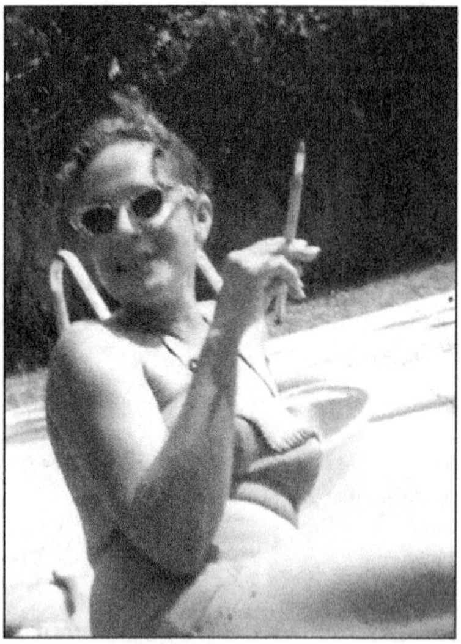

Gloria beside the swimming pool sporting the ivory cigarette holder Mickey gave her a few month's after Lucius's murder

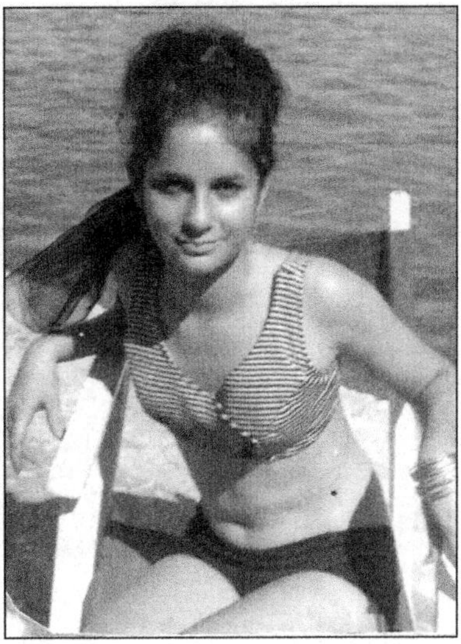

Libby at fifteen was too attractive for the competitive Gloria's comfort

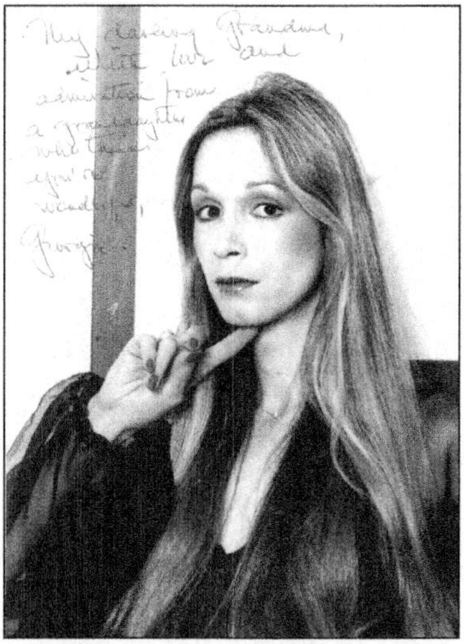

The author grew into another target for her mother's malicious vanity

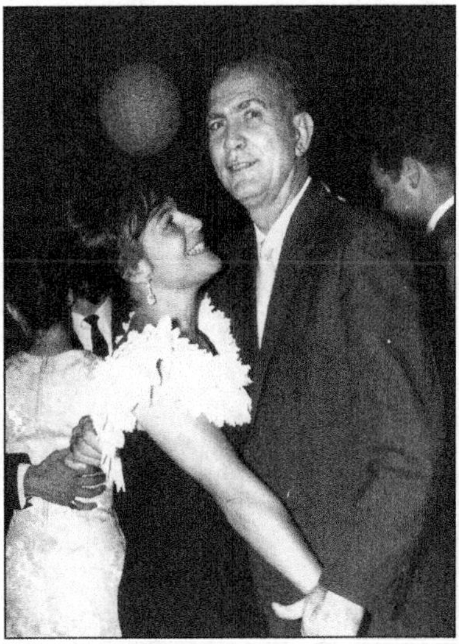

At forty Gloria was still exercising her sexual allure on husband and admirers alike

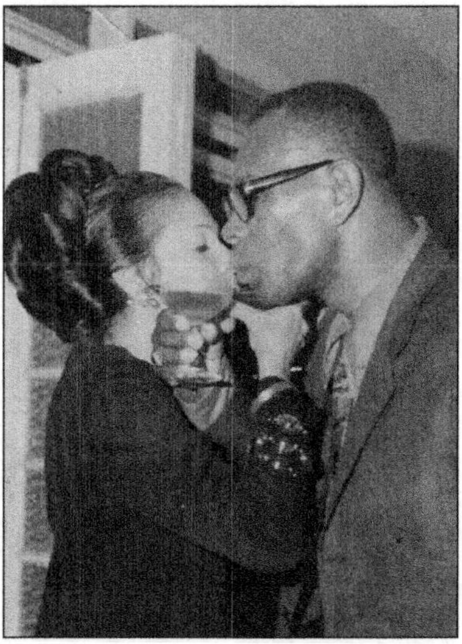

Although miscegenation was anathema to her, Gloria was happy to flirt with the Attorney General Victor Grant and anyone else who possessed political power

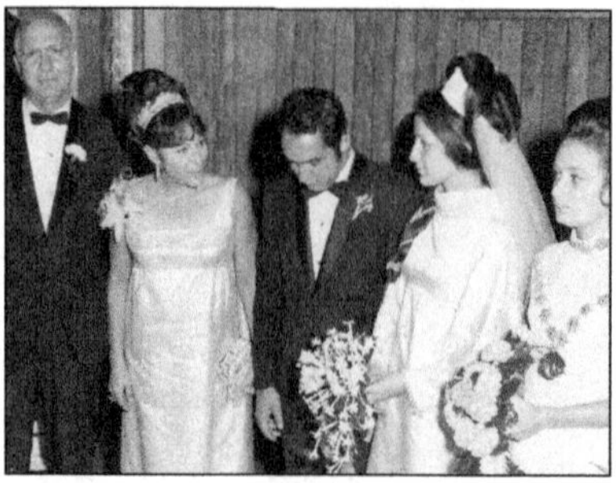

Michael, Gloria, Ben, Libby and Kitty might have appeared unified at the wedding, but behind the scenes Gloria had done everything in her power to usurp and minimze her daughter's big day

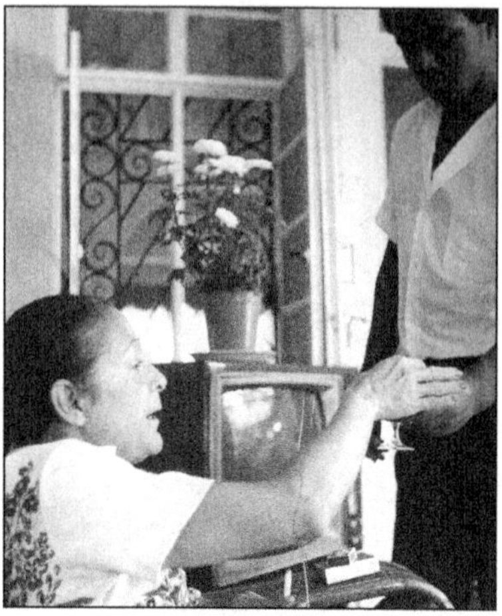

As Gloria's allure waned in her 40s, she turned to the raw exercise of power floated on a sea of booze to replace the highs her beauty had once brought her

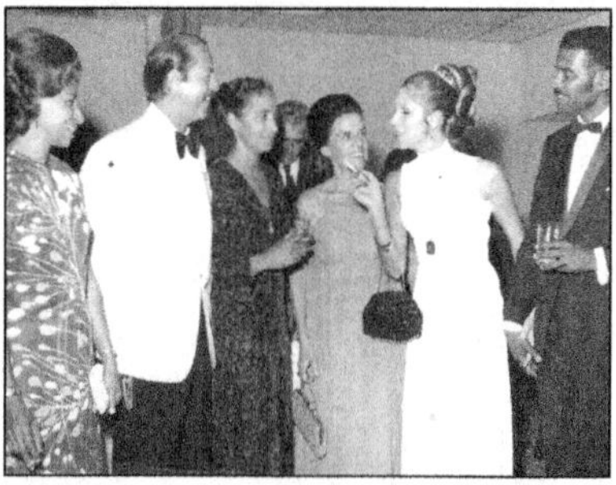

(L) The author (in white) between pianist Andree Juliette Brun and Dr Hugh Wynter, with (l to r) Dr Mavis Anderson, Jim Anderson,and Mrs Wynter at the Gala she organised which so infuriated her mother

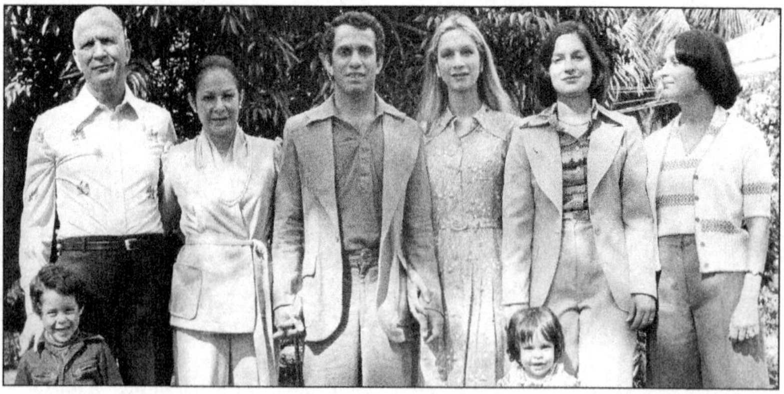

Richard Adeney photographed Michael, Gloria, Mickey, the author, Libby, Kitty, Andrew and Elizabeth (in foreground) within hours of Gloria refusing to ackowledge her drinking had become a problem

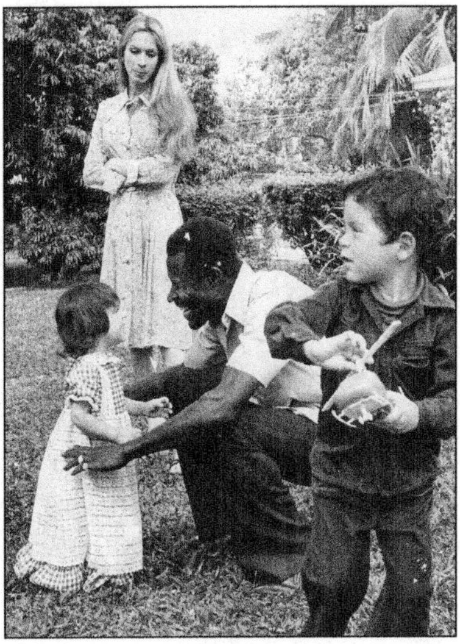

The author looks on as Owen, the head gardener and much reverred 'member of the family' plays with her niece and nephew

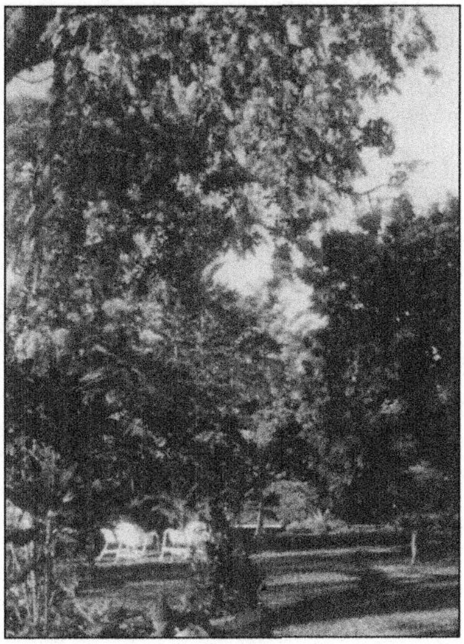

Gloria's orchid garden attracted viewers from all over the world

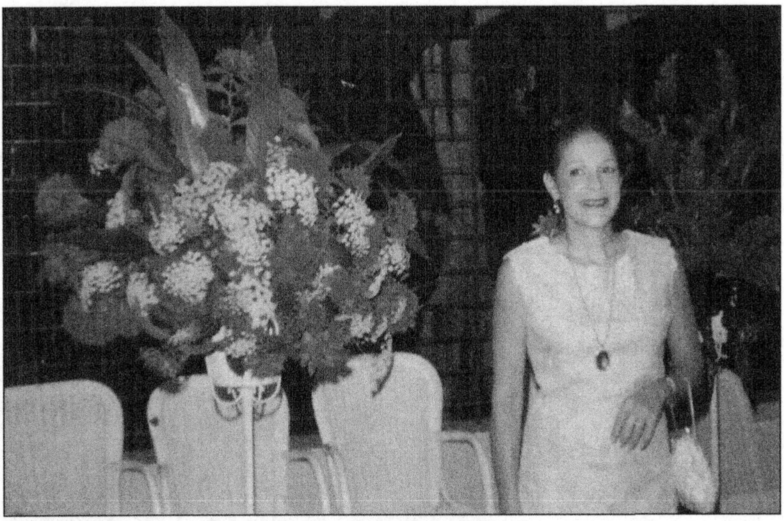

Gloria, dried out, on the fabled back verandah with some of the floral arrangements which brought her international recognition

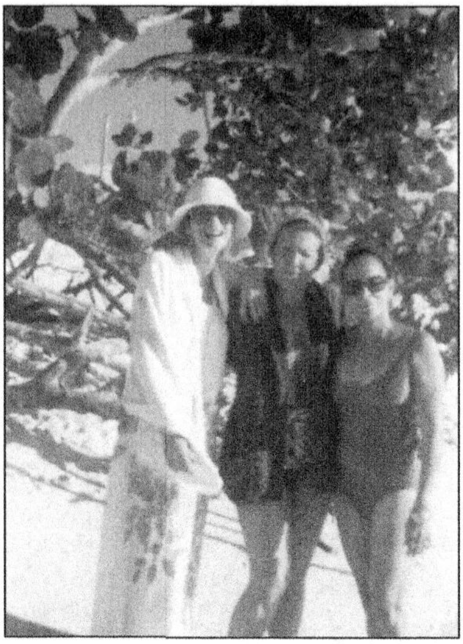

The author with Marjorie and Gloria in Grand Cayman the day before the major bust-up

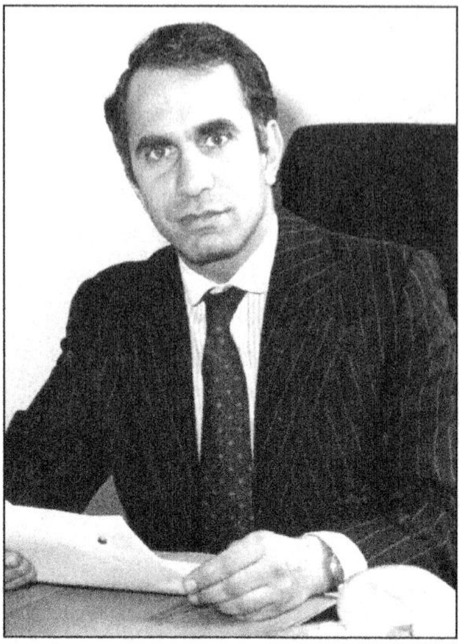

The 'Fool' had become a respected member of the legal profession in both England and Jamaica, photographed shortly before he was diagnosed with cancer of the mouth

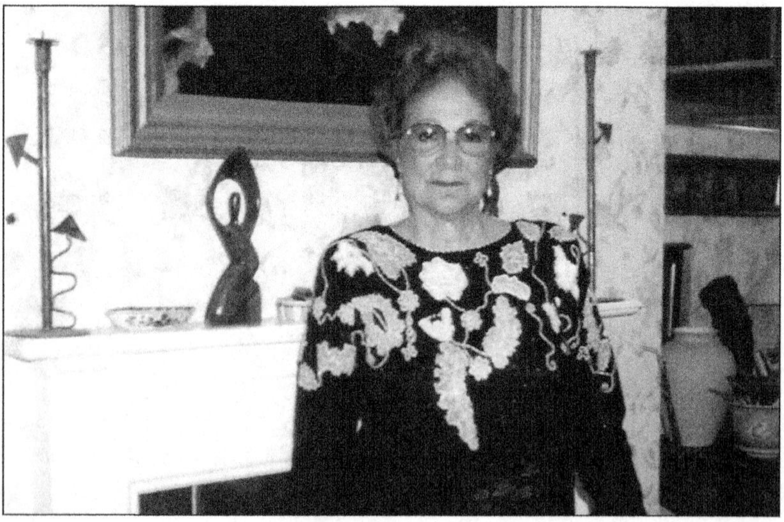

The widowed Gloria in London aged 70, when it appeared as if the leopard had dimmed if not changed her spots.

so eager to plunge the knife into me that she didn't even concern herself with Michael paying her off.

Of course, all the other servants knew that this was the precursor to the main drama, and as soon as the maid had departed, Gloria launched into a diatribe about how I had attacked her.

'You're a liar. You attacked me. You tried to burn me on my face with your cigarette. I only defended myself,' I said.

'Did you touch your mother?' Michael asked, suddenly switching into his 'macho-protector-of- the-delicate-wife posture'. Really, I thought, this is too preposterous. On some level, he is as deluded as she is.

'Do you know a way of preventing someone from burning you on the face with a lighted cigarette that involves not touching them?' I asked.

'You touched your mother,' he erupted accusingly.

'I defended myself against her, yes, but, before you surrender yourself to your baser instincts, let me remind you that she is my mother and she has no right to try to burn me on the face. You surely don't think I was going to stand by and let her burn my face without making every effort to stop her, do you?'

'This is my house and I am the only person in it with any rights,' Gloria announced. 'What I gave, I can take away.'

I could hardly believe it. Gloria, the quintessential denier of the undeniable, was admitting what she had done.

'She's actually admitting it,' I jubilantly shrieked to my father. 'She's actually admitting having tried to disfigure me. I implore you, for once in your life, to use the brain God gave you and think before you act. Is there ever any justification for a mother disfiguring her child's face?'

Michael, clearly torn between his higher and baser natures, looked from me to Gloria and back again.

'You really did that?' he asked her.

'Not only did she do it, she did it without any provocation,' I said, answering for her. 'I was in my bedroom minding my own business after she'd fired the maid, when she burst in, ranting and raving about me thinking I'm so beautiful. Before I knew what was happening, she was trying to stab me in the face with her lighted cigarette.'

'You must be mad,' Michael said to Gloria.

'Mad or sane, I rule this roost. I have ordered her out and you'd better pitch the little shit out with her belongings if you know what's good for you,' she said as coolly and unemotionally as if she were talking about discarding a useless piece of paper.

'Let me warn you,' I said to Michael, sick to death of his weakness in the face of her abusiveness. 'Mummy's abusiveness is now beyond what anyone, even an ostrich like you, can find acceptable. You have an obligation to yourself, to me, to everyone who comes into contact with her, to say "Enough is enough." If you don't draw a line in the sand now, you will live to regret it for the rest of your life.'

A man who condoned such behaviour was in part responsible for it; and even if I could not stiffen his backbone, I could at least prick his conscience since he, unlike Gloria, had one.

'The nutty buddy is at it again,' Gloria said disparagingly, 'chatting her pontifical rubbish.'

'The only nutty buddy around here is you,' I said to Gloria before turning back to Michael. 'If I leave this house this afternoon,' I continued, 'I will never live under your roof ever again. Someone has to make a stand, and I'd suggest you join me in making one.'

'You think your leaving this house is any loss to me,' Gloria piped up. 'I want you out. Out! I've ordered you out. Out! Out! I can't wait to see your back. I want to be rid of you. Your leaving this house will be no loss to me, I can tell you.'

'No. I know it won't be to you, but it will be to Daddy. No matter what has happened over the years, his children matter to him and he doesn't want to lose any of us,' I said, giving voice to a truth each of us was aware of. 'Don't think on some level he isn't going to hold it against you if you deprive him of any of us, for he will. He may not have the guts to tell you, but you know it, I know it, and he knows it.'

'Are you going to stand there like a damned *mumu* and let this whippersnapper run rings around you with her silken tongue?' Gloria said to the pained-looking Michael. 'Get her off my premises this instant.'

'Maybe you ought to go and stay with your grandmother for a few days,' Michael suggested, walking with me towards my bedroom.

'I've already arranged with Aunt Hilda to stay with her,' I said.

'Stay for a few days until things die down,' he said.

'No, Daddy. If I leave this house this afternoon, that's it. I will never live here again. Mummy has to be taught a lesson, and if you won't teach her, I don't know how she'll ever learn it.'

'She really tried to burn you on your face?' he asked, clearly struggling to believe the unbelievable even though he already knew it to be a fact.

I nodded.

'I don't know what I'm going to do with your mother,' he said impotently.

'Stop her or share responsibility for her behaviour,' I said.

'I wish life was that simple,' he said.

'It is, Daddy. It may not be easy, but it is that simple. When are you going to start facing facts?'

Crestfallen, he left my bedroom, to fetch Owen to help move my stuff into my car. Gloria had not only proven how viciously destructive she could be. Her proud, obviously sincere, admission that having me out of her house left her unmoved bore out psychiatrist S C Ekleberry's observation that narcissists' 'relationships must have potential for advancing their purposes or enhancing their self-esteem. Without any apparent payoff, a relationship has no purpose and is unlikely to be sustained.' Even though she was my mother, and I her daughter and supposedly her favourite child, she had shown that when the chips were down, her feelings for me were even more inconsequential than a decent person's are for a total stranger.

This attempt to burn my face was the most serious interfamily incident since Gloria had orchestrated depriving Mickey of Scrammy and Audrey's Beetle some years before. No one could quite get their head around what she had tried to do, though her unapologetic and remorseless failure to deny it meant that they could find no excuse to explain away her conduct either.

Maisie was particularly upset. 'You shouldn't have raised your hand to your mother,' she kept on saying, ignoring, like Michael, the realities of defending oneself against a crazed beast. 'But I cannot for the life of me comprehend how any mother, much less a child of mine, could try to disfigure another human being, and her own daughter at that.'

When Maisie raised the subject with Gloria, her unrepentant daughter could find no excuse or explanation. This still didn't stop her from abusing her mother for 'interfering' and making out that Maisie was therefore responsible for what had happened as a result of 'always interfering'. The consequence was that Maisie, incensed at being blamed for something which could not rationally be placed at her doorstep by any stretch of the imagination, stopped speaking to Gloria.

Mickey also stopped speaking to our mother. Michael had telephoned him to come up to the house to help move me out, and when he arrived and Gloria tried to stop him taking away a television set I had bought in New York with my own money on the grounds that it was hers, he snapped.

'You are a terrible human being. Vicious, spoiled, evil. If I never see you again, that will be fine by me.'

He pushed past her, put the television set in the car and exchanged not another word with his mother for the next few months.

When Gloria complained to Michael and tried to get him to defend her against his son, even he had had enough.

'For God's sake woman,' he said, 'are you going to drive away every one of my children?'

The answer, as it would turn out, was yes. Gloria was heading down a new path. With her looks on the decline, her circle of admirers diminishing, her political influence waning, she was intent on stripping her husband of every interest and link to the outside world. His role, although none of us knew it yet, was to be her anointed attention-giver. His existence was to be valid only insofar as it related to her. She had found herself a new companion, a new pair of ears, even though this was information she had not yet imparted to him, or indeed to anyone else.

Libby, in Canada, did not even know about the face-burning incident until weeks after it had taken place, but Kitty, who was at home, attending The Priory School, was in the thick of it. She quietly sympathized with me, keeping well out of her mother's way, lest she find herself in the line of fire, and proved – for neither the first nor the last time – an invaluable supporter. She was Aunt Hilda's favourite niece, and when she backed up my account of what had happened, Aunt Hilda, armed with corroboration, quickly spread the word throughout the family of how 'that madwoman has gone too far this time'.

Marjorie, in Grand Cayman, also had her part to play, sending me her sympathies and the offer of money if I needed it. I declined, as I had already found a job running a boutique. In fact, all the aunts and uncles and cousins who heard about the incident – and it flew around the family circle like wildfire – bemoaned Gloria's latest outrage. But no one except Maisie and Mickey actually challenged her directly.

Chapter Seventeen

Some things are so terrible that no relationship can recover from them. My relationship with Gloria had suffered such a severe blow that on one level, it was well and truly over and would remain so forever. It doesn't matter how you dress it up. When someone is so malevolent that they seek to ruin your looks because theirs are in decline, they have given you a snapshot of their soul which tells you in unmistakable terms that this person is not worth knowing. As far as I was concerned, the fact that the individual in question was my mother made the matter worse, and I was not tempted, for even a nanosecond, to justify or excuse her conduct.

From then, until Gloria died in 2005, the events of that terrible day in 1972 froze my heart. She was not a luxury I could afford. Had she been repentant or remorseful, there might have been room for healing, but because her attitude was one of absolute entitlement, she made it impossible for me to heal the breach. And it never really did heal, even though there were times when it looked as if it might have been papered over.

I have to say, in the early days, I was both outraged and upset by what Gloria had done, but on another level, I immediately accepted it with a serenity that I found surprising. Indeed, I queried why I was not having more difficulty coming to terms with what had happened, little realizing that she had liberated me from the obligation of having to cope with such a perverse mother figure. Some burdens are simply not worth the effort, and she was one. It would take me half a lifetime and years of therapy to figure out that this was why I had accepted the loss of my mother so readily. But even as I was trying to come to terms with what I was going through, I knew that she was now dead to me on a profound level.

Had she died then, I have no doubt that she would have spared me years of torment and questions. Instead, she now hurtled off down a new track, resourcefully obtaining for herself all the attention and sympathy which the real narcissist requires. In the process, she instilled doubt and distress the way wedding guests scatter confetti on newlyweds.

At this point, it is important to address the narcissistic personality and narcissistic personality disorder. Narcissism comes from the fable of Narcissus. As students of Ancient Greek mythology learn, he was a beautiful youth who did not think any of his female suitors worthy of his beauty. Extreme vanity being a sin, the gods condemned him to fall in love with his own reflection in a pond. Captured by his own image, he finally withered away and died.

The categorization of extreme narcissism as a personality disorder is relatively recent. Indeed, it is only in the last two decades that it has received the medical attention it deserves, having been registered as a mental disorder in the Fourth Edition of *Diagnostic Statistics Manual of Mental Disorders* (*DSM-IV*) in 1980. Until then, narcissism was seen more as a character flaw rather than a severe medical disorder and dismissed accordingly.

Gloria's serious personality disorder was always going to be difficult to treat even if it had been recognized for the real problem it was. Narcissists are notoriously unamenable to treatment, if only because they disdain anyone who is dumb enough not to appreciate them for the special individuals they are; and a doctor who is trying to cure them of the delusion that they are ultra-special is therefore inevitably regarded as the stupid one for not appreciating their true worth.

However, as the problem had not yet been recognized by the medical profession for the disorder it was, there was no prospect of us as a family receiving adequate medical guidance much less Gloria receiving appropriate medical treatment, even if she had been inclined to change – which she, like most other fully-fledged narcissists, was not.

Dr Martin Kantor describes in *Diagnosis and Treatment of the Personality Disorders* the clinical characteristics of Narcissistic Personality Disorder, all of which Gloria possessed in marked degree, as: inordinate self-pride; self-concern; grandiosity; exaggeration of the importance of one's feelings and experiences; ideas of being the perfect person; reluctance to accept criticism or blame; absence of altruism although gestures may be made for the sake of appearances and deficient level of empathy.

In *DSM-IV Handbook of Differential Diagnosis* Frances, First and Pincus complement those characteristics with the following, which Gloria also possessed in reams: entitlement; shallowness; preoccupation with status, renown, wealth and achievement; a craving for attention, admiration and praise and the placement of excessive emphasis on the display of beauty and power.

Narcissists have an exaggerated sense of their own importance. They routinely overestimate their abilities, inflate their accomplishments and are arrogant. Their belief in their own superiority is the bedrock of their self-image. As far as they are concerned, their belief in their own superiority is sufficient proof of its existence. Whenever others provide them with the external validation they need, they feel proud, vain, self-sufficient, self-righteous and contemptuous of others. They seemingly have little awareness that their conduct can be irrational and objectionable to others, as Drs Millon and Davis confirm. They are often envious of others and consider others to be envious of them. They begrudge others their successes and possessions.

Narcissists assume that anyone will submerge his or her own desires and interests to facilitate their comfort or welfare. They believe that if they want something, this is all the reason they need to have their desire gratified. In their view, anyone is – or should be – as concerned with gratifying their desires as they themselves are. As Millon and Davis put it, they consider that they deserve special consideration from others, while in *Narcissism: Personality Characteristics of the Disordered Personality* Paul Wink makes the point that narcissists use others to fulfil their own psychological needs and to maintain their sense of self, and that they value others according to how well those individuals provide comfort and emotional stability.

According to Martin Kantor, narcissists find it difficult to cooperate with others as their attention is always focused on themselves. Aaron Beck, however, takes the view that they regard other people as vassals or constituents and seek admiration from them to shore up their grandiose self-concept and to affirm or preserve their status of superiority. Such empathy as they possess is always directed at manipulating other people to gratify their own desires or needs. They seldom genuinely commit themselves emotionally and view others as 'feeding grounds' that must at all times provide them with the admiration and approbation they desire. The destructive consequence of their limited capacity to recognize the needs of others is, according to John Oldham and Lois Morris, their tendency to regard those needs as signs of weakness or vulnerability; and, as John Birtchnell and Charles Costello observe, in such circumstances they behave coercively or dominatingly.

Within their personal relationships, narcissists expect admiring deference and often behave contemptuously towards their 'loved ones'. Although they inflate their own achievements and exaggerate their own contribution, they devalue the contributions and achievements of others. Their natural state, as observed by Lorna Benjamin, is being pleased with themselves: they expect to be noticed and acknowledged as special.

They have no regard for their own personal integrity or for the truth or facts, and these failings manifest as pathological lying, according to Salman Aktar, or compulsively exaggerating traits which are incompatible with personal integrity. Millon and Davis also argue that they have a self-important indifference to the rights or needs of others. They are easily offended when others do not provide them with the required response, and thereby frequently feel mistreated, as Elan Golomb observes in *Trapped in the Mirror: Adult Children of Narcissists in Their Struggle for Self.* As far as they are concerned, the rule of reciprocity governing social responsibilities does not apply to them. They expect others to oblige and serve them without giving much if anything back. They are often abrupt, abrasive and lacking in gratitude; as Beck notes, they will throw temper tantrums, verbally harangue and physically, emotionally and, in extreme cases, sexually abuse others, because of their belief that others should be mainly concerned with making them happy or comfortable. They use self-deception to preserve their own illusions and are sufficiently ruthless to do whatever is required to reinforce their self-ascribed superior status. They display an uneven command of moral values and readily shift boundaries, inventing, reinventing or distorting existing values to achieve their goals.

Narcissists are susceptible to alcohol or drug abuse and addiction. This can be to achieve experience of wholeness and vitality, according to Gary Rodin and Sam Izenburg; as a mistaken and erroneous means of achieving significance and avoiding painful clashes with reality, according to Sperry and Clarkson; to fulfil their need for a high level of external stimulation, according to Dr Henry

Richards; for the feelings of dominance, euphoria and well-being they provide, according to Benjamin; to reduce personal discomfort and provide a sense of self-importance and power, according to Beck; or because of the self-involvement and self-indulgence which are fundamental features of their disorder. Unfortunately for all those concerned with narcissists, their belief in their own unique and special qualities insulates them from recognizing that they have developed a reliance on drugs or drink. As Aaron Beck observes, this also permits them to hypothesize that they can escape from the negative effects of addiction and can quit without any problems if they want to. Being so convinced of their innate specialness, they can maintain this delusion in the face of extraordinary evidence to the contrary, according to Richards, remaining firmly convinced that they are in charge of their addiction. In Leon Salzman's view, they possess an inflexible belief in being exempt from both the consequences of their own behaviour and from the laws of nature.

According to the Mayo Clinic, Narcissistic Personality Disorder is one of the rarest forms of personality disorders, limited in their opinion to less than one percent of the general population. In my experience, that figure rises exponentially with the degree of wealth and status people possess. Narcissists are rife in the upper reaches of society. Indeed, many of the character traits required for worldly success fall well within the bounds of the narcissistic personality spectrum, which is the healthier, reduced version of Narcissistic Personality Disorder. More men than women suffer from the disorder.

Because the basis of narcissism is an exaggerated love of self, the very traits which narcissists possess to such an exaggerated extent are, when reduced, shared by healthy people, positive self-image being a requirement of mental health. According to Len Sperry, they can be socially facile, pleasant and endearing, but they are unable to respond with true empathy and can be disdainful and irresponsible. Indeed, many of the traits which become so insufferable in those who suffer from Narcissistic Personality Disorder have great appeal in reduced quantities. According to John Oldham and Lois Morris, self-confidence is the hallmark of the narcissistic style. People with just a touch of the narcissist about them have self-respect; they believe in themselves and their abilities; they are ambitious; they take advantage of their own strengths and abilities; they see themselves as successful, usually the first step up the ladder to success; they are self-possessed and poised; they are outgoing, energetic, competitive, with instinctive political aptitude and an adeptness at understanding power structures; and with an ability to hear and accept criticism. Many of them have a gift for leadership and have personalities which make it possible for them to work effectively and comfortably with others. In short, they are the sort of people you want on your side if you want to get things done.

All those qualities, however, become deadly when allowed to run riot. Self-respect becomes arrogance. Self-regard becomes self-adoration. Self-interest ceases to be something positive and becomes destructive. If narcissism is allowed to flourish unchecked until it becomes a disorder, it usually spills over into other personality disorders. The most common are Histrionic Personality Disorder, self-promotion, attention-seeking and bullying being features of both disorders; and Antisocial Personality Disorder, which shares lack of empathy and amorality as features, making the ghoulish opportunism and fundamental dishonesty of narcissism escalate seamlessly into a complete lack of conscience.

Gloria already exhibited all the fundamental features of Histrionic Personality Disorder, which included constantly seeking attention and praise; often interrupting others in order to dominate conversations; the inflation of everyday events through the use of grandiose language; exaggeration of illness; the belief that everyone loved or was as preoccupied with her as she was with herself, those who were jealous of her simply feeding the delusion of self-importance through malice rather than love; and strong manipulative tendencies.

Indeed, so much of Histrionic Personality Disorder is subsumed in Narcissistic Personality Disorder that one might almost conclude that the former condition is merely a less self-delusional and more stridently attention-seeking version of the latter.

In the case of Antisocial Personality Disorder, there are distinct differences between the other two conditions, even though there are also similarities which mean that those who suffer from one or the other disorder usually exhibit symptoms of the third. Like Narcissism and Hysteria, Antisocial Personality Disorder has only been recently accepted as a valid personality disorder by the medical profession. It is my view that narcissists left unchecked inevitably graduate to antisocial conduct, and while Gloria was undoubtedly a primary narcissist, she also exhibited sufficient features of Antisocial Personality Disorder to make any omission of it indefensible.

Antisocial Personality Disorder covers a wide spectrum of disordered conduct, all loosely antisocial, meaning that it is against other people. Paradoxically, antisocial personalities usually have excellent social skills, which they adeptly deploy to wreak havoc on their trajectory through life. So new is this concept of personality disorder, that there is relatively little medical literature available on it. Diagnosis is difficult, not only because of how little is actually known about it, but also because antisocial personalities are so adept at pulling the wool over the eyes of just about everyone they come into contact with that many of them are misdiagnosed as being mentally ill when in fact they are not.

The medical profession now agrees upon a few defining characteristics of Antisocial Personality Disorder. They have no conscience, which does not mean that they do not know the difference between right and wrong, but that they do not think that it applies to them. Remorse is alien to them. They are never wrong and nothing is ever their fault. They are responsible for nothing, although paradoxically they feel they are always deserving of praise and approbation for everything, whether or not any of the credit is rightfully theirs. Rules are for others and for them to use to their own advantage against others. Like narcissists, they do not relate to other people as equals or indeed even recognize them as the same species of being. This lack of empathy, allied to their lack of conscience, gives them tremendous freedom to be as cruel and callous to others as they please. It also prevents them from having any real affection for anyone or anything. This does not mean that they altogether lack emotions. They can experience sensations such as 'love' and 'romantic love', but their experience of those is lesser in degree and intensity and is invariably self-serving. Certainly, they would never associate love with willingly sacrificing anything for a loved one, unless to do so provided them with a greater reward, in which case they might make the quantum leap and come up with a self-aggrandizing show of sacrifice that was actually anything but. Because they actually have fewer feelings and feel less intensely than others, their lives are devoid of the emotional wealth that a depth of feeling gives to those who truly care. This causes them to experience fundamental emptiness; and feelings of futility, pointlessness and boredom being inevitabilities which they then try to counteract with excessive external stimulation. Paradoxically, this very paucity of emotion, and the way they try to get away from it, gives them a superficial intensity which makes them appear to be more vivid, energetic, potent, powerful and charismatic than others. The result is that they initially appear far more attractive to others than either their emotional content or degree of interest warrants. They also frequently present themselves to others as possessing unusual sexual attractiveness, which, allied to the superficial charm most of them possess, sucks many victims into their orbit.

Most antisocial personalities suffer from varying degrees of other personality disorders along the antisocial spectrum. It is fairly standard to find that a sociopath is also a narcissist and a hysteric, as Gloria was, or a dependent, possibly borderline personality. In their youth, at the peak of their sexual attractiveness, they are often successful; but, no matter how successful they are, as the years pass and their basic emptiness renders all experience futile and unrewarding, they invariably start to behave in a destructive way that wreaks havoc in their own lives as well as the lives of everyone around them. It is a truism that no sociopath dies happy, surrounded by loved ones. Their end is always lonely and unhappy, unless of course they die young, before the cycle of destructiveness has run its course.

Because sociopathic personalities have poor impulse control, they surrender to their basic impulses with a relish that healthier people would find unthinkable. For instance, if they feel angry, no matter how inappropriate or uncalled-for anger is as a response to a particular situation, they will embrace it, act upon it, then justify their self-indulgence by turning it into the fault of their victim. This surrender to impulse is what makes sociopaths so dangerous; a murderous sociopath will have no more compunction about avoiding murder than an irate but non-murderous sociopath will have in slapping someone who doesn't deserve it when the urge to strike out grips them – as Gloria frequently did throughout her life.

Fortunately for humanity, most sociopaths are not murderous. Some are quiet, some noisy. Some are shy, some expressive. Some are physically violent, some physically timid. Some are aggressive, some passive; some dynamic, some lazy. In fact, sociopathy follows the range of human expression along with just about every other human condition, with the extremes such as murderousness being as rare as extreme self-sacrifice is with most people. This is just as well, for the medical profession estimates that one in every twenty-five people is sociopathic. Of that four percent of the population, three percent is male and only one percent is female. While many sociopaths are created by childhood experiences, the data suggests that such externals are never present in the upper-class female sociopath. For whatever reason, she is born rather than created by her external circumstances, which made Gloria's sociopathic tendencies a very disquieting fact for those who were genetically related to her. The very paucity of data – and the reality that the upper-class world is alien to most medical professionals – meant that there was every likelihood that they were missing the link between the upper-class sociopath who has graduated from fully-fledged narcissism to sociopathy due to the degree of indulgence that can only come with hyper-privilege.

It is now believed that fully sixty percent of all alcoholics and drug addicts are sociopathic personalities who are medicating themselves to escape from the deadness within. That is not to say that all alcoholics or drug addicts are sociopathic, or indeed that all sociopaths become alcoholics or drug addicts, any more than all narcissists become drug addicts and alcoholics.

Unfortunately, antisocial personality disorders, like narcissistic ones, are virtually untreatable. This is not because the medical profession does not know how to treat them. It is because antisocial personalities, like their narcissistic brethren, never think that anything is wrong with them. It is always someone else's fault, never theirs; and on the rare occasions when some personal experience or tragedy compels them to seek medical help, they invariably abandon treatment as soon as their symptoms of discomfort are alleviated, long before the underlying disorder, and the havoc it creates, can be addressed.

According to psychiatrists, psychologists and psychotherapists, antisocial personalities are, along with narcissists, the most thankless personalities to treat of anyone with a psychological problem. These two categories of disorder are far more resistant to treatment than even the clinically insane. They use everyone, abuse everyone and discard everyone as soon as they perceive it to be in their interest to do so. They might form alliances, even lifelong ones, but these are always exploitative. Indeed, one of the ways therapists diagnose the two disorders is by the degree of exploitation both the antisocial and narcissistic personality displays.

The antisocial personality, however, is no madder than the narcissistic personality. Although much of what they do might be termed 'mad' in the popular vernacular, in psychiatric terms, they are not clinically insane. They do not suffer from any of the psychoses such as schizophrenia or paranoia which are the province of the truly insane. Unlike primary narcissists, primary sociopaths are not really delusional or even self-delusional. They don't hear voices or see sights or have the highly inflated self-image of primary narcissists, even though they might well pretend to be delusional if they consider it to be in their interest to do so.

Above all, the antisocial personality has two features which aid diagnosis. They are invariably pathological liars, and they have a need for sympathy that goes above and beyond what ordinary people possess.

In 1973, when Gloria was about to embark upon her next foray into attention-seeking, Antisocial Personality Disorder didn't exist as a medical condition any more than Narcissistic Personality Disorder did. Otto Kernberg's theory, outlined in *Aggression in Personality Disorders and Perversions* – that hatred is the core affect of all personality disorders, deriving from childhood rage which once served to eliminate pain but later in life became a useful tool with which to eliminate obstacles to gratification – had not yet been propounded. Therefore, all that followed in our family life happened within the narrow parameters of the time, sending all of us hurtling down byways where we had no business being. In the process, Gloria obtained licence to run even wilder and create more havoc than she had hitherto done.

Gloria's new game started in September 1973. I had been living in England since May of that year. Although she and I were still estranged, we had been exchanging greetings in public ever since April of 1973, when Michael had forced her to host a dinner party in honour of my good friend Lady Sarah Spencer-Churchill. But we could hardly have been said to be speaking, nor indeed did I even care to hear what she was up to. I had reached saturation point and, as I said to Mickey: 'I don't want to hear one more word about her until you tell me she's dead.'

The deck was cleared for Gloria's new game when Kitty left home for school in England in September 1973. For the first time since the second year of her marriage twenty-five years before, she had Michael all to herself.

Now, normal people, even crazy people, don't set about devouring their nearest and dearest in methodical manner, but Gloria was neither normal nor crazy. For years she had been trying, by hook or by crook, to get her husband to give up every interest and activity which did not directly relate to or concern her. In this, she had been remarkably unsuccessful. No matter how she ranted, raved and blackmailed; no matter how much she moaned and groaned about how lonely she was when he left her to play poker and dominoes or to attend the race track, he ignored all her attempts to tie him up with marital ropes with a studiousness that showed just how much spine he could summon up when it was his skin on the line. 'I'm not your babysitter,' he used to tell her as he forced whichever one of their children was living at home to fulfil that role.

With Kitty out of the way, Gloria now played a new and inventive hand. Harkening back to her foray some years before when she had gone to the psychiatrist and declared herself mad, she came up with a variation which actually frightened all of us rigid, even though it also misfired spectacularly upon her. Two weeks after Kitty's departure, Michael came home to find Gloria cowering dramatically in their bedroom. She slipped him a note she had written. 'Don't say anything,' it said. 'There's a man in the linen cupboard monitoring our activities. Get rid of him for me.'

Anyone can imagine the shock Michael must have felt when he saw the note and, looking from it to his wife, witnessed her quivering theatrically, displaying something which was totally out of character for her: fear. He went to the linen cupboard, where of course, there was no man. Thinking that Gloria was finally off her trolley, he telephoned Mickey to come up to the house and help him. It says a lot about his relationship with his wife that even at this juncture, he was so afraid of doing anything to displease her that he needed to hide behind their son's shirttails.

Mickey arrived and duly telephoned Dr Charles Thesiger, the country's most eminent psychiatrist and someone who had treated many members of our family, though not Gloria up to that point. He rushed up to the house, diagnosed a psychotic episode of schizophrenia and paranoia exacerbated by excessive alcoholic consumption and arranged for her to be taken away, literally by the men in white coats, to Nuttall Hospital.

If, as I now suspect, Gloria had thought she was going to manipulate Michael into giving up all his outside interests to pay her the unending court she required now that she had him all to herself, she had miscalculated. Once Thesiger was called in, things spiralled out of her control. In the hospital, they derailed in a way she could never have anticipated. Thesiger, being a psychiatrist, was not as malleable as Jimmy Burrowes, the gynaecologist who had overseen her other recent 'breakdowns' but who had by now joined the exodus of decamping Jamaicans. He treated her as a psychiatric case in need of psychiatric treatment, not as a socialite to be indulged and, in so doing, wrested ultimate control from her. In doing so, he turned the tables on her in a way no one else had ever done before.

This was a new game: one where she was not calling the shots for the first time in her life. The first thing Thesiger refused to allow was Gloria's usual supply of champagne. Instead, he diagnosed alcoholism and prescribed a course of detoxification drugs to wean her off the alcohol she had been consuming with such relish for decades. Gloria, distressed to find that someone else was in command of the game she was playing, protested that she did not want the drugs he prescribed for her. She turned to Michael, Maisie and Mickey for help, hoping that they would convince the psychiatrist to restore her alcohol supply and terminate the detoxification procedure, but they, believing that she had had a genuine psychotic episode brought on by alcoholic hallucinosis, were in no mood to enable her. All her protestations of having not really seen someone in the linen cupboard fell on deaf ears as they encouraged Thesiger to continue the detoxification process.

Gloria was nothing if not resourceful. She now took to playing the loony for all it was worth, maintaining that Dr Theisger was sending her mad with the drugs he was giving her. 'One afternoon I went to the hospital for my usual visit,' I was told by Maisie, who did everything by the clock, making it easy for Gloria to time the scenes she wanted her mother to witness. 'When I got to her room, I noticed she did not have on her bangles. "Gloria," I said, wondering if one of the maids had made off with them, "where are your bangles?" She threw up her hands like a little girl and started to giggle. The nurse pointed to the flowers. The room was always awash with flowers. Your mother had hung them from the arrangements. Another time, when I got to the room, she was on the way to the garden, where, in full view of everyone, she squatted and urinated on the grass, for everyone to see. I sent the nurse out for her and when she brought her back I said, "Now Gloria, why did you do that? You surely know that there's no need to urinate in public when you have your own bathroom?" Do you know what her response was? "You've all decided that I'm mad to shit, so I can do what I want. And if I want to pee in public, I will." I was so worried that she'd never regain her mind that I don't know how the stress and strain didn't kill me.'

For the first two months of Gloria's hospitalization, Michael kept what was happening from both Kitty and me. My cousin Toni, rightly feeling that we deserved to know, finally informed me in November over Sunday lunch at the Connaught.

'Your mother has gone mad,' she said. 'She's been in the Nuttall for over eight weeks.'

I cannot tell you how shocked I was by that news. I promptly burst into tears and couldn't stop crying. When it became apparent that I could not calm down, lunch had to be adjourned to our friend Tom Gallagher's suite of rooms upstairs while he and Toni tried, unsuccessfully, to console me.

Toni's information was that Gloria might never recover. The prospect of Mummy being in an insane asylum for the rest of her life was too horrifying for words. I felt wave after wave of sympathy, compounded by grief. Guilt followed swiftly with the thought that all along she hadn't been bad, only mad. I started to think that maybe, just maybe, if we'd all been a little more attentive and a little less dismissive all the times she'd been crying out for attention, she wouldn't have gone crazy. Poor Mummy, I wailed, engulfed by the horror of what had happened to her, little realizing that I was responding in just the way the narcissistic, antisocial personality requires its victims to respond.

When I got back to the flat where I was living, I telephoned Jamaica, finally tracking Mickey down at the hospital. 'She's much better than she was,' he said. 'She's due to leave in mid-December. She'll be fine by then.'

'But Toni said…'

'That's all settled down now. She's given us all a warm time, but she's no longer acting up the way she was doing. Dr Thesiger says she'll be fine, but that she should give up drinking and seek treatment for her underlying medical problems. He says she's been medicating herself with alcohol and had a psychotic episode, but it's passed now.'

'So she's not insane.'

'No.'

'What a relief. I had visions of Mummy spending the rest of her life in a lunatic asylum.'

'Not only you,' Mickey said. 'Daddy and Grandma were so terrified I wondered how they'd cope.'

'You weren't worried?' I asked, picking up something unspoken in his manner.

'Not as worried as they were. You know what Mummy is like,' he said, alluding to her acting ability.

'You don't mean…?' I started to say.

'Let me put it this way, Georgie. Mummy gave us all one heck of a scare and she definitely has a drinking problem, as you, Libby, Kitty and I have been saying for years and Daddy and Grandma didn't want to acknowledge. But I'm not taking the "man in the cupboard" nonsense as seriously as they did. She was a bit too quick to backtrack on it, when she saw it wasn't yielding her the dividends she thought it would, for me to be convinced of her sincerity.'

I rang off, reassured but still sympathetic to Gloria. I was not as cynical as Mickey and did not dismiss the 'man in the cupboard' business as readily as he had done. I was prepared to give her the benefit of the doubt and even made plans to return home for Christmas, something I would not have done the week before.

I arrived in Jamaica a few days after Gloria was released from the hospital. She was certainly more subdued than I had ever seen her; but then, she had been drugged up to her eyeballs for the previous three months, so that was to be expected. What was not, however, was the fact that she was sipping sherry from a silver goblet. After greeting her with a kiss, I went inside to Michael.

'I thought she wasn't allowed to drink anymore,' I said.

He threw up his hands in the air, as if to say: 'What can I do?'

In the days and weeks to come, I could tell by the way Gloria behaved that she had been through something of an ordeal. Although she did not say so in so many words, it was apparent that she had had one hell of a shock finding herself detained in hospital with someone else calling the shots. For a control freak like her, that must have been traumatic indeed.

I was now firmly back to being the sympathetic old Georgie. Even if I could no longer summon up the warmth or trust I had once felt for my mother, she knew just how to play my compassionate streak to get me to sit with her endlessly, keeping her company as of old.

Early one evening we were talking in the drawing room when Gloria said, *apropos* of nothing: 'You know, I always knew even as a little girl that I wasn't really like other people. I wonder what the difference is.' At that moment, I knew she had given me a glimpse into her soul. She had come clean.

'What do you mean?' I said.

'It's nothing I can put my finger on. I've just always known I'm not really like everyone else,' she said.

Had I known then what I know now about personality disorders, my blood would have run cold. Without that knowledge, however, I did not realize that she was confessing the secret of all those who have a propensity to personality disorders: from an early age, they know they're *different*. This difference is as much a puzzle to them as it is to everyone else. It is also something with which they have to live and, I daresay, contend. To that extent, they are deserving of our compassion, which does not mean, of course, that we have to excuse or accept the grosser manifestations of their disordered personalities.

If I was blissfully unaware of the significance of Gloria's confession, I was only too aware that she was now reeling Michael in the way a fisherman reels in his catch. Hereafter, every time he left her alone to go to a race meeting or a poker game, he did so with the knowledge that his 'sick' and 'delicate' wife might be tipped over the edge into another 'psychotic episode'. So he dramatically reduced going out and, in the process, gave her the payoff she had sought all along.

Frankly, by the time I left Jamaica early in March 1974, I could hardly wait to breathe the polluted air of New York. It was fresh compared with what I was leaving behind. You could tell that the events of the last few months had taught Gloria no lessons. All the indications were that she was well on the way towards restoring all her old, destructive habits, from drinking like a fish to abusing everyone and everything. So I fled as soon as the book, which I had written in longhand over the last few months, had been typed up by a secretary.

Chapter Eighteen

In New York, I stayed with Jeanie Campbell, daughter of the eleventh Duke of Argyll and granddaughter of the Canadian newspaper magnate, the first Lord Beaverbrook. She was something of a character, which is typified by an anecdote she used to relate about her marriage to Norman Mailer. Norman, unconvinced that she really loved him, dared her to allow him to dangle her by the feet from the eleventh floor of her New York apartment building. Accepting the dare, Jeanie gave no thought to Norman being short and slight, while she was hefty and large-boned. Nor did she feel a moment's fear as Norman held her by the ankles, though she did feel triumphant, after he pulled her back inside the apartment, for she had provided him with indisputable proof of love. The fact that he might well have dropped her simply didn't enter into Jeanie's reckoning. Love was all.

Love or no, the marriage did not last; but Norman remained a part of Jeanie's life, because he was a devoted father and they had a daughter together, an adorable girl named Kate.

Jeanie was a genuinely kind and decent person who was always offering a bed to people like me or Prince Alexander of Russia, to name but two. We slept on Napoleon I's (surprisingly comfortable) camp bed, with the famous sketch Graham Sutherland had done of her Beaverbrook grandfather looking over our shoulders. A devout convert to Roman Catholicism, she tried to make her everyday life a cathedral to her beliefs, especially after she gave up drinking and acknowledged how destructive her family's alcoholic tendencies had been.

I would learn, once I had married her brother, that Jeanie was haunted by her family's heritage. 'There is something very dark about my family,' she used to say, using the polite word for evil. In particular, she alluded to past atrocities such as infanticide, murder, incest and the 1692 Massacre of Glencoe, when her ancestor the Earl of Argyll had orchestrated the slaughter of the rival clan, the MacDonalds, murdering in their beds the men, women and children who had given them refuge in keeping with Highland traditions of hospitality. To this day, there are people in Scotland who will have nothing to do with the ducal family of Argyll, whom they regard as the forerunners of the Himmlers and Goerings of a later age.

Jeanie was also haunted with guilt about the infamous divorce of her father and stepmother and the part she had played in destroying Margaret's life. She had helped Big Ian to break into Margaret's townhouse and steal her appointment books. He then used a series of innocuous entries about lunches and dinners with male socialites, mostly gay, to 'prove' that Margaret had not only kept a written record of her lovers but had also rated their performances numerically. As homosexuality was then illegal, and the men named would have gone to jail if Margaret had exposed them, honour gave her no choice but to endure in silence the persecution she suffered in the Divorce Court as she was 'unmasked' as a rampant harlot.

As luck would have it, who should come to stay with Jeanie while I was there but her half-brother Colin? He was *en route* from Fiji to Paris and made an impromptu stop in New York for two days.

Romance with Jeanie's brother was the last thing on my mind. I was having the time of my life being feted by beaus such as David Koch and Jimmy Clarke while I investigated the possibilities of having the book I had written published. Then Colin Campbell – tall, dark and handsome, charming, dynamic and four years older than me – burst upon the scene like a meteor. He was something of a hippy and was, unbeknownst to me, eager to marry the daughter of a rich man. 'The Argyll family only marry great beauties with money,' he used to boast to all and sundry while we were together, and having decided (with typical hyperbole) that I was the most beautiful girl he had ever seen and knowing from his sister that my father had money, he zeroed in on me with the tremendous energy he had at his disposal. He charmed me utterly. Proposing the first night we met, I accepted after Jeanie talked me out of my initial reservations of waiting and seeing. I then found myself being swept along on a wave of romanticism up to the altar.

In fairness to Jeanie, who was a romantic, she didn't think my interests conflicted with her brother's, although those were what she primarily had in mind. As far as she was concerned, Colin was lucking out. He was marrying a nice girl from a moneyed family who was well connected socially and known in Society as a 'great beauty'. Although she was aware that Colin had been a 'disturbed' child, being his half-sister and eighteen years older than him, she did not know him so well that she was aware of his history of violence. They had never lived together and indeed knew each other only in passing. 'Had I known what Colin was really like,' she would subsequently say to me, 'I would never have encouraged you to marry him.' Indeed, in the years to come, she would express her feelings of guilt for the part she had, albeit inadvertently, played in furthering a union that was by any interpretation disastrous.

Blissfully ignorant of the mess I was getting myself into, I stepped out of the frying pan of my family life into the fire of the Argyll family's. If ever a family was more appalling than mine, it was theirs.

If I was hurtling into a fool's paradise, at least I had sufficient good sense to keep my parents out of the loop. I knew from the way Gloria had behaved when Libby was getting married that she would have ruined any pleasure I might have had in my own wedding, had I been ill-advised enough to unleash her onto the arrangements. Michael, I knew, would never approve of Colin, because he would deem him to be 'penniless', worth a paltry $225,000 *in toto* with an income of only $12,000 per annum and, worse, no job. Indeed, he had never had a job. So, making sure I said nothing to anyone in my family, lest they talk me out of the reckless but romantic course upon which I had embarked, I eloped with Colin, Jeanie, her daughters Kate and Cusi to Elkton, Maryland, where Jeanie had been married before and where Colin, anxious to close the deal before I got colder feet than I already had, would have to wait two days instead of the eleven demanded by New York State's residency requirements.

Only after I was married did I contact my parents. I telephoned home to give them the news, speaking to Gloria, who, without missing a beat, said, 'Well, I suppose congratulations are in order.' If she felt slighted, she was too canny to let on to me or to anyone else. I conjectured that having a lord as a son-in-law would appeal to the English snobbery which was so much a part of her makeup and would compensate for the exclusion from the wedding arrangements I had foisted upon her. Michael I expected to be trickier to work my way round, but as I had presented him with a *fait accompli*, he too would have no option but to put a good face upon things, which is precisely what he did.

Colin and I flew to Jamaica five days after our marriage so that I could introduce him to the family. Needless to say, my father paid all our expenses.

All my new husband's worldly goods fitted into one small, cheap, battered suitcase, which didn't faze me at all, for I had never cared about money, and the fact that we would have to make our way in the world was something I actually found exciting.

As I had suspected, Michael was deeply unimpressed by Colin. In fact, as I would learn from my brother when the marriage was breaking up, Daddy had discounted Colin within twenty minutes of meeting him. 'Georgie has picked up a drunken bum who hopes I'll support them,' he told Mickey. 'I won't.' Unlike Gloria, who lapped up all Colin's boasting about his family heritage while dishing up her own share with a trowel, Michael was also unmoved by Colin's attempts to impress him. When Colin bragged that he could trace his ancestry back to the 1100s, Michael responded dismissively, 'We've been Christian since the sixth century and I don't think that's any big deal.' Indeed, so cool was my father about his own ancestry that it was many years before I learned that he was descended from the Emperor Charlemagne and from William the Conqueror, the French Duke of Normandy who wrested the English throne from the Anglo-Saxon King Harold in 1066.

Gloria, however, warmed to her new son-in-law as only a fun-seeking and status-obsessed tippler in love with pleasure, who has found her mirror image, can. Day in, day out, she and Colin used to sit down on the back veranda, knocking back the booze and shooting the breeze. I was delighted that they were getting along so well, though I used to be transfixed by how they managed to spend so much time talking about absolutely nothing at all. More my father's than my mother's daughter in many of my tastes, I could no more have stood so much aimless pleasure-seeking than contemplated a life without books: something both Gloria and Colin managed without any effort whatsoever.

Within days, my competitive mother was crowing about how she had my new husband's ear more than I did. In her mind, if not in his eyes, I had been relegated to second division, and as she set about organizing our wedding reception, I let her believe whatever she pleased. For all I knew, she might even have been right, for Colin and I barely knew each other; and the truth was that she had far more in common with him than I did. However, as I was neither jealous nor competitive by nature and found too much attention onerous owing in large part to the excessive amount, much of it negative, which I had received over the years, I was only too happy to let them chatter away while I retired to my bedroom to read a good book.

'From the womb to the tomb, men love me', Gloria was always saying, so it was inevitable that her sons-in-law would have to be the living proof of this, as indeed all four of them would become. 'I get along better with my daughters' husbands than they do,' she was always boasting, failing to realize how silly she was being when she indulged in such vanity. However, as she was the real power in the family, and I needed all her help – financial and otherwise – in my new life, I would have been disposed to let her get away with her harmless vanities, even if I had not been schooled from childhood to indulge them.

All things being equal, Colin's absorption into my family could not have gone better. Although I would later discover that my father's acceptance, more apparent than real, was echoed by a large proportion of the family as well as by various friends, who suspected that I had married someone with real personality problems, I was blissfully ignorant of any of their reservations until the marriage was breaking up.

At first, Colin behaved like the proverbial cat that's got the cream. The rule of primogeniture decreed that all second sons were substantially poorer than their elder brothers. Even if his family had been rich, which it was not, he was never therefore going to be 'in the money'. In fact, he was one step away from the poorhouse. He had already made several little asides to indicate how impressed he was by the way my family lived, as well as by the amount my parents were giving us as a wedding present. For the only time in my life, Michael and Gloria actually pushed their hands deep into their pockets and came up with a large enough sum so that we could afford to get ourselves a decent apartment in New York and furnish it stylishly. Maisie and Marjorie also gave us hefty sums as a wedding present, which meant that we had a comfortable margin within which we could set up our first home and supplement whatever we earned when we started working. This was more than most young couples get, and I for one was appreciative, while Colin, who had never possessed such a large sum of money before, acted as if he was in heaven.

Never one to miss an opportunity to gain ascendancy over someone she regarded as a social equal, Gloria now set about bedazzling her poverty-stricken son-in-law so that any advantage he had as a duke's son was eroded by her greater wealth, especially after he let it drop that the ninth duke's wife had been Queen Victoria's daughter Princess Louise and his family were therefore connected to the Royal Family.

Those who dared to outdo Gloria normally found themselves fighting rearguard actions against this wily guerrilla whose resourcefulness in redressing the balance in favour of her superiority was truly amazing. But, I reasoned, even she couldn't come up with anything to top the royal connection, little realizing how adept she was at switching fields of battle until she emerged victorious.

The fight back was actually amusing to behold. Shifting the balance of power away from background to money, she started to drop a comment here, pick up a large bill there with the disdain that gave him the message that what was heavyweight to him was a feather to her, and otherwise present a façade of casual munificence that on the one hand impressed him while on the other hand sent the message that he was the poor relation and therefore of inferior status.

The afternoon before our wedding reception, Gloria issued the *coup de grace*. She arrived home in a huge flurry from the bank, where she had gone to take out the jewels she needed for herself as well as those she was giving me as a wedding present. Calling out to Colin with uncharacteristic urgency, she said, 'Son-in-law, come into my bedroom with me. I want to show you something.' Then, almost as an afterthought which I could tell was calculated for dramatic effect, she added, 'You can come too, Georgie.'

Colin and I looked at each other, wondering what she was up to. Following her into the bedroom, we watched as she closed the door quietly, thereby enhancing the air of mystery and drama she was creating. To my surprise, she then threw down an array of jewels onto her marital bed: a specially made and intricately carved monstrosity which was a good two feet wider than the conventional imperial-sized bed and as awful in its splendour as she herself could be.

'I've brought a few things to give your wife, so she can start life as a married woman should,' she said, not so subtly making the point that he and his family couldn't provide me with such offerings. She picked out a yellow gold and diamond necklace; a pair of diamond earrings; and a ruby and diamond ring, nonchalantly throwing them towards me. It was so out of character that this alone alerted me to the fact that she was up to something. 'Here. These are for you,' she said, not even bothering to look at me.

As I thanked her, and Colin mumbled his appreciation, his eyes were on stalks, ogling the jewels scattered over the bed. 'Go on, Son-in-Law, you can touch as well as look, you know,' she said in her most maternal tone, inviting him to rummage through them. I myself would have been deceived into thinking what a caring person she was, had I not been provided with ample proof to the contrary over the years.

Colin, however, thwarted her by limiting himself to examining my presents. While he was making all the right cooing noises, she needed him to turn his attention away from the trinkets she was giving me to various parures of diamonds, rubies, sapphires and emeralds, which she had brought home from the bank purely to deliver the message to the man who had outstripped her in the family-connection stakes that if he thought he could beat her overall, he was sorely misguided. So this most independent-minded of women lapsed into the role of the helpless female, and with saccharine dripping off her tongue, inveigled him into examining the really valuable portion spread before him. 'Help me decide what to wear to your wedding reception,' she said. 'We girls always need the help of the men in our lives to make the most of ourselves.'

As Colin handed me my diamond earnings and started working his way through this truly impressive array of jewels, you could tell by the way he was drooling that Gloria had succeeded in making her point. Afterwards, when we were alone, he said, almost disbelievingly, 'They were real, weren't they?'

'Of course,' I answered.

'Jeanie said your family had money,' he marvelled, giving me the first inkling of his main motive for marrying me, 'but I didn't think they had this much. Fuck, your father's seriously rich.'

Gloria, of course, had pulled off another one of her tricks and in the process had stoked my husband's ambitions in ways that would create unforeseen problems for me. Thereafter, any chance I might have had to get this most workshy of men to find a job, excited the inelegant comment, 'Your father's got plenty of dosh. He should be supporting us, the cheap fuck-face.' While I agreed that my father was indeed unnecessarily parsimonious with me and my brother and younger sister, I nevertheless did not accord with my husband's view that Michael ought to be supporting us. As far as I was concerned, we were both young and able-bodied and could work for a living. Since I had given up the possibility of marrying several rich beaus for him, the least he could do was pull his weight and try to make something of himself.

For five months following this incident, our different approaches to our respective marital responsibilities were masked because we were on an extended honeymoon, first in New York, where I found us an apartment to rent on the fashionable Upper East Side while Colin stayed at Jeanie's apartment all day claiming to be too ill with stomach trouble to do anything useful – but never too ill to avail himself, Gloria-like, of whatever pleasures were on offer, alcohol, grass and various substances included – and thereafter in England and Scotland, where his brother Ian, then the current duke, organized wedding receptions for us in both places and we met each other's friends. When we weren't travelling around the country staying at his ancestral home, Inveraray Castle, or with friends like his half-sister Jeanie's cousin Alan Ramsay, we stayed at the cottage off the Kings Road near Sloane Square in London that Charles Delevigne, a chum of mine, found for us. This lifestyle was made possible entirely due to the generosity of my family, who had added to my parents', aunt's and grandmother's stockpile by coming through for us splendidly at the wedding reception Gloria had organized. Most of them came armed with cash after I got my Aunt Hilda to ring everyone up and tell them to give US dollars instead of the hodgepodge of silver, crystal and china which were the staples in those pre-wedding list days, when newlyweds were liable to end up with four silver water jugs; various platters and salvers that would be of no use to anyone without an army of servants; three different patterns of Spode, none in a full enough complement to ever be functional unless you then went and spent your own money to complete the set; and so many different bits and pieces of Waterford and Baccarat that you could scratch your head for the next fifty years and still not invent a way to put most of them to any use.

Being a great aficionado of uniformity, my idea had been to get the cash so that I could buy sets of everything. My husband, however, had other ideas. Never having had access to any money before, he fell upon it like a Roman foot-solider plundering Parthia. Suddenly this man who had never before been able to afford taxis, much less a car and had always had to use public transport, now became too consequential to travel anywhere except by limousine. The amount of money he wasted on a weekly basis on car hire alone was enough to keep two families. Between the thrice weekly visits to the trichologist Philip Kingsley to get his head massaged and his flowing locks treated with expensive in-house potions, his lunchtimes standing rounds of drinks for people he would never see again, and the wardrobe he now found it necessary to acquire in expensive shops, our china, flatware and crystal were being washed away on a tide of wastefulness.

In those days, I was far gentler than I now am. I hated hurting anyone's feelings and would find ways of getting across criticism so diplomatically that no one could take offence. Although I started advising caution, pointing out that we really shouldn't be staying in Britain living the high life when we were burning our way through funds which we would need to set ourselves up in the marital home in New York, Colin wanted to hear none of it. Playing the 'poor me' card, he made me feel like such a party-pooper that I let him do as he pleased, rationalizing that it was only a matter of time before we both had to knuckle down , in my view, to the real fun of building a solid life together.

A psychologist would say that I had been well trained by a self-indulgent parent to enable a self-indulgent spouse, but that would only be half the story. The other half was that I had bitten off more than anyone could chew. My husband was not only a constant tippler like my mother, but was also as self-obsessed as she was. From morning till night, he had only one subject of conversation: himself or, to be more accurate, his sad fate. As he told it, his life had been one long struggle against a cruel world with the odds stacked firmly against him. According to him, everyone in his life had always taken advantage of poor Colin, except his father and his stepmother Mathilda. He loathed his mother, who had favoured his elder brother Ian because he was going to be the duke, while he, poor baby, had only been the spare – a mere lord – and therefore overlooked. He also hated his brother, not only because he had been his mother's favourite, but also because he was the duke and therefore had all the privileges such as being the chatelain of the castle; holder of a variety of titles and hereditary positions such as Master of the Queen's Household in Scotland; and therefore the person of whom the shallow made a bigger deal. He said Ian was a conniving, pompous, jealous, drunken and self-important sod who enjoyed causing trouble for people, no one more so than his younger brother; and, as Jeanie confirmed the veracity of at least some of that, I was on my guard about this dreadful brother before I had even met him.

Although I had been fortunate not to have siblings like that, I knew only too well what it was like to be marginalized. I therefore empathized with Colin, seeing parallels between our pasts where none existed, and missing the truly salient point: he was whining and full of self-pity while I counted my blessings and felt no self-pity whatsoever.

Although I tried to avoid making the connection, I nevertheless could not help seeing that my husband was very much like my mother. The world began and ended with him. He was as jealous as she was. Like her, he held the floor as if no one else had a right to be heard. Even worse, he had her proclivity for drama, whipping himself up into frenzies which often as not ended with him calling the doctor to medicate him in the Colin Campbell version of Gloria Ziadie's nervous breakdowns. Even more than her, he would alight upon nothing, whip it up into something, ride the hobbyhorse for all it was worth for a few days, then abandon it as if it had never existed. This trait made it very difficult to know what did and did not matter to him; and with the passage of time, when I could come up with nothing that did consistently matter to him except his need for sympathy and attention, I stopped listening. This was just as well, for I had also discovered that his attitude towards facts was as malleable as Gloria's. I simply couldn't believe a word he said.

Although this caused me considerable disquiet at first, with time my sense of humour came to my rescue. I not only made a joke of this failing but even started to affectionately call him 'Conning': a nickname he seemed to regard more with pride than shame. This, I saw, was because he too shared her contempt for the constraints which fact placed upon his desires, and which he too ignored whenever they interfered with his gratification.

I consoled myself with the thought that at least he did not share Gloria's arrogant presumption that she was the cleverest person on earth, or the consequent disdain she expressed for everyone else. Mercifully, he also lacked her need for constant praise, though like her, he required constant sympathy. It was already painfully obvious that he possessed the same degree of determination as she did in charming, cajoling or hectoring others into agreeing with him, and when they failed to do so, his reaction was even more petulant than hers for, unlike her, he was not particularly intelligent or socially skilled, so failed to mask his feelings the way she did.

By this time, I was desperately trying not to ask myself what I had got myself into. As I looked at Colin Campbell, knocking back booze from eleven o'clock every morning, bobbing and weaving by midday like a coconut tree in a high wind, I tried not to think that he was a lush, and failed to make the connection between his medical history of childhood disturbance and his patently bizarre conduct.

Like the children of most alcoholics, I naïvely thought that if you removed alcohol from the equation, you would get a more reasonable person. Not that I actually thought that Colin had a drinking problem. In fact, I consoled myself instead with the observation that as he didn't start drinking until eleven, he couldn't be an alcoholic – otherwise he'd be like Mummy, who drank with breakfast.

I also tried to tell myself that he did not have a drug problem, that there was nothing wrong with him taking the amount of uppers and downers he swallowed on a daily basis, because these were prescription drugs given to him by doctors who appreciated his need to sleep, to rest, to relax, to gain a release from anxiety, to get over jetlag etc, etc, etc. 'You're uptight about drink and drugs because of your mother,' he used to say, not without an element of justice, while we both consoled ourselves in our respective ways with the denial of the obvious.

When he insisted on prolonging our honeymoon to a truly regal length, it became increasingly difficult for me to avoid facing the fact that real problems existed within the marriage. Not only was Colin workshy and lazy, childish and self-centred, histrionic and irresponsible, but he did not believe in what he called 'physical contact'. That meant no affection. No touching. No kissing. No intimacy at all. Our sex-life, if you could call it that, was a travesty. Once every three or four weeks he would click his fingers and indicate that I should go into the bedroom, where I would be expected to service him while he lay down on the bed like a cadaver: stiff, immobile and passive beyond belief. I was used to men who couldn't wait to manfully take charge in the bedroom and express their desire, so having this impersonator of the dead with an erection the size of a lipstick was something of a perplexity to me.

At least I knew his inadequacies had nothing to do with me. Every man I had been involved with prior to him couldn't wait to get me into bed, then keep me there, so there was no question in my mind where the fault lay.

Indeed, until I got married, I had never had a lousy lover. But Colin had an explanation for his profound inadequacies which tore at my heartstrings and might, or might not, have been true. 'Ian,' the ducal brother who was nine years his senior, 'used to abuse me sexually when I was a little boy. He used to force me to do things I find so upsetting I can't go into,' he'd claim, explaining away his singularly unmanly performance in such a way that only the heartless would not have accommodated his inadequacies.

As I tried to adjust to circumstances I could never have envisaged prior to my marriage, I found myself isolated by my discretion and sense of loyalty to my husband and by the fact that I did not want to give my parents, my mother especially, the satisfaction of being able to crow about my mistake in having married so precipitously. Although I resumed writing them the weekly 'duty' letters I had written to my father alone during the period of estrangement with Gloria, I was as careful as ever to follow the prescribed form and give them only 'good' news. This was not only a matter of pride on my part. It was also the knowledge that neither parent really wanted to know what any of their children's problems were. Needless to say, Gloria never replied to any of my letters, though Michael did occasionally.

On the other hand, my siblings and I had always been mutually supportive, so I was not entirely on my own in London. Kitty was at college in Surrey, and Mickey returned to live in London that summer, so I let them in on the secret that I was finding Colin's drinking and behaviour difficult to cope with. I swore them to secrecy and made sure that I kept the greatest problem away from them: Colin's violence.

This burst upon me with the suddenness of a tsunami on the Monday afternoon of the May 1974 Bank Holiday. We were in London and had gone, at his behest, to the pub at the end of Sloane Avenue for a midday drink. Despite us not having exchanged a wry word, at two-thirty in the afternoon he rounded on me while denouncing Mathilda, the stepmother he had claimed to love until he had gone up to Inveraray a week or two before and been influenced by Ian, who was suing her for some of their father's possessions which he felt should have come to him by right as the duke. 'She's a bitch,' Colin echoed Ian, and when I pointed out to him that he shouldn't let the brother, whom he said hated him, influence him adversely against the stepmother he used to say had been consistently good to him, he muttered that 'all women are bitches' and manhandled me out of the pub. As soon as we were in the sitting room of our rented cottage, he began pounding the right side of my face (the same side Gloria had aimed at two years before) in an attack that was as unprovoked as Gloria's had been. When he had finished his assault this side of my face was sunken, the bones having caved in under the force of his blows.

To say I was shocked would be to put it mildly. Not only did the attack come out of the blue, but it also left me a crumpled, disfigured monster, where only minutes before a proportionate and well-constructed face had existed.

I had married an exaggerated amalgam of my parents' worst features. Unfortunately, with none of their redeeming virtues, for he had none of their wealth, sophistication or generosity (no matter that it was only social and superficial.) He lacked my father's intellectual prowess and my mother's wit. He didn't even have Michael's testosterone-fuelled rampancy, or the deceptive sexual accommodation of my mother, otherwise I might at least have got some sexual satisfaction amidst all the bile and brutality. Indeed, he was the first man I had ever encountered who thought that his penis should point to the South Pole as a matter of course, and on the odd occasions when it did not, God forbid that any woman should get any consideration, much less pleasure, out of the phenomenon. The only redeeming virtue of my parents that he possessed was a smattering of their veneer of charm, but even there, he was no better at maintaining that than an erection, and few people wanted a third meeting with him.

Yet Colin Campbell had in spades the knack of making you feel needed by, and sorry for, him that Gloria also possessed. Even though we had been married for only six weeks when he smashed in my face, he had already made me feel that I was absolutely essential to his very existence. This profound sense of usefulness, together with the fear that I would look ridiculous if I ended the marriage when the newspapers had been billing us as the aristocracy's Romeo and Juliet of 1974, provided the motivation for me to give our marriage another chance. Therefore, when he proffered a heartfelt apology, explained that something like this had never happened before, that it wouldn't have happened if Ian hadn't unsettled him at Inveraray about their stepmother Mathilda, that it wasn't me he had been hitting out at but his mother and 'all other women who are bitches' and swore that 'it won't happen again' with all the sincerity of the truly insincere, I accepted his apology and explanation that the event had been an aberration.

I would, however, later discover from the author Michael Thornton and the socialite photographer Brodrick Haldane how Colin had beaten up his brother severely the night of their father's funeral in 1973, which was only one of many other serious physical assaults.

Of course, I should have left there and then, but I was twenty-four, not the woman of the world I now am. In my defence, I also suppose a girl, whose husband has smashed in the face her own mother tried to deface, has already been presented with a sufficiently distorted concept of what constitutes imaginable behaviour to render it likely that she will make the wrong decision. Doubtless, I would have taken a far sterner view and might never have considered Colin Campbell's conduct forgivable if Gloria hadn't paved the way two years before. But I was viewing his apology and assurances in the light of the fact that my own mother had refused to apologize for what she had done. At least he had the good grace to do so and to admit the wrong he had committed, which was more than could be said for her. Colin's apology somehow made the crime more forgivable than hers had been.

What also contributed to my willingness to forgive if not forget was that I was lucky enough that Mr Warner, the plastic surgeon, and Mr Murdoch, the dental surgeon, at St George's Hospital, Hyde Park Corner, London, managed to piece me back together so ably that there was no visible disfigurement. Within days I had resumed our busy social life, my hair covering the swelling on the right side of my face.

Even if I was displaying rather too many Pollyanna characteristics for my own good, I was nevertheless not gutless like my father. I knew from his errors with Gloria that a softly-softly approach to drinking and the bad behaviour people blamed on it would only result in a continuance of the same. And I was quite clear about one thing: if there was more of that, I would depart. So once I decided to give Colin Campbell and our marriage another chance, I did so with the understanding that he had to get help for his drinking and drug-taking. Either he sorted himself out and became the man I thought I had married, or I wanted out. 'If you ever raise a hand to me again, except lovingly,' I also told him, 'I'll be right out that door quicker than you can say "boo".'

I had no idea, as I recovered from the reconstructive surgery, that trying to preserve my marriage was a pointless exercise. Colin Campbell could no more become a positive and constructive person than Gloria Ziadie could. Cut from the same cloth, they were both personalities whom it behoved one to avoid unless one wanted all the punishment and misery which were the only things they had to offer. Not that I knew that then.

As the summer of 1974 rolled around, it was hardly a time of joy for me. I could already see that my marriage was sterile and might well not last, and I would need all the friendly faces I could muster to help me through what was likely to be a difficult period, whether we remained together or not. Colin Campbell was being patchy at best about giving up drink and drugs, but at least he agreed to cut our seemingly endless honeymoon short and return to New York to settle down to married life.

To say the least, I had mixed feelings about moving to a city I did not want to live in, where I had few real friends but many acquaintances (New Yorkers 'do' alliance far better than friendship), and where I would be without the support of friends as well as my brother Mickey and sister Kitty. London was a far more liveable city, not only in terms of its people and practices, but also physically, with green spaces and parks just about everywhere. Colin, however, was adamant that we would not live in London. 'I hate England and the English,' he often said, even though he barely knew either, having been born in France, raised in New York, and except for a couple of years at public school in the United Kingdom, was a virtual stranger to the country. And of course in England he was one of many lords, while in New York he was a rarity.

Whatever my misgivings, I had never been one to give way to despair when I could employ courage, so I returned to New York intent on putting a brave face on things and doing all I could to maximize the chances of my marriage surviving. I therefore swallowed hard and hit the streets running, looking for furniture, curtains etc. in August 1974, while Colin Campbell hit the bars on First and Third Avenues.

Within weeks, my husband had spiralled out of control with a totality that made Gloria seem like the very paradigm on rationality, even when she was at her most outrageous. His fulmination at the world at large was even worse than Michael in full flow during one of his daily eruptions down at the store. And at least Daddy was never drunk or spaced-out while giving vent to his demons.

Colin Campbell would say he was coming back home for lunch, then pitch up at five or six in the evening so drunk he could barely stand. Whether he was trying to be pleasant and jolly, indulging in the moroseness which was his specialty or vituperating about the cruelty of life, for which he of course was too good, he was always so insensible that it was impossible to follow the thread of logic which ought to have been running its way through his argument. 'He's like an egg beater in my brain,' I used to say to myself, wondering how much more of this I could stand.

Matters weren't helped by his habit of taking so many Valium *per diem* that he needed three doctors to keep him supplied with that drug. The Valium combined with the alcohol to have a potentative effect, which meant that he was four to six times higher with the combination than he would have been with only one of those substances. When one factored in all the other substances that he was also taking, and the fact that his grasp on rationality had clearly been tenuous even as a little boy, when his parents had consulted various psychiatrists in the hope that someone would be able to instil the power of reason, the wonder was that his feet ever touched the ground at all.

From my point of view, this situation had degenerated into absolute unacceptability. I didn't see how any rational person could relate to someone who took so many substances that there was no mental meeting point between them. Even if they had not prevented him from 'coming down' to a state of lucidity, I was painfully aware that the police could raid our apartment and cart us both off to jail for drug offences simply because we were cohabiting. I would then be placed in the invidious position of having to prove I had nothing to do with the stash of illicit drugs my husband was keeping in our apartment. America in those days was certainly not the place to fall foul of drug laws; and the idea that I was being exposed to such danger by my husband frightened me. Finally, I decided that I had to put my freedom above my marriage, and demanded that he get rid of all the drugs he had there. Whether he did or not, I will never know; but when he saw that he couldn't jolly or bully me out of my inflexible stance, he agreed to do so. I slept easier in my bed as a result, knowing that if ever there was a raid, at least I would be able to pass the lie detector test.

The worst thing of all, however, was the extreme pressure my husband started applying upon me to get a well-paying job so that I could make enough money – since I had refused to approach my father to replenish what he had squandered – to keep him in the style to which he had now become accustomed. Although I was still expected to be out and about on a daily basis furnishing our apartment while he went to the 'pub', and of course I had to have both lunch and dinner ready for him whether he then ate them or not, I was also supposed to instantly gratify my childishly impatient husband's need for money by coming up overnight with a job that paid me six figures.

Never before nor since have I been subjected to so much pressure from another human being. Gloria at her worst was nowhere near as bad a nag as he was. 'You know people. Get in touch with them. With your connections and brains and my name you'll coin it in,' he used to repeat several times a day, every day, as if there was something wrong with me and the world, because in the hour or two since he had last expressed the desire, I had not managed to pluck the job he required me to out of thin air.

Nor was there any question of the delicate flower I had married becoming a breadwinner, for he had decided that he was too 'free a spirit' for the constraints of a job. Instead, he would write a book. I felt my soul slither towards the netherworld as the childhood bugbear of Gloria's 'nerves' transferred itself into my married life as Conning's 'free spirit'.

By this time, I had telephoned Bill Paley, then the head of CBS TV, whom I knew would help me find the sort of job Conning required me to have. He happily agreed to see me and made an appointment for September 11, following his return to New York. Everyone in New York goes away in summer. He also indicated that he had no doubt his people would find something suitable for me in his organization, which came as a great relief to me and Conning as well – at least for half a day.

Despite Bill Paley being one of the most influential men in the US, this timescale wasn't good or quick enough for Colin Campbell. No amount of reasoning on my part would appease him. Even though we were not in danger of running out of money right away, he was doing a Gloria and demanding that I satisfy his desires there and then. This, of course, was neither reasonable nor sensible, for there was no way I could land a good job except through connections. So he started seriously suggesting that I contact Jackie Onassis and get her to find me a job 'because she's the Queen of America and you know her'.

'I can't do that. I don't know her well enough. And even if I did, I wouldn't feel comfortable using someone like that.'

'You and your precious sensitivity,' he sneered.

'Bill Paley is far more likely than Jackie to come up with what we want,' I said to the ignoramus who, despite having spent most of his life in New York, hadn't even known who Bill Paley was until I told him. 'A wait of a few weeks isn't going to make a scrap of difference one way or the other.'

'It will, you stupid bitch. I need the money. Now. Why do you think I married you? I married you for your father's money…stupid bitch. And because you have a reputation for being a great beauty, and we Argylls always marry famous beauties with money. Your father should be giving me the money we need, and if not, you should be earning it. *Now*,' he said even more aggressively than Gloria would ever have done.

'Well, you didn't think this one out, did you?' I riposted, stung to the quick. 'Because everyone knows I have no money. If you wanted to marry someone for her money, you should have married someone with it. You don't marry the daughter for her father's money. His money isn't hers. Surely you thought of that simple little fact?'

'You're a stupid bitch, and your father's a cheap fuck-face. He's fucking supposed to be fucking giving us fucking money. What's the point of marrying you if you don't deliver the goods?' Colin sneered in as grotesque a fashion as Gloria at her worst.

No one wants to believe a bitter truth when it is presented to them in unvarnished form, and I was no exception. Although Colin Campbell was speaking the simple truth about why he had married me, I chose not to believe it. Rather than accept it as a fact, I preferred to think that he was only saying such cruel things because he was drunk and stoned out of his mind.

Only too soon, however, he would provide me with proof of how truthful his admission was – and how naïve I was not to believe it. In the process, he taught me that the parents I had considered as rarities, owing to their aberrant behaviour, were not only a lot less rare than I had previously believed, but also no worse than some of their peers. It was quite a lesson to learn. It made the world I would have to occupy a far less desirable place than I had thought of it as being.

Chapter Nineteen

If my parents' negligence of their children's emotional needs had one positive effect, it was to make each of us self-reliant. On the other hand, the inevitable consequence of their mistreatment was to accustom us to ways of behaviour that were detrimental to our welfare. The result was that we all possessed excellent coping mechanisms for situations in which we should never have been.

But no adult is totally the product of his or her environment. Each of us has our own soul, our own heart and our own will. If we cop out of our responsibility to ourselves and blame our parents for what we make of our lives, we do not learn the lessons we need to in order to avoid perpetuating negative patterns, and we run a greater risk of ending up messes. I was absolutely determined that no matter what happened in my life, neither it nor I would become a mess.

No matter which way I looked at it, my marriage was nevertheless a mess which threatened to spread into all the other areas of my life. I was painfully aware that this raised a host of issues around which I had to carefully navigate my way if I were not to cock things up so gloriously that I would never be able to look back on this period of my life without lasting self-recrimination.

Unlike my mother, I had no illusions about being perfect and felt that a mark of good character was not only to admit one's fallibility but also to learn from it. Like most young girls, I nevertheless fell into the trap of thinking that my marriage would work if only my husband would change. Turning the proverbial sow's ear into a silk purse didn't seem to be too much to ask. I genuinely believed that everyone wanted to be a nice and kind and good and happy person; and when they failed, it wasn't through anything intentional so much as having inadvertently lost their way. In my mind's eye, no one – not even Conning or Mummy – chose destructiveness over constructiveness, negativity over positivity, evil over good, or misery over happiness. Once the bright light of enlightenment shone upon their problem, and they became aware of the error of their ways, all people would want to rectify them. All I needed to do was what Michael should have done with Gloria years before: find a way for my errant spouse to see the light. I was sure that once I did, Conning would be eager to pursue the path that led to harmony and joy rather than chaos and problems. Then we would be on track to have a happy and enduring marriage.

If only.

While youthfulness might have led me to unrealistic hope, it couldn't blind me to the very real problems that were right under my nose on a day-to-day basis. Conning's failure to contribute in any way, shape or form to our void of a relationship was what was preventing it from becoming a viable entity. He was not fulfilling even one aspect of a husband's role. Financially, sexually, emotionally, spiritually, sensually, affectionately, practically or constructively, he was utterly remiss: a total failure. More to the point, he had no desire to even try to function as an adult male. I realized getting him to see the light would not be easy. Whenever I tried to point out to him that there were two of us in the marriage and that he should occasionally make a contribution if it were to become a worthwhile, living, satisfying entity instead of a sterile shell, I was met with as much biting disdain as I had seen my mother display. Sometimes I even got the impression that he had no idea what I was getting at. This incomprehension opened up a whole new and frightening dimension: how do you reason with someone who is so lacking in feeling for others, so devoid of understanding of the basic requirements for a relationship, that he doesn't even know what you're talking about? At least Gloria knew what she should be doing, even if she didn't do it.

It is a fact of life that people left to their own devices soon reach their true level. Shorn of the friends and relations who had surrounded us in Britain, within three weeks of being on our own in New York, our relationship sank to a new depth. Conning quickly cast me back into the isolated figure of my teenage years: condemned to act out a role I did not want while being treated as an inanimate object. My husband, like my parents before him, had no interest whatsoever in me as a person, though, like my mother, he expected me to be both willing servant and adoring audience. He made it as clear as Michael and Gloria had each done in their different ways that he had no concern for, or interest in, my thoughts, feelings, pleasures, likes, dislikes, moods and ambitions, save for how these affected him – at which point he cared intensely. I was back to being a commodity, the way I had been used by my mother and ignored by my father. I had to ask myself: did I really want to go through something similar to what I had done while growing up? Why should I endure being treated like a disposable object whose relevance only kicked in when I could be of use to a selfish and self-centred husband who had neither heart nor conscience? The answer was no: I did not want this. On the other hand, nor did I want to walk out on the marriage just because it wasn't satisfying. So I decided, rather than up sticks and depart there and then, I would stay as long as I could and let circumstances force me out as and when they became unbearable.

On September 11 1975, I got a helping hand when Colin Campbell burst into our apartment in the early evening after a heavy day out drinking and drug-taking and, for the second time in our marriage, launched an unprovoked physical attack upon me. This time, however, he did not hit me on my face. As the blows and kicks rained down all over my body, he kept on saying almost proudly: 'I'm not going to touch your face.' If he thought such self-restraint was laudable, that was not a sentiment I shared. As far as I was concerned, a man who can refrain from providing visible proof of his abuse can also refrain from beating his wife altogether.

When the attack started, I expected it to be over as quickly as the first one. This was not a case of history repeating itself, however, but of my husband giving free rein to desires I did not even know he possessed. Over the next six hours, he beat me with a ferocity and intensity that seemed more appropriate to a bad Hollywood movie than real life. Time and again he renewed his attack, battering me until physical exhaustion forced him to take a break. He used his hands, his fists, his arms, his legs, his feet, the whole weight of his body. Naturally, I tried to escape. Once I even made it to the door of the apartment and tried to get it open, but he wrested me to the ground by grabbing my ankle in his very own version of rugby as played by the Campbells of Argyll.

Then he dragged me by that same ankle through the apartment to our bedroom, where he pummelled me until he ran out of breath.

At this point he muttered darkly about what bitches all women are and went into the living room, doubtless to have another drink and recoup his strength for yet another onslaught.

Finally, after yet another wave, I managed to escape into the bathroom and lock myself in while he was taking another of his breathers. If I hoped this would deter him, I soon discovered how wrong I was when he started to hammer at the door, threatening to kill me if he obtained access before I gave it to him voluntarily. My sense of self-preservation getting the better of my reluctance to endure further physical pain, I opened the door, figuring that blows, or even broken bones, would be preferable to death.

Gloria and Michael at their worst had been nothing like this un-caged beast; and frankly, I was at a loss as to how to bring it to a close. Although I had hardly been passive throughout, trying everything from charm and reason to silence and compliance in an attempt to bring it to an end, I had not yet sought to wrest control of the situation from him, save on the one occasion I had locked myself into the bathroom. With a flash of clarity, I saw that there was one and only one way out. I needed to dupe him into thinking that I had taken enough of his Valium tablets to kill myself. He wouldn't want people to blame him for having beaten his wife until she committed suicide, and would doubtless come up with a remedy to save his own skin. In doing so, he would inadvertently save mine as well, for if this abuse were to go on much longer, he could well kill me whether he intended to or not. So I sprang out of bed, went to the medicine cabinet in the bathroom, swallowed about four or five of his Valium tablets – which I knew would safely render unconsciousness thanks to having spoken to one of his doctors about his level of consumption of that drug only days before – flushed down the lavatory the remainder of the hundred or so tablets he had in the three bottles he collected from his three separate doctors, and lay back down on my bed waiting for the drugs to take effect.

I say 'my bed' because we had separate beds, if you can believe something so unnatural for young people in their twenties – his choice, not mine. I wish I could also say that I waited for unconsciousness with a sense of ghoulish amusement. I was not blind to the situation's ridiculous aspects. But I was so benumbed from what had happened in the previous six hours that the smile couldn't travel from my brain to my lips, even though I was gratified to note that Conning hadn't managed to beat me into losing my sense of humour.

I awoke to find myself in the Lenox Hill Hospital. Sure enough, when Conning realized what I had done, he swung into action, telephoning Patricia Fleischmann, a mutual friend of mine and his sister Jeanie's who had been my matron-of-honour. She suggested that he telephone an ambulance and get me to the hospital as soon as possible, warning him that he would be in big trouble if I suffered lasting harm.

In New York in those days, it was against the law to try to commit suicide, and hospitals would not release you unless they were certain that you were no threat to yourself. I was therefore duly interviewed by a psychiatrist prior to being released. When I told her what I had done and why, she commended me for my resourcefulness and referred me to Al-Anon, an organization for the friends and relations of alcoholics which I had never heard of before. Then she released me with the suggestion that I get help for his drinking immediately, otherwise I might not be so lucky the next time.

In some ways, this doctor's advice was a Godsend, because once I started going to Al-Anon and to open meetings at its collateral organization, Alcoholics Anonymous, I gained valuable medical knowledge about alcoholism and drug addiction. But in another way, it kept me involved with a problem that was not mine for four years longer than I would otherwise have been entangled by it, for I kept on attending meetings hoping that somehow they would relieve the anguish I had endured. Only when my good sense returned, and I decided that the best way to leave the pain of the past was just to leave the past in the past, did I actually begin the healing process. Nevertheless, thanks to Al-Anon and AA I acquired sufficient knowledge to see that alcoholism was neither Conning nor Gloria's primary problem, though their alcoholic consumption exaggerated the underlying personality problems they had.

With me in the hospital and Patricia and Jeanie knowing how badly he had abused me, Conning now swung into action to protect himself, as he himself informed me on the way back from the hospital when he came to pick me up the following day. He telephoned my parents to tell them that I had 'tried to top' myself 'for no reason at all'.

Kettle did not miss the opportunity to fry her vulnerable daughter by informing Pot, 'Don't you worry, Son-in-Law. I know from my own experience what a piece of work that child can be. Attempting suicide is her favourite trick to get attention. Don't give into her and let her have her own way. Hold fast and make sure she doesn't get the better of you. You have our support. I've had a warm time with her too, so I can sympathize with you.'

'But why would she have done something like that for no reason?' the more reasonable and less vicious Michael wanted to know, according to Conning, who proudly recounted the whole sorry conversation.

'You know what she's like, you old *mumu*,' Gloria had said, evidently silencing Michael. 'Son-in-Law, if I followed your father-in-law, I'd have all my children and half the world running rings around me the way they do with him. You hang in there and don't let that little hussy prevail. And if you have any other problems with her, you let me know. I know how to deal with her even if her father doesn't.'

As the taxi was taking Conning and me the short distance from the Lenox Hill Hospital to our apartment on 83rd and Third, I could not help feeling that my vain and competitive mother had yet again found a way to place unnecessary obstacles in my way rather than help to remove them. I could tell that Conning was speaking the truth, because I knew the way Gloria phrased things. There was no way my self-centred birdbrain of a husband would have had the intelligence, much less the powers of observation, required to mimic her with the accuracy he was doing. The disloyal way she managed to undermine my position, turning the innocent party into the guilty one, cut me to the quick; and I would have railed at the injustice of being given such a faithless mother had I had anyone who was interested in listening. But there wasn't.

Gloria only managed to crow for another day, however. Richard Barker, a friend of Conning's mother who had called to visit while Conning was out drinking to get over the trauma of what I had done to him, took one look at me, and seeing how badly beaten up I was, said, 'I see Colin's been up to his old tricks. Get your passport.'

The following morning, Dick put me on a plane to my sister Libby and brother-in-law Ben in Canada. Upon examining me, Ben telephoned my parents. 'I have Georgie with me. In all my years as a doctor I've never seen a worse case of wife-beating. She's bruised from her neck to her ankles. Ninety percent of her body is literally black and blue.'

'I suppose you want us to believe that she didn't do anything to provoke him?' Gloria said aggressively, leaving no room for error as to where her sympathies lay.

'There are times when I think you really must be mad,' Michael snapped at his wife. 'Can any man ever jus…jus…justify beating any woman like that?'

Gloria, her fun spoiled, showed her total lack of concern for her own daughter by announcing that she had had 'enough of this extra *pazevie*' before slamming down the receiver, leaving Michael to show that at least one of my parents had a heart and some interest in my welfare.

'Georgie, when Colin tel…tel…telephoned and told us what you'd done, he never sa…sa…said a word about why you'd done it,' Michael said, so upset on my behalf that his tongue was loosened and he barely stammered. 'I don't want you to go back to that monster. Get a lawyer and divorce him. No woman should live with a man like that.' For a Catholic who was the brother of a nun and the nephew of an archbishop that was advice which so went against the grain of the Church that it showed the extent of his disapproval as nothing else could have.

As regards who would pay for this divorce, the man, who was so quick to pick up expensive bills for his friends in chic restaurants all over the world but was equally slow to put his hand in his pocket for the first three of his four children, remained silent. Once more he was giving me the message that I would have to fend for myself, which showed me the limited extent of his regard. Obviously I would need financial assistance if I were to seek a divorce; but Michael didn't offer it, which made leaving my abusive husband an altogether more difficult task than it would otherwise have been had my father cared enough to push his hand into his well-lined pocket and give me a sum that would have made all the difference to me, but none to him.

As far as Gloria's response was concerned, it cleared up any lingering doubts there might have had about the veracity of Conning's account of the conversation he had with her. After this, any temptation I had to confuse the veneer of civility that had been emanating from Gloria's quarter since my marriage as a substitute for maternal feeling, was eradicated instantaneously. Although it would take me several more years to accept the degree of malice, competitiveness and envy that motivated her, in that instant I understood that she was still no more reliable and feeling towards me than she had been since the incident when she had tried to burn my face. In effect, I should continue to regard her with as much suspicion as my other siblings had employed. I should also remember that when she said, as she often did, that we should 'abandon people to their fate,' this was no idle figure of speech but the living verbalization of her *modus operandi* and confirmation of her utter heartlessness.

Had Michael offered me financial help, I might well have been more motivated not to return to my husband. As it was, I was too depleted by my physical and emotional ordeal, which now included cracked ribs and pleurisy, to deal with moving my clothes and chattels out of the matrimonial home and finding another apartment. I could therefore hardly consider seriously fulfilling his recommendation that I divorce Conning. So, when my errant spouse started telephoning, begging and pleading with me to return to him, blaming alcohol for his violence and swearing that he would cut down on the booze, I agreed with a marked lack of enthusiasm to give the marriage one last chance. However, to keep him in line I issued what I hoped was a well-judged caveat just as I had done after he had smashed up my face in May, 'If you so much as lay a finger on me ever again in any but a loving way, I'll be out the door quicker than you can say "boo".'

I wish I could say that I returned to New York with hope, but I did not. I did not see how anyone who so relished violence could change into a gentle and loving person. I felt it was only a matter of time before Conning's violent streak got the better of him again, so I resolved to use whatever time was left to prepare for my departure. I got a job and squirreled away every spare cent for the day when Colin Campbell's violence would make a divorce inevitable and in the meantime prepared myself mentally, changing my goal from that of a lasting marriage to that of a friendly divorce. Preparedness, I hoped, would reduce some of the pain of this failed union.

It was at this juncture that Conning and Ian tried to get me to approach my father to settle outstanding debts they had in England. They were being threatened with lawsuits: Ian by Manufacturers Hanover Trust Bank which had a loan on his London house at 79 Park Walk, Chelsea, and Conning by The Priory, the famous drying-out clinic at Roehampton outside London, where he had run up bills for a series of stays before our marriage. Of course, there was no way my father would have come to their rescue, and I told my husband this. Although I did not realize it then, my failure to solve their problem cooked my goose in ways I could never have imagined.

It's just as well that I did not expect to hear from Gloria or Michael during this period. I knew that my father would feel satisfied with having fulfilled his duty by advising me to leave 'the monster' and would avoid further contact lest I ask him to make a financial contribution, while my mother, never one to write even at the best of times, would be too busy having a good time to actually do anything for any of her children, her erstwhile favourite included.

Nevertheless, I maintained the practice we had all been reared to fulfil by writing them weekly letters, taking care as always not to burden them with anything troublesome or negative. I knew my place in the scheme of things. If I could not shine brightly, I was not to disturb them with what Gloria referred to as 'botheration'. So I kept my counsel and did not allude to my problems, writing letters that appealed to their vanity and fulfilled their need to consider themselves as marvellous parents whose children adored them because of their innately splendiferous wonderfulness. This innately splendiferous wonderfulness was not based upon anything as mundane as actions, however, but was entirely due to the special people they were by virtue of being Michael and Gloria.

Towards the end of October, Michael telephoned and said that he wanted Kitty, Libby and me to spend Christmas in Jamaica with him. One of the more touching things about him was his desire to be surrounded by his children at Christmas. Because Mickey had just left Jamaica yet again, there was no question of his returning so soon; but Michael was otherwise happy to spend a small fortune on our plane fares and the fares of our spouses. 'I'll have to talk it over with Colin,' I said, who leapt at the opportunity to return to Jamaica for the second time that year.

Once Michael bought the tickets, Conning's behaviour, which up to that point had been tolerable, took a sharp turn for the worst. It was as if he felt that now that I was committed to spending Christmas with him, I couldn't leave him until after the holidays, so he had license to do as he pleased. Where previously he had been relatively abstemious, he now hit the bottle with renewed vigour. Within a fortnight, he was back to being as alcoholically pugnacious and vitriolic as he had been in the last weeks of August and the first weeks of September.

A few evenings later, I returned home from the job I had got to bring in some money to find that my husband, who was supposed to be working on a travel book, was doing research yet again in the bars of New York City. Throughout this time, he completed no more than fifty sentences, and finally, four months later, he would give up all pretence of actually bothering. In those early days, however, I tried to have faith, and had to jolly myself out of the dispirited feeling that settled over me. I ate supper in solitude, then went to an Al-Anon meeting around the corner, leaving Conning's dinner for him on top of the stove.

Because women cooked no matter what in those days, it did not occur to me to question why I should have to work all day, come home and cook dinner for someone who never worked and was out all day boozing. Had he polished off the food one left, I might have derived some satisfaction from that; but, as it was, his appetite was as birdlike as my mother's. He seldom ate for, like most alcohol guzzlers, he was getting all the calories he needed from the vast quantities of booze which he consumed. Those very quantities filled his stomach and gave him a sensation of satiety. Unlike Gloria, however, whose erratic bouts of eating resulted in moderate consumption of food, whenever Conning did eat, he overate so grossly that the last thing anyone could derive was satisfaction, either from witnessing the repellent quantity he packed away or from having prepared the food. He would wolf down his dinner and everything else he could lay his hands on, scattering food everywhere like a pig at the trough. He never took the time to cut and chew before swallowing, often even dispensing with cutlery. As one looked at him, it was difficult to believe that one was looking at a human being, much less one who was supposed to be a gentleman. In Alcoholics Anonymous and Al-Anon they called this gluttonous practice the 'chuck-hors', and I was just glad that my mother did not share it with my husband. Not only was it repellent to observe, but afterwards he would inevitably be ill, thrashing about in pain until he brought up much of what he had downed.

When I returned from my Al-Anon meeting that November evening, I found Conning lying on the sofa thrashing about groaning. Food, forming a trail from the kitchen, was scattered all over the floor in the living room. What he hadn't gorged upon he had dropped, leaving it for me to pick up – as usual. Normally, I would have swung into action, cleaning up after I had fetched and carried his medicines, including the kaolin and morphine which he took for his 'stomach trouble' and which I had tenderly fed to him countless times. However, the subject of the meeting that evening had been about the very thing I was now witnessing, so I put the advice into action. I did nothing to help, though I did commiserate. 'I'm sorry to see you like this,' I said in Al-Anon speak before stepping over the food and heading towards the bedroom.

'Aren't you going to clean up the mess?' Conning demanded with all the irritable entitlement of my mother. Unlike us, however, he did not come from a heritage of hot-and-cold-running servants, so he had absolutely no justification for expecting to be waited upon hand and foot. In the few months that we had been married, however, I had spoiled him rotten, and he now acted as if he had a right to be served, quite forgetting that I was his wife, not his maid.

'No,' I said pleasantly. 'I didn't help you to abuse yourself, so helping you to escape the consequences of that abuse will only prolong your agony. It would be cruel to assist you, now that I know the damage I've caused by trying to help in the past.'

Before I could even make it to the passage leading to our bedroom, I felt him grab me by the arms and swing me around.

'You stupid bitch,' said the miraculously recovered hulk of six foot two, glowering at me menacingly. 'You're my fucking wife. Clean up the mess, you stupid bitch. Bitch.'

As my husband's fingers dug into my arms, I knew that this was the moment I had been waiting for. It was the death knell of our marriage.

'I am neither stupid nor a bitch,' I said calmly and quietly, 'and I would thank you to release me from your grasp, as you're hurting me.'

Conning looked at me, curled his lip, seemed to reflect momentarily upon whether he should proceed or retract, and, having made his decision, let go of my arms. He muttered about how awful Al-Anon and AA were, 'filled' as they were with a 'bunch of losers and no-hopers'.

This was a bit rich coming from someone who knew little about those organizations, having been to only two meetings under sufferance. He, not they, was the paradigm of the loser and no-hoper, having never in his twenty-eight years accomplished anything or indeed ever finished anything he had ever started except mayhem. But I kept my counsel and went to bed early.

As I lay in the dark, I could see no alternative but to ask for a divorce. I had no doubt that this incident was the start of the cycle of physical abuse which would end in my battery or death. The moment for departure was upon me.

The following morning, I telephoned Conning from the office to say that our marriage was over. He listened quietly then telephoned me later to ask me to stay 'as a friend' to help him 'beat drink'. This was clever of him, for he knew I was a great believer in harmoniousness and wanted us to remain friends, no matter what. He now played me so well that he obtained my agreement to help him until we returned from Jamaica in early January 1975.

However, to show that I meant business and was not prepared to be the only party who was contributing to the marriage, I resigned my job, fully aware that that would put pressure on him to deliver or depart. Quite where I would get the money from to divorce him, I did not know.

It was at times like these that one could not help noticing how much more difficult one's life was for having a financially-mean father and a generally-mean mother.

Confronted by my resolution, Conning stopped drinking. He still continued to take Valium in vast quantities; but without the alcohol, he became far kinder and more decent. Within days he was begging me to give him one last chance to prove that he could be the sort of husband I wanted, and though I held out no real hope, I nevertheless agreed to give him until our return from Jamaica. 'Otherwise I want a divorce as soon as we come back,' I said. 'We can remain friends. We're both young, and it will be better for us if we part sooner rather than later, while there's still a measure of affection between us. That way we can remain friends and at least our marriage will have been a force for good even if it didn't last.'

Two days before we were due to leave for Jamaica on Sunday December 15 1974, a reporter named Jolyon Wilde came around to interview us on behalf of the *Sunday People* newspaper in Britain. Up to that point, I had never even heard of this publication, but I would discover in a matter of weeks that it had great significance, especially where the Argyll family was concerned.

Although the purpose of the article was supposed to be about how we liked living in New York, once he was in the apartment, Wilde abandoned all pretence and started to quiz me about my medical history. While Conning went and fixed himself the first drink he had openly had in weeks, I refused to play ball and threatened to sue if the paper printed anything untrue. As soon as Wilde left, I telephoned Barbara Taylor Bradford, who offered to kill the story. This, I would subsequently discover, had been set up by Ian Argyll with the connivance of Conning, as a money-spinner, to discharge the debts they still had hanging over their heads. They – and by 'they' I mean Ian, as Conning simply did not possess the intelligence to think up such a wily plan – had come up with the idea of realizing Michael's and my own worst nightmare in an attempt to raise enough money to pay off all their bills by putting the most salacious spin they could upon my medical history, and selling the story to the newspaper with which the family had a history of doing business. Ian was the prime mover, but Conning – who had a duty to be loyal to me – went along with it. I have consequently never excused either brother for what they did.

Little realizing that my husband was as treacherous as my mother, I flew to Jamaica with him thinking the story had been killed stone dead by Barbara's good offices. I had no idea that he was actually telephoning his brother behind my back, using my parents' telephone to revive the deal.

It is just as well I was ignorant of what was going on behind my back, for to my face, my mother was doing her level best to live up to her oft-repeated boast of being the biggest bitch in the world. She didn't even attempt to be civil with me while going all-out to embark upon another charm offensive so that one and all could see that she and 'Son-in-Law' got along famously, even if he and I didn't. Most days they sat around sailing on a conversational sea of booze, once more showing their capacity for trivia by chatting from morning till night about nothing at all. I left them to their own devices as much as good sense allowed, hoping that in my absence this self-regarding daughter of Narcissus from whose womb I had sprung would resist the temptation to further undermine my position by telling any of the lies she so enjoyed retailing about others when she wanted to boost herself at their expense.

My one consolation during this period was that Conning and I were not sleeping at my parents' house but at Helen Ziadie's. This gave me a measure of respite I would not otherwise have had. Though Helen and Gloria remained firm friends, she so disapproved of the way I had been treated during my childhood, and of her friend's present attitude towards me, that she always provided me with moral support while I sounded off about Gloria. As she laid great stress upon loyalty, taking my side they way she did was a real boon, I can tell you.

By Christmas Day, though, I had had all I could bear. No matter how well Conning and Gloria got along, or how often she delivered the bitchy message that he needed a 'good strong woman to take care of him and make better all that had gone wrong in his life', meaning someone like her not someone like me, there was no way I wanted this drunken oaf as a husband. So I called him up to the swimming pool and informed him, 'Enough is enough. I'm not going back to New York with you. I want a divorce. I'll see lawyers here,' my brother having been a respected member of the Bar I would have access to the best legal brains there, 'and you can sort things out at your end. I'm happy to reconfirm that I don't want any alimony,' I said, alluding to how he had cannily got me to waive all my rights to it prior to our marriage, something I had been happy to do. 'And we can remain friends,' Polyanna finished up saying.

Conning's reaction was surprising. He merely asked me not to tell my family until he was about to leave. Little did I know it, but Conning had not been trying to preserve our marriage, but to keep it intact until he and his brother could achieve their objective of getting the *Sunday People* to publish the story Barbara and I had managed to stop. They saw that there was a richer vein to mine if we were still together when the story broke.

I would subsequently learn from my guilt-ridden sister-in-law that her family had form where stitching up wives in the press was concerned. 'Big Ian' – as their father, the eleventh Duke of Argyll was known – was the father of cheque-book journalism. With the help of his son Little Ian and Jeanie herself, who was a well-known columnist as well as granddaughter of the press baron the first Lord Beaverbrook, and therefore possessed an insider's knowledge of how to maximize press interest, he had instigated the longest, costliest and most scandalous divorce action in Scottish legal history when his third wife Margaret had refused to give him a pay-off of £250,000 to end their marriage in 1959. Their rationale was simple. The family needed the money and since Margaret would not cough it up – she had already re-roofed Inveraray Castle and redecorated it at the cost of millions of dollars in today's money, they would raise a commensurate sum from the press by selling stories about his marriage. With that objective in mind, Big Ian, Little Ian and Jeanie spread the rumour in Fleet Street that he would cite eighty-eight co-respondents. This, of course, grabbed the press's attention in a way nothing else could have, and set the tone for the most salacious divorce of the century, though when push came to shove, there were only three co-respondents cited when the papers were served. A fourth would subsequently be added towards the end of the hearing, when it became apparent that the divorce action was bound to fail unless Big Ian came up with at least one co-respondent who could be seen to have had the opportunity to commit adultery.

Having sown the wind, Big Ian exploited the whirlwind of interest he and his children had created by selling stories about the supposedly nymphomaniacal Margaret, Duchess of Argyll to the *Sunday People.*

By any interpretation, this was a resourceful way to obtain the money Margaret had refused to hand over to Big Ian. Of course, once they undertook such a devious and amoral enterprise, they had to demonize the unfortunate woman to justify their own inexcusable behaviour, and though Jeanie would subsequently repent the part she had played, neither Big nor Little Ian ever did. As far as father and son were concerned, they had been the injured parties.

As I would discover for myself when my own turn came, with people who were playing such a skilful game of persecutor as victim, malice wasn't even their primary motivation, though they quickly retreated behind that unworthy sentiment to justify their unjustifiable conduct rather than admit that their motivation was money, pure and simple. .

Everyone now knows about cheque-book journalism; but between 1959 and 1963, while the Argyll divorce took place, or in 1974, when mine started, the practice was virtually unheard of – certainly in polite circles. People, whether ordinary or privileged, simply did not stoop to such depths.

Or so I thought.

I was about to learn differently.

On December 29 1974, the *Sunday People* published a front-page story under the headline 'Sex Change Secret of a Peer's Bride'. The first I knew of this was when my brother Mickey, who was in London, telephoned to tell the family about it. Michael's and my worst fear had come true; and, though I was dreadfully upset to be characterized in such terms, at least Conning was good about it. Indeed, he was supportive even in the body of the story, saying that I was 'the most beautiful girl he had ever seen' and 'as much a woman as any and more than most'.

Although I wanted to sue, Gloria and Michael refused to bankroll me, so once again, I found myself being cast back on to my own too-slender resources.

If I was expected to be self-reliant whenever I had to endure life's downside, Gloria had a different attitude when I tried to implement my right to choose when I left my violent husband. As soon as she discovered that I had no intention of returning to New York with him, she turned the full force of her persuasive powers on me. 'Don't worry, Son-in-Law,' she assured him right in front of me. 'I won't let you face the music on your own.' Then, hopping onto the moralistic high horse which was the favourite vantage point of this amoral hypocrite, she launched into a diatribe, accusing me of being an 'ingrate,' a 'selfish so-and-so who doesn't think about anyone but yourself'. 'Colin has been loyal to you,' she announced. 'He's standing by you and supporting you during this scandal. You *have* to go back with him. It's the only decent thing to do.'

Michael, however, was firmly behind me. 'Don't go back to New York with him,' he said once Conning was out of earshot. 'You're not a pu…punching bag. His behaviour is worse than any sa…savage. Don't lis…listen to your mother. You never ki…killed or stole from anyone so you have nothing to be a…a…ashamed of. You can stay here as lo…long as you want.'

I knew Michael deplored his son-in-law's conduct, which was so bizarre and out of control that he was a caricature of the textbook drunk. I also knew he loathed his child being on the front pages of the gutter press worldwide after the story had been picked up everywhere, but he had swallowed his distaste and had the good grace not to allude to it. For that, I was grateful as well as touched. It showed that Daddy basically did care about me, which was one of the few positive things to come out of an otherwise insufferable situation.

Gloria, however, was the antithesis of anything positive. She was her usual dominating self, nothing if not persistent. Once she had decided to assert herself at my expense by concluding that I would return to New York with Conning, on and on she went, like a dog with a bone, for the four or five days that remained of our trip. At first, I tried to argue rationally, pointing out the danger I would be in physically if I returned during this phase of Conning's drinking cycle. This earned Gloria's sneering comment that 'it's a woman's duty to control her husband. If you can't control yours, you can't be very much of a woman.' Then, when I still refused to agree to go back, she started on about how 'people will say that he doesn't want you, now your "matter" is public.'

'Ah, so I'm supposed to go back and run the risk of being beaten to a pulp just to silence gossip. Pray, tell me, how can they say that he dumped me when it is I who am refusing to go back to New York with him?'

'You know that. I know that. But not everyone knows that. People will talk, and I for one am sick and tired of the scandal surrounding you. It's worse than the stench of a rancid nigger, and if you don't have enough pride to think of yourself, think of your father and me and the rest of the family,' Gloria continued tenaciously, clearly intent on pressing my buttons.

However, I had known her a little too long to fall for that line of twaddle.

'Then they'll just have to talk,' I said. 'For I am *not* going back with him.'

'You are a selfish little so-and-so, and I rue the day I ever gave birth to you. It's my fault though. You see, Son-in-Law, I spoiled your wife rotten. That's the root of all my problems with her. And for all I know, the source of yours too.' She kept the bit firmly between her teeth until I finally relented and agreed to go back with him – but only for a few weeks.

The night of our return to New York, Jolyon Wilde arrived at the apartment uninvited; or so I thought, until I realized that the only way he could have known when we were due back was if Conning had informed him. He said he was there to conclude his dealings with Conning for my life story. This was the first I had heard of any such proposition, and I went ballistic. Conning, living up to his nickname, denied having entered into any such arrangement with Wilde, and continued to pretend that the story had come about by unknown forces. The reporter, however, was having none of that. He kept on insisting that they had an agreement and Conning had to honour his part of it, while I, Gloria-style, stood on the sidelines shrieking invective. One thing led to another, and within minutes, they were slugging it out on the floor. Finally, Wilde, though smaller, got the better of the drunken Conning, and after delivering a few choice punches, fled while I was telephoning the police.

This was too good an opportunity to miss. I demanded that Conning file assault charges against Wilde. 'You will stand up in court and tell everyone the lies he has told about us. That will be a much better way of getting the truth across than suing, and it won't cost us a penny,' I said, the taste of vindication sweet in my mouth.

The police duly came, listened to out accounts and, the following day, picked us up and took us downtown to the precinct to take our statements and start the process which would provide us with the platform for rectifying the awful story Wilde had written about me.

The morning after, still disbelieving of my husband's complicity in the article, I bounced out of bed bright and early to go on a job interview. I would need something to do as well as an income for the duration of this stay in New

York. When I was about to leave, Conning, in true Judas style like my devious mother, kissed me goodbye on the cheek, which was very uncharacteristic for someone who didn't like touching feminine flesh. He said, 'Don't worry. Everything's gonna be all right.' And as soon as I was out the door he telephoned Wilde and arranged to sign a contract with him for an account of what his life had been like with the woman whom he had kicked out when he had discovered her secret!

I returned home to find a belligerent Conning howling about how he wanted me out of 'his' apartment. Of course, I had no idea that he had to have me out to make the money Wilde had signed him up for, or that he had even signed a contract with Wilde, and refused to go when he could furnish no reason that made any sense. I pointed out that he could leave if he wished, but that, unbeknownst to me, would not have dovetailed with the story he had signed for: that he had already kicked me out.

He then made sure I would leave by flashing his fists a few times under my nose. So I telephoned my good friend Mary Michele Rutherfurd and went to stay with her at her parents' Park Avenue apartment.

Once there, I got in touch with my parents to bring them up to date on this new development. 'I war…warned you not to go…go back with that lunatic,' Michael said, while Gloria couldn't resist implying that it was all my fault that her advice had rebounded by sneering, 'If you're going to lay claim to being a woman, you'd better learn how to act like one and control your husband.' For sheer, unadulterated viciousness, I thought that was pretty unsurpassable, though I wasn't stupid enough to say so.

Being caught between a Colin Campbell and a Gloria Ziadie gives a whole new meaning to the devil and the deep blue sea, I can tell you. Two days later, Stephanie Bennett, my literary agent at the time, telephoned to tell me that things were a lot worse than I had hitherto thought. Conning had personally arranged to sell a story to Wilde about kicking me out prior to actually doing so.

'The Judas,' I said and felt myself being catapulted down the darkest hole I had ever been thrown into. Not even Gloria's treachery over the years was anything to compare with this.

'Jolyon Wilde is doing a story this Sunday about you based on Colin's interviews,' Stephanie revealed. 'It's another front-page story. Like the other one, it will be picked up by other publications worldwide. He wants your comments. My advice to you is to give him an interview.'

So that Friday afternoon Stephanie and I duly showed up at Wilde's office. Doubtless in the hope that my reaction would give him a better story, Wilde even played me sections of his taped interviews with Conning. Thereafter, I would never be able to delude myself that he was the innocent I had previously thought him to be, or that he was anything but a calculating, unconscionable opportunist. With each word, I felt more and more lights within me being doused until finally there were few if any left. It would take another twenty years before my spiritual luminosity shone as brightly as it had done prior to that.

How could anyone be so low? I kept on wondering, struggling to come to terms with the way my husband had betrayed me, in the days, weeks, months and years to come – and all for a few paltry thousand dollars. I still did not know about the part he or his brother had played in the first story.

When 'Peer Kicks Out Sex Change Bride' was published, my father suggested that I return home. He duly bought my plane ticket, and I set off home with my spirits somewhere in my boots.

Although Michael and I had never been close, by this time I felt a lot more warmly towards him than my mother. Her attitude towards me had been 'as cold and impersonal as the grave' to use her oft-repeated phrase to describe the way she projected her feelings when she wanted to freeze people out.

'Well, you made your bed, now you've got to lie in it,' she would endlessly repeat in the days to come, as if she were reading off a laundry list, while I lay collapsed on the *chaise longue* in the drawing room, crying inconsolably. Quite why she sat with me mystified me, though I now suspect it was partly to crow over my distress and partly for want of anything better to do. I, who had dared to eclipse her in the beauty stakes by being written about in the world's press as this supposedly great beauty and had compounded my offence by marrying a lord with connections to the English royal family, had been brought low; and she certainly wasn't going to deprive herself of the pleasure of witnessing my agony. Or maybe she didn't have enough of a heart to care. Either way, she was no consolation at all, though my beloved aunt Marjorie, who – unusually for her – was staying for a few days when I arrived, gave me all the love and comfort I needed.

Only after Marjorie's departure, when Conning started to telephone begging me to give him another chance, did Gloria bestir herself. Once she came alive, she cast herself in the role of chief *directrice*, raining unwanted and inappropriate advice down upon me as if I were an Indian field in the middle of the monsoon season. Determined not to have this egotistical busybody muck up my life any more than she already had with her gratuitous advice, I ignored it all, though I was tactful enough not to let on that this was what I was doing.

Then things took an unexpected turn when Conning's brother Ian jumped into the ring, telephoning me to offer help if I wanted to hospitalize my husband. 'As long,' he added, 'as you pay the bills.'

I was aghast when Gloria hopped into the conversation uninvited. 'Ian, this is Gloria, Georgie's mother. You may be sure that nothing that happens will take place unless I agree to it. I call the shots around here, and I shall be monitoring all future activity. I trust I make myself clear and you will be cooperating to prevent further scandal. My husband and I are sick to death of it all, and I hope you are too.'

'I've been telling Colin to keep out of the papers,' Ian, who I would soon learn had orchestrated the whole scandal, said with breathtaking hypocrisy.

As I tried to explain to Ian that I could not agree to hospitalizing Colin or paying for his treatment, if only because my actions could be misinterpreted, Gloria kept on interrupting so much that I finally had to ask her to please get off the line so that I could make my point without further interruption.

Although I did not know it at the time, I now had the onerous task of dealing with three, not two, devils and the deep blue sea, for Ian was far cleverer and even more malign than his younger brother. How I ever got through the succeeding days I will never know. To say that I felt like I was living in the middle of an insane asylum does not begin to approach the way I felt. I had one consolation, however. Gloria having awakened, all I had to do was sit back and listen – or pretend to listen – while she showered me with instructions as to how 'you can get yourself out of the hole you've dug for yourself.'

The difficulty with the Glorias of this world is that one is liable to fall for their act, even when one knows from past experience that it is love of drama rather than love of the individual that is motivating them. They are so focused, so potent, with all the sincerity of the truly insincere, that even if you try to resist, these forces of nature eventually wear you down. As I really needed someone to bat on my team at that juncture, she had an easier task of convincing me than she might otherwise have had. It also has to be said that I was predisposed to fall into the old trap, because the progeny of seriously disordered personalities usually want to believe that those parents basically love them, are interested in them and have concern for them. And when they shine the bright light of their attention upon the said progeny, the silly chump usually takes a benevolent view when what is really called for is a more measured one. So, while not exactly basking in Gloria's concern, I allowed it to warm the cockles of my heart and started to think, 'Mummy does care, even if she doesn't always express herself the way one would like.'

Maternal love or not, there was no way I was going to stay in Jamaica one day longer than I had to. Impatient to resume my life in whatever form it would take after my divorce, I agreed to go back to Conning but only to sign divorce papers and wrap up our New York life.

Gloria and her 'Son-in-Law' alter ego both expressed the view that I might change my mind about the divorce, but I knew better than either of them.

Although I was careful not to remove Conning's hope for a future with me, I had no such reservations about expressing my determination to be rid of him to my mother. This was an error on two fronts. Firstly, she liked Son-in-Law and wanted a divorce no more than he did. Secondly, once she realized that it was inevitable, she tried to keep me with her in Jamaica, doubtless so that she could regulate the divorce proceedings the way she had regulated Libby's wedding while at the same time having me as a captive audience.

There was no way I was going to let her wear down my determination a second time. I could see what the end result would be if I did. Once she had got bored with this latest source of amusement, she would turn her fusillade upon me personally. It would be 1971 and 1972 all over again, except that this time I would have the handicaps of a failed marriage and worldwide tabloid publicity for her to use against me. The bumbling if violent drunkard seemed a far preferable alternative compared with her. I therefore explained that I had to return to the apartment in New York to gather evidence against Conning for the divorce and had to do so immediately.

The one thing you can bank on with the Glorias of this world is their insensate lust for intrigue. At my mention of the 'evidence' I would 'amass' 'against Colin', Gloria opened her eyes wide at the possibility of a new drama afoot. Those huge brown eyes, which would have been beautiful had they been set in stone but were, in my opinion, always too glazed to be anything but repellent, now glistened as much as two stagnant brown pools can. I saw that I had inadvertently hit the bull's eye. 'What do you mean?' she said, saccharine dripping off her tongue. Whenever Mummy was sweet, you knew she had something up her sleeve. 'Evidence? What evidence?'

'Well, my literary agent said she's seen the contract Colin signed with the *Sunday People*. It's in the apartment. I need to get hold of it. It takes no imagination to see the effect it will have in the divorce court. I'll purloin it and give it to Charles Dismukes for safe keeping,' I continued, alluding to Lady Sarah Spencer-Churchill's lawyer and a friend of mine. 'There are also all the letters he has in his possession which show that he has a history of violence, drug-taking and drunkenness as well as long police records in Australia and New Zealand. You should see some of the things people wrote over the years to his father. And some of the letters his father wrote to him. I need to have the evidence of what he's like in case I have to use it in a divorce. I can't afford a my-word-against-his scenario.'

'You're up against a thousand years of bad blood,' Gloria said melodramatically. 'My advice to you is to tread very, very carefully unless you want to end up like Margaret, Duchess of Argyll, who is reviled and discredited. I'm not sure I would return to him if I were in your shoes.' I could see she was trying to undermine my game plan so that hers, whatever it was, would prevail.

'Believe me, I intend to tread very carefully indeed,' I said, intent on returning, irrespective of how much she undermined me.

In the days before my scheduled departure, she made a variety of attempts to convince me to stay with her, but when she saw that there was no way I would be obliging her, she hopped onto a new bandwagon. 'The first thing you have to do,' Gloria would begin, before throwing up all sorts of rubbish advice which might have seemed good to her, but were wildly inappropriate for me and my circumstances. Because response was as futile as reason, I simply let it all wash over me and allowed myself to become the silent pair of ears she preferred to any rebuttal. In the process, I also managed to acquire some brownie points from her, for when I was leaving, she handed me some much-needed US dollars and made me promise to write and telephone 'whenever there are any new developments'.

Although I was relieved to leave before Gloria turned, as she always did, my heart was nevertheless warmed by the display of motherly love. It therefore struck me as ironic that I was almost hopefully expectant about facing the man I so wanted to be rid of.

At first, Conning, still trying to get me to stay with him, could not have been sweeter. Gloria, of course, had trained me well. I was predisposed to accepting intentions at face value, but not even Conning could explain away his betrayal of me to Jolyon Wilde as having been 'misquoted'. Though I did not let him know that Wilde himself had played enough of the tapes for me to know that he had been only too accurately quoted, I absolutely refused to back down. I wanted a divorce. To drive the point home, I told him that there was no way I would ever sleep with him again, then took off my wedding ring and revealed that I intended to start going out on dates. If he did not like us leading separate lives, he could leave the apartment.

Luck undoubtedly plays a part in life, and I was fortunate enough to come home early one afternoon shortly after this conversation. Conning, who could never speak at a modulated pitch when a bellow would do, was on the telephone to Ian. My ears perked up as he prattled on about how 'they won't go along with that'. What, I wondered, wouldn't 'they' – presumably me and my family – go along with? Deciding that discretion is the better part of valour, I let myself into the apartment quietly. Still not suspecting Ian of having played any part in the press betrayals, I tiptoed into the bedroom and picked up the extension. I then discovered Conning had actually been speaking the truth when he told me that he had married me primarily for my father's money. There he was, lambasting me for failing to get my father to 'cough up the dough', while Ian was doing a Colin on Colin and pressurizing him to find a way to force open the Ziadie purse, because they had not realized enough money from their forays with the press to satisfy both Manufacturers Hanover Trust and the Priory. I cannot describe the shock I felt when I realized that my brother-in-law was involved. He, a gentleman, a duke, Master of the Queen's Household in Scotland and, I had thought up to that point, a far more civilized person than his over-the-top brother, was in cahoots with my husband.

Fortunately for me, both brothers were in love with the sound of their own voices. As I listened, I discovered that Colin's disaffection with me had set in early, up at Inveraray the previous year, when he had realized that I would not ask my father for money. I had then compounded my failure by expecting him to fulfil the role of husband in a responsible and meaningful way, namely by bringing bread to the table and being a man in the bedroom as well as out of it, instead of a leech. Ian displayed a loathing of me which was at odds with his avowed posture and was also reminiscent of the pathological hatred he felt for their stepmothers Mathilda and Margaret. He was still furious with me for having refused to restore the original Campbell stronghold, Innischonnel Castle, and for refusing to get my father to bail them out of their present indebtedness. He couldn't get over the fact that I had got something out of the marriage, namely the title Lady Colin Campbell, while neither of them had achieved the financial rewards for which they had hoped.

As they fulminated, I discovered that they had actually come up with an earlier plan to make money out of me. The original idea had been to induce me to commit adultery, after which Colin would divorce me on those grounds, and they would sell stories about me during the divorce the way Big Ian and Little Ian had done during their father's divorce against Margaret. It was only after I had failed to oblige on the grounds of infidelity that they had alighted upon my birth defect as the next source of revenue.

However, the two stories had not earned the brothers as much as they had hoped. They still had debts to clear – and now wanted to see a profit for all their efforts – and Ian was arguing strongly that the most profitable course of action would be for Colin to institute annulment proceedings. It was clear to me, as I listened, that this was not the first time this subject had been discussed. I hardly dared breathe as Ian said, 'It will be an absolute sensation, old boy. Pa's divorce amalgamated with the April Ashley spectacle. It will have the punters hanging from the rafters. Just think of all the stories we can sell. The whole world will want to know what Georgie is like in bed. How does she piss? What's it like having sex with her? She'll be the most notorious woman in the world by the end of the annulment.'

To his credit, Colin was baulking at the suggestion. 'It would destroy her,' he said. 'She's been a good wife to me. She's stood by me and tried to help me with my problems. I can't do that to her. She doesn't deserve it.'

'Old boy, don't be such a sentimentalist,' Ian replied; and I knew there and then that I would be presiding over my own destruction if I didn't take matters into my own hands.

Sometimes having Gloria Ziadie for a mother has been an advantage. This was one of those occasions. Taking a leaf out of her book, I snuck out quietly, 'arriving' back home with much ado, slamming the door shut noisily, then, innocent as a lamb, cheerfully saying hello. Conning quickly concluded his telephone conversation, then, possibly because he could think of nothing else, said: 'Ian really has it in for you.'

'I can't see why,' I said in mock innocence.

'I don't know. He just does,' he said.

'You yourself are always saying he's jealous of you and doesn't want you to be happy. As you put it, you're tall and he's short; you're a strong personality and he's a conniving little worm; he's a secret poof who used to force you to have sexual relations with him and he's worried I know about it – which of course any wife would – and he wants to eliminate me before other people find out about his filthy incestuous practices. If he's as jealous of you as you say he is – and I have only your word to go on where this is concerned – of course he would have it in for me,' I said, secretly delighted to be stoking the fires of sibling rivalry even if every word was also just and true.

The moment had come for me to demand movement on the divorce. I therefore insisted that Conning make an appointment with Richard Steele of Cusack and Stiles, his mother's lawyers, to draw up divorce papers. 'I want a divorce and I want it sooner rather than later. You will have to be the Petitioner. That way no one can say I tricked you into a divorce. And you, I fear, will have to pay for it, otherwise I can be accused of connivance.'

Later on, after Conning had been to see Mr Steele and the divorce was not progressing as he saw fit, since he wanted me to turn over all my chattels to him, he came clean about Ian trying to persuade him to annul the marriage. If he thought that would terrify me into making any concessions, he was wrong. 'Go along with that treacherous little shit if you want to lose your liberty,' I said. 'Because, believe me, you will. You cannot annul this marriage, as it is valid and has been consummated. When your annulment fails, I shall have you committed to an asylum and make sure you remain there.'

'Ian wouldn't let you.'

'What's he going to do to stop me? As your brother, he's not your next of kin. I am. And I will exercise my rights fully, of that you can be sure.'

'You can't do that,' Conning riposted, no longer the big bully but a frightened little mouse.

'I can and I will. And I would recommend that you don't take my word for it. Check it out with your lawyer. He'll tell you that that's the law. So, buddy boy,' I continued, deliberately goading him with an expression I knew he loathed, 'the choice is yours. You either give me an uncontroversial divorce or drag me through the courts in sensational fashion, at the end of which you will lose and I will have you locked up for the remainder of your life. Oh, incidentally,' I said, in a tone of voice that was straight out of my autocratic mother's book and conveyed the impossibility of opposition, 'you can also tell your brother that neither of you will be selling any more stories about me as long as you and I are married. And you had better sober up. Otherwise you'll have to find somewhere else to live. Oh,' I then said, as if this were an afterthought when in fact I had been waiting for an opportune moment to drop that pearl of poison in Conning's ear, 'you can thank your brother for putting the idea of hospitalizing you in my head.'

'How did that bastard put that idea in your head?' Conning, sucking deeply on his cigarette, asked, always happy to strike out at anyone, even – maybe especially – his brother-in-arms.

'I certainly didn't telephone him in Jamaica to ask him to hospitalize my brother. My brother is sane and lucid and decent and would never sell a story about an enemy, much less a friend or a wife. You are both so dishonourable you make a Bowery bum look like an elevated form of human life. If you want money so badly, why don't you get off your lazy arses and work for it? What makes you think you're so important you can't work? If you didn't have an utterly skewered system of values, you'd know that the ultimate in treachery isn't stealing from a stranger but betraying a friend. I've not only been a good wife to you but also a good friend. You are beneath contempt, but push me any further, and I'll have you locked up – and then I'll throw the key away.'

It is amazing how even the biggest jerk comes to his senses when it's his skin on the line. I could tell from the horrified look on Conning's face that he thought I meant it. Which I did. Not only did he cut way back on the booze, but when his drinking started to escalate again, he actually took himself off to spend a week with a friend until he felt more able to control himself again. Of course, I heard nothing further about him and Ian selling any more stories about me or of Ian's cockamamie plan to annul the marriage.

Shortly after this, I happened upon a letter Ian had written his brother still preaching the merits of a sensational annulment. Now that I had something in black and white instead of a snatched conversation over the telephone, I went to town. First I wrote Ian a letter informing him that I knew exactly what he was up to and that I never wanted to see him again. Then I informed Conning that I would not tolerate Ian's presence in any property I owned, rented or occupied. I did not want to hear about him, discuss him or have anything at all to do with him. As far as I was concerned, Ian Argyll had ceased to exist. If Conning wanted to see him or speak to him, he could do so. I did not believe in standing between siblings, but I could no longer tolerate that evil little weevil in my life.

Getting rid of vermin is easier said than done, however. I was about to discover just what Jeanie Campbell meant when she talked about how 'dark' her family was. I returned home early in the evening of Saturday March 23 1975 to find Conning even more tanked up than usual. Ian was in New York, and the brothers had met for lunch. He was obviously agitated, but whether this show was genuine or simply calculated to manipulate the viewer was not something I could figure out. Nor, frankly, did I care any more. I was sick and tired of the constant and never-ending histrionics; and when he started in on what an awful person Ian was, I didn't even want to hear what he had to say. Then he informed me that Ian had seriously suggested that they hire a hit man to eliminate me. That revelation grabbed my attention, for I had discounted too many of Conning's ravings in the past as nothing but verbal diarrhoea, only to discover that they might have been ravings, but they were also warnings that could and did come true.

I wasn't about to take a chance on my life, so I marched straight over to his desk, picked up the telephone and informed my parents of this latest development. Knowing the importance of having Conning hang his brother with his own words, I made him tell them chapter and verse about this latest scheme.

'I'm glad you had the good sense to let us know,' Michael said to Conning. 'You do realize that you'll both b...be in a lo...lot of trouble if anything ha... happens to my daughter.'

'I don't want to go along with it,' Conning said. 'That's why I told Georgie and you.'

'Colin, this is Gloria. My advice to you is that you get right back to your brother as soon as we hang up and tell him what I have in store for him. I am going to telephone Rudolph Greene. You might remember him. He's the

Chief of Staff of the Army whom you've met here. I'm going to tell him what you have just told Michael and me, and ask him to pass on our concerns to the British authorities. You can be sure that you and Ian will either face the executioner or then spend a lifetime in prison if any harm comes to our daughter.'

'But I don't have anything to do with Ian's plans,' Conning said, seeking to be excused from punishment in the event that Ian did do something.

'Then you'd better get your brother to back off,' Gloria said, clearly relishing playing the lioness protecting her cub.

'I'm as appalled as you,' Conning started to say before Michael cut him off.

'Well, Colin, if th…that's all, I'll leave you and Gloria to ta…talk.'

From the time I had returned to New York in February, Gloria, who had never before been known to write any of her absent children anything but a short letter once or twice in a lifetime, had turned into a latter day Saint Paul. Epistle after epistle rained down upon my letter box at 340 East 83rd Street as if I were an Ephesian. One day she would be analyzing, the next remonstrating, the third planning for the future. My divorce had become like Libby's wedding. However, while Libby had been on the spot and had no escape, I was in another country, so I pretty much ignored her instructions, though I must admit the receipt of those letters was a moral boon.

Confusing with love Gloria's need to be central to whatever was the sensation of the moment, I had by this time concluded that I might well have misjudged her. Could the last few years, troubled as they had been, have been a misunderstanding? Had I misread her character and motivations? Was she really loving and not the hateful, conniving, destructive bitch I had come to think of her as being? No one would have been happier than I to discover that I had been wrong and that she really was the attentive, loving mother half her world believed her to be.

As the weeks turned into months, and Gloria's charm and superficial concern worked their magic, I was lulled into hoping that she might really be as misunderstood and put-upon as she believed herself to be. 'Who knows?' I would say to myself. 'Maybe adversity really can be the catalyst to rescuing and reshaping relationships.' Maybe Conning had done me the ultimate favour by returning me and my mother to the supposed intimacy we had once shared.

Chapter Twenty

The problem with disordered personalities is that they are fundamentally contradictory. While you think they are being constructive, the other part of their personality pushes both them and you into destructiveness. Every act of love, every sign of loyalty, every indication of fidelity that would be, in a more ordered personality, another brick in the courtyard of genuine affection, is as transient and meaningless as writing on the air.

It is hardly surprising that people who are involved with disordered personalities end up feeling as if they have been mangled in a wringer, for in a very real sense they have been. Nothing is constant except turbulence, nothing permanent except instability. However, even disordered personalities need a break from their abusiveness, not only to recharge their batteries or to further their hidden agendas, but also to be true to the more positive parts of their personality. Few of them are purely destructive, even though they and their victims are all prey to the more destructive aspects of their personalities.

In the run-up to my divorce, both Conning and my mother started to behave with unexpected benignity. I had no idea that my snobbish mother was basically entertaining herself with the latest Society *cause celebre*, milking it for all it was worth in social and egotistical terms, or that my husband was similarly looking around for a way to further exploit me financially and was in the meantime biding his time in the hope that a show of togetherness would achieve what treachery hadn't so far been able to. What I did know, however, was that Gloria and Conning still 'got along like a house on fire', as she herself used to put it.

A case in point was the furniture in the New York apartment. Conning telephoned my parents thirty-three times over the last weekend of March 1975, using his revelation about Ian's death plan as the cover for his new stance of protectiveness, and pleaded with them to get me to relinquish my claim to the chattels as a part of the divorce settlement. He claimed that the only way he could get Ian off his back would be if he could present the chattels as a sop to his avarice, failing which Ian would either place more stories in the gutter press about me or make him cooperate in selling them against his will.

So Michael and Gloria joined forces with my errant husband to convince me to sign over ownership of the contents of the New York apartment. As these were worth enough money to keep me afloat for quite a time after the divorce, I was reluctant to part with them, not only because they were mine by right, but also because I would need the money to live on in the near future. Experience had taught me never to trust in my parents' generosity.

'It's blackmail, and one should never give in to blackmail,' I said to my parents, but they were desperate to avoid further scandal – a desire with which I sympathized – and seemed to believe that palliating Ian through Colin was the way to achieve that objective. I thought their stance was silly, counterproductive and irresponsible and told them so in gentle terms. I argued that they were allowing Ian to strip me of assets I needed to survive after the divorce. This attempt to buy silence was at best a temporary respite, unless they financially backed my ambition to sue the newspapers. 'The only thing that will assure zipped mouths is a show of strength. A show of weakness will only encourage further forays into blackmail,' I said.

'Child, we know better than you. You will do as we say. Sign over the damned furniture to Colin so we can all have some peace. You wouldn't want your father and me to lose patience with you at a time like this. Just remember you need us more than we need you,' Gloria barked.

I have to say that I signed over those chattels at Mr Steel's office with a leaden heart. Although I hoped against hope that my parents would replace what they were strong-arming me to surrender, I had no more confidence that they would do so than I had in Conning's claim that his hounding of them was to spare me from Ian. By this time, I knew my husband well enough to suspect that he was most likely blaming his brother for something that he wanted. Ian, I realized, might well have nothing whatsoever to do with this plan, and this view received confirmation when the chattels were sold and Colin pocketed the proceeds without sharing a cent with Ian.

Now flush again, Conning became relatively benevolent. This told me that I could have had a compliant husband if only I had been prepared to bankroll him. But I would sooner have had no husband than one I had to buy. I was enough my mother's daughter to believe that men should support women and not vice versa.

I looked forward with very mixed feelings to the first week of May 1975, when my marriage was scheduled to end. On the one hand, I would be supremely relieved to be rid of the threat that Colin Campbell and Ian Argyll posed as long as I remained Conning's wife. On the other hand, I was sad to see my dreams of a happy marriage dissolve. I also had serious misgivings about how my parents would respond once they realized that I would be going to live in England after the divorce, rather than returning to their house in Jamaica to become Gloria's babysitter, as they were both inveigling me to do.

Conning jetted off to Santo Domingo early in May. The following morning, after the hearing, he rang to inform me that we were divorced, then stunned me by telling me that he was flying on to Jamaica the following day to stay with my mother. Madame Magnanimous was going to console the Son-in-Law who had caused the breakdown of his own marriage. Whatever next? I had to ask myself as I hung up the telephone.

Delighted as I was that we seemed to be achieving a friendly divorce, I nevertheless felt that the visit was inappropriate, so telephoned my mother, only for her to tell me how much she was looking forward to seeing Son-in-Law. 'I told him, you're still my son-in-law whether you and Georgie are married or not, and of course I'm always happy to see you whenever you want to come and stay.' I could not be sure whether to feel pleased or betrayed. It was obvious Gloria was intent on keeping in with His Lordship no matter what, but I could also see how her opportunism could work to my ultimate advantage, so rather than choosing between feeling pleased or betrayed, I settled for bemusement.

Within the hour, Conning rang back to say that the flight was going to cost too much and he would be returning to New York the following day as planned. I breathed a sigh of relief, for I suspected that the combination of those two might well have caused me unforeseen problems.

Once Conning was back in New York, the sticky question of where I would be living in the future arose. Getting rid of him would prove to be as difficult as letting down Gloria and Michael, who wanted me back in Jamaica. Although I had led Conning to believe that I would entertain the idea of staying with him after the divorce, I never seriously had any intention of doing so. Once I had the divorce papers in my hands, and Charles Dismukes confirmed to me that they would stand up in a court of law, I informed the three of them that I would be returning to London to live.

'You do as you please,' snapped Gloria, who hated being denied anything. Michael was more reasonable. 'You have a ho...home here whenever you want,' he said.

'What about me?' Conning wailed.

He had evidently forgotten that we were now divorced and such responsibility as I had had for him had ceased along with the marriage.

It was no surprise to me that my parents, having more or less twisted my arm into surrendering my chattels to Conning, now elected to retreat into silence rather than make good the financial loss they had inveigled me into suffering. Mr and Mrs Generosity, who were always delighted to throw large sums of money at entertaining friends and who thought nothing of losing a year's allowance for one of their children on a race at the racetrack, were once more making absolutely sure they would not have to push their hands in their pockets. I tried to squelch the feelings of disappointment along with the knowledge that people are mean with money when the degree of love they possess is also insignificant.

Gloria, who had been peppering me with letters and telephone calls, now reverted to type. She immediately stopped writing letters or making telephone calls. At least Michael continued to write occasionally, providing me with letters if not financial assistance. Although Gloria's attitude brought me no joy, I was no longer a child but a big woman of twenty-five. I had my life to lead, and I really couldn't allow my mother's waxing and waning to affect me too much. Nevertheless, it was disappointing and hurtful to see, yet again, that Gloria's interest and sincerity, although occasionally apparent, were never real or lasting.

By this time, I was seriously dispirited by the callousness and selfishness which I had encountered not only from my husband but from my parents as well. I had, at least in the early days of my marriage, expected better from

Colin Campbell. And I had allowed myself to be taken in by Gloria's display of interest over the previous months. I was truly upset that I had allowed her to dupe me yet again; that I had failed to remember the lessons of the past; that I had allowed myself to open up only to be discarded by her if I were of no more consequence than a cigarette butt, once she had nothing more to gain from the scenario.

Despite being down, I was not out. I had a life to live, so I set about cleaning up the mess Colin Campbell and Ian Argyll had so resourcefully made as soon as I arrived in London. If Mary Anne Innes Kerr, John Pringle and Princess Elizabeth of Yugoslavia were to be believed, I had suffered no damage socially. Nevertheless, I had practically no money and no means of earning any in the short term. I was too ill from all I had been through to work, and I also wondered what effect the publicity would have upon my employability.

The way ahead, I decided, was to try to restore my reputation. Ignoring Gloria's chilliness, I telephoned her and appealed to her to convince Michael that the £1,000 or £2,000 it would cost to institute proceedings for libel against the newspapers would be a small price to pay, not only because the offending bodies would have to pay damages to settle the suits, but also because an apology and retraction of the misrepresentations would give me a better chance of finding another husband. 'You will just have to rely on your much-vaunted reputation as a beauty to see you through,' she said with all the sweetness of strychnine.

Ah, so there we had it: the admission of what was motivating her. Although both she and Michael were tight-fisted where I was concerned, my competitive mother had seen that the damage my ex-husband and brother-in-law had wrought on my reputation could be made to work in her favour in the contest she ran against me – and everyone else she regarded as competition – to remain the most desired and desirable object in her orbit. She might not have succeeded in destroying my face with her lighted cigarette, but she was taking full advantage of circumstances that would provide a similar effect, for my reputation would reduce the advantage my looks had in my life thereafter.

To say that I was sickened by this realization is to minimize how utterly stomach-churningly dreadful I found it. The one thing the daughter of a narcissistic mother knows, however, is the futility of fighting against her extreme vanity. Gloria's pathological lust for admiration and attention was equalled only by her lack of scruples in seeing off competition; and it mattered not one jot to her whether it was a stranger or her own daughter. She had found the perfect way to eliminate me as a competitor in the beauty stakes. So I swallowed hard, dusted myself off, tried to come to terms with yet another atrocious betrayal of motherly care from my atrocious mother, and fell back, as I had been doing for most of my life, on my own meagre resources.

Once the newspapers knew that I was in London, they all wanted my 'side of the story'. When I baulked at providing it, they all went on and on about how important it was for me to do so. The way the journalists made it sound, everyone wants to be in the public eye, and all those who are in it pant to have the general public know them better. I was frankly uninterested in telling my side of anything, except to have Conning refute the lies he had told about me. Although I had never sought fame nor wanted it – much less notoriety – I did see where it was necessary for my future marital prospects that I be fairly represented in the press. I was therefore somewhat relieved when Conning agreed to my selling a joint interview with him to the *News of the World* in which he would recant the lies he had sold to the *Sunday People*. In the same article, I would provide a more balanced version of my life story than had hitherto been published. While I hated having to speak about myself, my distaste in doing so was less than my distaste in having to go through life with an inappropriate Mark of Cain.

Once the interview was set up, Conning showed how appropriately I had nicknamed him by backing out of the enterprise. 'Why sell them one interview when we can sell them two?' he said, causing my stomach to churn with frustration. My objective was to bring the press interest to a close, not to perpetuate it, as he seemed intent on doing.

Despite Conning reneging on our agreement, I nevertheless went ahead with the interview. I had two strong motives for doing so. Not only did I have a desire to set the record straight, but I also needed to raise enough money to sue the other publications which had written libels about me. As I saw it, the only way to rectify the false impressions was to sue the newspapers which had peddled the tall tales.

So I sold 'my side of the story' to the *News of the World* and, in so doing, not only raised the money with which I then sued several newspaper companies, but also soft-pedalled the atrocious behaviour of my parents and ex-husband in the hope that we could maintain civil relations.

To their credit, Michael and Gloria appeared to understand that I had spared them when I did not have to. They glossed over my explanation that they had been embarrassed by my medical problems and had sought to sweep them under the carpet, and never once alluded to the article for the remainder of their lives. Conning, however, freaked out when he read that I had stated that the marriage had collapsed because he was 'moody' and 'sometimes took out his moods on me'. Notwithstanding the fact that those comments were hardly pejorative, especially in the light of the tremendous physical and emotional abuse to which he had subjected me, he ranted and raved and telephoned me about forty times to issue threats that he was a Campbell and that their motto is '*Ne Obliviscaris*', meaning 'Forget Not'. 'I will get you for this,' he ranted. 'I will have vengeance! Vengeance! Vengeance! Vengeance! Vengeance! You will be crushed by the might of the Campbells, you stupid bitch.'

Anyone else would have had the good sense to realize that he had got off lightly, for I could easily have alluded to the broken bones, hospital stays, beatings and batterings I had endured during the fourteen torturous and tortured months of our marriage. But Conning was not anyone else. No matter how many times I pointed out to him that I was well within my rights to make the comments I had in the newspaper article, and that it was a bit much for him to expect that I would not countermand his lies with a mild hint of the truth, he refused to give way. Finally, after about the fortieth telephone call, I snapped. 'You surely didn't think I was going to accept any blame for the failure of a marriage that was entirely your own fault?' I said.

'I'll show you,' he shrieked, as punitive as Gloria at her worst. 'I'll show you the way we showed those fucking MacDonalds. No one crosses the Campbells of Argyll and gets away with it. No MacDonald and no fucking wife.'

And show me he did. Within days, he had sold a story to the *Daily Express*, a newspaper then owned by his half-sister Jeanie Campbell's uncle Max Aitken, stating that the reason why he divorced me was that he needed to have an heir and I couldn't give him one. That was the final straw. He, not I, was the one who had not wanted children. Indeed, he often told me that one of the reasons why he 'knew' our marriage would work – and why he had proposed so quickly – was that I couldn't have children and he didn't want any. Now here he was using the very thing that had appealed to him to lay the blame for the failure of our marriage at my doorstep.

Some things in life are unforgivable. This was one of them. As far as I was concerned, that story ended the possibility of any friendship between us. Aside from the fact that it was untrue, there are some things people simply do not say unless, of course, their purpose is to wound and to destroy the possibility of any future relationship. I had never told him what a pathetic inadequate he was in and out of bed; nor how his penis was a turn-off, being misshapen and the size of a lipstick, because, in life, there are some truths you never utter unless you want to finish off any possibility of amity for the future. Intent on doing just that, I wrote him a letter reminding him of the real reasons why our marriage had failed, and ending by telling him never to get in touch with me again.

To make my position as unmistakable as possible, I then announced in the Court Circular of *The Times*: 'Lady Colin Campbell wishes in future to be known by her maiden name, Miss Georgia Ziadie.' This was calculated to put distance between myself and my ex-husband, but if I hoped the press would have any more respect for my wishes than my ex-husband did, I was wrong. Not one British publication ever referred to me by my maiden name.

In October, the man whom I had asked never to get in touch with me again telephoned, asking if he could come around and collect pictures of his which had arrived with my possessions while he was away in Scotland for the summer. Although my brother Mickey had arranged that Conning would collect these items from him and not from me, my determined ex-husband had clearly decided that he would use them as a Trojan horse. So now he refused to pick them up from Mickey.

'Christ,' I thought, 'what does it take to get these people to respect your wishes?'

Like Gloria, however, he could persuade the Pope that Judas was a good Christian; and as he begged, pleaded and promised that he only wanted to collect the pictures and depart on cordial terms, after which he would respect my desire not to see him again, I heard myself relenting.

However, no sooner did I let him into the flat and hand over the pictures than Conning brought up my refusal to use the Campbell name any longer. After the usual pleading and cajoling had not elicited my usual sympathetic response, he hit the bull's eye. 'You're doing yourself no favours,' he said. 'You've played right into Ian's hands. He's banging around Scotland telling everyone you were forced to give up the name.'

Although I had no means of knowing if Conning was speaking the truth, I was definitely prepared to be manipulated into changing my practice if there was even an outside chance that his malevolent brother was saying things like that.

'Is that a fact?' I heard myself saying as I felt my blood pressure rise. 'Well, it looks as if your brother's resourcefulness has won the day where your persistence failed.'

Thereafter, I resumed styling myself Lady Colin Campbell, although I must admit that I envisaged being rid of the moniker within a year or two when I remarried, as I had every expectation of doing. It never occurred to me that I would not remarry, but then I was not aware of how badly scarred by my marriage I had been. It was a real case of 'once bitten, twice shy'.

If Conning scored a victory over me that October afternoon of 1975, I achieved an even more decisive one over him early that same evening when James Adeane, a beau whose uncle was then the Queen's Private Secretary, arrived to take me to dinner at his Ennismore Gardens flat. What would become one of the most decisive exchanges of my life started out simply enough when I introduced James to Conning. 'What do you want with a bitch like her?' Conning demanded of him rather than opting for a more conventional greeting. This was word for word what Gloria had asked a beau of mine in 1973, and I could not help but think that my ex-husband was as malicious as my mother had been.

James shot me a compassionate look while Conning declared that he wanted 'a quiet word with my wife'. As James stepped aside, Conning said, 'I don't have any money to get home. Can I borrow a quid?'

With blinding clarity, I saw that this might be the moment to get rid of him once and for all. So, measuring every word, I replied in a tone of voice I had never used before with anyone. 'You'll have to walk home,' I said, ice and rock jostling for pride of place. 'I'm afraid. I do not have a pound to lend you. Goodbye. And good luck.'

I could tell that Colin Campbell had got the message. The only problem was: would he remember it in the morning?

Evidently, he did. Since that October evening in 1975, he has never made an attempt to see me again. Of course, that does not mean that he hasn't popped up like the proverbial bad penny. Every time one of my books is published, he purveys yet another version of why our marriage ended. None of his versions accords with any other, which illustrates his actual level of truthfulness. He has threatened my life and that of my children, as he was stupid enough to confirm to the journalist Michael Thornton in 1995. But at least I have never seen him again. And, with a bit of luck, I never will either.

By now, I had become well and truly enlightened as to what I was up against when dealing with the Argyll family, because I had met Conning and Ian's stepmother Margaret, the notorious Duchess of Argyll. We hit it off immediately – largely, I suspect, because we had suffered similarly at the hands of the same family, though what she went through was infinitely worse than anything I endured. When she told me about the part Little Ian had played in her divorce, there were such resonances with mine that I knew she was not exaggerating one jot. The venom she described both father and son as being capable of was also something that I recognized as having been inherited by his second son as well. We used to talk far into the night at her Upper Grosvenor Street house opposite the American Embassy, swapping stories about the family's extraordinary behaviour.

What emerged was not only how unjust the whole thing had been, but how terribly wounded Margaret had been by it. Although I did not yet realize the full depth of my own wound, I certainly had compassion for her and hoped that she was right when she displayed faith that the outcome for me would be better than it had been for her. 'I was a dumb bunny,' she used to say, 'but you are intelligent, and they haven't been able to run rings around you the way they did me.'

I was not so sure. I suspected that the real difference between our circumstances was that times had changed radically between the early 1960s and mid-1970s. If I turned out to have got an easier ride, that accounted for it.

I also saw that the sexual and cultural revolution of the 1960s, of which her divorce was such a cornerstone, had swept away much of the awe with which people viewed dukes and duchesses, lords and ladies. Although we were all still newsworthy, it was now as mere figures of interest rather than semi-deities who had been cast out of Valhalla.

Margaret agreed with me that my best chance of achieving a life of relative normality was to litigate to prevent the press from repeating the slurs the brothers had propagated. She even introduced me to David Napley, the well-known solicitor, and when his costs proved to be beyond my slender means, to Radcliffes, her other solicitors, who prosecuted the matter on my behalf over the next two years.

Chapter Twenty-One

While my suit for libel trundled on through the London law courts, I tried to get back on my feet in that city. Beneath a supposedly glistening social life, I was struggling not only financially but also emotionally. Although Michael would write occasionally and every Christmas paid for me to go back to Jamaica to play my part in the family production, Gloria had reverted to suffering from paralysis of the writing hand and general coldness of the organ which passed for her heart. With no drama to sustain her interest in our relationship, it had returned to the empty shell it used to be. I still wrote them nice, chatty and agreeable letters once a week, and they still telephoned me briefly on my birthday, which was cheaper than sending a present, but that really was the full extent of the relationship.

Things might well have gone on indefinitely as they were, and I might well have never examined the profound lack of positive or sincere feelings that emanated from my mother, continuing to delude myself as to what sort of person she really was, had Gloria not pushed her luck every time I returned to Jamaica.

Christmas in 1975 was bad enough. I arrived, and she brought up so much material from the store for me to sew evening dresses for her that I felt as if the family home had become a bazaar. These were not good days for Jamaica or Jamaicans of any complexion, but especially not for families like the Ziadies, who were on the List of the Twenty-Two Families the Manley government was targeting as it pursued its ambition to turn Jamaica from a multicultural democracy into a black semi-communist state. So I kept my counsel and allowed my opportunistic, exploitative mother to trap me behind a sewing machine in the study as the decades rolled back and she chattered non-stop, pouring out all the venom she had about everyone and everything.

Not once during the whole time I spent there did she display any interest in what I, or indeed any of her other children, was up to. She asked no questions, wanted no answers, desired no information. Had she shouted from the mountain top that she couldn't have cared less what the four of us were up to, she could not have conveyed her utter disregard more clearly. But it wasn't her egotism alone that was the problem. Her drinking was also getting out of hand again. It was now two years since she had been dried out, and she was back to her previous, awesome level of consumption. A bottle of gin and a bottle of port a day were nothing for her to get through, and although she was reasonably civil and pleasant first thing in the morning, by midday she would be her customarily acerbic self, and by dinnertime she was the proverbial 'bitch on wheels' she took such pride in proclaiming herself to be.

Michael, justifiably concerned, turned to us children for help. All of us were at home for the Christmas season, and it struck neither him nor any of us as odd that our pussy-whipped, pusillanimous father should be turning to the children, whom he had failed to protect, to rescue him and our mother from the mess she, with her drinking, and he, with his cowardice, were once again making of their lives. We had endless discussions about the best way of proceeding, always in whispers when Gloria was at home, and in more normal tones when she wasn't. Once more, I had cause to reflect, we children, whose parents never allowed us to have problems of our own, were being sucked into their problems in a neat inversion of traditional parent and child roles.

At that time, I was still attending Al-Anon, trying to make some sense of my dreadful marriage and, in the process, learning how to deal with my marginally less appalling mother. The family knew of my experience with that organization, so everyone was only too happy to alight upon me as if I possessed the solution to Gloria's problem, meaning their problem, especially as she had made it plain that she had no intention of being dried out again. As we all mistakenly associated her toxicity with the quantities of alcoholic toxins she was pouring into her system, we thought things would improve if she could be persuaded to lay off the booze. Little did we know that she was not one of those alcohol abusers whose problems can be solved by removing alcohol from the equation; she had a far more severe, underlying personality disorder, which could be neither cured nor treated.

I could see that there was a measure of fear and desperation in the family's willingness to defer to my supposedly superior knowledge on the subject of alcoholism. We all knew how much Gloria loved her booze, how vicious she became when crossed over things that didn't matter, and therefore how likely she was to turn ultra-vitriolic if her supply of alcohol was being threatened. Mickey and Michael wanted her dried out again, and were prepared if necessary to bring in the men in white coats to cart her off, but Gloria was defiantly insistent that she would never go willingly.

If there was one lesson I had learned in Al-Anon, however,it was that you cannot force addicts to give up their substances. They must want to do so. So I advised trying to obtain her consent.

With that objective in mind, I tried to locate a local Alcoholics Anonymous meeting. I was pleasantly surprised to see that there was indeed a chapter of that organization in Kingston, and that it consisted exclusively of upper and upper-middle class Jamaicans. Gloria would not be able to object, as Colin Campbell had done, to mixing with the rabble as an excuse for having nothing to do with that excellent twelve-step programme.

If this might seem a petty consideration to the onlooker, it was actually of crucial importance when dealing with someone as snobbish as my mother. I was further encouraged when one of her distant cousins, a high-ranking army officer, offered to act as her sponsor. I became absolutely beside myself with relief and hopefulness when he went one better and offered to meet her and to 'intervene', which meant that he would come along and try to encourage her to seek treatment.

I duly reported all of this back to the family, who all agreed that the best way forward was to be led by this successfully recovering alcoholic. He recommended dropping in early enough one morning to catch her before she had started pouring gin down her throat. He would try to interest her in giving AA a chance, and if all went well, it would be the start of a new way of life for all of us.

It is really quite touching how optimistic people can be in the face of overwhelmingly negative odds. Of course, none of us knew that Gloria was not primarily an alcoholic, but was actually a histrionic, antisocial narcissist who was using alcohol to self-medicate. Narcissism and histrionic personality disorder had not yet been categorized as medical disorders, and the definition of what constitutes a sociopath had still not been expanded to include the more privileged elements of the population. As far as the medical profession was concerned, sociopaths were still being wrongly indentified as exclusively criminal lowlifes, so the idea that a well-bred socialite could be amongst their number simply hadn't occurred to anyone. In the decades to come, of course, the medical profession would realize that fully sixty per cent of all alcoholics and drug addicts are sociopathic and/or narcissistic and the reason why they are drawn to substance abuse is that it helps them to escape from the voids within their personalities.

As you can imagine, if the medical profession itself was in the dark when dealing with my problematic mother, there was scant hope for our family. We had no idea we were dealing with a hopeless case. None of us knew that her disorders were incurable and, moreover, that narcissists, hysterics and sociopaths never look inwards to solve their problems. As far as they are concerned, there is never anything wrong with them. All problems stem from outside of them. As far as the narcissists are concerned, they are such self-idolaters, worshipping at the altar of their own perfection, that a classical narcissist like Gloria was hardly liable to listen to anyone who admitted to fallibility.

Although I did not relish being put in the frame for trying to help my mother, and although I could see that the rest of the family was only too happy to place me in it, hoping that they would spare themselves the odium of dealing with her vengefulness, I nevertheless agreed to spearhead the intervention. As I saw it, if a problem exists and there is a chance of a solution, you do what you have to, even if the consequences are not pleasant. Not, it has to be admitted, that I thought I would have as much of a problem with Gloria as I turned out to. She was so obviously off the rails that I could not imagine how she could fail to realize it. I did not yet know that lack of insight is a characteristic of the personality disorders she possessed. Nor did I consider it a possibility that she would hold my good intentions against me to the extent she did. So, with the approval of my father, grandmother and siblings, I arranged with the 'sponsor' to come and see her early one morning.

Although they were distant cousins, they did not actually know each other, so after I had made the introductions, I left them alone. Later, he would tell us how he had broached the subject of alcoholism with her, telling her how his drinking had damaged his life and how much better and happier this had been since he had been following the twelve-step programme. Gloria listened politely, then when he suggested taking her to an AA meeting, she informed him that that would be most inappropriate as she did not have a drinking problem, was not an alcoholic, and in classical narcissistic mode, indicated that she despised people who suffered from such weaknesses. Gloria then dismissed him by saying that she had to get dressed, as Richard Adeney – the flautist and great friend of my bother Mickey who was also an amateur photographer – was coming around to take group photographs of the family, something of a rarity as we were normally scattered all over the world and seldom were assembled together under one roof.

'I tried, but I don't hold out much hope for a change in her attitude for the foreseeable future,' her proposed sponsor told us later. 'She's inflexible and heavily into denial. She's convinced she doesn't have a problem and that all her problems originate elsewhere. Maybe when she hits bottom, there'll be a chance, for I can tell that she is extraordinarily determined. If she brings even a small portion of that determination to living a twelve-step life, she'll be incredible.'

Later that afternoon, Richard duly came around and photographed us. By then, Gloria was well oiled, but the one thing that never deserted her no matter how much she had had to drink, was the veneer of social control; and, though obviously tanked up, she performed as well as if she were cold sober.

Afterwards, Richard and the rest of the family sat around talking. Gloria for once was uncharacteristically quiet and remained so for the remainder of our visits. Although none of us realized it, she had gone to ground to head off criticism of her conduct and, with it, criticism of her drinking habits. Her introversion would yield no insights, though they did focus her attention on me as a target. 'Georgie sic'ed AA on me, and I am after her blood,' she informed Kitty later that year when Michael said that he wanted me to return home for Christmas.

Blissfully ignorant of the venom I had unleashed in my viper mother, prior to leaving Jamaica I sold some jewellery so that I could afford to live and fund my libel suits.

Although I thought I was coping well with all the emotional strain induced by Gloria's problems, when I returned to London I realized that all the poison I had absorbed, with no commensurate outlet, had left me feeling pretty low. Hopeful that I would be able to shrug off the mood quickly, I was surprised that it took the better part of four months. It was then that I realized the spiritual price I was having to pay for being a dutiful daughter, so I resolved never again to allow Gloria to put me in the position of being a captive pair of ears without a voice or the right to any feelings. 'She is a real user,' I decided, a conclusion I might not have arrived at so readily if I had not just seen off another user in the shape of my ex-husband.

When you are dealing with disordered personalities, the truth can become obscured by the hopefulness you feel. This, I would come to realize, was the trap into which I fell, along with pretty much the rest of the family, after Gloria was dried out later that year.

Her so-called sobriety coincided with Mickey and Kitty returning to live in Jamaica, the former to become a partner in Jamaica's leading law firm, the latter to stay at home and take up a teaching position at The Priory School, having just graduated from college in the United Kingdom. They were back only weeks before Michael prevailed upon them to assist him in dealing with his recalcitrant wife, whose alcohol consumption was matched only by her maliciousness and her determination to continue floating on a sea of gin and port. I shouldn't actually use the word 'assist', for our pusillanimous father turned over all of the actual arrangements to Mickey. Meanwhile, he leaned heavily on Kitty for emotional support, terrified that Gloria would hold against him the stay in the rehabilitation unit of the hospital that he had in store for her. But her conduct had become so dreadful that even he could see that something had to be done.

Mickey duly went to see Dr Charles Thesiger, who had been in charge of Gloria's last spell in rehab. After explaining how adamantly she was refusing help, Mickey was reassured when the doctor wrote out a prescription of drugs. 'They'll knock out a horse,' he said, advising Mickey to have the servants administer the dose first thing in the morning before she had had a chance to hit the bottle. The men in white coats would then come and scoop up the unconscious Gloria, who would be carted off to the hospital for detoxification. Or so the plan was supposed to go.

'The first attempt was a non-starter,' Mickey reported. 'We poured the drugs into her orange juice, but she said that it tasted funny, so she sent it back. Knowing how suspicious she is, I decided not to try to convince her to drink the draught and got Dr Thesiger to change the potion to something more tasteless. This she did drink, but remained fully conscious, despite his assurances that it was as strong as the other knock-out drug. When the attendants came for her, instead of an unconscious Mummy who would be stretchered into the ambulance without any fuss, there was a very belligerent Mummy whom they had to chase around the house to catch and restrain. It was pure farce and would have been funny if it hadn't been so sad. When they finally caught her, they held her down while she kicked and screamed. They had one hell of a time to inject her with the knock-out drug so they could get her into the ambulance and take her to Medical Associates,' the hospital which was actually more like a five star hotel. 'Even after they'd managed to inject her, she continued to scream invective and kick out, flailing and trying to run away while at the same time demanding they let go of her as she wasn't going anywhere with them. They were utterly astonished that the dose hadn't knocked her out, and they had to give her a stronger one of whatever it was, before they could finally get her onto the stretcher and into the ambulance. It was not a pretty sight, believe me.'

Despite the rocky start, this spell in rehab went smoother than the previous one, possibly because Gloria knew she was well and truly caught in a vice and had better cooperate unless she wanted to run the risk of being detained against her will the way Aunt Flower and I had been. She therefore did not play the lunatic in an attempt to gain sympathy or manipulate the family, nor did she pretend to have any adverse reactions to the drugs. Charles Thesiger, however, held out little hope for a trouble-free future, as Gloria was declaring that she intended to start drinking again as soon as she was out of the hospital. 'You can't help people who don't want to help themselves,' he told Michael, Mickey and Kitty, 'and she doesn't want to help herself.'

It was at this juncture that Michael, the coward who had always allowed his indulged and self-indulgent wife to ride roughshod over everyone and everything except himself and his pleasures, summoned up the backbone none of us believed he possessed. 'If you touch alcohol again,' he informed her, so seriously that she believed that he meant it, 'that is the end of our marriage. Your drinking has made all our lives, your own included, a misery, but I have had enough. Not even one drop ever again.'

The boundaries being drawn, it was a more compliant Gloria who was released from the hospital after a relatively short stay.

Blaming her drinking instead of her character for the sort of person she was, I forgave everything she had ever done and mentally started our relationship afresh. Although she was still as unresponsive and uncommunicative as ever, I nevertheless wrote affectionate letters, intent on making her feel loved. I even looked forward to going home for Christmas, full of hope that now the rot had been stopped along with her drinking, we could all have the nice, loving, happy relationships we were meant to be having.

Talk about a fool.

The first hint that happy days were never going to appear came the first evening I was back in Jamaica. I arrived from the airport after dinner, to find that Michael and Kitty were in their bedrooms, and Gloria was reposing in the study in darkness. 'Come and sit with me,' she said once the servants had brought in my luggage and deposited it in my bedroom.

'Why are you sitting in darkness?' I enquired.

'You know lights bother my eyes,' she responded, as if sitting in darkened rooms were a normal habit of hers, which it had not been up to this point. Rather than make an issue of it, I said nothing about how much I loathe the dark, or how discomfiting it is to sit in a darkened room speaking to someone you can't see, and instead just reclined on the *chaise longue*, open to all the good that would now surely come forth.

I didn't even have time to warm the cushion before Gloria said, 'I want you to remember that no one but me has any rights in this house.'

'I haven't flown halfway across the world to have you pick a fight with me,' I replied, my hopes of a happy mother-daughter relationship dashed on the rocks.

'Pick a fight with you? Pick a fight with you?' she said scornfully. 'Who are you for *me* to pick a fight with?'

'The person you're picking a fight with, that's who,' I said, getting up. 'The one who you've just told has no rights in this house...along with everyone else but you. Except that every human being has rights. You can't strip people of their rights even when you fail to acknowledge them. Now, if you have no objection, I think I will retire. Goodnight.'

'I can see that you've come intent on making trouble. This house has been totally peaceful without you. I'm not going to have you come here and cause trouble,' retorted Gloria, the past-mistress of shifting blame.

'Good night, Mummy,' I said with supercilious politeness through gritted teeth, walking out and heading straight to Kitty's room, where I recounted what had happened.

'I'm not surprised,' she said. 'She blames you for having to give up drinking. She says you sic'ed AA on her.'

'She what?'

Kitty repeated what she had just said; and we looked at each other, silently acknowledging the preposterousness of our mother's position, then resorted to the ultimate defence against insanity. We laughed.

'She didn't really!' I said as Kitty and I cackled uproariously.

'She most certainly did,' Kitty managed to splutter between gasps.

For the next five or so minutes Kitty and I could not stop laughing. Humour really was our ultimate defence against Gloria's bizarre thought processes. Without it, we might well have ended up killing her, but with it – and with each other - we managed to derive at least some amusement out of something that really wasn't particularly funny at all.

'Fun and jokes aside,' Kitty finally said when we had both stopped laughing, 'you need to be careful. She says she's after your blood. And you know what she can be like.'

'Thanks for the tip,' I said, instantly regretting having come home for Christmas and feeling something of a fool for having dared to hope that my mother might actually turn into a nice person once alcohol had been removed from the equation. 'I'll make sure I factor her attitude into the way I deal with her.'

The political situation in the country had deteriorated, and in the days to come it was apparent that Michael was worried that Michael Manley intended to nationalize his assets. Although one would have thought that Gloria would reserve her hostility for the ex-boyfriend who was intent on destroying her class as a whole while he experimented with a Cuban-style Jamaica, she seemed to have none towards Michael Manley but an excess for her husband, whom she blamed for not getting the lion's share of his money out of the country when it was easy to do so. On and on she banged day and night: which at least meant that so far she had avoided 'taking me on'.

Finally, I was forced to conclude that her rage lay in the fact that she was going to end up with less money than she had expected, after marrying and staying with Michael for financial reasons. One didn't know whether to laugh or cry at her predicament, and to this day I sympathize with her while also feeling that she got her just deserts. It was as if God was paying her back in some measure for all the times she had hurt people – herself included – with her ruthless, cold-hearted, self-aggrandizing materialism.

Having resolved never to be trapped again by my mother as a captive audience the way I had been the previous Christmas, and having been warned by Kitty that the vampire intended to suck my blood if she could, I was ready and waiting to head off her suggestion a few days after my arrival that 'we have a nice, companionable time together while you make me a few of your fantastic designs and put to good use the fortune you cost your father and me to send you to the Fashion Institute in New York, instead of wasting your talent and education the way you normally do.'

By this time, I had formulated a plan, which was to use my fundraising talents to benefit charity and get me out of the house rather than allow Gloria to trap me there and turn my dressmaking skills against me. So when she made her suggestion, I said that I could not do so, as I was already committed elsewhere.

My brother had paid for a girlfriend, an opera singer, to come to Jamaica with him. She was trying to crack the London scene and needed money, so I suggested organizing a recital for her, with the proceeds of the gate going to her and the proceeds of the programme going to charity. She was enthusiastic, to put it mildly, as was Hugh Wynter, the head of the Department of Obstetrics and Gynaecology at the University of the West Indies, for which I had previously raised funds in 1972. So I was able to tactfully avoid being stuck in the study behind the Singer sewing machine while Gloria turned on her oral tap and drowned my spirits in her venom.

Also in the interests of tact and in the hope that by including her Gloria would not feel left out and consequently resentful of a success she actually had had no part in creating, I suggested to her that she become my co-chairman. 'You won't have to do anything,' I said, pandering to both her aversion to work and her proclivity to glory-seeking. 'I'll do it all.'

This time Gloria was more than willing to jump aboard a vessel she knew would float to success. The previous time, when there had been room for doubt as to whether a neophyte like me had the ability to pull off a successful event, she had made sure she kept herself aloof from it.

'As long as I don't have to do anything,' she graciously consented, as if she were doing me the favour and not the other way around. Then she did absolutely nothing except make one, and only one, suggestion: that I ask Rudolph Greene, her good friend and the Chief of Staff of the Army, to be the treasurer.

I should have known that my mother would never make a suggestion unless she had something up her sleeve. But I had lived away from her for years; was still hopeful that by giving up drink she was on the road to giving up being poisonous. Moreover, I had not yet arrived at the conclusion that she was an utter and vicious manipulator whose favourite sport was intriguing against others. So Pollyanna agreed to ask Rudolph, who of course agreed readily; and though I did not yet know it, I was now hurtling down the path Gloria had set me upon.

From that moment until the evening of the recital, Gloria took no part in any of the arrangements, activities or work. While I happily beavered away, she reposed at home, doing nothing. Christmas lunch passed off as uneventfully and pleasantly as possible. Afterwards, the whole family, save Michael and Gloria, decamped for the new year to Newcastle, the army training camp which was inaccessible to the general public and where there was no threat of crime from criminal or political elements, political shootings and beatings then being an everyday occurrence. Michael and Gloria came up for a day, and, to my surprise, my normally indolent mother even agreed to go for a walk with us. That, coupled with the fact that she had not been overtly hostile since the evening of my arrival in Jamaica, led me to think that maybe she had turned over a new leaf and that her first night's aggression was simply a slip back into the past.

I only realized how wrong I was towards midday on the day of the recital. Gloria came home from the hairdresser and the bank, and marched up to the pool, where I was sitting with the photographer Cookie Kinkead, an old friend of mine. 'I've just been to the bank,' she said in her haughty, accusatory tone of voice, 'and my ruby bracelet is missing.'

'I'm sorry to hear that,' I said, not appreciating what she was implying.

'Well, what have you done with it?' she demanded, as if she were sane and I was cracked.

I looked at her blankly. It took me a good few seconds to grasp her implication.

'What do you mean, what have I done with it?' I replied, as calmly as I could muster. 'How could I have done anything with it? I have never even been to the bank with you, much less to your safety-deposit box, so how could I have done anything with it? One needs access to do something with an item.'

'Well, the bracelet is missing, and you're the one person who has always wanted it,' she persisted.

The bracelet was the most important part of the ruby and diamond parure she had promised at the time of my marriage to hand on to me ultimately, when she had given me the diamond and ruby ring which was a part of it. Now she was accusing me of stealing the bracelet rather than waiting until I was given it.

'You fucking bitch!' I exploded. 'You goddamned money-grubbing cunt! How dare you accuse me of stealing your bracelet? Who the fuck do you think you are? You are nothing but a fucking lunatic and a *rass* bitch. You think you're so clever, but you're as transparent as glass. You're obviously up to one of your plots and schemes, and while I may not know what your objective is, I can see that you're hoping to discredit me and knock me out of the running. You are a vicious cunt, and I rue the day I passed through your legs. You're not fit to have a bowel action, much less children.'

'Get out. Get out of my house right this instant,' Gloria ordered.

'Get out of *your* house?' I said as contemptuously as I could, knowing how she hated anyone speaking down to her. 'This isn't *your* house, you deluded piece of shit. This is my father's house, and I'm going nowhere. You want to get me out. Try to throw me out, and see if I don't break every bone in your body.'

For the next four hours I let rip, dragging up everything I could remember that she had ever done to anyone. I surprised myself with some of the things I came out with. I had not even remembered them until they spilled out of the dossier of my unconscious. Gloria, worried that the neighbours would hear because we were outside, in the grounds beside the swimming pool, tried to manoeuvre the action into the house. But I was having none of it. Gleeful to be enlightening anyone who was listening behind the ten-foot-high walls dividing our house from the Canadian High Commissioner's Residence to the left, the Hendricks family (with whom she had been on the outs for twenty years) behind us, or Michael's cousin Philomena de Aloma behind the Canadian High Commissioner, I shrieked even louder.

'You're only worried that the neighbours will discover what a fucking cunt you are...if they don't already know. Well, I'm not budging from here, and if you think that taking refuge in the house will force me to go there, forget it. I'll simply stand up in the driveway and scream at you from whichever vantage point allows the most exposure.'

Towards the end of my tirade, Michael came home, and the scene shifted inside.

'Get this lunatic out of my house,' Gloria ordered him.

'What's happened now?' he wanted to know, with more resignation than annoyance.

'That fucking cunt you're married to had the gall to accuse me of stealing her ruby bracelet,' I spat with all the contempt I could muster. I hadn't had Gloria as a role model all these years without learning a thing or two about inflection, I can assure you.

'Don't speak about your mother like that,' Michael said.

'Why not? Because she doesn't deserve it? It certainly can't be because she deserves respect, so it must be because you don't want to hear the truth,' I said in a voice laden with sarcasm and challenge.

Realizing that I had no intention of backing down and fully aware that what Gloria had accused me of was so preposterous as to not even warrant consideration, Michael said, 'Gloria, you can't seriously think sh…she took your bracelet?'

'Of course she doesn't,' I said. 'How could I have when I don't live here; I have no access to her safety-deposit box, and I've never even been to her bank? All of which that fucking cunt knows only too well.'

'Throw the hussy out of this house. This is my house, and I will not have it here,' Gloria demanded of her husband, as if by referring to me as an inanimate object she could downgrade me from being human to something lifeless. I knew only too well, she would also hope that she was killing two birds with that one stone and press my button about my neutral past by referring to me in the neuter. However, I had heard her refer to too many people as 'it' for me to fall prey to such pointless sensitivity.

'I am going nowhere as long as you want me out of here,' I announced to Gloria, more for Michael's benefit than hers, as a warning to him not even to try to kick me out.

'This is my house, and I want her out of here,' Gloria persisted.

'I would not have condescended to stay in the same country, much less the same house, as you, you fucking bitch,' I spat, 'except that I am going nowhere now that I know you don't want me here. You see, my dear woman, two can play at the game of "Whatever You Want, You Can't Get". I would recommend that you telephone the police and ask them to remove me the way they're always removing domestic servants on your behalf. Let's see how that little scenario pans out when they discover that it's me they're supposed to be removing. I can just see the headlines now: "Lady Colin Campbell removed from that fucking cunt Gloria Ziadie's hell-hole after the manipulative bitch had the temerity to trump up accusations of theft against her own daughter to fulfil some so-far-unknown Machiavellian scheme of hers." Shall I get the telephone for you, or will you get it yourself?' I sneered sarcastically, knowing that I had well and truly trumped her.

'I'm going to my bed to rest,' Michael said, having chosen not to get involved, and thereby leaving me to continue slinging the mud that Gloria had hurled at others over the years back into her face. Nor did I even pause for anything but breath until it was time for me to get dressed for the concert. Then and only then did I stop – some four hours after I had started.

As I would never have expected to find myself in the situation I was in, I had never imagined what my reaction to such a diatribe would be. But once it was over, I was surprised to see that I felt good about it. I had spoken – or rather screamed – the truth for several hours. I had not exaggerated once. I had not been unfair. Every word I had said, stretching back over some twenty-two years, was just and measured, if delivered heatedly. The truth had set me free, and I felt a deep satisfaction that I had been the only person, in the whole of my mother's life, who had actually confronted her with the monster she truly was. I didn't expect it to change her, but at least she now knew that at least one person on this earth had her measure.

For the three or so days that remained of the holiday, I purposely neither avoided nor sought out Gloria. Having spent much of the earlier part of my life ignoring my father, I found it surprisingly easy to treat her as if she did not exist, even when we were in the same room together or partaking with others of the same conversation. I simply cut her dead. If I was saying something and she interrupted, I continued talking as if she had not opened her mouth, and persisted until she had to shut up or make whoever was present aware that there was a problem between us. As her audience mattered more to her than the reality of our relationship, she backed down and, in so doing, threw me the victory. Once or twice, whether deliberately or accidentally, she ended up in my line of vision. I looked straight through her while looking directly at her. Because she was acutely attuned to the behaviour of others, she knew that I was cutting her far more effectively than I would have done had I averted my gaze or glared at her, and I detected the faintest glimmer of embarrassment the last time I did it.

I had one and only one message for my mother. 'You no longer exist. To me, you are neither living nor dead. You are nonexistent.'

On the day of my departure, she did an uncharacteristic amount of hovering, as if she were hoping to effect a *rapprochement*, though one could not rule out the possibility that she was laying a trap, and if one offered or accepted what appeared to be the olive branch, she might very well turn it around into the bitter chalice of repulsion and sail off with some cutting comment about you being an ingrate of whom she had had enough.

Either way, I had no interest in engaging with her. She had killed stone dead any residual affection I had previously harboured for her. Because she had effected her accusation without the protection of alcohol, I could no longer blame booze for what sort of person she was. She, not drink, was the problem. She was the bitch, as she used to announce proudly; and if she was no longer a drunken bitch, she was still as much a bitch as she had ever been. With drink removed, she no longer had an excuse, nor would I give her one.

I had no regrets about having hurled a lifetime of abuse at her, nor did I regret the fact that she no longer existed for me. It felt good to be rid of her. Relating to her had been like swimming in a sea of faeces; and truthfully, I was glad that I would no longer have to deal with her.

Chapter Twenty-Two

All families have their myths and unique structures. Ours was no exception.

Because I was the latest in a long line of relations who had severed links with Gloria, everyone seemed to think that I would behave as they had all behaved previously, and return to the fold when things had quieted down. Any temptation I might have had was removed when Mickey informed me a few months after his return to England that our mother had telephoned him to tell him that she was sending his girlfriend a fraction of the proceeds of the concert's gate as her fee. 'I don't care what arrangement Georgie made with her. I am not giving the general public the chance to say that any member of my family uses charity to benefit their friends. She's no star, and she'll just have to be satisfied with a fee that's more in keeping with her stature,' Gloria decreed.

'So now we have the motive for why she had the gall to accuse me of taking her ruby bracelet. That woman is so conniving she is almost beyond belief. Has she "found" the bracelet yet?' I asked mockingly.

'Funny you should ask. She found it last week.'

'Transparent as glass,' I said.

'Not even Daddy believed that you took it,' Mickey said, making her isolation clear.

My resolve, already hard, now became granite-like. I would never again allow my mother into the inner circle of my life. Never again would she occupy a place in my heart. If I could help it, I would never speak to her again either. As the weeks became months and the months became first one year, then another, the family began to apply pressure on me to forgive and forget.

Gloria's mother Maisie and her sister Marjorie were especially keen for me to start speaking to her again. 'The woman is every bit as big a bitch as she claims to be,' I said to both of them. 'I see no reason to speak to her unless she turns over a new leaf.'

Although I wrote to my father once a week as always, I never once included Gloria in the greetings, nor did I ever ask after her, and on the few occasions he telephoned me, I declined to speak to her when he asked me if I wanted to.

I might well have never spoken to her again had Kitty not then announced her engagement and asked me to be her matron of honour. Because she was getting married in the grounds of the family home, and I would have to stay there if I were to be a part of the bridal party, I found myself in a quandary. It was one which I resolved effortlessly, for I was not about to have my negative feelings about my mother sully my beloved sister's wedding. Nor was I prepared to allow those sentiments to prevent me from playing my rightful role in such a happy event. Gloria had deprived all of us of enough joy over the years. So I flew back to Jamaica, cloaking myself in the mantle of civil but aloof good manners, and dealt with her the way one deals with undesirables one has to endure: politely and distantly, making her well aware of my lack of affection and regard but doing it so civilly that she had no come back.

Maisie and Marjorie, indulging in the futile hope that is so characteristic of dysfunctional families, breathed a sigh of relief and seriously expected that now that the ice was ostensibly broken, the water would warm up. I, however, knew differently. I had come to the conclusion that I justifiably loathed my mother because she was a loathsome individual and nothing short of a personality change on her part could alter or improve such reality-based facts. As this was about as likely as turkeys becoming kings of the jungle, I was not about to permit the well-intentioned but ultimately self-deluding hopes of mutual relations to catapult me back into the morass. False hope, I had come to realize, was every bit as dangerous as having no hope at all when realistic hope was warranted. So I kept my emotional distance and left Jamaica, glad to be out of such a conflicted and oppressive environment.

A few months later, Michael was shot and nearly killed by the gunman from whom Mrs Powell saved him when she threw herself over his prone body. Of course I telephoned home and received progress reports from my brother and sister about our father's recovery, and when he was out of the hospital, I spoke to him and wrote him. I was studious in addressing letters only to him, however, and never once sent love for my mother, who remained *persona non grata*.

Needless to say, the days of my returning home for Christmas were now a thing of the past, and though my father kept on inviting me back each year, saying that the family wasn't complete without me, I kept on declining.

'Why don't you just ignore her?' Mickey asked me in 1979 while trying to convince me to go back with him for Christmas.

'I'd sooner take a shower with Zyklon B gas than play happy families with *her*,' I said.

Although I had absolutely no interest in discovering what Gloria was up to, I could not escape being provided with information by other members of the family. Mickey was especially assiduous in keeping me abreast of our mother's activities. 'She's really turned over a new leaf now that she's got used to not drinking. She's taken up orchids in a big way and has become quite a force in the Orchid Society and the International Horticultural Society,' he said. He was clearly enjoying having a positive relationship with the woman who had made the first two decades of his life a misery, and while I was pleased for him, I only needed to hark back to that afternoon when she, stone-cold sober, accused me of stealing her bracelet, for all my acquired scepticism to surface.

Despite this, Gloria being interested in anything outside of herself seemed like a harbinger of good. Without realizing that even her interest in orchids allied her love of beauty with her rampant narcissistic snobbery, no flower being more special than orchids, I opened up to the possibility that she might have improved somewhat. So when Michael telephoned me and told me that she was *en route* to the Far East to participate in orchid shows in China – which had just been opened up to visitors – as well as Japan, Hong Kong and God knows where else, and he would like it if I had her for tea at my flat on West Eaton Place in London's Belgravia, I agreed. Nevertheless, I made sure I protected myself against the possibility of things spiralling out of control by having a German friend, whom she did not know, present.

Renate, of course, found her charming and beautiful and all the things strangers always did. For my part, I found the whole experience decidedly uncomfortable. It was as if I were giving tea to a total stranger and one, moreover, with whom there was no underlying emotional connection. After about an hour and a half of strained chitchat concealed under a slathering of social grace, she rose to say goodbye, and I breathed a sigh of relief, glad that at least nothing unpleasant had taken place.

Shortly after that, Mickey returned to live in England. Although he had been firmly in the first circle of Jamaica's legal profession, he could no longer take the atrocities that were everyday occurrences for those who lived in our once-idyllic country. Giving up a partnership in the island's leading law firm, as well as a lavish house which he shared with his great school friend, David Boxer, he showed his mettle by seeking to replicate in his adopted country a degree of the professional flexibility and influence he had enjoyed in his native land. Because the Jamaican legal profession was fused while the English was not, with barristers appearing in court upon the instruction of solicitors, who effectively employed them to be their voice-boxes, he announced that he was going to become a solicitor. 'I see no merit in waiting for employment from solicitors when I can be one and give barristers employment,' he explained. Mickey therefore duly found himself a studio flat in Notting Hill, got himself a part-time job and took whatever exams he needed to switch professions. This was, of course, all done without the help of our parents, whose largesse extended no further to their only son than it did to two of their three daughters.

Aside from admiring Mickey for chucking over an illustrious career in Jamaica with such alacrity, I was thrilled to have him back in London. We had always been close, with many shared interests, including music – which played a huge part in his life – and art, which was the equivalent in mine. Through him, I met all the leading musicians of the day, from Richard Adeney and Willard White, who were his close personal friends, to the great Russian pianist Shura Cherkassky, who was more of an acquaintance but nevertheless still a firm part of his circle.

Mickey had a quiet dignity which prevented him from taking advantage of the social world the way many other young men about town with limited funds did. Unless he could pay his way and reciprocate on equal terms with any hospitality proffered, he refused invitations. Until he finished his studies and set up his English law firm in 1981, with gifts from our grandmother, aunt and a loan from our parents, and began to earn good money once more, he limited the extent of his socializing. As I took part in the social peregrinations which had already resulted in me being written about as one of England's leading socialites, there was many an occasion when I would have preferred to share the experience with my brother than with one of my walkers. But I knew that was out of the question, so I respected his attitude and never tried to undermine it.

Nevertheless, I was delighted when Mickey finished his mature student days and started up his law firm, for that meant that he could now lead a life more in keeping with expectations. And I could share more of my life with him.

Ironically, starting up his law firm was what led me back into the family fold in a roundabout way. I had recently left my job at Lloyd's, the insurance market, after nearly four years there, and, knowing my abilities, Mickey said, 'Why don't you come and work for me?'

'I can't think of anything I'd like less,' I said, being a firm believer in keeping business and pleasure separate.

'Well, let me put it this way. I could do with your help. I can't think of anyone whom I trust more or who is more capable. I never cease to be amazed by how fast you type, and with your social skills, you'll be just the ticket for the firm.'

Put that way, how could I refuse? So I went to work for Mickey for the remainder of the year and, in so doing, gradually found myself being influenced by him and the rest of the family to give Gloria another chance by returning home for Christmas 1981. 'This year we're spending Christmas in Cayman with Auntie, so you won't even have to spend much time in Jamaica. Just a few days,' he pointed out.

Although I had no real hope of my moribund relationship with my mother coming to life, I could see the wisdom of returning to the fold in the way he was suggesting. Our grandmother was not getting any younger, and though we all expected her to live to a ripe old age like her father, who died at ninety-four after a lifetime of drinking, smoking and womanizing, I was eager to see Maisie again. The year before, she and Uncle Perez had been badly beaten up by gunmen during a raid on her house in Jamaica. She had popped a diamond ring in her mouth rather than surrender it to them, and after she was released from hospital, she flew out vowing never to return to the country in which her Jewish ancestors had first settled in the early 1500s, at a time when the Inquisition was at its height. Nor did she ever go back to the land of her birth.

To me, there was something sad about circumstances forcing an old lady to sever links with a country after a familial connection of half a millennium, but what made it especially poignant was that Michael Manley was then voted out of power a few months later in a landslide that was more akin to a rout than an election. He had been so confident of victory that he had not even bothered to rig the polls or intimidate the electorate the way he had done prior to the previous election. Eddie Seaga, the Anglo-Lebanese scion of the family many thought was related to ours because the Ziadies and Seagas had been friends for generations, was now prime minister. Our cousin Senator Arthur Ziadie was now one of the new political powers in the land. Within days all the racist rubbish to which families like ours had been subject for eight years was at an end; and, with a white prime minster and various white ministers, white Jamaicans were once more acknowledged as having the right to live in and contribute to the land of their birth.

If Eddie Seaga's victory came too late to save my grandmother from a move she made out of fear, it was timely in terms of the position families like ours occupied in Jamaica's national life. Not only had Michael Manley intended to strip my father and people of his background of their citizenships on the grounds that they were white oppressors of black people; but, like the French aristocracy after the Bourbon restoration, they now found that overnight they were once more given respect. It is in situations like that that you understand how true it is that a week is a long time in politics.

Although my father was relieved that the nightmare of the Manley years was at an end, Gloria's reaction was more complex. Still furious with her husband rather than her ex-boyfriend for the loss of all the assets that the latter had nationalized, she was even more openly contemptuous of Michael's skills as a businessman than she had ever been. At the same time, however, she paradoxically enjoyed with relish the reflected glory that the Ziadie family and the other Lebanese families were enjoying with these latest changes to the political landscape. As a socioeconomic entity, they were now right where the English had been at the time of Gloria's marriage to Michael: at the very top of the national heap. It was ironic that she had ended up where she had started, her personal circumstances reflecting the changes within the national life. One could not help but notice how appropriate she felt this was, even if one was painfully aware how little she deserved such approbation.

Flying into Jamaica that Christmas of 1981 with Mickey was like flying back in time in both good and bad ways. Of course I was as mightily relieved as everyone else to see that the old, more tolerant and civilized Jamaica had replaced the doctrinaire Castroism of the Manley years, and of course it was good to see the family home looking as beautiful and well-staffed as ever. Its chatelaine, however, was still Gloria; and no sooner had she induced me to join her in the darkened study that first night of my arrival than she sent yet another shot across my bow the way she had done on my previous Christmas visit five years earlier. 'You know,' she said brightly, having perfunctorily dispensed with the niceties of asking about my flight, 'it's been absolutely wonderful having no children at home. Children are such a burden. Your father and I get along far better now that none of you is underfoot here. You were all nothing but a disruption, and I cannot tell you how wonderful it is having none of you getting in my way. Frankly, I never could stand *pickney*.'

'*Pickney*' was the word the servant classes used to describe children; and though I would notice in the days to come that Gloria was doffing her hat to the new upper-class fashion of interspersing her sentences with the vernacular in an attempt to show that she too was keeping apace of the changes within the new Jamaica, I detected that in this instance she was using the word as a putdown.

I felt like pointing out to her that if she thought I had flown halfway across the world to see her, she was wrong. However, I let it pass in the interests of harmony, though I did notice, as she continued in like vein, that she was clearly trying to wound me by making me aware that she had never wanted any of the four of us. Ever.

What to do? Should I go to bed, the way I had the last time she had greeted me so callously, or stay? I really didn't feel up to any conflict, so I decided to change the subject to something that would deflect her. I therefore started telling her about a new beau of mine. Seamlessly, she started milking me for information of how he was in bed. So I told her.

'You are a Ziadie and a Burke. You're just like your grandmother and aunt. They have debased themselves on the altar of penis. But I am a Smedmore. The whole palaver leaves me cold,' she said, communicating her distaste for carnal pleasures for the umpteenth time, while conveying how much she despised those of us who had more normal feelings than hers.

'Maybe it's your loss more than ours,' I said, my earlier phlegmatic attitude now replaced with the determination that she would not get the better of me. As I was talking, I rose, crossed over to her chair and kissed her goodnight, brushing cheeks the way one had been brought up to do. 'But it's late and I'm tired so I'll say goodnight.'

'Stay with me a little longer,' said Gloria, who never let anyone go without a fuss.

'I'm really very tired and I must go to bed,' I replied, intent on departing from that dark and depressing environment before I was totally rattled by it.

The following morning, my brother and I flew to Cayman with our parents. Michael was his normal self; and so, unfortunately was Gloria. Although she took care to keep her hostility covert, she made sure I didn't miss it. 'The Look' that we had all dreaded as children had lost none of its potency, and she kept on darting me poisonous looks. 'I'm not going to let her dirty looks upset me,' I told Mickey, but they certainly ensured that I avoided her as much as possible.

On the other hand, the delight I felt in seeing my aunt and grandmother more than compensated for having to endure the unpleasantness of being near my mother. They were both as much a pleasure to be around as ever. I was also interested to note that Marjorie had really come into her own. Armed with her backing, her husband Alex had set up the most profitable customs brokerage firm in a country that had to import everything from water and lavatory paper, through furniture, clothes, shoes, building supplies, even concrete, to vegetables, fruit and meat. Virtually every item imported was cleared through customs by their company, with the result that they had made millions of dollars in the space of a decade to add to the money Uncle Ric had left her.

Marjorie and Alex now enjoyed a lifestyle that was sumptuous without being vulgar. They had bought a seaside club on the Ironshore at West Bay and recently finished converting it into their house. It might have looked like a comfortable beach house from the outside, but was more akin to a Fifth Avenue apartment in Manhattan on the inside. The floors, unlike most West Indian or North American houses, were not tile or marble but two-by-five inch blocks of parquet covered with splendid Persian carpets. Stuffed with antiques, 'Blue Horizon' – as the house was still called, despite its change of usage – was a testament to Marjorie's good taste. It was also exceedingly comfortable, with large guest suites and a guest apartment in one wing that could be fully self-contained if one wished it to be. However, why one would have wanted to use its kitchen when one had a cook in the other kitchen in the main body of the house was a mystery none of us ever solved, although we used it as a talking – and laughing – point.

Blue Horizon's drawing room was furnished with huge wing-backed chairs and ottomans for putting up one's feet, and antique *chaises longues* upon which to recline inherited from the Smedmores and Burkes. When Marjorie had one of her parties, guests ate off the most marvellous Spode plates and drank from the finest Waterford or Baccarat crystal cut-glasses in the vast dining room, which was dominated by a huge dining table and sideboard which were also family heirlooms.

As far as my siblings and I were concerned, Blue Horizon was a much nicer home than our parents' house, not because the house itself was nicer – it wasn't, and whatever benefit its seaside location gave it was lost compared to the splendour of Gloria's garden – but because one could actually relax and be happy in it.

As I unwound and basked in the love that my aunt and grandmother gave all of us, I was glad that Mickey had inveigled me into spending the Christmas holidays *en famille.* Though Gloria and I were hardly on the cosiest of terms, the atmosphere, if one overlooked Gloria's dirty looks, was so benevolent that I actually allowed myself to lower my guard.

Fatal mistake.

One talent the Glorias of this world have is an uncanny sensitivity to the emotional states of others. It is both their trap and their strength. Like a shark who can detect a drop of blood miles away, they can sense exactly when is the most propitious moment to strike – and when better for an attack than when your guard is down and you are therefore most vulnerable?

I was sitting on the covered swing on the front porch having breakfast with Auntie and Mickey when Michael came out on the morning of New Year's Eve. As he walked by, he grunted loudly.

'What's the matter, Mike?' Marjorie enquired good-naturedly of the brother-in-law with whom she got along well.

'That one is the biggest dis...disappointment of my life,' he stammered, referring to me.

'For God's sake! We've all been having a perfectly nice time,' Marjorie spluttered impatiently, implying that he was threatening to ruin it.

'It's true,' he said rather less assertively than before. To me, it was obvious that Maxi Mouse was tucking his tail between his legs and preparing to flee back to the safety of his other and even more critical half.

'What brought that on?' Marjorie said when he had slunk back inside.

'Mummy's been dropping poison in his ear about Georgie,' Mickey said.

'Oh, she has, has she?' I said.

'I beg of you, please, let this evening pass off without incident,' Auntie implored, referring to the large dinner party for about sixty she and Alex were having.

'Don't worry, Auntie. I promise you, no matter the provocation, I will do everything in my power to avoid Daddy and Mummy wrecking this Christmas season for you the way they always wreck it for us,' I said.

'Thank you, darling,' she said, leaving me alone with Mickey.

Within seconds of the good sister's departure, the bad sister showed up. Mickey mumbled something under his breath and shot off before I even had time to exhale the cigarette smoke I had just sucked in. Gloria headed straight for one of the antique wooden armchairs which were so characteristic of eighteenth- and nineteenth-century plantation life in Jamaica. Supremely comfortable as well as practical, they had deep seats and backs covered by cushions and wide arms which were convenient for reading, drinking, even working or playing cards. While she was plunking down her manicure paraphernalia, I calmly gathered up my packet of cigarettes and lighter and rose to leave.

'Don't go. Stay and keep me company,' Gloria said pleasantly.

'I really have to get myself dressed in case Auntie needs me for anything,' I said equally pleasantly and equally hypocritically.

'What could she possibly need you for?' Gloria demanded waspishly. 'With a house full of servants and half the population of Cayman brought in to help out today. Sit with me for awhile. I haven't had a chance to have a proper chat with you since you came.'

Foiled unless I was willing to create an atmosphere, I sat back down and lit a new cigarette from the butt of the old one.

'What happened with your father?' Gloria said in her most innocent tone of voice. This was always a dead giveaway that she was up to some mischief, and even if Mickey hadn't just told us of her impersonation of Iago, I would have known she was up to something because of her mantle of innocence. I answered Gloria's 'innocent' question as neutrally as I could manage, feeling my spirits sinking as I said, 'Nothing really.'

It really was frankly demoralizing to have to participate in such sick games, but that made me even more determined not to let her suck me into her manacle.

'You can tell me,' she said, opening her big brown eyes innocently and pretending to be agog with interest. Her displays of interest were always another dead giveaway that she was up to no good, for she never had any interest in anyone or anything unless it was to her advantage – and certainly, where we, her children, were concerned, her displays of interest were either to gather information to use against us in the future, to trap us in a web of her weaving in the present, or to milk us for emotional sustenance.

'It really wasn't anything,' I said, again neutrally but still resolved not to tell her about Michael's attempted outburst, though I had no doubt that he already had. Indeed, I suspected – as did the rest of us – that she had pumped him up so that he would initiate an eruption to which I would respond. Her favourite game was to nag Michael until he did her dirty work by attacking whomever it was she wanted to target, after which that individual would respond, and you would find yourself in the middle of the most dreadful melee.

I would actually have been amused by Gloria's disingenuousness if I didn't deplore it so completely. I could see that any adverse reaction on my part would hold a double advantage for her. On the one hand, she would have the pleasure of tormenting me, and on the other, she would love nothing better than ruining Auntie's New Year's Eve party. But I wasn't so stupid as to turn into the Trojan horse she could use so mischievously. I could also see that, if I fell into that trap, she would not only ruin the evening for all of us, but would also – at least in her own mind – manage to escape the blame for it, for she would then say that Michael and I were at fault. Of course, she didn't know that Mickey had already blown the whistle on her behind-the-scenes mischief-making, so to an extent she was functioning exposed while thinking her scheme was concealed.

'Of course it was something. If it weren't, you wouldn't all have been talking about it. What happened?' she said imperiously, switching to her customarily demanding and dictatorial tone of voice, as if her desires were irresistible and we had all been put on this earth to gratify her as and when she felt like it.

'It really was nothing,' I said, almost sweetly and certainly more sheepishly than I had intended.

Gloria looked daggers at me. You could see the rage pouring out of her. How dare I thwart her? How dare I refuse to gratify her? Mindful of how my competitive mother would damage my adored aunt's evening if I let her, I said nothing but looked at her, took another puff of my cigarette, inhaled, smiled wanly, then exhaled. All non-threatening on one level but decidedly threatening on another for, by holding my ground, I, the snivelling little worm to which she had given birth, was defying the great puppet-mistress. For about thirty seconds, the air was heavy with unspoken tension. I decided to make my escape while things were superficially pleasant and so gathered up my cigarettes and lighter prior to standing up. I can still see Gloria glaring at me with a profusion of hostility over the rim of her glasses as she continued pushing back a cuticle with a wooden stick.

'Child, you could make an attempt to return to normalcy, you know,' she said viciously, intent upon roping me into a slanging match by pressing my buttons, and thereby instigating the chaos which would ruin Auntie's party and assure her of the malevolent satisfaction that chaos-creators so love.

At that juncture, I realized that much of my life had been a preparation for this moment. How I handled it would not only determine whether I was free from some of the psychic scarring one endures at the hands of the sadistic parent, but might also allow me to beat her at her own game and thereby wrest some of her power to dominate all of us away from her. Would I remain a victim, or would I effectively challenge the conqueror and maybe even dent her crown? I saw that the only way I had a hope of succeeding was if I remained absolutely calm, if I didn't allow myself to become emotional. This was not such an easy task for someone as passionate or as emotionally engaged as I am, for though I no longer had any love for my mother, I certainly had a plethora of loathing. Nevertheless, I was determined to vanquish her if I could.

'Normalcy?' I said as calmly and bitingly as possible, which, to my surprise, was quite a lot. 'You want me to return to normalcy? Now do pray tell me, how can I return to something I have never known? Where would I learn to be normal?'

'Your father and I brought you up to be normal,' she said, ignoring the fact that there is nothing normal about bringing a child up in the wrong gender, and thereby hurtling right into my trap.

'*You* brought me up to be normal. *You and Daddy*,' I said mockingly but still so calmly and quietly I was aghast at how self-possessed I was remaining. 'Are you trying to lay claim to being even approximations of normalcy? Or are you being your customarily immodest self and demanding to be recognized as a paradigm of something when you are its antithesis? You brought me up to be the opposite of normal. If you're laying claim to normalcy on those grounds, you are truly laughable, along the lines of Hitler wanting to convince the world he was doing it a favour by getting rid of the Jews, or the Marquis de Sade wanting people to believe it was acceptable to torment people.'

If I had opened up my hand and slapped Gloria across the face, I could not have evoked greater surprise. Never before had I ever seen her flounder, but then again, no one had ever spoken to her so witheringly in her whole life. As her look of shock gave way to confusion as to how this could be happening to her, I let her flounder while she unsuccessfully tried to reclaim control of herself and the situation.

'You…your father…I…we…'

'What? Cat got your tongue? Or are you back on the gin?' I said pointedly but still quietly and calmly, turning the tables on her by using her ploy and striking at her weakness the way she had tried to strike at mine. 'After all,' I continued sarcastically but still the essence of quietude, 'it is ten o'clock in the morning, and that's surely several hours past the time for the first drink of the day for lushes like you.' Gloria gasped for air as I rose from the swing. 'Yes,' I said lightly, 'I can well see why I never had a hope in hell of achieving, much less returning to, normalcy. With role models like you and Daddy, was there ever any possibility of any of us even knowing what the word "normal" meant? Normalcy? Hah!' I spat, mimicking Gloria mocking others. 'Normalcy indeed. What a joke. You look as if you left the remnants of your mind in Medical Associates when they dried you out.'

With that *coup de grace*, I swanned inside, still mocking Gloria by mimicking her walk.

I suspected that this woman, who hated anyone getting the better of her, would soft-pedal our *contretemps,* as no one had overheard it, so quiet had I been. And sure enough, she did. While normally she would have been barking for Michael to come and finish off her dirty work, this time she remained 'still as the grave', as she would put it, intent on keeping silent about how I had turned the tables on her. I, on the other hand, was exultant. I had succeeded where no one else had ventured. I therefore rushed inside to give Auntie and Mickey verbatim accounts of the encounter, with every gasp and nuance enacted as it had happened. Then I hopped into Alex's car and went around to Grandma's house, where I once again recounted my victory. The reactions of each of my relations were interesting. Mickey was filled with admiration, Auntie with relief that I had declined to allow her sister to ruin her special evening, while Maisie wondered aloud for the umpteenth time what motivated her cruel and recalcitrant daughter to behave the way she did.

Although the remainder of my stay in Cayman passed off without further incident, I cannot say I felt either comfortable or happy being around my mother. Indeed, being in the same room as her made my skin crawl, more so that it ever had done with Daddy during our turbulent years when he used to scapegoat me regularly. Although he had been quite brutal and loathsome at times, one could sense that she was more potently and calculatingly malevolent than he had ever been.

However, I had compensations in the form of my beloved aunt and grandmother, with whom I spent much of each day. Not knowing when I would see Maisie again, I indulged as fully as possible in the pleasure of her company.

One afternoon, after we had been to the beach and I had taken her back home, Maisie said to me, 'I want you to know that I am leaving you this house.'

'I don't know what to say, Grandma,' I replied, wondering how my siblings would react to the news. 'Do you think Mickey and Libby and Kitty will mind?'

'Not at all. I've already spoken to Mickey and Kitty. Mickey even helped me with legal advice. I made up my mind to do it after what that beast, your husband, put you through. And after what has happened here with your mother, I can see I've done the wise thing. You're the softest of you four children. I'll never forget how you came down to Fairway Avenue twice a day every day to rub in ointment into my scalp for weeks when I had that problem.'

'For goodness sake, Grandma, anyone else would have done the same,' I said, touched by her appreciation.

'Oh no, they wouldn't,' she said, wagging her finger at me. 'You've always been kind-hearted, and I for one intend to make sure that you are protected when you're older. Kind-hearted people always have harder lives than toughies, because toughies take advantage of the kind-hearted. Between the problems you were born with and your mother, I would never rest in peace unless I knew I had done all in my power to make sure that you have the security you deserve.'

Maisie then went on to tell me the dynamics of the bequest, which moved me more than I can say. Then, as if that were not enough, she ended up by asking me if I needed any financial assistance. She knew I had already informed Mickey and the rest of the family that I would not continue working for him when we returned to England. 'I'll stay until he replaces me,' I had said. 'He's as demanding as Daddy, even though he doesn't carry on like a lunatic. But he's had me doing the work of two people, and frankly, now that his firm is up and running, I want out.'

I declined to accept Grandma's help, not because I could afford to turn it down, but because, although asset-rich, she was cash-poor compared with my father. And I felt if it was anyone's responsibility to subsidize me, it was his.

Finally, the day of our departure for Jamaica dawned. I drove over to Grandma's house to say goodbye. As I was driving off and giving her a last wave, the thought flashed through my mind that I would never see her again. Shrugging it off as being a fear-given voice, I felt sadness engulf me, and can still see her waving back to me from the doorway of the front door.

It would actually be the last time I saw her alive.

If I had enjoyed being in Cayman because of my aunt and grandmother, I enjoyed being in Jamaica because of my friends. Indeed, they were what made being in that country bearable. I could not abide being near my mother, and though relations with my father were cordial, I did my utmost to be out of their house as much as possible to escape from her.

Three days before Mickey and I were scheduled to depart, one of the servants called me to the telephone. It was my cousin and godmother Cissie. 'Hi, I just heard on the bush telegraph that you're in Jamaica. So am I. If you're going to be in, I'm coming down right now to see you.'

I cannot convey how delighted I was. I had always loved Cissie and seldom saw her, for she came very infrequently to Europe while I had never been to Houston in Texas, where she lived. That meant that we only saw each other at weddings, funerals or by accident, like now.

As good as her word, Cissie showed up within minutes; and we were happily sitting in the study talking when Gloria, who had been out somewhere, burst into the room, arms flailing and tongue wagging, 'I'm here, Cissie,' she said, then pulled her usual trick and started to talk at her audience.

'I'm awfully sorry, Mummy,' I interrupted, 'but Cissie was in the middle of telling me something, and I'd really like to hear the end of it.'

'That can wait,' she said dismissively, picking up her thread.

Determined not to be shunted aside as usual, I interrupted Gloria again.

'What can it wait for?'

'What are you on about?' Gloria said irritably, giving me one of her 'don't-you realize-I-am-the-centre-of-the-universe-and-you-are-nothing-but-an-insignificant-flea?' looks.

'Cissie was in the middle of telling me something, and I want to hear the end of it,' I repeated.

For the second time in less than a fortnight, Gloria looked profoundly shocked. She was having a hard time believing that anyone, especially a child of hers, would have the temerity to challenge her. And, to add insult to injury, this was now the second time in as many weeks that I had done it.

'It's okay Georgie,' said Cissie, picking up on the mood of the moment and trying to pour oil on troubled water. 'It's not important.'

'Maybe it isn't important to you, but it is to me. I want to hear the end. Please continue,' I said pleasantly.

No sooner had Cissie picked up the thread of her story again than Gloria, who had no powers of concentration when anyone else was talking, interrupted again, stopping Cissie dead in her tracks.

'For God's sake,' I snapped. 'This is too much. Where are your manners?'

'My manners? My manners?' Gloria said haughtily. 'Who do you think you're interrupting? I was in the middle of telling Cissie something.'

'No you were not. Cissie was in the middle of telling me something,' I said firmly but calmly, once again holding my line as I had recently done at Blue Horizon. 'It may not have occurred to you, but Cissie did not come to see you. She came to see me. You have many more occasions for seeing her than I do, and I don't think it's asking too much to have her finish what she was saying.'

'How dare you speak to me like that?' Gloria snapped icily.

'Because it's the truth. Now are you going to give Cissie a chance to finish, or are you going to have this degenerate into a slanging match? For, I can assure you, there is no way you are going to dominate this conversation the way you always dominate everything else. Cissie is here to see me, and this conversation is going to resume its natural flow, or it's going to be dashed onto the rocks.'

'You really look as if you're mad,' Gloria said disparagingly, trying to recapture some control.

'Madness, my dear mother, is something you are rather more of an authority on than I am. Let's remember who is always in and out of the loony bin versus who was policed by psychiatrists for years in the hope that you and Daddy would turn up some psychiatric reason to prevent me from having a proper identity. The fact that they couldn't come up with one thing wrong with me says all that needs to be said.'

Cissie laughed nervously.

'Why don't we all just calm down?' she said, taking a sip of her Red Stripe.

'Can you believe, after all I've done for this little ingrate, that she would speak to me like this?' Gloria said to Cissie, rather cleverly trying to claw back the advantage by making herself into the victim.

'And just what is it that you've done for me that deserves undying gratitude?' I asked caustically.

'Cissie knows only too well,' Gloria said

'No disrespect to you, Cissie,' I said to my cousin, 'but you haven't lived in Jamaica since I was a toddler, and I can bet my bottom dollar that much of what you think you know about our family life is Gloria and Michael propaganda. If you really want to know what a poisonous bitch your good friend Gloria is, why don't you ask Audrey what Dearest Mama did to Mickey over the VW she gave him?'

'That,' Gloria spat dismissively.

'That,' I mimicked, 'was only one of the most awful things a mother could do to a son.'

'I'm sure that was long ago,' Cissie said, trying to be conciliatory.

'That may be so, but she's not got better with time. If anything, she's refined her bitch skills,' I said.

'Come on, Georgie. You know you love your mother,' Cissie said, still trying to be conciliatory but inadvertently giving me the one opening I would never have expected anyone to provide, to issue the *coup de grace*.

'Love?' I trilled in astonishment. 'Love? Love that poisonous bitch? You must be joking.'

'But you were always her favourite,' Cissie said, looking from me to Mummy with an expression of frantic appeal, as if to say: 'Please kiss and make up and let this dreadful situation end.'

'A poisoned chalice if ever there was one,' I replied. 'Do you know what being her favourite involved? Being trapped here in the study day and night, year in year out, listening to her go on and on about poor Aunt Juliette, Aunt Doris, Aunt Hilda, Auntie, Grandma, even you. Endlessly spewing forth venom about all the people I loved. Let me tell you something, Cissie, if I ever loved that thing that passes itself off as a mother, I haven't for many a year.'

'You love your mother. I know you do,' Cissie, still hopeful, said, giving me yet another unexpected opening to launch a second onslaught.

'Hate. Hate. I hate her. That's what I feel for her. Hatred. She's a low-down poisonous bitch who's spent her whole life fucking with everyone – possibly because she can't enjoy the act of fucking itself, despite her vampish behaviour – but whatever the reason, she's nothing but a lowdown cunt, and I loathe her. Loathe,' I said, switching my gaze from Cissie to Gloria, who had up to this point been under the mistaken belief that everyone just absolutely adored her.

You could see that Gloria was visibly surprised by the way I felt.

'You see what I have to contend with?' she said, making yet another play for the sympathy vote when she had recovered her composure.

'I'm sure Cissie sees what we've all had to contend with over the years where you are concerned. You may think you're so clever that no one can see through you, but I can tell you that you are a lot more transparent than you think. You're no candidate for sympathy and have never been. You're no victim. You're a vicious cunt and so full of shit that if anyone ever gave you an enema you'd disappear off the face of this earth without trace,' I said hotly.

At that, Cissie started to laugh despite herself, partly I suspect through unease, but also because she had been amused by my comment about Gloria disappearing if given an enema. Gloria looked daggers at her, and as Cissie struggled to regain her composure, I let rip.

That was the start of another tirade of several hours' duration. This time I not only dredged up what Gloria had done to all and sundry for Cissie to hear, but also informed Gloria exactly how everyone felt about her. I was determined to put a mirror to her face, for her to see herself as others saw her, not because I hoped to help her, nor even because I wanted to hurt her, but because I felt that the time had come for her to know the truth of how others regarded her. 'Your problem is you think your shit is chocolate ice cream,' I told her, 'and everyone must not only swallow it willingly, despite knowing it is shit, but they must also enthusiastically shriek "Geronimo" as it clatters down their throats, because you have decreed that it is so. Well, let me inform you, you delusional self-idolater, your shit is shit. It is not chocolate ice cream. And no one likes swallowing it.'

Michael returned home from work at the height of this scene.

'I want this stinking ingrate out of my house,' Gloria said to him. 'She's been stinkingly rude to me in front of Cissie,' who had fled by that time. 'Get her to pack her knapsack and pitch it – and her – out.'

'What's happened now?' Michael asked wearily.

As Gloria launched into a self-justifying account, I kept up a chorus of, 'That's a lie', 'That's another lie,' or 'Liar.'

When Gloria had finished her account, Michael said, 'Apologize to your mother.'

'What for?'

'I said ap...apologize to your mother,' he growled.

'You have got to be joking,' I said. 'Only in this house is the truth fairly told regarded as something for which to beg forgiveness.'

'Apologize to your mother,' Michael erupted so angrily that he no longer stuttered. He raised his hand as if to hit me, but before he could extend it properly, I had bolted from the drawing room, where we had been standing, rushed through the dining room and breakfast porch into the kitchen, where I grabbed one of the large kitchen knives and returned brandishing it.

'You will remember that I told you, the week before I turned twenty-one, that you would never touch me again after my twenty-first birthday,' I said pointing the kitchen knife directly at my father's gut. He had slapped me across the face for no reason in front of our cousin Toni de Acevedo at the time. 'Well, that was eleven years ago. Put me to the test, you big bully, and see if I don't spill your cowardly guts all over this rug.'

Michael blinked, nervous as to what I might do. With that pause, I flew into his face. 'Come on,' I said. 'Be a hero, Hero. Beat me up the way you used to when I was young and vulnerable. What? Not so courageous now that you see that there'll be consequences? You are pathetic. Pathetic. I have more balls than you, and I have none,' I spat as he backed away.

'Gloria, why is it that every time this child comes out, you have to cause trouble?' Michael said to my astonishment.

'Ah, so you do see the light of day,' I said to my father.

'I will not endure having this stinkingly impertinent freak in my house for one instant longer. Throw it out,' Gloria ordered Michael.

'You cannot refer to the child like that,' Michael said, yet again astonishing me.

'I can and I will. I gave birth to it and I can do anything I want with it. I should have closed by legs when it was passing through the birth canal, that's what I should have done,' Gloria said, her eyes blazing with fury because things were not going the way she wanted.

'Listen, woman, I've had a busy day and I'm going to my bed to rest,' Michael said, directing his comments to Gloria as he made off for their bedroom. 'Can't a man ever have peace when you're around?' Then, he turned around, looked directly at her, and said, 'You are something else.'

This scene, I could see, had taken a far more unexpected turn than I could ever have predicted. Michael had not only crumpled against me with minimal resistance, but had openly left Gloria in the lurch by taking my side.

Once he had left us alone, I decided to give her a dose of her own medicine. 'I simply cannot understand, dearest Mamma,' I said mockingly, 'how it is that I am still here. Do please explain to me how is it that the great Hero whom you've always mobilized to batter and bully us hasn't pitched me out along with my knapsack? Has the great Gloria lost her magic touch? Surely Hero should have done your bidding instead of taking my side, which, make no mistake about it, he has done. Very wisely too, if I may say so, if only because it shows that morality isn't completely dead in this hellhole. But do tell me, dearest Mamma, how ever are you going to manage, now that all your marionettes seem to be acquiring minds and tongues of their own? The natural order of things in Gloria Ziadieland seems to be rather turning on its head, don't you think?'

'You must be mad,' was the best Gloria could manage.

'But I am mad. Mad as hell. Not quite as mad as you, and certainly not mad in the same way, for I am mad as in angry, which is exactly the reaction everyone else should be having with you, while you are both mad and angry because the world refuses to revolve around you the way you think it should. Shall I tell you something? I'm cutting you no slack whether you're sane or not, for either way, you are every bit as big a bitch as you used to boast of so proudly, and I for one have your measure. Anyway,' I said, terminating the encounter, 'I have had more than enough of you, and hereafter you no longer exist for me. I would therefore advise you to keep out of my way for the few days that remain of my visit. After all, you wouldn't want me to knock into you now that you are invisible as a result of not existing.' And with that, I turned on my heel and walked off.

Those were the last sentences of any length I would utter to my mother for over a decade. I returned to England with Mickey and was so shattered by what had transpired that I began exhibiting signs of clinical depression. I cried at the drop of a hat. Anything and everything set me off. I could barely function, even at the office; and Mickey's law partner finally told my brother that they would have to find a way to manage without me before my two replacements had been fully broken in. He also insisted that I go to see my GP; and when I did, the doctor said I was indeed exhibiting symptoms of clinical depression and prescribed me a short course of antidepressants.

This was a real turning point in my life. My encounters with Gloria were the figurative straw that broke this camel's back. I had finally reached a crossroads that meant I would either continue down the road my parents had set me on, as I had been doing all my adult life, and remain as vulnerable and victimized as I had hitherto been, with all the attendant pain that such a way of being brought, or I could turn off it, find a new way of being and cease being an ideal target. This new way would not guarantee a life free of strife, trouble or pain, but it would mean that I would no longer have to put up with the deliberate cruelty of my sadistic mother. I had always tried to turn both the positive and negative in life into life-enhancing experiences, but each time I made any real progress emotionally, Gloria had found a way to drag me back down. The result was that I was always waiting for the other shoe to drop with everyone else, the way it did with my mother and had previously done with my father and ex-husband. Although I tried to fight it, underneath my cheerful and open façade lay real dread as to what would happen next. With an attitude like that, I no longer enjoyed having people close to me, which set up a vicious cycle, for that in turn made me feel more isolated than my naturally warm and sunny disposition inclined me to be. It made relating to people a real discipline requiring breaks from them rather than the joy it should have been. As the therapist who would subsequently help to salve my wounds put it, I was 'one of the walking wounded'.

Of one thing I was now sure. My new life could not include my mother. I could see only too clearly that I would never be free to have a good life unless I was free of her. She was too malign an influence, too disruptive, destructive and malicious to have around, even peripherally. I had to expel her the way I had expelled Colin Campbell. The choice was clear. Good or Gloria. Once I saw what the choice was, I was determined to excise her with the same finality that I had excised my ex-husband.

The next thing I decided to change was my career. Up to this point, I had been waiting, the way all of my single or divorced friends were, for a loving husband who would provide me with a way of life that gave me all the interest and variety I needed. The result was that I had never bothered to develop my artistic talents professionally, for marriage was ultimately the only worthwhile career open to women of my generation and social background. I decided, however, that the time had come to break the mould. I would develop my artistic talents, at least until the husband of my dreams came along. After all, it had been nearly eight years since I had left Colin Campbell; and though there had been possibilities for marriage and some of the men had been really nice, I had opted to remain single, unaware that I had developed an antipathy to being tied down because my marital experience had exacerbated the underlying mistrust I had of close relationships. This was as a direct result of the parental abuse my siblings and I had been subjected to over a lifetime.

There was no way I wanted to return to dress designing. I had found it too boring and insubstantial when I was younger, and I did not expect that to change now that I was older. Nor could I model any longer. Writing, however, was something else again. I had always found that intellectually as well as emotionally satisfying, and was cognisant that the only reason why my book *The Substance and the Shadow* had not seen the light of day in 1974 was that I had chosen my privacy over Howard Kaminsky's offer of publication.

Rather than dusting it off and trying to get it published, I decided to turn my hand to something new. Operating on the premise that the best works are written by those who stick to what they know, I started a play based upon my bizarre family life. I made it a four-hander, the characters being my parents, my brother and me. When it was finished John Whitney, then the head of Capital Radio, asked if he could see it. Could he? You bet he could. I duly took it to him at his office in Bowater House in Knightsbridge, then sat back nervously waiting for the feedback. I was gratified when he said he liked it and that I had a real gift for dialogue. I was even more pleased when he said he was going to try to have it put on at the Duke of York's Theatre, which his group of companies owned.

Mickey, however, was not exactly thrilled at the prospect of being featured, even as 'Nicky Aldobani' instead of Mickey Ziadie, though he generously did not stand in my way in the event that the Duke of York's decided to do it. I knew from him that Michael was indifferent, while Gloria didn't mind in the least being portrayed as the flagrant bitch she was, as long as she was the star of the show.

'It's interesting to see that, her lust for admiration notwithstanding, Mummy's vanity is so great that she will sooner be reviled than ignored,' I said to my brother, who laughingly agreed.

Months later, John informed me that the accountants, whose control of all entertainment companies is absolute save when these are one-man operations, had decided not to run the risk of putting on a new production and had opted instead for a revival of a musical. I duly shelved the play, only to take it out again a few years later when John was heading up The Really Useful Company and wanted to have another go at having it produced. Once more, the accountants prevailed, but by then it didn't matter, for I was well on the road of my new life, and John's interest had at least provided me with the fillip I needed to continue writing.

If utilizing my creativity was a step in the right direction, it was not the most significant step I took at that time. That was going into therapy. I cannot exaggerate how fortunate I was when a friend put me in touch with the most wonderful psychotherapist. Austrian by birth, international by persuasion, Basil Panzer turned out to be the perfect 'fit' for me. Wise, intelligent, sophisticated, civilized, sociable, decent and kindly, he had an understanding of the upper classes that many other therapists lack. This was of fundamental importance where I was concerned. A therapist who is in awe of a patient socially – as an earlier therapist of mine had been – or who does not understand the world being spoken of, and the values within it, can only be of limited help and can sometimes be a real hindrance. But Basil, with his sophistication counterbalanced with true wisdom, real heart and genuine intelligence, was able to help me unburden myself of a lifetime of anguish. In the process, he became the good Mummy and the good Daddy I had never had, and he re-parented me in the most life-enhancing way, without my needing to be a burden to my friends or relations.

It is a sad but true fact that friends and relations, no matter how interested, really are not adequately equipped to relieve someone of a lifetime's pain The process is too arduous; and frankly, so few people possess the psychological skills needed to cope with real emotional distress that even when they are trying to help, untrained friends and relations can hinder unintentionally.

Of course, I was no stranger to the therapists' couch, even if my earlier experiences had hardly been conducive to assisting me in relieving myself of the emotional baggage with which my parents and ex-husband saddled me. Because of those experiences, however, I knew that Basil was good, and could moreover see that the process would ultimately work, even if it was also evident that I would be reaching the figurative light at the end of the tunnel in years, not days, weeks or even months. Rome, after all, had not been built in a day, and it certainly couldn't be dismantled and rebuilt too quickly either.

Often I would come home from a most enjoyable afternoon or evening out and start to cry for no reason at all. These jags would last for anything from five to twenty or so minutes; and the interesting thing was that they were not sad, although one would hardly have called them pleasant either. At first, I wondered if I was still depressed and this was a symptom, but I quickly realized that I was no longer depressed, and it was simply a mechanism by which I was releasing all the tears that had been unshed for years.

It was in the middle of this period, in summer 1982, that I received a telephone call from my brother to tell me that Gloria had rung him to say that our grandmother had just died. She had developed pancreatitis suddenly and been taken to the hospital, where the doctor had warned Marjorie that she would most likely expire the same day. Marjorie had telephoned Gloria in Jamaica, but she could not get a flight to Grand Cayman until the following afternoon.

'Mamma hung on until your mother got here. You could tell she was determined not to die until she saw her,' Marjorie told us when we four grandchildren congregated in Cayman three days later for the funeral.

As I observed my mother's behaviour, I was struck by the irony of how much my grandmother had loved her, yet how that love had been soaked up as a right without ever being returned. Although the rest of us were pretty cut up, especially as how none of us had expected Maisie to die for years to come, extreme longevity being a Burke family trait, Gloria remained unmoved and dry-eyed. Even during the funeral and afterwards, at the grave, she was the only member of the family who behaved as if nothing untoward, much less sad, was happening.

We went back to Blue Horizon where all the family and friends had congregated for the reception. 'Mummy's behaviour is too odd for words,' said Mickey, who had delivered the eulogy and managed to do so without shedding one tear, though he had shed many others elsewhere. 'She hasn't cried once. Is she human?'

'I daresay she's thinking of all the money Grandma's left her,' Kitty quipped.

'Still, you'd think a daughter would shed even one tear for her mother,' Mickey said. 'Especially when you stop to consider the morbid and protracted expressions of grief she gave vent to after Grandpa's death.'

By this juncture, I was so indifferent to, and detached from, my mother than I did not even have a take on her lack of a reaction. I cannot say that I was surprised by her cold-hearted response, for I had given up having expectations of her. Unlike many of the family, who were still trapped in hopefulness, I had shifted to absolute acceptance, with the result that I was never taken unawares the way the others were. I did, however, note that it was chilling in the extreme to react so coldly to a mother's death, and was indicative of someone who was truly heartless. Even if you had had a troubled relationship with a parent, that individual was still your parent and you would have to have a freezer for a heart not to experience even a drop of grief at their passing. Yet, from the day of Maisie's death until Gloria's own death, she never once shed a tear nor expressed any grief, remaining supremely indifferent, except to the money she inherited.

In the way of families who do not wish to face the truth about a loved one, several members of ours tried to dress up Gloria's lack of emotion as something it was not and to explain it away as innocuous. I, however, took the opposite view and decided that it provided me with incontrovertible and significant evidence of why I should keep her out of my life.

Throughout the time Mickey, Kitty, Libby and I were in Cayman, I remained on cordial terms with everyone, with the exception of my mother, who still had a talent for delivering the subliminal message. She made sure that she let me know in a variety of unspoken ways that she still had me 'in her sights'.

'Did you see Mummy cut her eye at you just now?' Kitty asked me on one occasion when Gloria was looking daggers at me across the table until I looked up and caught her eye.

For my part, I thought Gloria was being infantile and declined to be engaged. I could tell that she was annoyed that I was not rising to the bait, and was not surprised when she came up with her next ploy, which involved cruelly but cleverly playing upon my sensitivities regarding my birth defect. She did so under the guise of giving a present to each of the four of us, her children.

'Girls,' she announced, directing her comment to Libby and Kitty, who were sitting at the top of the breakfast table, while Mickey, Auntie and I were at the bottom, 'tomorrow I'm going to take you to the bank and give you both a piece of jewellery. And you two,' she said, looking right at Mickey and me pointedly and lumping us together so obviously that it was clear she intended to make it clear that she was refusing to acknowledge my gender, 'I'm going to give the two of you two hundred dollars for you to buy something for yourself.'

I wish I could say that I wasn't aghast at the viciousness and malice of the woman. However, I was. Was there any depth too low for her? Any cruelty too debased to resist?

Poor Mickey, he was also being cheated out of a present of commensurate value to what Libby and Kitty would receive, just so Gloria could needle me. But at least our two sisters were getting more valuable presents than they otherwise would have received – the only way Gloria could create a hurtful contrast. I was tempted once more to tell her exactly what I thought of her but realized that, if I did so, I would be playing right into her hands and giving her the satisfaction of knowing that her cruelty had wounded me. Instead I ignored her, at least until Auntie and I were in her bedroom. Then I let rip.

'Sometimes I have to wonder what is wrong with your mother,' Marjorie said, distressed on my behalf, for she too had picked up the innuendo, as indeed anyone but a fool would have done. 'What have you ever done to deserve the way she treats you? Or Mickey and Libby before you for that matter? I just don't understand it.'

I had to confess that I didn't either. Although I could readily accept that my mother was a bitch, that was hardly an adequate explanation for her conduct or its motivation. Something was clearly profoundly wrong with her; and frankly, I was of the opinion that no one had ever got to the bottom of it – not her parents nor her friends or her family, not even her doctors.

Once more I was faced with the dilemma of how to handle a situation I wanted no part of. I was sorely tempted to tell Gloria to convert the two hundred dollars into one dollar bills, roll them up and stuff them up her arse one by one. However, if I did so, she would have the satisfaction of knowing that she had hurt me. Rather than give her that satisfaction, I decided to deprive her of it. The only way to do so was to act as if I had not understood what she meant, and though she knew me well enough to guess that I had understood it only too well, as long as I did not provide her with confirmation, a sliver of doubt would hopefully exist. So I pretended that there was nothing out of the ordinary with her 'present', and looked her dead in the eye when she handed Mickey and me four fifty-dollar bills each. 'How very generous,' I said, politely but with just enough of an edge that there could be no doubt that I too was delivering a message. 'I fully appreciate this, as you can imagine.'

Certainly, Gloria would pick up the jibe of being mean, but I would never know whether she had understood my full meaning. There was little doubt in my mind that she was bright enough to know that once more I had the last word. It was a small victory, but a victory all the same. The one thing I had learned with the Glorias of this world is that one must never, but never, allow them to walk away from an encounter feeling victorious.

Nevertheless, I could not escape the realization that there was something fundamentally sad about anyone who was so debased that she had to play such pathetic games. By this time I had accepted that there was no way of changing Gloria, and, since I couldn't change her, I really didn't want to see her or deal with her unless, as in this case, I absolutely had to. Though Maisie had been my adored grandmother, she had also been Gloria's loving mother, and Gloria had at least as much right to be there for her funeral as I did.

For the remainder of the 1980s, I was very much the odd one out where the family was concerned. Although everyone else also accepted that Gloria was an incorrigible problem, I was the only one who had stepped outside the family circle and refused to become a part of it whenever she was around. For their part, they dealt with her by accepting her bizarre behaviour and pretending to her that they had not noticed it, then complaining behind her back to each other. I could see the merit of that coping mechanism, for it allowed for an approximation of normal family life. But I also felt that it enabled Gloria to continue behaving as she had always done. By refusing to confront her with how awful she was, and thereby letting her get away with the consequences of her actions, the family perpetuated a situation that could only change if everyone refused to accept the unacceptable.

There was, however, another reason why I had to step aside. I was the one she was targeting specifically, the way she had targeted Mickey and Libby while they were growing up, Kitty still being exempt from her line of fire. This allowed my three siblings to function within her sphere without the acute discomfort two of them had once experienced but I now suffered whenever I was around her.

Michael, however, did not give up hope of reincorporating me into the family circle. Year after year, he still offered to pay for me to return to Jamaica or Cayman for Christmas, while I preferred to stay in England alone and miss out on the dubious joys of Ziadie family life. In the mid-1980s, shortly after Kitty left her first husband, he asked me to join him, Kitty, Mickey and Gloria on a trip he wanted to make *en famille* throughout Europe. The prospect of Paris and Florence etc with Gloria was as inviting as swimming across the shark-infested Caribbean waters from Devil's Island to the Guyanese seashore, and I declined without a sliver of temptation.

Then Mickey came back from Christmas in Jamaica one year and confirmed for me how right I had been to give Gloria a wide berth. 'You will never believe what Mummy did to Owen,' he told me.

Owen was our head gardener and an exact contemporary of Gloria's who had first worked for Marjorie before switching to Gloria when I was about four years old. He was as much a part of our family life as any of the Ziadies, Smedmores or Burkes, and when he developed glaucoma and started to go blind towards the end of the 1970s, it was understood by one and all, Gloria included, that he would keep his job even when he could no longer function in it. This was the patrician way, the right and decent way, the way people of our kind behaved; and it would have been unthinkable to deprive Owen of his livelihood after a lifetime of service. So Leslie, the under-gardener whom Gloria shared with Michael's sister Hilda, did the lion's share of the gardening as Owen's sight failed.

'She got rid of him,' Mickey said.

'How do you mean?' I said, aghast.

This was worse than any cruelty she had ever devised to entertain herself at Mickey's, Libby's or my expense, for at least we were able to continue eating.

'She pensioned him off. Or so she put it,' Mickey said disapprovingly.

I knew I would not have long to wait to hear the details from my brother, who was not only kind-hearted and decent, but also 'the BBC and the Jamaica Broadcasting Corporation rolled into one,' as Gloria used to put it with more accuracy than charity. 'If you ever want news to travel, just confide in Mickey, and you can be sure it will hit the streets.'

'According to her,' Mickey continued, 'she gave him a lump sum payment of a few thousand Jamaican dollars for him to invest and live off at home, instead of having to go to the trouble of being helped to work every day. I said to her, "But Mummy, how can you do this to Owen? He's worked for us all his adult life. He can't get another job, and that's hardly going to be enough for him to live off for the rest of his life." You won't believe what she said,' Mickey, related, visibly distressed.

'I'd believe anything of that woman God cursed us with as a mother,' I said.

'"It will be more than enough for him to manage on. And he has his family to help him out." I tell you, Georgie, I'm still reeling from the shock. But Libby and I have stepped into the breach. We got in touch with Owen's daughter and have told her that we will provide an income for him every month. How could Mummy do this to Owen?' he wailed plaintively, at a real loss to comprehend such heartlessness.

'She's certainly excelled herself this time,' I said, also at a loss.

'At least she still has Leslie,' Mickey said, clearly nervous that Leslie would be the next member of staff to hit the scrapheap. The former under-gardener was mad – really mad. An alcoholic who suffered from hallucinations, he was more than merely eccentric. He would come to work and spend hours lying down on the swing. Then, all of a sudden, he would jump up, as if a light had gone on in his head, grab the machete, and start to wield it with the force and fury of ten demons, all the while babbling to himself.

When he had first started working for us, I was worried that he would one day turn his cutlass on us, but with the passage of time I had come to realize that Leslie was harmless. Indeed, he liked all of us, including Gloria. Every evening, when he was ready to leave work, he would come to say goodbye to her. Their interchange was a set piece which never varied.

'Bye, Mama,' he would say.

'Mama? Mama? How could I be Mama to an ugly *nayger* like you?' Gloria would reply.

Leslie would laugh, Gloria would harrumph, then he would be off.

'Have no fear, Leslie's job is safe as long as he does his work,' I said.

'She likes him,' Mickey said.

'I suppose she does,' I said. 'Not only because he's such a good gardener, but because she's finally run across someone who makes her look sane by comparison. Though that is not an attribute that would outlast uselessness, I'm sure.'

Gloria's treatment of Owen gave me yet another chilling insight into the sort of person my mother was. However, that was not the end of the story. From this time until Mickey died in July 1994, he and Libby faithfully paid Owen the pension Gloria and the pussy-whipped Michael should have. Then, when he died, my sisters, aunt and I decided to use the several hundred thousand Jamaican dollars he left in a bank in Kingston as a source of revenue for Owen. Gloria, being one of Mickey's five beneficiaries, could, of course, have taken her fifth share out, but always mindful of how others would view her, she pretended to go along with our scheme and even agreed to withdraw an agreed-upon portion of the interest each month for collection by Owen's eldest daughter.

At first, all seemed to go swimmingly. Then, in 1996, when I was in Jamaica and asked after Owen, Gloria the ever-resourceful aggressor yet again presented herself as being a victim when I asked her how Owen was.

'I have no idea how he is,' she replied. 'You know how impertinent those damned niggers are now that they think the country is theirs and they're our equals. I had to liquidate the account because his rancid daughter was stinkingly rude to me and accused me of being a patronizing white woman. So I said to her, "Then let me stop patronizing your father. Come back next week, and I'll have the proceeds of the account for him to do whatever he wants with. But just make sure neither you nor he crosses my threshold ever again." You know what they're like,' Gloria said, appealing to class and colour solidarity.

'But Mummy, suppose she doesn't give Owen all the money,' I said, yet again aghast at what she was doing.

'That's his problem, not mine,' she said dismissively.

If Gloria expected me to buy into her version of events, I did not. I was pretty sure she, who was laziness and self-centredness personified, had simply decided that she couldn't be bothered to administer Owen's pension account and so had taken steps to terminate it. She was now coming up with a justification for doing so which she hoped I would understand. Not only did I not do so, but I was also only too aware that she had acted without reference to her sister or any of her daughters, the other owners of the money. This was a denial of our right to decide for ourselves what to do with our share of the money. Also, we couldn't even be sure if she'd actually handed over all of it to Owen's daughter, and frankly, I for one had no great confidence that she had done so. However, the only way of finding out would have been to ask the bank manager, and that would have been unacceptable for two reasons: Firstly, he might have said something to Gloria, which would have created a wealth of animosity between her and the rest of us; and secondly, asking him would have alerted him to the fact that there were problems with Mummy, and it would not have been correct to knowingly reduce her in the eyes of someone like her bank manager. So I tried to find out from Gloria how to contact Owen.

'I really don't know. I had his number written down somewhere on a piece of paper. If I haven't thrown it out, I'll let you have it,' she said irritably, giving me the brush-off and thereby preventing me from ever getting to the bottom of what had really happened, for she was the only person who knew how to contact Owen.

After I had written the first draft of this book and was speaking to Kitty about this incident, she said, 'She didn't give Owen's daughter any money. She told me she'd closed out the account and kept the money for herself because it was her money and she was sick of giving it away to Owen. "But Mummy," I said to her, "it's not your money. It's our money." Do you know what she said? "Whose name was on the bank account? Mine. So it was my money." "No Mummy," I said. "Even if your name was on the bank account, it was Mickey's money and there are five of us who were left his money. You were administering that account on our behalf." She remained adamant that it was hers and hers alone to do with as she pleased. I can remember as if it were yesterday saying to my husband Michael when I rang off that I may love Mummy because she's my mother, but I cannot say I like her at all.'

Gloria's first machination regarding Owen's livelihood confirmed for me yet again that I was wise to have cut her out of my life. By doing so, of necessity I saw less of the rest of the family, except for Mickey who, like me, lived in London. Because I would not go wherever Gloria was, I missed all the family Christmases that Mickey, Libby and Kitty still attended. The family, however, was slowly splintering through death and other external forces. First to go was Uncle Perez, Gloria and Marjorie's stepfather, who died in 1987. Shortly after that, Alex sold his and Marjorie's customs brokerage business against her wishes for so many millions that even she, who disliked boredom, felt compelled to limit her objections, though only too soon he would also regret his actions when the boredom of retirees replaced the novelty of freedom. In the meantime, he bought two houses in Victoria, British Columbia, 'One for us and one for Michael and Gloria, as an incentive for them to leave Jamaica, if only for part of the year,' he announced.

Michael, however, had been diagnosed a year or two before with Parkinson's disease. It was progressing at an alarming rate, partly because he was too undisciplined to take his medication regularly. 'It makes me feel sick,' he would complain, taking it only as an antidote to his symptoms, despite the protestations of his doctors as well as of his son-in-law and great-nephew Ben, who is an excellent physician and kept on telling his 'Uncle Mike' that it was the worst thing he could do.

'Let him do whatever he wants,' was Gloria's oft-repeated comment. I do not believe that she had discovered the virtues of stoicism or acceptance. She had always been too lazy to bestir herself on her children's behalf when we had been young and needed to go to the dentist or doctor; and I have no doubt that hiding behind a cloak of noble *laissez faire* acceptance was, to her mind, easier than encouraging her weak and wet but undisciplined husband to follow an exacting medical regimen. Yet she was, for all her faults, extremely disciplined and could easily have influenced him to medicate himself properly, especially as the more ill he became the more dependent on her he became. Which may well have been her payoff, for illness reduced him to a captive audience for whom there was no escape from Gloria.

In my view, that was the real reason she stood by and let him decline so rapidly. Attention was one of her great motivating forces, and having him available as and when she wanted him was her idea of heaven. The child she had trained up to be the lifelong companion had escaped from her clutches, but now she had the perfect substitute: the husband who still claimed to worship her and who was very much under her thumb. While a healthy Michael had always proven frustratingly elusive at providing her with the pair of ears she required, an infirm Michael would have little choice but to sit and listen.

Gloria also used Michael's illness to avoid availing herself of her sister and brother-in-law's generosity in buying her and Michael a house in Victoria. She had never been interested in any show but her own, and while she was only too happy to turn Christmas festivities over to Marjorie for celebration sometimes – thereby relieving herself of a responsibility the irresponsible Gloria would have tolerated only for the cachet of being the social lynchpin she was – she was hardly about to allow her less flamboyant sister to rope her into spending one day, much less several months a year, upon a scene that wasn't of her own making. She therefore declined to even look at the house, and it eventually had to be sold.

During this period, I went to Jamaica twice for Christmas. On both occasions, I stayed with friends, while my parents – thank God – were away, so I managed to escape the duty visits that would otherwise have been necessary. I cannot say I missed either of them. Although I was on cordial terms with my father, the past was laced too thoroughly with pain for me to have anything but the husk of a positive relationship with him. I was aware that we would have been able to have had a closer and fuller relationship than we did, had he been married to a different woman. He too was aware of that fact, and not only where I was concerned, for he expressed this view to friends. 'Daddy would have been a much better and more involved father if Mummy hadn't stood between him and us,' even Mickey once said. 'That woman has a lot to account for.'

Be that as it may, the fact was that Gloria had stood between him and three of his four children; and I for one could not escape from the fact that the overriding sensation I experienced when left alone with my father was awkwardness. Although I would discover when Mickey was dying that my brother had similar feelings, my reaction was less accepting than his. Bolting after a decent interval was my favoured way of coping, while Mickey's view was more tolerant. 'Daddy is the most reserved man I have ever met,' he would explain. 'He sits so uneasily in his own skin that it makes talking to him an uncomfortable experience. But if you persevere, it gets better.'

Despite the way I felt about being in my uneasy father's presence, I nevertheless possessed a greater degree of affection for him than I had for my mother. I had long since forgiven him for all that had happened while I was growing up and held none of it against him. How can you blame someone who inadequately handles an extraordinary situation beyond the limits of his capabilities? Michael, I knew, held no real malice towards me or anyone else. Sure, he was hot tempered. Sure, he let his passions and impulses get the better of him. He was weak and lacked self-discipline, but these flaws were matters of character rather than of heart or conscience; and that, ultimately, made them more acceptable and forgivable.

Gloria, on the other hand, was a walking, talking calculator. Indeed, she was organized in every aspect of her life. If you opened one of her cupboards, perfect order reigned. Even her hosiery was neatly packaged, folded in plastic bags one on top of another as if her chests of drawers were display cabinets in Bergdorf's or Sak's. She was an avid note-maker, as I would discover when she died and ran across reams of notebooks, all neatly annotated with her thoughts, observations, plots, schemes, desires, plans. If you checked anywhere in her house, you could see that the only time there was disorder was when it had nothing to do with her. Her garden, so famous in horticultural circles, was the same. An incomparable control-freak, she oversaw an empire of what she regarded as perfect order. That took organizational skill, discipline, energy, force of character and ability. Her flaws were not matters of character or self-discipline. She had no passions or impulses to give way to, beyond a lust to be the centre of attention and a determination to prevail at all times against all people, and to utilize any tool in her rich fusillade of manipulation to do so. Unlike Michael, Gloria did not really have a heart, nor did she have a conscience; and while she was a more superficially charming person than he was, and she lived very easily – too easily – in her own skin, which never prickled with conscience or the discomfiture of human fallibility, there was something so inhuman and inhumane about her that she chilled my blood. She was actually the perfect malice machine, identifiable to the uninitiated as such only after she had wrought her havoc, but until then superficially desirable.

One could almost say that I was afraid of her, except that it wasn't fear of what she could do that motivated me, so much as a horror of what she was. On an atavistic level, she so took my breath away that I never wanted to spend even a minute in her company.

Chapter Twenty-Three

By the dawn of the 1990s, I had put enough emotional and psychological distance between my mother and myself to know that I was no longer vulnerable to her games or the mess I had been brought up to be a part of. I was, in short, free of her. Although much of this liberation was due to Basil Panzer's excellent therapeutic work, another part was also due to the maturity which aging brings. I was now forty years old and had taken appraisal of what I had, what I wanted and what I didn't want for the future.

Even though my life appeared to be glamorous from the outside, it had been anything but a picnic, although that is not to say that it wasn't pretty good by this time. I had a devoted boyfriend I loved and who loved me; two gorgeous black-and-white Springer Spaniel daughters called Tum Tum and Popsie Miranda, whom I loved utterly and whose importance in my life cannot be exaggerated; many good and interesting friends on both sides of the Atlantic, some famous, some not, but all apparently devoted; and a rich and full social life which meant that I had come across some of the most interesting, eminent or famous people in the world. This I had turned to my professional advantage by writing a social column, 'Out and About with Lady Colin Campbell' in the glossy magazine *Boardroom*, which sat in every boardroom in the City of London and brought me far more prestige than the paltry salary I earned. I also received the occasional journalistic assignment from publications such as the *Mail on Sunday*'s *YOU* magazine; and while no one would have accused me of being a literary heavyweight, I had also published a book, the critically acclaimed *Guide to Being a Modern Lady* in 1986.

Whenever I wasn't writing, I still spent a great deal of time on my alternative, unpaid occupation: the spiritually-enriching business of raising funds for charity. I had a nice if modest two-bedroom flat in the most prestigious apartment complex in the United Kingdom, namely the Duke of Westminster's Cundy Street Flats in London's chic Belgravia. Although I still had no money of my own and an income that meant that I had to watch my pennies at all times, I nevertheless had a lot to be grateful for. I was fully aware that I could continue on the same path and be counted lucky by many of my peers as well as a quantity of the unseen people who read about me but knew me not at all.

However, if there is one lesson the daughter of a narcissist learns, it is that the opinion of onlookers is of slight consequence. Did it really matter, in the deepest recesses of my heart or mind, whether I had a glamorous life, and whether strangers or friends thought it enchanted and enchanting? The answer was no. Sure, admiration was more pleasant than revilement, but neither actually amounted to fulfilment, which was the truly important thing in life – at least to me.

I had now reached the age where stocktaking seemed sensible, so I asked myself if there was anything I lacked that I still really wanted. The answer was 'my own family'. I was very family-orientated and had always been. Even as a child, I had adored my dolls and would spend hours mothering them. My experiences with Michael and Gloria might have turned me off my own parents, but they hadn't turned me off family life in general. Indeed, I loved family life. I was from three large families and was happy to be a part of them.

Despite my reputation as a renowned international socialite, I was also very domesticated and loved the creature comforts of home. I was as happy curling up in bed with a good book or having a friend over for supper as I was attending one of the balls or premieres which so excited the gossip columnists and paparazzi. I was also a good enough cook for two separate publishers to have approached me to write a cookbook.

Anyone who knew me well was of the opinion that I was a stable, sensible, loving woman with a strong enough character to stand up for what I believed in rather than following the herd, without being so overpowering that I gave no one else a chance. As the Honourable Clare Pennock put it, 'Georgie has a big heart.' This was a view even my father supported, for he told Judy Ann

MacMillan when I had adopted my sons, 'Getting two instead of one might seem crazy, but at least it shows she has a good heart.' By inclination as well as qualification, therefore, motherhood seemed my ideal calling.

Although it was not yet the done thing for single women to adopt, I had never been afraid to break new ground, and decided that that was the route I would pursue. I saw – correctly as things turned out – that motherhood would prove to be the ultimate in fulfilment, and when the English system proved to be hopelessly geared against the adoption of infants, I turned my attention to Russia. There, good sense prevailed. The authorities understood that it was preferable to have children adopted as young as possible, a view antithetical to the doctrinaire megalomaniacs who had hijacked the English system. There, adoption was an option only after children had been damaged by years of being shunted between foster carers – usually just before they were old enough to leave the fostering services. I could not escape concluding that the English social services were far more concerned with keeping their vast horde of social workers in jobs by ensuring that there was always a ready stock of children in care, whom they would have to police, than in solving the problem of those children needing homes.

There was no way I intended to take on a child who had been emotionally damaged. I had had quite enough of emotionally damaged people to last a lifetime, thank you very much. 'I've cleaned up enough of other people's messes,' I revealed to one of the few sensible social workers I came into contact with. 'If I make a mess of motherhood, I want to be quite sure that the fault was mine and mine alone. I am only interested in babies.'

In furtherance of my objective, I turned my attention to the dual task of obtaining a baby and the funds to support us. As luck would have it, the Princess of Wales now entered the picture in a most unexpected way. I had floated the idea with her as well as with three of my charities, which were three of hers, that I write her official biography with the focus being on her charity work as opposed to her personal life, which we all knew, in the circles within which I moved, was disastrous. Although she ultimately pulled the plug on the book and withdrew her cooperation, preferring to go instead with Andrew Morton, who was an altogether more malleable and willing Mercury than me, and was prepared to trash her husband when I was not, she did not do so until after I had gone some way towards agreeing a publication deal with a publisher. As both my agent and the publisher felt that my book would become an international bestseller – which it did – and I wanted the money so that I would have sufficient funds to adopt and bring up a baby, I decided to proceed without Diana's cooperation and wrote *Diana in Private: The Princess Nobody Knows*. This lovers-and-all biography created an absolute sensation when it was published in 1992, bringing me the financial rewards that made motherhood possible.

Coming from a background as social and royalist as mine, there was every likelihood that my family would be embarrassed by the book. But since none of them was contributing to my support, I decided to give their potential disapproval the weight they gave my penury. I therefore ignored the clucks of disapproval which only too soon disappeared when the Morton book came out, as Diana's royal stock went crashing down in Establishment circles while both our books flew off the shelves, and the public availed themselves of opposing versions of her life.

I was now an authoress with an international profile. I was frequently on American television channels, especially CNN, all of which were beamed via satellite to Jamaica, where my parents still lived. I was gratified to learn that I was now referred to in my native land by such sobriquets as 'the celebrated Lady Colin Campbell' and that Jamaicans of all kinds, always nationalistic, had embraced me as a figure of pride now that I was so visibly successful.

Insofar as the majority of my friends and relations were concerned, my new profile was a source of celebration and, at times, humour. My parents, on the other hand, were 'still as the grave', to use one of Gloria's favourite phrases.

Although I would later learn from the servants prior to my mother's death and from cousins of hers afterwards that Gloria would sometimes tell them how proud she claimed to be of each of her children's accomplishments, she took great care to keep any pride she might possess away from me – or indeed from anyone close to me who would be liable to repeat it back to me. With me as well as with potential repeaters, she was determinedly silent. This was not so puzzling on reflection for, by behaving as she did, she managed to accrue to herself the benefits of my accomplishments as and when they suited her without ever giving me the satisfaction of providing the recognition any normal parent would gladly give a child.

Although I did not know it at the time, this was typical narcissistic behaviour. Narcissists are intensely jealous of anyone else's successes or accomplishments and will do anything to neutralize the positive benefits of those accomplishments – unless, of course, they can take advantage of those same accomplishments.

On the other hand, the pussy-whipped Michael, more firmly in Gloria's clutches than ever now that he was incapacitated by Parkinson's disease, grabbed the only opportunity open to him to break ranks and get across the delight he felt in my newfound success. I had been flown out to Jamaica by *YOU* magazine, who were doing a cover feature on me and 'That Book', as they billed it, on the North Coast, where I had spent summers as a child. Knowing that Gloria was not in Jamaica, I telephoned Michael and arranged to drop in to see him prior to boarding my flight back to London.

This was the first time I had seen my father for years, and I was horrified to see how Parkinson's disease had reduced him from a towering and imposing man into a wizened, crippled shadow of himself. He could not walk without assistance. He could barely talk. His face was frozen in the Parkinson's glower, and he shook like a tree being battered by hurricane force winds even when he was sitting or lying down.

He was on the back veranda when I arrived, sitting waiting to receive me. I bent down to kiss him hello, then sat opposite him. 'So how are you, Daddy?' I asked, my tone of voice as open as if we had always had a good relationship. This, after all, might be the only chance we'd have to hold a conversation of any significance unsupervised by Gloria.

'As you see me,' he said, his once-booming voice – the Voice of God, as a friend once put it – reduced to a whimper.

'Mickey says you haven't been well.'

'Mustn't com...complain,' he said, the stoical resignation which everyone had admiringly told me about being immediately apparent. 'If you want anything to eat or drink, get Bir...Birdie,' the housekeeper, 'to get it for you.'

'I'm okay,' I replied.

'Do you mind if we go...go into the bedroom? I need to lie down.'

After I had called his nurse to help take him into his bedroom, and after she had settled him in bed, I sat on the sofa facing him.

'You look well,' he said.

'I am,' I replied, feeling as awkward as one always did when speaking to Daddy.

'Your mother and I saw you on television the other day,' he said. 'You were good.'

'Where is she?' I asked, not because I did not know – Mickey had told me – but because one needed to oil the conversation to avoid it becoming too stilted for words.

'She's with Dolly,' her cousin in Florida.

'How is she?'

'Same as ever,' he replied, looking at me poignantly. Although I did not yet appreciate the full significance of that look and would only discover it on the evening of his burial, when Birdie told me and Kitty how Gloria used to beat Michael up when the mood took her, I could tell that it was laden with significance.

'I want to ask you something,' I said, having decided to grab the bull by the horns while the picador was out of the arena. 'Do you regret having married Mummy?'

'That,' he said levelly, 'is a very go…good question.' He paused, looked at me with an expression suffused with unspoken emotion, sighed, then continued. 'I met your mother when she was fi…fifteen. I was her uncle John's go…good friend and I was with him when she wa…walked into the room. I took one look at her, and that was it. I loved her then, and I love her now.'

'What was it about her that appealed to you?'

'She was a very pretty girl. Pretty and vivacious. And mad.'

'Mad?' I repeated, hardly able to take on board what I was hearing.

'Mad. She's given me a wa….warm time, but she's been a loyal wife, and she's given me four good-looking, intelligent, decent and successful children. I'm very pl…pleased with the way all of you have tu…turned out. No ma… man can ask for more than that. But it's a pity your mo…mother couldn't have been an easier sort of person.'

'She certainly has stood between you and us,' I said.

'I know,' he said. 'But what could a man do?'

The time had come for me to leave for the airport, so I said goodbye, wondering if I would ever see my frail father again, but so glad that I had taken the time to look in on him. I was only too mindful, as he must also have been, that none of this would have been possible had Gloria been present.

For the remainder of the year, whenever I wasn't crisscrossing the globe from England, America and Europe to the Far East, promoting my book, I hunkered down to write my next book. I was very aware that I would soon be a mother, as my agent in Russia was keeping me abreast of how close to realization my adoption papers were. I therefore capitalized upon whatever free time I still had, before I lost it in the welter of diapers and sleepless nights that are inevitable when you have a baby, to earn yet more of what I called 'baby money'.

Although many of my friends and just about all of my relations, with the exception of my cousin Enrique and my aunt Marjorie, could not understand why I would wish to burden myself with a baby when I had such a 'good' life, I ignored their misgivings. I knew that what I was doing would turn out to be the best thing that I could ever do, and when my brother Mickey, who was particularly agitated lest I make a mistake, remarked, 'As Daddy says, you don't know what you're getting when you adopt a baby,' I could not resist replying: 'I don't see how I could ever do worse than if I gave birth myself. Our genetic pool, despite its supposed good breeding, has just about every flaw known to man, and I would suggest you and Daddy remember that. And let me also remind you that you didn't want me to get a dog. Remember what you said about me tying myself down? Well, look at the joy Tum Tum has given me. What you need to realize is that responsibility is spiritual wealth. It is not necessarily a burden – at least, not to me.'

Gloria, meanwhile, made it obvious to all and sundry that she could not have cared less whether I adopted a child or not. We were still pointedly estranged, and her only comment, oft-repeated, was, 'Let Nutty Buddy do whatever it wants as long as it doesn't look to me to take care of any *pickney* it picks up. I never took care of my own, and I certainly won't be taking care of anyone else's.'

In June 1993, right after the launch of my latest book, *The Royal Marriages* in America, I went to Russia to pick up my son. While there, I was given the choice between him and another little boy and, unable to choose, decided to have them both. This, it would turn out, was the best decision I could have made, for everyone who makes the choice between two babies is evidently haunted for the remainder of his or her life by the child he or she left behind, while I now have two glorious sons, and they have had the benefit of a 'twin'.

To my family's credit, once I returned with my two sons, they all accepted both babies without reservation. They made absolutely no distinction between my two sons and Libby's children, or four years later, when Kitty had her daughter, between them and Gabriela. Believe me, if there had been even the slightest inflection, I would have picked it up, but there never was any. As a result, Dima, Misha and Gabriela have grown up being treated exactly the same by everyone in the family; and, by one of those odd quirks of fate which make life so fascinating, Misha and Gabriela have always looked so much alike that strangers often think they are brother and sister.

The presence of my boys changed my life in unforeseen ways. Amongst those was the relationship with my mother. Until their arrival, I had not wanted to see her again. But once I had them, even though I still had no more regard for her than I had previously had, I could see how much richer their lives would be if they were a part of an ostensibly cohesive family. As things stood, they were already being cheated by having only one parent, and I simply could not allow them to miss out on having grandparents as well. No matter how awful Gloria had been as a mother, I had seen, from her contacts with her three grandchildren by Libby, that they had not been damaged by her but rather enriched by this attractive if rather oddball grandmother. I would gladly have made a far greater sacrifice for my boys than the odium of enduring my mother for their benefit, and when my father, always the more family-orientated of my two parents, expressed a desire to see the boys, I promised to take them out to see him in Jamaica in February 1995.

By then, of course, my immediate family was reeling from the shock of my brother Mickey's death at the relatively young age of forty-six in July of the year before. He had been diagnosed as suffering from cancer of the mouth in December 1993. Prior to that, he had planned to fly to Jamaica for three weeks just after Christmas. Upon consulting with his doctors and being told that a few weeks would make no difference one way or another before starting treatment, he proceeded with the visit. A strong motive for his doing so was to tell Michael and Gloria in person that his prognosis was not particularly promising and also to see his beloved Jamaica one last time, if things turned out as the indications led him to suspect they might.

Mickey, always a powerhouse of energy, duly flew to Jamaica, where his strength, which had already been declining in the last few weeks, evaporated so utterly that he was bedridden for much of the time. This, for someone whose idea of a little light exercise after lunch had always been to take a two-hour hike, should have been frightening for anyone who cared to look; but Gloria, as self-absorbed as ever, did not even notice that her son was ill.

By Mickey's own account, he was waiting for the right moment to tell our parents the news which he imagined would distress the both of them. The only problem was that Gloria was perpetually drunk, having started to drink again sometime at the end of the 1980s or the beginning of the 1990s. No one knew precisely when, for in a large house full of servants, concealment was easy. Evidently little had changed since the halcyon days of the 1970s, when I had witnessed her terrorizing all and sundry from her favourite chair on the back veranda, which she still occupied while ranting and raving as much as ever.

Nor had she lost her talent for lying in deed as well as word.

'Mummy never once came in to see how I was until David came to see me,' Mickey told me, referring to David Boxer, the well-known artist who was then curator of the National Gallery of Jamaica and Mickey's best friend from school.

Kitty, who was there as well, takes up the tale. 'David, Mickey and I were in the bedroom talking when Mummy came in and started to fuss, playing Florence Nightingale. You know how she can be. Mickey waited until she'd left the room, then said to David, "Don't believe a minute of it. She hasn't come in to see me once since I've been here."'

Finally, when Mickey could no longer wait for the opportune moment that was evidently never going to present itself as long as Gloria continued her drunken reign of terror from morning till night, he seized the first chance that presented itself and told both Michael and Gloria that he was gravely ill and might die. Not surprisingly, Michael was devastated, but Gloria was not having anyone steal any thunder from her. She, the hypochondriac who had never endured a day's physical ill health but nevertheless had never been known to do anything but bitch about her imaginary aches and pains, was hardly going to be outdone by a little thing like her son possibly dying of cancer. So she launched into a tirade about her ills and about how much more difficult her life had been than Mickey's ever could be, letting him know in no uncertain terms that she was supremely unmoved by his news and any sympathy or concern should be reserved for her and not wasted on him.

This was too much for Mickey. Finally taking a leaf out of my book, he lambasted her in the same way I had done twice before for about three or four hours. According to him, and to Kitty who witnessed the scene, he dredged up everything she had ever done to him or to anyone else he could think of. He told her exactly what a dreadful person she was, and spelled out precisely how everyone regarded her. By the time he had finished, he had reduced her to tears – though whether these were of impotent frustration or the intense humiliation that narcissists are prone to, when people present them with a picture contradictory to their self-image, is not something I can assess. My own suspicion is that she was indulging in maudlin self-pity while hoping that by crying she would silence him, but if that was her objective, she failed spectacularly. He only stopped when he had said everything he had to say. 'He gave her no possibility of escape', was how Kitty put it. Then, having delivered his message, he declined to speak to her until he departed for England, fully aware that he might never see her again.

Mickey came back to London appreciating for the first time in his adult life just how dreadful a person our mother was. 'I never want to see her again. Never,' he said, recounting the full horror of how callously she had behaved.

'I'm really sorry,' I said to my brother, who was obviously extremely cut up by what had happened. 'At least you have the consolation of knowing you reduced her to tears, even if it's scant consolation.'

'The woman is a complete monster,' he said, and though I agreed, even I, who already had such a low opinion of Gloria, was dumbfounded. How could she have turned the possibility of his death into a contest? This was yet another unbelievable experience to have to work through and incorporate into the already bulky dossier of motherly misconduct; and I was furious with her for having hurt Mickey at such a vulnerable time. But he was adamant that he was now beyond pain as far as she was concerned – something with which I could identify – and he quite determined never to see her till he was dead.

It was against this backdrop that I found myself cast as the bearer of news for the rest of the family. Despite what had happened between Mickey and Gloria, I took the view that, since she was his mother, she still deserved to be kept informed. Michael, I knew, was worried sick and avid for news, so I would telephone our parents, our aunt Marjorie and our sisters with regular updates, and in so doing, my relationship with Gloria changed for the better superficially, as I had to speak to her rather than Michael, who would listen in on an extension but had difficulty making himself understood over the telephone now that Parkinson's had severely weakened his vocal chords.

Gloria had always been a lover of drama who rose to the occasion as and when circumstances required her to come up with a good act. Whether

Michael had said something to her, or she had simply had enough time to see that anything but a display of maternal interest would be ruinous to her standing within the family, she now started to behave relatively normally. Although there was no warmth between us, nor was there any conflict as I relayed the news.

While Mickey's chemotherapy was working, being the liaison was not unduly upsetting. But when, at the end of the second session, Mickey's cancer was growing quicker than the toxins were killing it, the oncologist switched the treatment to radiotherapy. This, I knew, was a mere palliative, a precursor to death, for I had already had a quick word with Professor Stuart, the oncologist. He had revised earlier medical estimates of years into a matter of two or three months 'if he's lucky. But he could go at any time if he catches a cold or anything like that.'

Trying to get across the message to the family that Mickey was dying quicker than everyone feared was no easy task. Both our sisters were heavily into denial, as was Marjorie, who had always said, even to her husband, 'I love Mickey more than anyone else in this world.' Ironically, the one person to whom it was relatively easy to get through was Gloria. Unencumbered with the emotional baggage of caring, she had no defences to knock through, so took the bad news on board with an alacrity that made the task amazingly easy. Insofar as the others were concerned, however, they only accepted the reality of what was happening when Libby's husband Ben had spoken to Professor Stuart and spelled out the ramifications to them.

Libby and Kitty flew over to see Mickey as soon as they could make the arrangements. So too did Marjorie, who came with Alex. Michael was too ill to travel, but Gloria certainly was not. However, rather than get on a plane and come and see her son and mend fences before it was too late, she took off for America, where she went shopping. Mickey seemed unperturbed, but I was having trouble getting rid of Pollyanna, and from time to time would check to see if he had softened in his determination not to see Gloria again. The answer was always the same, although a curt 'no' gave way to 'I don't want her up here. I couldn't cope with her behaviour. Not at a time like this.' Then, in June, just before Marjorie was due to return to Grand Cayman, Professor Stuart dropped the axe while Mickey was in St Mary's Hospital, Paddington, for a transfusion. The cancer was spreading so wildly that the frequency of the radiotherapy sessions would have to be increased substantially. But even then, it was only a matter of time. Mickey, however, hated those radiotherapy sessions, not because they were so dreadful in themselves but because of the hours of waiting involved. Right in front of Marjorie and me, he therefore informed Professor Stuart, 'The time has come to stop treatment.'

'I'll arrange for palliative care, so you'll be comfortable,' Professor Stuart said before telling Mickey how sorry he was at the way things had gone. With that, he departed, leaving the three of us to face the fact that Mickey had only a few weeks left to live.

Mickey displayed notable courage as well as dignity in the way he told Auntie and me what arrangements he wanted us to make once he was dead. We, of course, were beside ourselves, but he broke down only once, when he was instructing us what to do with his body. 'I'd like to be cremated and my ashes buried at home, under the macca tree,' he said. 'But I leave the final decision up to Mummy.'

I now found myself in a delicate predicament. I was Mickey's next of kin as well as executrix. I was also his sister and the daughter of our parents, and though I didn't want to exert any pressure upon him to do anything he didn't want to, nor did I want to leave unsaid or undone any of the things one ought to deal with while there was still time. So I waited until the next time Mickey was in the hospital, a week or so before he died. It was now obvious to even Mickey himself that he would be dead very soon 'I'm not trying to suggest anything you don't want to do,' I said to him, 'but if you want to see Mummy again, now is the time to get me to phone her.'

'Um,' Mickey said, indicating that he would think about it.

Later, as I was walking through the door to go home, he said, 'Phone Mummy. Tell her if she wants to come, she can.'

This was hardly an expression of desire, but, preferring to believe that Mickey secretly wanted to see Mummy and hopeful that they would kiss and make up before it was too late, I put a spin on things when I got home that would have made Tony Blair or Josef Goebbels proud. 'Mummy, I've just left the hospital. They don't think Mickey has more than another week or two. He's asked me to phone you and tell you he'd like to see you before he dies,' I said.

'What? And leave your father alone at a time like this? It's out of the question,' snapped the woman who had returned to Jamaica only a day or two before from her latest trip abroad.

'I'll be fine,' advised Daddy, who was on the extension. 'You can go, Gloria.'

'Absolutely not,' she said imperiously. 'Mickey will just have to manage without me. There's no way I'm leaving your father alone here.'

'Didn't you just get back a day or two ago?' I said without side, though I can assure you that the acid was choking me.

'That's different,' she said.

'Gloria, you can go,' Michael said again.

'My duty is to be by your father's side,' said Gloria, who always hid behind nobility when she was being low.

'Mummy,' I said, still pleasantly, taking another stab at implementing what I interpreted as my brother's wishes, 'I don't think you understand. Mickey is going to be dead in a week or two, maybe three if we're lucky. He wants to see you. What am I supposed to tell him?'

'Tell him whatever you want, but there's no possibility of me leaving your father here on his own,' she said as coldly and imperiously as if I were telling her an enemy wanted to cross the road.

I heard the click of the extension hanging up. Daddy, knowing the futility of trying to get her to do anything she didn't want to, and doubtless suspecting that I would let rip when I had had enough, had got off the phone before the fireworks started.

'I want to know how it's okay for you to leave Daddy to go shopping and to parties abroad, but all of a sudden, when your only son wants to see you before he dies, you can't tear yourself away from him,' I said cuttingly.

'I don't need to account to you for my actions,' she said, still coldly and even more imperiously than before.

'You are the most selfish, self-centred piece of shit that ever existed,' I said furiously, giving vent to my anger and to the pain I felt in sympathy for my dying brother, whom I would have to disappoint. 'You have only ever thought of yourself. Daddy doesn't need you, and you know it as well as I do. You simply can't be bothered to bestir yourself because there's no pleasure to enjoy as a payoff. How can you do this to Mickey? You tell me. How?'

'You can say any damned thing you want, my mind is made up,' she said coolly.

'You are a horrid, horrid human being and I curse the day God ever inflicted you upon us. Why it isn't you dying instead of Mickey is something

I will never understand. Fuck off, you filthy piece of shit,' I screamed, banging down the receiver.

I was so distressed that I promptly telephoned both Marjorie and Kitty.

'Maybe she can't face losing Mickey,' her sister said, attempting to explain away her callous sibling's heartlessness by attributing sensitivity where none existed. Kitty took a more realistic view, but even I, who knew in my heart of hearts that Gloria would have hopped on a plane at this very moment quicker than you could say 'boo', if she had been asked by the President of Peru's wife to join her on an orchid-gathering expedition at Machu Pechu (as she had once been), still found it difficult to get my head around the fact that the real reason she didn't want to see Mickey was that it simply wasn't going to be fun. It wasn't that she loved him so much that she couldn't face him dying. It was that she loved him so little that she preferred to avoid the unpleasantness. This was nothing more than the ultimate variation on the theme of 'I'm-too-nervous-to-cope-with-the-children-going-to-the-doctor-or-dentist' from the mother whose strong constitution and nerves of steel could always cope with anything arduous as long as it was socially desirable, but nothing tedious or responsible unless there was pleasure or image-enhancing feedback attached to the enterprise.

'Mummy says that as much as she'd love to come up,' I said to Mickey the following day when I went to visit him, determined to keep what had happened from him, 'she can't leave Daddy. You know how devastated he is by what's happening with you.'

'Poor Daddy. For all his faults, he really does love his children,' Mickey said. He looked at me, I looked at him. 'It's just as well she can't make it,' he then said. 'She'd only create havoc.'

I understood then what I had not appreciated before: Mickey did not want to see Gloria. He had simply done the decent thing and given her the chance to see him on the off-chance that she wanted to. I was absolutely gutted that my dying brother could have the generosity of spirit to make the potential sacrifice of his peace of mind in the last days of his life for the mother who was so selfish and shallow that she couldn't even consider making a far lesser sacrifice for him.

Less than two weeks later, Mickey was dead. I arranged a funeral service for him in London, which Libby and I attended, followed by a cremation. St. Mary's Hamilton Terrace was packed to the rafters, and afterwards a multitude of strangers came up to Libby and me and told us of many unknown acts of charity Mickey – who gave away ninety percent of his income to others – had done for them. Knowing the respect and regard others had for our truly altruistic brother, and the good use to which he had put his life, was a great consolation to us.

Because Mickey had died in one country and was being buried in another, the rest of the family agreed to fly to Jamaica for the burial service Gloria was organizing there a week or so later.

When I arrived in Jamaica two days before the service, I found everyone in a state of agitation because Gloria had decreed that the occasion would be by invitation only. Although no one was prepared to confront her directly, she was trivializing Mickey's burial by turning it into a purely social event. He had been an eminent member of the legal profession, but none of his colleagues, save the two or three she chose to invite, could attend. He had enjoyed a wide circle of friends, none of whom could come unless they measured up to her exacting social criteria. She hadn't even bothered to ask many of the family, decreeing that she was not going to have her garden trampled by a marauding horde. The result was that the hundreds of people who wanted to pay their respects were unable to do so, while social luminaries with whom Mickey had not associated either personally or professionally for thirty years, were in attendance. For years afterwards, I kept on running into people who bemoaned the fact that they had not been able to say goodbye to Mickey.

In fairness to Gloria, who was a superb organizer and had an eye for beauty as well as a fine sense of occasion, his burial service was lovely, as was the setting. She had got the servants to place a semicircle of chairs between the lychee tree and the macca tree on the front lawn, where Mickey had wanted his ashes buried. The focal point was a damask-covered table containing his ashes, a nice photograph and a sumptuous floral arrangement which she had done in his honour. But lovely isn't fitting when something should be more substantial, and the whole family was furious with her, even though she remained oblivious to the offence she had caused.

She was oblivious as well to how utterly she had let Mickey down at the moment of scattering his ashes. Marjorie, Kitty, Michael, Gloria and I had all agreed that the most appropriate people to scatter them were those who had given him life. However, when the moment came, Michael, who, aside from needing help to get up and walk, was so bereft that it was obvious the task was beyond him, pointed the urn in Gloria's direction. She waved it away. 'You do it,' she said to Kitty, who was sitting beside her, as if she were graciously endowing her with the privilege of entering a ballroom before her.

Kitty took the urn, turned to me with an expression that was a mixture of bemusement and disbelief and mouthed under her breath for us to scatter our brother's ashes together. We rose as one, screwed the lid off the urn together, then took turns to scatter his ashes where he had wanted them to be buried, cognisant of the fact that even that wish had not been fulfilled, for Gloria had refused to countenance it.

'There's no way he's going to be buried here,' she had decreed. 'Not when old *nayger* is so superstitious. If word ever got out, we'd never be able to sell the house if we want to in the future. Scattering ashes is another matter altogether. They're so ignorant they won't mind that, little realizing that a corpse is a corpse whether its ashes are scattered or buried.'

Nor was Gloria's refusal to scatter her son's ashes the only astonishing turn events took during the service. The only dry eyes belonged to her. Everyone else was upset, even the socialites who had seen practically nothing of Mickey since our teenage years together, but who were nevertheless moved by the death at only forty-six of a man who loved life and had everything to live for.

After the service, there was a reception, as there always is. I did my utmost to avoid Gloria and cannot communicate how relieved I was that I had been wise enough to stick to the decision I had made in 1982 never again to spend another night under my mother's roof. At the conclusion of the reception, I was glad that I had somewhere to go rather than to stay and listen to this deluded bitch congratulate herself on the lovely send-off she had given her son. 'Christ,' I said to Marjorie and Kitty, who were also upset by the trivialization of the occasion, 'doesn't Mummy ever connect with reality?'

From then, until my departure from Jamaica, I did my utmost to avoid Gloria. Once the overseas relations had all left, she made this easy for me, as she was never at home. From morning till night, this supposedly devoted wife, who had shirked her duty to her son under the guise of supporting her husband in his hour of need, was on the street. She left him to his own devices, with only the servants or whoever might drop in, to cope with his grief alone.

Michael never recovered from having to witness his son's funeral. He now started to say that he wanted to die too, though I doubt that his desire was based solely on Mickey's death. He could no longer read, which was a severe loss to someone who was as omnivorous a reader as he had always been. He could barely talk and, when he made the effort, was virtually unintelligible to anyone who did not know him well, what with his speech-impediment and the inaudibility Parkinson's brought with it. He could not walk without assistance and, even with it, could only shuffle for a few yards before collapsing from the exertion. He spent most of his time lying in bed, but even there he was a prisoner of his disabled body, for he could not turn without the assistance of his nurse. He used to watch television for short snatches but did not have the strength to sustain longer viewing, with the result that his life had been reduced to a limbo-like existence of boring nothingness somewhere between life and death.

To give Gloria her due, she still slept with him every night in their specially-made bed which was larger than imperial size. 'If I didn't,' she said, 'those damned nurses would never turn him when he needs to be turned. I can count the number of times they've been awake when he rasps out the request. Even though they're supposed to be awake on the sofa in case he needs them, they're always fast asleep.'

To what extent Gloria's claims were her typical self-dramatization, one will never know, but what Kitty and I did discover, the night of his funeral, was how Gloria used to slap him around when she felt in the mood. Birdie, the housekeeper, told us how she would 'box him up when the spirit take her.'

Ironically, Michael never said anything to any of us, though this abuse was a well-established feature of his infirmity by the time he passed away in December 1994. I suspect he remained silent because he knew that Gloria would only deny it if he complained, then, once the fuss had died down, she would be even worse.

It would subsequently emerge after the funeral that Birdie had tipped Libby off some time before Michael died, but she had decided not to intercede as long as Gloria did not do him actual physical harm, because doing so would only result in the staff being dismissed. And Michael wanted to be surrounded by people he knew and liked.

For my part, I cannot help feeling that our father had another motive for bearing Gloria's abusiveness with the resignation he did. For most of his married life, he had stood by silently while our mother abused us, always uttering the same refrain: 'Whether your mother is wrong or right, she is right.' He had also permitted her to abuse relations and staff, and only very rarely had he objected, though these intercessions had invariably resulted in her backing off, which made his silences all the more unacceptable as a result. Because he did have a conscience, I suspect that he bore his cross with the knowledge that what he was called upon to endure was infinitely less terrible than what he had so cavalierly allowed many of us, his children especially, to suffer.

The chickens, so to speak, had come home to roost. Wasn't it only just and right that he should allow them to crap all over him? At least they weren't pecking at his innards the way they had done with us. But maybe his motivation was even simpler. Maybe he felt that he deserved the abuse Gloria was giving him because he had somehow let her down. She was always very adept at getting her victims to feel guilty about her or to sympathize with her. Or maybe he just loved her, abusiveness and all, and if this was the price he paid for being with her, then so be it.

By the time Michael died, Gloria was as eager for him to go as he said he was. 'On the day your father died, your mother went up to the hospital and kept on saying to him, "What are you hanging on for? Let go, for God's sake. Let go. Just let go, old man." She was really fed up with him but he couldn't die until his time came,' his nurse, whom I later inherited as a nanny for my boys, told me.

Of course, dealing with long-term infirmity is difficult; and Gloria had seen that Michael was given fine medical and personal care from the nurses and staff over the years. None of us could decry her right to be relieved on his and her own behalf, though the hypocritical way in which she immediately turned their relationship into something that it wasn't, was remarkable. Narcissists, however, always revise relationships to support their self-image. 'Isn't it funny?' observed his nephew Eddie. 'When Uncle Mike was alive, Gloria didn't have a nice word to say about him. But now that he's dead, he's become a saint.'

Little knowing what we were letting ourselves in for, Kitty, Libby, her husband and children and I flew into Jamaica for the funeral. We could hardly believe it when Gloria announced to us that she intended to have another private funeral. 'Absolutely not,' we said. As one, we siblings argued that he was our father and that gave us a right to have a say in how his send-off was managed. A private occasion would trivialize him and deny those who wished to pay him their last respects the opportunity to do so. Marjorie, who had flown in from Cayman with her husband, backed us up. This, however, did not stop her silly sister from continuing to argue for a guests-only event. 'Daddy's funeral is not one of your parties,' Libby snarled, curling her top lip in a dead giveaway of scorn, while Kitty screamed, 'I'm not allowing you to ruin Daddy's death the way you ruined Mickey's.' Knowing how much our vain mother cared about public perception, the three of us then announced that we would be boycotting the funeral unless it was open to the public.

'For God's sake, Gloria!' Marjorie interceded. 'Michael isn't even in his grave yet, and already you've started the squabbling. Let him rest in peace. Acknowledge that his children have the right to see their father buried in a manner that is in keeping with the dignity of his life.'

Reluctantly, Gloria gave way, and Michael got the send-off he deserved, not that his pathologically energised widow was going to miss any other opportunities to give full rein to her narcissistic tendencies.

Narcissists are both laughable and frightening if only because their disconnection with reality allows them to twist and turn everything, even the most obscure aspects of history, into something you would never imagine it could be. I was now about to discover just how resourceful Gloria could be.

The first inkling I had that my father had been a saint was when my sisters, mother, and aunt were sitting in the front pew at Sts Peter and Paul Church waiting for his funeral service to begin. To fill time, I read the oration Gloria had composed at the back of the Order of Service. Articulate and moving, it was a dignified acknowledgment of his virtues, and showed what a talent Gloria had for writing. She pointed out his undoubted kindness and generosity in the face of need: he had educated many of his clerks' children as well as assisting with the education of some twenty nephews and nieces, and had also helped many others out financially when they needed it. He had even started friends up in business without seeking recompense. But then she couldn't resist ruining a splendid accomplishment by tipping it into fantasy, stating, rather pointlessly as I then thought, that Michael was a devout son of the church who had gone to Mass every Sunday.

Libby and Kitty had also been reading the Order of Service at the same time, and, when they reached the end, Libby and I both said at the same time how beautiful Gloria's reminiscences were. 'Church every Sunday?!!!' we then added jokingly. Gloria, who was known for her wit and sense of humour, could easily have done what Marjorie or anyone else would have, and said something like, 'Well, you know, it's a eulogy.' Instead she demanded that we accept the lie as a fact, asserting seriously, 'Your father went to Mass every Sunday of his life until he was too ill.' We shot each other a look, as if to say. 'What's the point of sticking to our guns?' and in so doing acceded to Gloria's reshaping of history yet again. Only later, when she said, 'Monseignor has agreed that I can be buried with your father when my time comes,' did I realize that this Pope-hating Anglican had manipulated the poor man into a concession based entirely on a series of lies concerning both her status and Daddy's.

At least on this occasion Gloria gave a loved one a suitable send-off. Michael's funeral turned out to be both beautiful and tasteful, with his many friends, relations, colleagues, former employees and a host of other people I had never seen paying respects. Back at the house afterwards, I saw friends and relations I hadn't seen for over twenty years, for funerals and weddings are the big bonding events for international families. While the former are poignant events, they also afford people, who lead divergent lives in a variety of places, an opportunity to come together to celebrate not only the departed life but also life itself.

Everyone who knew Michael and Gloria well wondered how she would cope with widowhood. She had been so indulged for half a century that this was a reasonable supposition. While ill health had ruined the last years of his life and shown her to be a conscientious overseer, theirs had been a turbulent union in which he had played the spoiling if selfish adorer to her spoiled and self-centred adored. To a large extent, he had made it possible for her to remain not merely a child but an *enfant terrible*, and everyone in the family had a great deal of sympathy for her.

For my part, I had put past differences to one side and been as kindly as possible ever since Michael's admission into Intensive Care in October 1994, when it had become likely that he would die this time, even though there had been other close calls in the past. As a result of my attitude, something of the old ease which Gloria had enjoyed with me, while I was growing up and being the endlessly obliging nurturer, had re-entered our relationship. The others, noticing that, had immediately cast me in the old role of favourite, thereby absolving themselves of the burden of having to deal with Gloria and ensuring that she would look to me to lean upon, which, of course, is precisely what she did.

It has to be said, I was not surprised by this. I had always said to Mickey, who constantly wondered how long Mummy was 'going to keep up her malice' regarding me, 'Have no fear. If Daddy dies on a Tuesday, she'll be on the blower to me on the Wednesday, trying to reel me back in.'

The question was: how did I feel and what did I want to do?

I cannot say that I trusted Gloria any more than I had previously. I liked her a bit more, because she was undoubtedly charming when she wanted to be, but even then, I did not like her so much that I would have gone out of my way to see her, had she been anyone but my mother.

But she was my mother. That was the sticking point. That was what made our relationship unique. That was what gave it spiritual overtones that other relationships lacked, for God in his wisdom had ordained that we were mother and daughter. I also wanted my children to be part of an extended family, and with Michael dead, she might prove to be more amenable to good behaviour than she had hitherto been. Although I did not kid myself into thinking that she was going to turn into a wonderful person, I was prepared to give her a chance to be a part of my life as long as she behaved in a positive and constructive manner.

She, seeing the opening, took it. At first she seemed to be turning over a new leaf and becoming a nicer, kinder, less demanding person, not only with me but with everyone else. She seemed to drink less, or at least no longer came across as aggressively drunk as she had before.

The following year, Kitty remarried, appropriately enough for Michael's favourite child, another Michael. Gloria, who might have had a reputation for generosity in the world at large but actually had a tightly closed fist where her children were concerned, surprised us all by insisting on paying for the wedding. Charming though the occasion was, it was also bitter-sweet for us, our loss driven home by Marjorie's husband giving Kitty away instead of her own father or brother. 'We're now a family of hens,' Marjorie quipped poignantly and only too truthfully, voicing what was in all our minds.

Hendom, however, seemed to have humanized Gloria in a way nothing else had in the past. She made an attempt to muck in with everyone and to be just another member of the family, rather than the Queen Bee who would buzz around making everyone's life a misery as she picked fights or demanded attention. She got along with Marjorie rather than taking pot-shots at her sibling, and also had smooth, un-contentious dealings with Libby and me. Her conduct was so amiable that we all commented upon it. The only disquieting note she struck was when she laid claim to being so close to Mickey that 'he told me everything. He never ever made a move without first consulting me.' This about a son who would have preferred to have his tongue torn out by pliers without anaesthetic rather than tell our mother anything of note, even when they had been ostensibly getting along, was almost too much to bear. But bear it we did – in silence – little knowing that she was simply being true to the narcissist's need to find a use in death for those they had also used in life, tailoring the relationship to her self-idolizing needs.

Of course, no one is perfect and if we want to have relationships with others, we have to accept them with their faults. As Gloria's self-promotion shrank to more tolerable levels, I was happy to reward her – and myself – with a closer relationship. I therefore started to telephone her once a week, just to check in and see that she was okay. I also used to telephone Marjorie as well, and the difference in tone and content could not have been more pronounced. With my mother, the conversation, no matter how pleasant, was always stilted, always revolved around her, and always consisted of her complaining about everything, especially how 'lonesome' she was. Marjorie, on the other hand, always wanted to know what I was up to. When she asked after the children, you knew she was genuinely interested and not just being polite. And complaints about the imperfect world were never a feature of our calls.

Nevertheless, my relationship with Gloria had improved no end, and if one had to exercise patience, at least the duty was not totally unpleasant.

The following year, I was asked to go cruising on a friend's boat in the Lesser Antilles. My boys' nanny was also due her annual leave in Jamaica, and Gloria actually offered to keep them for the week that I was going to be away. This, I saw, was a way of getting me to visit, which I was happy to do, for I was strongly motivated to have as good and positive a relationship with her as I could.

Before heading for Jamaica, I flew with the boys and a friend to Grand Cayman, where we spent time with Marjorie and Alex and had a lovely, relaxed time. Then it was on to Jamaica with the hope that Annette's presence would assure us of some protection in the event that Gloria's maliciousness came to the fore again.

At first, things went swimmingly, but by the end of Annette's stay, the leopard couldn't keep her spots dimmed any longer. Annette and I arrived home, the day before she was due to return to London and I to leave for Antigua, to find Gloria in high dudgeon. 'You allow those children to run wild. They have no discipline. They ran from the pool into the house naked,' my mother, who had never before espoused prudery, said waspishly.

I laughed.

'It's no laughing matter. They were naked. Do you think it's appropriate for children to run around naked, as if they're savages or wild animals?' she demanded.

'For goodness sake, Mummy,' I said, trying to reintroduce an element of proportion into the exchange, 'they're three years old. What could possibly be wrong with three-year-olds running around naked? It's not as if anyone but the servants can see them, and even if someone else could, they're too young for there to be any harm.'

Gloria looked at me with her most withering expression. 'You look as if you're bringing them up to be homosexuals,' she said as nastily as she could.

My blood pressure rose instantly. For a second, I was tempted to warn her to back off, but decided that I would ignore her instead. I didn't want poor Annette finding herself in the middle of one of those amazing rows for which our family was justifiably notorious.

Also, I couldn't help suspecting that my mother was deliberately trying to orchestrate a scene which she could then use to prevent me from going on the cruise. The children couldn't come with me because it was just too dangerous to take them on a sailing boat of under a hundred feet until they could swim properly. Although their nanny had returned from leave and would be taking care of them in my absence with no inconvenience to their grandmother, I saw how easily Gloria could scupper my trip if I gave her an opening. I could almost hear her refusing to allow the children to stay with her if I said anything, and this escalating into a full-scale row. Then I would be forced to make alternative arrangements in less than a day, which the children would find unsettling, or forgo the trip altogether.

Gloria would have known that there was no way I would relegate my children to *ad hoc* arrangements. Her intention was plainly to make me cancel the trip and, in so doing, condemn myself to spending an extra week with her. However, I was not prepared to do that under any circumstances, so rather than react to Gloria's provocation and give her what she wanted, I muttered something inoffensive and got Annette away before the conflagration took hold.

Although I was upset, I was nevertheless pleased that Gloria had given my friend a glimpse of how bitchy, vicious, argumentative, manipulative and malevolent she could be for no apparent reason. Seeing was always preferable to people having to believe a second-hand account.

The following day, Gloria offered to take me to the airport. This in itself was unusual, but the reason became apparent *en route* when she warned me not to interfere with her drinking. I was only too happy to provide her with the assurances she sought, for I sincerely believe that people have a right to destroy themselves if they wish to do so. My overriding concern was not to live her life for her, but to have as good and happy a relationship as I could, and I told her as much. This seemed to satisfy her, and I boarded the flight feeling that the conversation had clarified things from both our perspectives.

I returned from the cruise to hear from Gloria that there had been no ructions, though she had rather disrespectfully ignored the children's established routine and had made them go to bed at six o'clock every evening, despite the fact that the sun did not set until later. This I discovered the first evening I was back, when the boys came out to the front veranda, where I was sitting with her, to tell us goodnight. 'But it's bright daylight,' I spluttered to the nanny. Gloria quickly jumped in.

'They've been going to bed, as all well-behaved young gentlemen do, every night at a civilized hour,' she declared authoritatively. 'Haven't you, boys?'

Dima and Misha nodded sheepishly, planted decorous kisses on their grandmother's proffered cheek, then I kissed them goodnight. 'I take my hat off to you,' I said, not without a measure of irony, as soon as they had gone inside, 'even though I've never found it necessary for them to go to bed when it's bright daylight. What I want to know is: how did you accomplish the feat?'

'Oh, there was all hell to pay and a great battle of wills the first night, but by the second night they realized opposition was futile. Let me tell you something, you'd better look out. They're no more than three feet tall and already they wrap you around their little fingers. If you lack control now, how are you going to manage when they're six feet tall? You'd better take a leaf out of my book if you know what's good for you,' she said.

Even though I was miffed at my mother's usurpation of the boys' regimen, I decided it would be silly to make an issue of it. This was the acceptable face of mother-daughter conflict, and she had hardly done anything terrible. True, once I had left for Antigua she had ordered the nanny to keep them outside in the grounds from the moment they had finished their breakfast until they were ready for their late afternoon bath prior to having dinner and going to bed. But they had suffered no harm, even if they were now brown as berries thanks to having spent so much time outside. If she wasn't your ideal grandmother, at least she had leavened the loaf with humour when she was in a good mood, for the boys were perceptibly amused by her. The only sensible thing was for me to accommodate our differences, especially now that our relationship was more normal and constructive than it had been for over two decades. So I focused on being grateful that the boys were developing an acceptable relationship with their grandmother and that she had 'kept' them, thereby permitting me to go on a most enjoyable cruise.

Relationships being ongoing things in which all healthy people respond appropriately to the positive as well as the negative, my emotional response to Gloria's generally positive conduct was to reward it by becoming more positive in my attitude towards her. Quite naturally, I was lowering my guard, not enough to lose the reserve I had developed towards her over the years, but enough to believe that her benevolence ran deeper than it actually did. Almost despite myself, I was coming to trust her: an almost fatal mistake, as things would turn out, but one which I defy anyone with a heart not to have made.

I wish I could say that I was the only member of the family who fell for Gloria's benevolent act, but I was not. Marjorie, Libby and Kitty all fell into the trap, albeit in varying degrees. As Kitty was the only one of the four of us who had always had an uncomplicated relationship with her, her emotional need to have a positive resolution to a mixed past was less pronounced than ours. For that reason, Kitty was still freest from the pitfalls of false hope or unproductive tolerance and, as a result, was the first to see through the more acceptable façade to the destructive reality that still existed beneath it.

The catalyst was her daughter Gabriela's birth. Kitty had absolutely no experience with babies and was not going to have a nanny, so Marjorie, Libby, Gloria and I agreed to take turns giving her the benefit of our experience until she had adjusted to motherhood. Marjorie, ever the nurturing 'Mama' to each of her four 'children', as she called us, flew up to Boca Raton for the birth. Afterwards she settled Kitty and the baby at home, prior to handing over to Libby, who flew in from the Midwest to take over. By the time I arrived from London to relieve Libby, a pattern had been established. 'Take a tip from me, keep your mouth shut. Kitty is determined to do everything by the book,' Libby warned as soon as I landed. I hadn't been at Kitty's house for more than an hour before I saw what she meant. Kitty had read all the baby books which were then supposed to be the last word in mothering, and there was no way she was open to any of us making practical suggestions that went contrary to the experts' advice.

I could well understand her need to keep us at a distance. In a family such as ours, where everyone is opinionated and some of us are dominating, there is a thin line between assistance and interference, and if she wanted to demarcate rather more firmly than was otherwise necessary while she was in a fragile state, that was fine. As Marjorie and Libby had done, I therefore respected Kitty's choice to follow a literary rather than a practical maternal model. After making it clear that I was there to be called upon as and when she wanted me, I left her to her own devices, relieved to see that she was intent on being a good and conscientious mother. Only once, when Gabriela, who had colic, cried throughout the night until five o'clock in the morning, did I take the initiative. I went into the baby's bedroom and said, as gently as possible, 'Kitty, you must be dead tired. Here. Let me try.'

An obviously weary Kitty gladly handed the baby to me in a motion that said, 'Thank God.' I took Gabriela in my arms, spoke to her in my most soothing voice, and within minutes she was fast asleep.

'What did you do that I didn't?' Kitty asked as if she had somehow failed.

'She was picking up your anxiety. Just remember if she takes too long to settle, you'll become anxious, which will create a never-ending spiral of anxiety, with her feeding off yours and you feeding off hers. Then she'll never go to sleep. Always give yourself a break before you get too caught up in the cycle. No baby ever suffered because it was left to cry alone for five minutes. In that time, she might even fall asleep, and if not, when you return to her refreshed, there'll be a calmer you to soothe her,' I said.

'Why didn't I think of that?' Kitty asked.

'Because experience teacheth wisdom, and you don't have any experience yet. Give yourself another few months, and believe me, you'll know all the little secrets that only experience brings.'

In the days to come, I was most impressed with how attentive a mother Kitty was. The truth was, except for that one incident, she could have managed perfectly well without me. I was really there for moral support. This was just as well, because I was being replaced by Gloria who, despite having had four children, had never taken care of any of us. Though Gloria had laid claim to being fond of babies when she was younger, it was one thing to coo at an infant when it was bathed, powdered, dressed and fed, but quite another to undertake those four tasks without a maternity nurse and a nanny to assist you and hand the baby back to at the first sign of trouble. Quite how much experience Gloria actually had with infants was therefore a moot point, and I for one knew her too well to put reliance on any claims she made to expertise.

The day before I was due to fly back to London, I picked Gloria up at Fort Lauderdale Airport and drove her back to Kitty's house in Boca Raton. The harbingers were not good. She was in aggressive mode and went on and on about Kitty's husband Michael, to whom she had taken an aversion since the marriage. The problem lay in the fact that he was not as deferential as she would have liked. Although he was correct and polite on the few occasions they had met, he made it plain in his own quiet way that he was his own man and not someone she could wrap around her little finger. To a narcissist, that is like a red flag to a bull. The better she got to know him, the less she liked him. Since she couldn't very well say, 'I can't stand Michael because he has too much backbone for me,' she had started to criticize him on spurious grounds. Michael, she insisted, had married Kitty for her money and for social advantage. She refused to accept that his family had at least as much money as ours, or that they were every bit our social peers, his mother being a scion of one of Spain's greatest aristocratic families. She brushed away facts, like Queen Fabiola of the Belgians being one of his mother's friends from childhood, as being of no significance, and declined to acknowledge that it was far better for a family to boast a saint, as theirs did, than a politically important archbishop, which was the best we could do. 'I am going to whip him into line,' she decreed ominously, so I tried pointing out that she had come up to help, and her attitude would only cause trouble. 'He needs to be put in his place, and I am here to give him his Waterloo,' she replied stubbornly. Realizing that reason was never going to prevail, I shut my mouth. As Gloria was so fond of saying, you can take a horse to the water, but you can't force it to drink.

Even I could never have imagined, however, how quickly her stay would degenerate once I had left. Within forty-eight hours, Kitty, who could just about tolerate Gloria's bitchy provocation of her husband, had thrown her out of the house, because our dear mother kept on creeping into Gabriela's room and waking her up every time Kitty managed to get her to sleep. As babies with colic take hours to settle, one needs no imagination to appreciate why Kitty acted as she did.

However, Gloria being Gloria, she spun Kitty's justifiable action into a platform for martyrdom. She got in touch with Marjorie, Libby and me as well as her Floridian cousins and complained bitterly about Kitty. To hear her tell the story, our sister was a 'stinking little ingrate' who had spurned her help and was making a 'complete arse of herself over a man, humiliating herself at every turn'. She declared that she never wanted to see her again, ignoring the really vicious act of waking up a baby with colic every time its mother had managed to get it settled, and indeed, it was a year or two before things had quieted down enough for them to resume relations.

In the meantime, Gloria was careful to keep in with both Libby and me. She even started to telephone me occasionally, and when I mentioned that I was going to Cayman for Easter with the kids and my new boyfriend and his daughter, she proposed joining us there. This she did, and was as mild as a lamb throughout our stay.

That June my autobiography was published. One never knew what response Gloria would take to things, but she was anodyne. I was pleased to see that harmony continued to reign between us. Though I had made things easy for her by declining to criticize her in print and had actually managed to accomplish the apparently irreconcilable feat of fairly recounting my life story while ignoring the damage one of the leading participants in it had caused, had she had it in for me, she could have jumped on a myriad of things and whipped herself up into a frenzy.

There was no doubt that Gloria was lonely at this time of her life. Whenever one telephoned and asked how she was, a plaintive little voice always replied, 'Lonesome. Very lonesome.' She somehow managed to forget to mention the many people who dropped in to see her or asked her out. To listen to her, no one ever came to visit and she never received an invitation to anything. However, I knew better, not only because she was often out when I rang, but also because I received reports from alternative sources and had also seen, on my visits to Jamaica, just how full a life she led. She had many friends and acquaintances, some from Old Jamaica and some from New. She was still active in horticultural circles and travelled all over the world judging events when she wasn't travelling for its own sake. She was the First Vice-President of the Salvation Army, which is nothing like the Salvation Army in Britain or the US, where the charity lacks eminence. In Jamaica it is the nation's foremost charity and as a result is tremendously prestigious. It has always done excellent work amongst the poor, and Gloria had turned her organizational skills and dynamism to good effect for them since the 1980s, earning the respect of the organizing body in the process. Her life was not the desert she made it out to be, even though it was hardly as glamorous or exciting as it had been in the halcyon days when she was younger and Jamaica was the ultimate in chic.

For someone who had so angrily resisted the passage of time and the inevitable reduction of the seductive powers that came with the loss of youthful beauty, Gloria appeared to have finally made the transition to a useful and serene middle age with a degree of success that I, for one, was happy to witness. She seemed to have understood that life was about more than being the centre of attention and the cynosure of all eyes. Her activities suggested real progress along the road to profundity, and she no longer reacted viciously if someone else dared to snatch away some of the attention she had previously regarded as being her sole due. I concluded that she had finally sorted out her values and had chosen gold over glitter. This was a tremendous relief, for a relatively healthy and balanced mother is infinitely preferable to a sick and unbalanced one, and if there were occasional flashes of the *enfant terrible* of old, circumstances dictated that one cut her some slack and recognize that she was a much nicer person than she had ever been. All the signs were that she would continue to develop along the same lines, and I for one did not envisage a return to the past. How naïve I was.

Still not understanding that the leopard hadn't changed her spots but was merely concealing them, I continued telephoning Gloria regularly and provided her with as much emotional support as one could from across an ocean. Occasionally, she would even telephone me, and I was therefore happy to ask her to join the kids and me on a trip to Thailand for their half-term in 1998.

'I'll treat you,' she said.

'That won't be necessary, Mummy, but thanks nevertheless,' I said.

'No. I insist,' she said.

She arrived two months after *The Real Diana*, my biography of the Princess of Wales, was published in America, in time to take in the Chelsea Flower Show. While she happily toured the displays, I was caught up in some pretty unwelcome litigation with which I had to deal.

On the one hand, I was being sued for unpaid fees by a law firm that had represented me in various libel actions in the early 1990s, notwithstanding that I had entered into a contingency agreement with them and therefore should not be liable for fees. Indeed, the partner who had handled my matters at that firm had even confirmed this fact in writing as well as on tape; but that hadn't stopped the senior partner from issuing a writ once they fell out. On the other hand, a house I owned was being occupied by a crooked tenant, and I had instructed another law firm, which came highly recommended by the well known socialite Sir Dai Llewellyn, to get her out as well as to defend me against the other law firm's claims. While the 'fees' case was always going to be protracted, the 'crooked tenant' one should have been resolved by this time, but my current 'solicitor' had – mistakenly, according to him – served the court papers early, with the result that the crooked tenant, who should have been forced out by the court within three months, was still *in situ* after six.

In a situation such as this, dismissal is the usual response. However, I had not yet sacked the solicitor, whom I would later discover wasn't even a solicitor though I had been led to believe he was one, because he had agreed to absorb all additional expenses resulting from his error. This he characterized as over-eagerness on his part rather than incompetence or worse. Had I changed solicitors, I would have had to pay the new one, so it actually made financial sense to have the non-solicitor straighten out his mess free of charge.

However, because I could not trust the non-solicitor to do his job properly, I had to check everything he did, to ensure that there were no further slipups, especially as the crooked tenant was determined to stay in the house as long as she could spin out the legal process. Just before we were due to leave for Thailand, she had even had the temerity to make an application to the court to have the trial postponed till the end of the summer school holidays in September.

These preposterous lawsuits meant that I was buried in paperwork when I wasn't giving television and press interviews to promote my Diana book, with the result that I could not sit down all day and keep Gloria company the way she wanted me to, even if I had wanted to – which I did not.

To an extent, the woman visiting me was something of a stranger. While some things, such as her persistent desire to have you 'sit with' her were familiar, others were not. She had never been a houseguest of mine before, and I was pleasantly surprised to note that she was actually very respectful of one's environment. She moved nothing, or if she did, she replaced it exactly where she had found it. As I am the sort of person who places things precisely where I want them and expects them to remain there until such time as I move them, I was gratified to note that she was not so arrogant as certain cousins, who came to stay and moved everything that got in their way. She was also quiet and took care to fit in with what was going on around her, rather than imposing her presence upon the household, the way some other houseguests did.

Gloria had friends in London, some from her youth whom she had not seen for years. They were eager to entertain her, and I was surprised that she displayed so little interest in seeing them. Had I not made the arrangements myself, I daresay she might well have left London without seeing any of them. This struck me as perplexing, for the Gloria I knew and remembered had always been extremely sociable, and I was astonished by her attitude. Ultimately, it would prove instructive and lead me to conclude that the people whom she claimed to be so fond of actually meant less to her in reality than they did as figures in her own mental drama: another classic feature of narcissism.

All in all, however, her stay in London prior to our journey to Thailand was a success. Even though I had a feeling that there was nothing to relate to beneath the pleasant surface, I was just so glad that the superficialities had been pleasant that I overlooked the lack of depth.

In Thailand, however, I started to find this lack of depth disquieting. She seemed to have no real interest in me or the children, which made conversation at dinner, the one meal of the day we shared together, stilted. As often as not, this would result in us having a non-conversation about nothing, which was something of a strain. Nor did she want to see the sights of Phuket, which the boys and I did, or even to go on an elephant ride, despite never having been on one before. She said she was perfectly happy staying in her bungalow reading – something which she had never done before – or resting, while the boys and I swam in the pool or at the beach during the day. The one time she came alive was when we went shopping, which we usually did after dinner. Even then, she surprised me, because she insisted on paying for suits for the boys, despite the fact that I would happily have bought them.

But I noticed that, when the tailor was fitting her suit, the demanding Gloria of old was neither dead nor buried, because she was adamant that he fulfil her every wish so exactly that I ended up having knots in my stomach. Just like in the days of old when she used to do the same thing to me while I was fitting her.

That moment aside, the trip passed off so uneventfully and superficially cordially that I could hardly believe it. Beneath the surface, I remained unconvinced that it was the success she indicated it had been. Whether that was because I had learned, over the years, never to trust the face she presented to one, knowing that it usually concealed another, or whether it was because I was perturbed by the absence of detectable emotion beneath the surface, I did not know. What I did know was that I would not have been surprised if Marjorie, Libby or Kitty had told me that she had reported back to them that she had had the most dreadful and boring time of her life. Instead of which, I subsequently heard, to my utter astonishment, that she had said it was one of the most enjoyable holidays she had ever had. Not that I believed the veracity of her positive claims any more than I would have believed the negative. While it had been superficially pleasant, it had hardly been that great. Indeed, beneath the pleasant surface, there had been such a detectable void that it qualified as something less than satisfying. But if she wanted to make it out to be better than it was, that was fine by me.

We returned to London for me to be confronted by a legal mess. The non-solicitor had sent in a massive bill for the work he had guaranteed he would not charge me for. I promptly telephoned him to ask for an explanation. He denied having waived the fees and tried to blackmail me by saying that I could not afford to have two law firms saying that I had not paid their fees, for it would look as if I was in the habit of dodging my commitments to lawyers. 'I have a firm policy when confronted by blackmail,' I said. 'Resist it.'

When blackmail failed to elicit the response he desired, he said that he would refuse to hand over the papers for either action to any new solicitors I instructed until I stumped up the twenty-something thousand pounds he was demanding. 'You seem to forget that I am the one who did all of the witness statements and who has had to spoon-feed you every step of the way in both actions,' I said. 'I have all my work on disc, and I can reconstitute the files. I don't need you, you snivelling little worm, and if you don't hand over my files, I'll sue you for them.'

No sooner had I hung up than Gloria, who had hitherto been assiduous in keeping herself utterly uninvolved in any of my legal troubles in the two decades I had endured them, jumped up and started telling me what I should be doing. However, nothing she said was relevant.

The last thing I needed at that moment was to listen to the dominating egotist, who believed in her perfection and everyone else's relative inadequacy, and who could never resist regulating whatever drama was taking place around her. I had seen her hijack too many of other people's dramas, including my own marital woes, turning them into her own production and gratifying all her needs, without once giving a rational thought to the welfare of any of the other participants, to allow her to gain a toehold now.

'Mummy, please,' I said as pleasantly as I could. 'Much as I appreciate your concern, you don't know the ins and outs and have no experience of legal affairs.'

'Come and sit with me and tell me all about it, and we'll sort it out together,' she said, hoping to wheedle me into turning over control to her while at the same time 'sitting with' her.

'Much as I'd love to, I really don't have the time. I only have a few days to reconstitute the files and find another solicitor. I'll be doing in days what one normally does in weeks,' I said, a powerful sense of *déjà vu* overtaking me.

When she realized that I was eluding her, the sweet older lady, who had been radiating mildness for the last few weeks, suddenly dropped the mask. 'You can't expect people to give you good service if you accuse them of cheating you,' she snapped nastily. 'My advice to you is telephone him back and say you misunderstood.'

'And pay him the £20,000 he's trying to screw out of me?' I spluttered in disbelief.

'You can't expect him to work for nothing,' she said.

In a flash, I saw where she was coming from. She wanted me to be available to her for the week or so she had left in England, but I would be otherwise engaged if I had to deal with this legal mess.

'There is no way I am paying anyone for work he wouldn't have had to do if he hadn't cocked things up, causing me losses of several thousand pounds, and which he has moreover confirmed in front of a barrister he would not be charging me for. If you want to reward him for what is effectively extortion, you go ahead and do so. He'll turn over the files to another solicitor, and I'll only have to do a minimal amount of checking. Otherwise, I fear, you'll just have to entertain yourself while I attend to this, as there is no way I am succumbing to blackmail,' I said as calmly and pleasantly as I could force myself to manage.

'Child,' the Gloria of old rasped even more nastily now that I was frustrating her, 'you will clearly never learn.'

'And what does that mean?' I asked with just enough edge in my voice for her to know that I wasn't going to be quite the pushover she might have thought I would be. The rule in our world was that a hostess was never rude to a guest, and I suspected that she was hoping I would rely upon it, but there was no way I was going to abide by it in these circumstances.

'The way you spoke to that poor man,' she said, one shark intent upon extending courtesy to another, albeit one she didn't even know.

It occurred to me she might also be hoping that if she could convince me to buy his lie, not only would I be available for her entertainment for the remainder of her English stay, but also that the next time she wanted to pull the wool over my eyes, I might be more amenable to being deceived by her and spare her the tongue-lashing the truth warranted. I had over the years witnessed her chipping away at the carapace of other people's resistance, none more so than Michael's, with dogged relentlessness; and though I couldn't be sure that she was doing so in this instance, nor could I be sure that she wasn't. If there was one thing she had taught me, it was to be vigilant against her machinations and to block any route that could be potentially damaging to one's interests. She was just too effective a viper to be dismissed or let off the hook.

'That *poor* man is nothing but a shyster who is trying to extort money out of me and I am mystified as to why you are seeking to defend the indefensible actions of someone you do not even know, against your own daughter,' I said hotly.

Realizing that there was no way she was going to prevail, Gloria wisely threw in the towel. 'You have it your way,' she said neutrally.

'Believe me, I will,' I said. And I did. Not only did I sue the solicitor who wasn't even a solicitor, but his firm had to settle when their own barrister confirmed that they hadn't even paid his fees, despite me having sent them the money to do so. David Scutt also confirmed that the non-solicitor had indeed agreed not to charge me for the work he then tried to obtain some twenty thousand pounds for.

Confronted by the need to occupy herself, Gloria now started seeing the friends it was easy to see, though she did not extend herself to go and see the cousins of hers who lived in the country. I was so preoccupied with reconstituting the files that I had no time for anything else, but Gloria seemed to have assumed a more accommodating attitude now that she realized I was too busy to become the pair of ears she had hoped I would be once the children were at school and she would have me all to herself. Resuming the mantle of accommodation, she even remained equitable when Birdie, her housekeeper, telephoned to say that there had been a burglary at the house in Jamaica and thieves had stolen all the jewellery in the house. 'It doesn't matter,' she said to me so serenely that I was relieved that she was back to being benevolent instead of dominating. 'There was nothing of real value there. Just a lot of gold stuff with the exception of my really good diamond and ruby suite which I wore to a wedding just before I left. Otherwise everything of real value is still in Cayman.'

For all her faults, Gloria was an excellent judge of dubious characters. She had a nose for hidden stench like a tracker dog does for a corpse. As her friend Cecily Tobisch commented when she died, 'Even though she could be so negative about people, time and again she turned out to be right. Once or twice I had to wait fifteen years to see what she meant; but, lo and behold, something she warned me about all that time ago would happen, and I would be amazed at how she had detected that failing in the person.'

This trait now came to the fore in London. A good friend of mine brought around her boyfriend for a working supper. He was interested in acquiring the English rights to my latest Diana book, but since the evening was a mixture of business and pleasure, the tone and structure were sociable. Gloria therefore joined us right after Gary and Charlotte's arrival. Gary, who was crass but charming, with the ego of one of those banking masters of the universe which he had been until recently, started to question Gloria about herself in such a way that we could all tell he was trying to find out how much money she actually had, clearly to see if the information he could elicit might be of use to him sometime in the future. 'I'm really a very humble person,' she said with mock humility, using the word in its classical, and American, meaning, as a precursor to launching into what a wonderful person she was.

'But I thought Georgie was from this grand family,' Gary spluttered, mistaking her usage of humble for the British euphemism for 'common', and thereby showing his hand rather more clearly than he had intended.

As Gloria bristled, ready to strike swords with this man whom you could see, from the expression on her face, she regarded as a swine and peasant, I stepped in.

'Gary,' I said, intent on diverting the conversation into safer pastures. 'Mummy isn't trying to tell you she's humble in the English sense of the word. She's letting you know she has the virtue of modesty. A problem of semantics arising from the way English is used on different sides of the Atlantic, I fear, and nothing at all to do with background or money.'

Without missing a beat, Gary resumed his cross-examination. Charlotte and I noticed that Gloria now had a perceptible antipathy towards him, so I was not surprised when she called me downstairs to the kitchen, ostensibly to help her with refreshing the drinks, and said, 'Make sure you don't have *one thing to do with that man*. He is a real chancer, with worse manners than a hog.'

Despite her contempt for him, once the business side of things had been discussed, Gloria could not resist the temptation to assume centre stage. For the remainder of the evening, she was back to being the same old devourer of attention that she had ever been. No one could get a word in edgewise, not even Gary, who was used to dominating proceedings but had finally been trumped by an even more dominant personality. Thereafter, I was cast back to when I was aged five, ten, fifteen or twenty, as my mother hijacked the conversation, steering it wherever her impulses and urges took her. Good manners alone ensured that I put a good face on things, and while I would have dearly loved to shut her up, I saw how impossible that was, so, bowing to the inevitable, I just sat there, a pair of ears yet again.

Gloria in full flow was an awesome sight, even if it was one I disliked witnessing. I was sitting in my drawing room hoping to be anywhere else, when she informed Gary and Charlotte that the reason her father had been murdered was that he was a Knight Templar who had been liquidated because he knew too much about certain political machinations.

This, I fear, was too much for me.

'What are you talking about?' I snapped. 'Grandpa was murdered by Clifton Eccleston, a thief who killed him for five shillings and his watch. His death had nothing to do with politics.'

'What would you know? You were a child when he was killed. He was my father,' she asserted.

I was absolutely outraged that the daughter Grandpa had loved so dearly could use his murder as yet another device to keep herself the centre of attention while, at the same time, awing her audience enough to receive the doses of admiration and sympathy she required. Bad manners or no bad manners, I was not going to let her get away with such a betrayal. So I started a heated debate with her, which I only let go of when I had made the points I wanted to, namely that she might have her interpretation of her father's death, but I had mine, which was the official, more reality-based, version.

Thereafter, I allowed her to witter on while I analyzed her motivation for spinning Grandpa's murder into something it was not. I came to the disturbing conclusion that she had found a new way to gain ascendancy over others. Now that the world had moved on from the time when breeding was the perfect way to lay claim to superiority, and now that snobbishness was passé, political influence was the politically-correct way to get across how important she was.

This analysis was resonant of the time Mickey had come back to England in the late 1970s after Fidel Castro had been on an official visit to Jamaica. 'You will never believe what happened,' he had said. 'Castro was staying at the Italian Ambassador's Residence, opposite the Canadian High Commissioner's Residence beside our house. People were wondering why he hadn't been put up at Jamaica House or Vale Royal. Mummy said in all seriousness, "The Government has put him there so that they can watch me watch him." Sometimes I think she's really mad.'

I assured Mickey that one should never dismiss her bizarre claims as mere madness, for, if you looked behind them, you usually found a very sane explanation – one that boosted her image or sense of importance.

Or was I being unduly harsh? Was Gloria just paranoid? Although narcissists display symptoms that are uncomfortably close to paranoia, they are not actually psychotic. Rather, they suffer from the character flaw of extreme self-importance, which parallels the self-centredness of paranoiacs, but without its insane aspects. On reflection, I came to the conclusion that anyone who had such tight control over her actions, that she would indulge her 'crazy' theories only when she stood to gain a direct and desired payoff, could not be crazy. Real craziness was beyond the control of the mad, and often as not would result in loss rather than gain. Hers, however, was always within her control and always, except amongst a few people like me, resulted in her achieving the objective she sought. I concluded that, rather than being crazy, she was very deliberately and creatively pulling the strings. As she regaled Gary and Charlotte with her nonsense about the political reasons for Grandpa's murder, I concluded that she was still the old, competitive, attention-seeking, self-important Gloria who would say or do anything to boost herself using those in her life, dead or living.

Once I realized this, I was almost relieved, for at least it meant I knew the person with whom I was dealing. The mild, unreadable Gloria had been a total stranger, and while the old Gloria was less pleasant, at least one could 'read' her.

She was due to return home a day or two later. As if by silent consent, we both stepped back from the abyss, neither referring to the evening that had nearly derailed our newly established pleasant relationship. As she prepared to leave, I brought all my diplomatic skills to bear to convey appreciation without sounding hypocritical, for I wanted to be positive and hoped that by being so, we could lay down another brick in the courtyard of our burgeoning relationship. I remained truly grateful that the overall trip had been reasonably pleasant and relatively successful. If my mother wasn't perfect, and could still be a pill on occasion, at least she wasn't always one the way she used to be. Nevertheless, a little of Gloria went a long way, and I was glad to see her go. Things, I could tell, would have degenerated the longer she stayed, and that I did not want.

Throughout the following year, our relationship continued much as it had since our *rapprochement*. I called her once a week and listened while she remained consumed with self-pity and moaned about how 'lonesome' she was. One was always trying to come up with solutions to the problems Gloria said she had, but she wanted sympathy and attention, not solutions. At some point in every conversation, you would realize this and thereafter be reduced to making sympathetic sounds which might have made her feel better but solved nothing.

However, I never lost heart. I was not about to desist from furnishing solutions just because she seemed incapable of acting upon them. After all, who knew? Where there was life there was hope, no? And someone who was as intelligent, dynamic, energetic and capable as Gloria must, at some point, get bored with having the same problems year in, year out, no?

Of course I faced the fact that she might well never want her problems solved. But, even if she did not, I was not about to desist from providing solutions, for there was no way I was going to allow her to cast me in the role of enabler and make me complicit in the perpetuation of her problems.

Gloria certainly did have problems. She had not repaired the breach with Kitty, and though her relationship with Marjorie was superficially positive, beneath the surface it was anything but. The sisters had a vicious sibling rivalry going back to childhood, and Marjorie did not want to see Gloria in any but the most structured situations.

This could cause problems, such as when Libby's son Andrew was getting married in 1999. All of us planned to fly to the Midwest for the wedding. Then Marjorie announced that she would not be attending if Gloria went. 'I would shoot myself if I had to put up with your mother for a whole week,' she declared. 'Either she goes and I don't, or I go and she doesn't.'

I could not help sympathizing with Gloria, even though I also understood Marjorie's position. Her husband had recently been diagnosed with prostate cancer, and there was every possibility that this might be the last family occasion he would attend. Yet Andrew was Gloria's first-born grandson. She had always got along well with him, and it seemed almost cruel that she would be excluded from his wedding because her sister could not bear to be around her for any length of time. Although I tried to talk Marjorie into softening her stance, pointing out that she and Gloria would not have to come into much contact with each other and that everything had gone well at Kitty's wedding four years before, Marjorie refused to budge. 'There is no way I am putting myself through a week with your mother. It's either her or me.'

Gloria knew as well as the rest of us that Libby would prefer to have Marjorie at the wedding. To her credit, she gave way graciously. Whether she accepted that the chickens were coming home to roost and she deserved her exclusion, I do not know. She was intensely proud and would never have let on that she accepted that she was very much an 'also-ran' in the family stakes, while Marjorie was the favoured thoroughbred of all us children. But she knew it to be the truth and wisely stepped aside, possibly in case she was asked to do so, which she would have found deeply humiliating. I was sad for Gloria and wished that Marjorie had been less resolute, but the fact was, both sisters were getting their just deserts. Ultimately, Gloria had no one to blame but herself for the isolated predicament she now found herself in.

Chapter Twenty-Four

With hindsight, I can see that Gloria might well have kept up her act of being the benevolent old lady towards me, but for two unrelated events. The first was the financial reverses I suffered in the late 1990s, which wiped out the only foundation she had for respecting anyone. Simply put: if you did not have real money, she regarded you as a suitable object for contempt. These reverses began simply enough when a merchant banker friend since the mid-1980s said he was leaving Lazards to set up his own consultancy. Although I do not believe in mixing business with pleasure as a rule and, moreover, had an aversion to the stock market, having been through the crashes of the early 1970s and the late 1980s, he convinced me to sell my London house and turn the proceeds over to him for investment. He promised returns which were very attractive, even doing what few financial advisors do: he provided guarantees which meant that there was no real downside. I had a certain income and the capital was ring-fenced.

It was only after the house was sold that I had the first inkling that something might be amiss. He then informed me that he would take between fifteen and fifty percent of the profit in return for investing my funds. However, he was a very close friend and always going on and on about honour, and as everything seemed to go along swimmingly at first and he was making me money, I marked down the disquiet I had felt to my *naïveté* regarding how the financial world works.

Then the technological bubble burst, and he started to lie about the performance of the portfolio. When he could no longer conceal the losses, he turned to bullying, which was the worst thing he could have done, for I was by that time an old hand at protecting myself against such tactics. His behaviour became so appalling, there was no prospect of continuing a friendship with him. I started to tape our telephone conversations, and when I had enough incriminating material against him, I lodged a formal complaint about him with the Financial Services Authority. Too late, however, to retrieve my financial situation, which was now considerably less secure than it had been before I took his advice. Although I wasn't quite penniless, I was certainly no longer flush.

Meanwhile, the law firm which had sued me for non-payment of contingency fees, despite having lost five and a half of the seven complaints against me in a trial lasting a week, were awarded ninety percent of their costs by the judge. This flew in the face of the rule of proportionality by which judges were supposed to function, for the judge was allowing them to claim costs of some £150,000 for an award of £11,000. That excluded my own costs, which I would also have to bear.

Furious at such a preposterous judgement, I wanted to appeal, but my solicitors assured me there was no point, as the judge had protected himself in his ruling by stating that, notwithstanding the fact that Lord Denning had ruled that the word of a client should always take precedence over that of a solicitor when there was a disagreement regarding fees, he was opting for Lord Wigoder's ruling in the Botkin Adams murder case, namely that a judge should prefer the word of a professional over that of a lay person. In other words, he was using a criminal ruling to permit him to prefer the evidence of his legal colleague over my own, despite the fact that the Chief Justice had specifically ruled that no judge should do so in civil cases like mine.

My lawyers, whether through incompetence or collusion with the other side, took care to prevent me from appealing by also telling me that I had a longer period within which to lodge an appeal than I actually did. The result was that, when I got to Jamaica a few weeks later and discovered from Mickey's old friend David Boxer, who is a justice of the peace, that the judge who had made such an unfair award was a sworn enemy of my brother, it was too late for me to appeal.

Bad enough as that was, what made the situation infinitely worse was the fact that this very judge had kept his association with my brother secret for the first two days of the trial. Then, he had called in the barristers from both sides at the end of the second day and informed them that he 'had an interest to declare'. His interest? That he had acted for my brother in a professional capacity; was sorry to read in the court papers, all of which he affirmed he had read prior to the trial, that he was dead; and wished my barrister to convey to me that he had always liked my brother. Did either side have a problem with him continuing as the judge? Of course, if I had known his real status *vis-à-vis* my brother, I would have called an instant halt to the trial and demanded that my costs and the other side's be paid by the Lord Chancellor's Department. As I was ignorant of the true facts, however, I allowed my lawyers to talk me into agreeing to a continuance of the trial, especially when they argued that it would be silly of me to object, as that would mean having another trial, with me being liable for the costs of this trial so far. 'And he liked your brother,' they reiterated, as if that sealed things in my favour.

Of course, once I discovered from David Boxer how the judge had deceived me, I felt I had grounds for acting and came back to England intent on having his costs award overturned. I was looking at costs of over £200,000 for disputed fees of £11,000 – fees which I could not reasonably have said to have incurred if the contingency agreement whose existence the partner had confirmed did indeed exist. Good friends in the upper reaches of the legal profession warned me, however, that I would only be throwing good money after bad if I appealed, for the legal profession in England always closes ranks to protect its own, and there was no way another judge would unpick the stitch-up, especially as it had been done to protect the senior partner of the firm that had brought the action against me. He was a costs judge.

'It's a pity the press didn't cover your trial,' a friend of mine who is an eminent barrister and senior judge said. 'They couldn't have got away with it then.'

'But they were there for the first two days. You know how boring these trials are. The court reporter asked my solicitor to keep him abreast of the proceedings and warn him when things were coming to an end. He also wanted to see me testify. But my lawyers told me to avoid the press and refused to keep the court reporter in the loop,' I explained.

'Why not, when it was so clearly in your interest to have the bright light of publicity shining on the dark dealings of the court?' said the senior judge, who has a fine sense of theatrics.

'They said they didn't think publicity was in my interest,' I said.

'Ah, well, there we have it, my dear Georgie,' the judge said. 'Take my advice and always shelter under the glare of publicity. It provides a heat that prevents old boys from prevailing,' alluding to the 'old boy network' which has been a byword for corrupt protectionism in several of the professions for well over a century.

Meanwhile, my solicitors were milking the situation, now that the trial was at an end, to screw tens of thousands more pounds out of me than we had agreed upon as their fee. Once again, a law firm was running the same argument that the blackmailing non-solicitor had used the year before: 'If you don't succumb to our blackmail, we will argue that you have a track record of non-payment of lawyers' fees. And, judges always prefer the evidence of members of the legal profession over the lay public's, irrespective of Chief Justice Lord Denning's ruling.'

However, I wasn't any more amenable to their threats than I had been to the non-solicitor's or my mother's, and, despite weighing the risks, disputed their fees through the only venue that had jurisdiction: the courts.

Of course I was taking a big risk. All judges might well be corrupt. But I doubted it. My friend the senior judge was not. My grandfather's cousins, who had been Chief Justice of Jamaica and President of the Court of Appeals of East Africa, had not been. To make sure that I encouraged honesty or, in its absence, expediency, I decided to act as my own lawyer. 'I know that the litigant who acts for him - or herself is supposed to have a fool for a client,' I said to my aunt Marjorie, who was very concerned about what was happening. 'But I don't see what choice I have. The lawyers' game couldn't be more obvious. They overcharge you. You resist and turn to another lawyer for help. That lawyer also overcharges you, and then you have to go to yet another lawyer to rescue you. Except that it's likely he'll also overcharge you, setting up a never-ending spiral of claim and counterclaim, with each law firm emboldened by the prior claims of its predecessors. That's how my father-in-law and the legal profession managed to ruin Margaret Argyll financially. Except that I'm not Margaret. I have the intelligence to defend myself without recourse to any of them. I will beat those bastards at their own game.'

Truthfully, I doubt very much that I would ever have had the backbone or the ability to fight legal professionals on their own turf if I had not had to defend myself against my even more malignant mother. For the first time in my life, I saw how my success in refusing to be defeated by her had strengthened me. In doing so, I had not only liberated myself from her but also from everyone else like her. And by having beaten her at her own game, I could apply the knowledge I had learned to fight – and hopefully conquer – other equally unscrupulous individuals.

Although I cannot exaggerate how nerve-wracking it was to fight the good fight against those bastards, I refused to give way until both law firms either settled with me or withdrew their claims.

Lawsuits are procedural, and judges can throw out cases if you make even minor procedural errors. So I effectively had to learn overnight the legal procedures that all law students take years to learn. At the same time I also had to become proficient in the skill of how to present my case in court without ever having had any experience in doing so. But, I reasoned, if lawyers could do it, so could I. No matter how dreadful some of them were – the legal profession seems to attract a large percentage of aggressive and unscrupulous shits – not one of them could possibly be worse than my mother. All the same, I was to encounter one or two who were her match.

In England, law cases move at a snail's pace. What might take weeks or months in America takes years and sometimes over a decade in the UK. The result was that between 1999 and 2003, I spent a large portion of my time entangled in litigation.

At first, I dealt exclusively with the cases involving the two crooked law firms. The first one settled at the courthouse door when they read the witness statement of the barrister whom they had instructed to act on my behalf. He stated that the law firm had neglected to pay him his fees, even though I had put them in funds to do so, and that the non-solicitor had entered into an agreement with me, in front of him, not to charge for the work for which he had subsequently sought payment. The barrister's statement meant that they would have lost had they been stupid enough to go to trial.

The second law firm had an even more ignominious end. Not only did a judge slash the costs they were claiming by nearly fifty percent, but within a few months I was delighted to receive a letter from the Law Society informing me that the firm had been closed down and the senior partner struck off. So dishonesty hadn't paid off in the long run.

However, there was no doubt that the years of litigation had exacted a heavy price upon me financially. In that time I had not been able to write, therefore I had not been able to earn anything. I was now one step away from being flat broke. Then in a stroke of good fortune, a case I had lost was revived in a most unexpected way, and I stood to recoup a sufficiently large sum to keep the wolf from the door.

In 1995, a neighbour had flooded my property in the country and refused to make a claim on her insurance. As I did not know her, I could not discover her motive, though when the matter came to trial in 1999, I suspected class prejudice. This would be confirmed during the second trial in 2003, when her boyfriend made it clear in court that they disliked me because I was upper-class and they were working-class. During the first trial, however, she had been careful to play her cards close to her chest, with the result that we could not definitively come up with a motive for her malicious conduct. Nor could we prove that she was responsible for the flood, or that it had not been an accident as she claimed it to be. We therefore lost, and I was faced with paying out more costs on a matter where I was patently the injured party.

Then in the early 2000s, I discovered, much to my delight, that I had grounds for appeal. Because the damage she had caused had been extensive, and because I now had sufficient experience as a litigant-in-person to have the confidence to represent myself, I launched an appeal.

Many lawyers, I discovered yet again, were cut from the same cloth as Gloria. There was no trick in the book too low to pull, no depth too low to plumb. However, if there was one lesson that Gloria had taught me, it was that you don't need to be wily. You only need to use your opponents' wiles against them. All wily people think they're so clever that their tactics will never boomerang upon them. However, Gloria had taught me that the boomerangs she had hurled always fly back to their senders if you are adept at making sure they don't hit you. The important thing isn't to be a good tactician but to exploit effectively the tactics of your opponent.

Using my relationship with my mother as a road map, I sidestepped each projectile the other side sent at me, using their own ploys to further my case and to undermine theirs. For instance, at one point they got in touch with my witnesses and tried to cross-examine them before the trial. 'But they're not *your* witnesses,' the solicitor told me when I telephoned to remonstrate with him. 'They are the court's witnesses. I have every right to get in touch with them if I so choose.' This, of course, was absolutely opposite to what Brian Hepworth, a solicitor representing my ex-publishers, had once told me, so I checked with the Law Society and learned that yes, anyone can get in touch with a witness prior to a trial. As long as that witness agrees to speak to you, you can pump him or her for as much information as you want.

As luck would have it, the engineer who had been the insurance company's expert witness was known to a friend of mine, so I asked her if she would approach him to find out if it was okay for me to speak to him. This she did, and once he agreed, I telephoned him and could barely believe my luck as he started to provide me with technical explanations of why the other side's case was rubbish.

That May of 2003, I duly showed up in court. With my heart in my mouth but my courage intact from having seen off the biggest bitch of them all, who had done for sport and pleasure what the other side was at least doing for money, I presented my case. For two days, I examined my witnesses, cross-examined theirs, gave my evidence, was cross-examined, then summarized my case. I was up against the legal team of the Norwich Union, the largest insurance company in the country, but I hoped things were as clear to the judge as they were to me. I had not let their barrister twist and turn anything, even though he tried to do so with all the talent of Gloria at her most pernicious. I was jubilant when the judge rendered his verdict in my favour Quick as a shot Gloria-in-a-barrister's-wig jumped up and sought leave to appeal. 'This *is* an appeal,' the judge snapped, refusing him leave and awarding me all my costs, to include those from the beginning of proceedings in 1995, with a significant percentage of them to be paid immediately.

By this time, I was penniless, being too busy litigating to work as a writer. Had it not been for my sister Libby and Aunt Marjorie, who gave me enough money to help me pay my living expenses – Libby later lending me an even more significant sum to prevent me losing my houses – I would definitely have collapsed financially.

While this was going on, Libby appealed to Gloria to help me out. She chose her moment well, waiting until they were having a conversation in which our mother admitted that she had just discovered a bank account in Jamaica she had forgotten all about. It contained US$500,000. 'You know, Mummy,' Libby then said, having tactfully waited a few minutes, 'Georgie is having a really tough time of things right now. She could do with some help.'

'Help? Help?' Gloria trilled. 'I'm in no position to help anyone. I myself need all the help I can get. She will just have to manage without me.'

Libby was so upset that she telephoned Kitty as soon she had hung up from our mother. 'She wouldn't miss $20,000 or $30,000, and it would make all the difference to Georgie. I just don't understand Mummy. How can she refuse to help out her own daughter when she didn't even remember the $500,000 she had in that account?'

Although I did not yet know of Libby's intervention or Gloria's refusal – and one can well imagine how I felt when I found out – I had never once expected my mother to come to my assistance. My needs were still no part of our relationship. Except for that one occasion in 1998 when she had tried to convince me to stump up over £20,000 in fees so that I would be available to 'sit with' her in London, she had never once displayed any interest in my legal difficulties. Indeed, she had always gone to the trouble of letting me know that I should never consider asking for her help by constantly bemoaning how she was getting 'practically no interest on my money'.

Gloria had always been adept at bawling, rather than pleading, poverty – at least to her children. She took great care that the people she cared about knew all about her spectacular jewellery collection and the riches of the Ziadies, so from early childhood we had to reconcile the irreconcilable public and private faces of wealth with her declarations of penury. By the beginning of the new millennium, however, she had turned up the volume to such an extent that we would have thought she didn't have 'two brass farthings' to her name, as she used to put it, had we not known better.

Occasionally, she used to float the idea that she should marry one of her well-off 'boyfriends', but as we knew they were screaming queens, none of us thought that there was any prospect of her remarrying.

Then, in January 2001, she suddenly opted to sell the family home in Jamaica and move to Grand Cayman two months later. This was a hare-brained scheme that had been the idea of her brother-in-law Alex. He was something of a romantic, warm and generous when in a good mood, but the absolute antithesis when in a bad one - a control freak who had trained Marjorie so well that she lived in constant fear of his verbal abuse. She would sign cheques and important papers which he put under her nose without even looking at them, lest he regarded perusal as an act of mistrust for which she would have to pay dearly. He had been encouraging Gloria to think that his brother Anthony was keen on her. When he discovered that he had prostate cancer in 1999, he swung into high gear, telling her how she must come and live near him and Marjorie. 'You and Anthony would make a good couple. The two Smedmore sisters for two of the Stanton brothers,' he said, encouraging her to think in marital terms.

None of Gloria's surviving children found anything ominous in this. We knew she was lonely and would have been happy for her to marry Anthony. He seemed like a nice man, the one fly in the ointment being that Marjorie could not stand him, though she was careful to keep the reasons why to herself. So Gloria and Anthony as a couple became something of a family joke, all in an innocent and seemingly positive way.

Meanwhile Alex's health was declining, and it was becoming obvious as 2000 progressed that he would not make it.

Although he still did all within his power to encourage the Anthony-Gloria match, Alex now started to come out with some truly dodgy remarks. 'Marjorie and I have no one to leave our money to, and I intend to spend out all of mine before I die,' was but one of the more choice sentiments emanating from this six-foot-one fount of charm and fury.

I did not take any of this seriously. I was used to people in the family saying things they did not mean in the heat of the moment and could not imagine that Alex would really be as malicious as he now seemed intent on being. Then Libby discovered that he had used his influence to have Marjorie's name put on the title deeds of the house our grandmother had left me. Worse, he had had this done in the early 1990s, when Marjorie had been diagnosed with late stage-three Hodgkin's disease and we had all expected her to die. This was before my Diana book was published and therefore before I had the means to fight him in the courts for the return of Maisie's bequest. Had Auntie died then, my house would therefore have fallen into his lap, and I would have been at his mercy until he decided to turn it over to me. All of a sudden, the man I affectionately called 'Unks' seemed more foe than friend.

To my consternation, Anthony could not have been more helpful in acquiring the proof that I needed to confront Marjorie and have her rectify the situation. He went to the Land Registry and faxed me the entry which showed, as clear as day, that Marjorie was now the absolute owner of my house.

Her name had once been entered as trustee, but that important distinction had now been eliminated and, with it, my ownership. I must admit I was surprised that Anthony should be so helpful against his own brother. Not being paranoid, however, I never gave it another thought, though of course it made me even more in favour than ever of a match between him and my mother.

Once I had the proof of Alex's chicanery, I telephoned Marjorie and asked her for an explanation. 'You know I trust him with my life,' she said, obviously embarrassed to have to explain away her husband's conduct. 'He'd never do anything that wasn't above-board, of that I can assure you. I'm sure there's an innocent explanation.'

'Are you aware that Grandma's will has disappeared?' I asked.

'How could it?' she said, perplexed.

'You tell me. After all, it's your husband's nephew's law firm that probated her estate. They told me that they keep all wills until the bequests are concluded, yet when I asked for a copy of Grandma's will, they discovered it no longer exists, even though her bequests will only be finalized when you die,' I said.

'Are you saying that Alex might have done something he shouldn't?'

'I am saying that, as things stand, Grandma's house will be his if you die tomorrow.'

'But everyone knows Mama left you the house.'

'I know it. You know it. Alex knows it. Everyone who knew Grandma knows it. Yet somehow the Land Registry doesn't know it. You see the difficulty?'

'What do you want me to do?' Marjorie said.

'I don't mind if your name stays on the register as an owner in trust, but mine must appear on it as well as the absolute owner.'

'I'll arrange to have it done,' Marjorie said.

Although I was glad that we agreed upon a resolution to this problem as quickly as we did, I could not escape the sensation that Marjorie had discovered what Alex had done some time before I telephoned her. She was as honest as the day was long and would never have agreed to him doing anything so underhand. But he had cowed her so thoroughly over the years that I suspected she was hoping I would never discover the alteration, which she would rectify once he was dead, thereby avoiding the unpleasantness which it would inevitably cause if I found out.

Gloria, of course, was jubilant. 'I always told you he's one to watch,' she said of the brother-in-law who extended her endless hospitality, had been generous enough to buy her a house in Vancouver and was, even now, responsible for her selling her Jamaican house, even if he had also encouraged her and Marjorie to sell large tracts of land in Cayman at knockdown prices so that he could have the money to charter submarines for catered dinner parties and other such wasteful extravagances.

This, however, was only the tip of the iceberg. Once we siblings knocked heads together with our mother, we discovered that his arithmetic was peculiarly askew for such a successful businessman. For instance, there was the time he sold a large parcel of Grandma's land to developers; and the one-fortieth share my brother, sisters, our cousin Dolly and I received was different for each of the five of us and certainly proportionately smaller than the amount Marjorie and Gloria received for the thirty-five one-fortieth shares they owned equally between them. Tellingly, none of us ever saw the paperwork for the deal, and not even Marjorie knew how much she received. Nor did we have any way of finding out. If we had asked for a proper accounting, Alex would have been so outraged that it would have caused a rupture in relations between him and us, thereby putting Marjorie in a difficult position. So none of us challenged him.

One would have thought that Gloria would have had second thoughts about moving to Grand Cayman to be near her brother-in-law after incidents like that and the misregistration of my house. But she did not. She had found a purchaser who was willing to pay her in US dollars; and she was still locked into the pipedream of being Alex's double sister-in-law. So she sold the house without once consulting either of my sisters or me, acting as if it were perfectly normal for a mother to exclude her children from all dealings regarding their family home.

Despite feeling that courtesy alone required that we be kept in the loop, Libby, Kitty and I said nothing. This was partly because Jamaica had such a reputation for violence that we had always had it in the back of our minds that she could easily be murdered living all alone in that ambassadorial-sized house. Even the housekeeper, who lived on the premises, effectively lived in another house, for the servants' quarters were in a separate wing unconnected save by a walkway to the main house, and she slept further away from Gloria than neighbours in adjoining houses did in less prosperous areas.

Independent as Gloria was when it came to making decisions or effecting plots and schemes, she was quintessentially dependent where any form of labour or responsibility was concerned. Once she agreed the sale of the house, she promptly telephoned to ask me to come and help her move. Quite why she needed my help when there were professionals whom she was employing was something one was not allowed to ask. I therefore said I would not be able to go to Jamaica until the children's half-term in February, so that became her target date for leaving the home she had lived in for fifty years.

In January, I received a panicked call from Marjorie. 'You have to go to Jamaica to help your mother. She's sitting in that house all alone, staring into space day and night, wondering how to go about moving. She doesn't even know what to select to bring here.' Maisie's house was a fraction the size of Gloria's.

'All it needs is a tape measure and a piece of paper. She measures the rooms in Grandma's house and the pieces of furniture she wants to take, then figures out how or if they can fit. It couldn't be simpler,' I said.

'Maybe to you but not to her. She's overwhelmed and just sits down all day in the study staring into space.'

'Auntie, I can't just pick up and go like that,' I said. It was at the height of my complaint against my financial advisor and my two eight-year-old sons were in school. 'I have responsibilities here, and I'm already going out next month to help her with the move itself. Get Libby to go.'

'She doesn't want to, and Kitty is out of the question,' Marjorie said. 'You'll have to go.'

I must confess that I had a degree of compassion for my mother. She had only ever moved house once, half a century before. 'If you don't go and help her, she'll never be prepared when the movers come.'

'Let me get this straight. You want me to go to Jamaica, measure up Mummy's furniture, then fly to Cayman to see what will fit in Grandma's house. Is that right?'

'Will you?' she said.

'Why can't Mummy do it herself?' I said.

'You know what she's like,' she said. 'She'll come with you. But she can't manage on her own.'

I agreed to go, partly because I felt some compassion for Gloria but largely, I suspect, because I enjoy helping others, even though I could ill-afford to cross the Atlantic twice in three weeks when the air fares were at their peak and I knew there was no prospect of my mother offering to pay for anything.

This trip would ultimately be one of the events that showed me that

Gloria remained an unappreciative opportunist who had no compunction about using people, then acting as if they hadn't provided any of the help they had. Unaware of what I was letting myself in for, I duly flew to Jamaica. I took the measurements of the various pieces of furniture she wanted to take to Cayman, then flew with her to that island to assess what would and what would not fit.

We stayed with Marjorie and Alex, who looked remarkably healthy for someone who was about to die. The cancer, however, had spread to his bones and he was in pain. Even though we had almost fallen out over Maisie's house, by unspoken consent we agreed to let bygones be bygones, and I even accommodated him when he asked me to intercede with his doctor to get the painkilling dosage increased. But the doctor, who was English, remained unmoved by my implorations, explaining that Cayman, being a part of the Americas, functioned under American rules and he couldn't increase beyond the recommended dosage. 'In this part of the world,' he said with knowing Britannic wit, 'they can't have people becoming addicted to opiates. Not even when they're dying.' In Europe better sense and greater humanity prevailed, and though it was scant consolation to note that some governments were as crazy as my mother, in a funny sort of way I could not help feeling that Alex was getting his just deserts.

Despite what had happened over the house, I was nevertheless still sufficiently fond of him to regret that he was dying. Gloria, however, had now decided that he was a 'snivelling little so-and-so', that 'the sooner he dies, the better, preferably before I move to Cayman.' She was determined that she would extract a copy of Maisie's will out of him if it was the last thing she did. 'When I stop to think of all the land he's made Marjorie and me sell over the years just so he could show himself off socially, I could choke. Mama was my mother and even I have never seen a copy of her will.' That first evening, as soon as we had all finished dinner and had repaired to the den to watch television, Gloria announced, 'Alex, I want to see a copy of Mama's will. Please get it for me.'

'It's in the second drawer from the top of the filing cabinet in my study,' he said, as if he had known all along this moment was coming and was well prepared for it. 'You get it, Georgie. I'm not feeling up to moving.'

'And make sure you take a photocopy,' Gloria said in her most assertive tone.

When I returned with the will duly photocopied twice, once for Gloria, the second time for me, she snatched hers away from me and said to Marjorie, 'Have you put Georgie's name on the title deeds yet?'

'It's in hand,' Marjorie said.

'Glad to hear it. Make sure it's wrapped up before we leave,' she trilled, and I must confess, at that moment, I was mightily pleased to have a mother like her. She certainly knew how to get things done.

Although Marjorie and I ignored the issue that had arisen between us, there was an outside chance that it might have caused resentment on one side or the other. That seemed increasingly unlikely the longer we were around, for my aunt was evidently in more need of her family than ever. Alex's treatment of her was now so abusive that even the hospice nurses complained about it to Gloria and me.

'Auntie,' I said, feeling that I had to say something to make Marjorie feel better. 'I hope you understand that people who want to live go through a very angry phase. I wouldn't take any of it personally if I were you.'

Gloria, of course, had her own interpretation of what was going on, as I discovered as soon as we were alone. 'He's furious that he's leaving her behind when he hoped that she'd leave him alone to chase all those young men he's always taken such an interest in.'

'What do you mean?' I asked.

'Why do you think your grandmother took to her bed for a week when she married him? Because he has a reputation for *liking boys*.'

'But he and Auntie have always been so happily married,' I said, knowing, as we spoke, that for once Gloria was being truthful as opposed to gratuitously nasty, even if one could also detect the satisfaction she enjoyed in being able to bring her sibling rival down a peg or two.

'Oh, I admit she's made the best of a bad deal, but she's had her work cut out for her, believe me. You children don't know the half of it, because none of us wanted you to,' Gloria said smugly, warming to her theme and letting rip about her sister's turbulent second marriage.

In confirmation of the beans Gloria had spilled, a day or two later Marjorie discovered that Alex had spent every penny of the millions he had made, as well as a large tranche of her own money.

'What have you been drawing out $30,000 and $40,000 cash per week for?' she demanded to know right in front of us.

'It's my money, and I can do what I want with it,' he said so nastily that I wondered if Gloria had been giving him lessons.

'None of it was ever yours alone. I put up the backing for the business, and I worked in it with you. But even if you can lay claim to some of *that* money, you can't lay claim to one penny of *my own* money. What gives you the right to have torn through my money as if it's trees in a forest fire?'

Alex looked as if someone had opened up a hand and slapped him across the face. You could tell he was mortified to have Marjorie raise these issues in front of Gloria and me.

'Can't we discuss this later?' he said conciliatorily.

'There's nothing to discuss. You are not allowed to spend another penny of my money,' she said angrily. Like me, she had quite a temper when roused, though she was ordinarily a truly sweet person.

'What about my massages?' he asked.

'At a hundred dollars a time every day of the week, you will just have to do without them,' she said.

'They're the only pleasure left to me,' he said pathetically, presumably hoping to trade upon her sympathy.

'Then you'll just have to do without any pleasures at all between now and when you die,' Marjorie, whose birthday is three days before mine, said in true leonine fashion.

'We'll discuss this later,' Alex said as normally as he could manage.

'No we won't,' she said decisively. 'We will never discuss this again.'

'You see?' Gloria said to me afterwards, pleased to be vindicated. 'I told you. You know why she doesn't want to discuss it ever again? She knows he's been bleeding their accounts dry to give her money to his boyfriends. But she dares not confront him about it, for if he admits it, she'll never be able to face him again. She doesn't want to have to face the fact that for thirty-five years she's been living a lie. The things some women will do for a man,' she said contemptuously. 'Thank God I have never worshipped at the altar of penis the way my sister and all of you daughters have.'

Only too soon, we would discover that Gloria should have been reserving for herself some of the contempt she had for her sister and children. Although we suspected that her major motive for leaving Jamaica was to advance her relationship with Anthony, she was so secretive and canny that we could not determine the state or degree of the relationship between them. Libby, Kitty and I concluded that it was more of a fancy than a fact, but we could not be sure. Had we known what was – and wasn't – really going on, we might have been able to have a positive influence upon Gloria and prevent her from making a mistake that would affect the remainder of her life and very nearly result in the destruction of her relationship with her three living children.

However, one of the characteristics of her personality type is to keep everyone in the dark; and just by being herself, Gloria placed herself beyond anyone's help. Like all narcissists, the most vital parts of her life took place in her head, not in reality, which meant that she was never amenable to reason or indeed to help, both of which she seemed to regard as interference.

On a profound level, she not only accepted this fact about herself, but clung to it, irrespective of what she was depriving herself of. She made it clear she was not about to open herself up to anyone, one of her favourite adages being, 'You can't help people who don't want to help themselves.'

If Gloria was deliberately opaque about the nature and possibilities of her relationship with Anthony, she could not have been more transparent about how companionable she was finding the process of choosing furniture with me. Day and night all she wanted to do was discuss and re-discuss what to take and what to leave.

Nor was this the only rich seam for Gloria to mine conversationally. There was also the exhaustive question of what to do with the remnants of the furniture she was leaving behind. Had I been another sort of person, I would have got fed up, but I had come to help and was happy to do so, even if there were times when I could sense that she was using the move as an excuse to tie me to her. But then, I had known for many years that no one ever left Gloria without her trying to extend the duration of their visit. 'Don't go yet' was one of her most overused expressions. As she had not been unpleasant even once, however, I focused upon that positive and hypnotized myself into accepting the 'Glorianess' of it all.

Within a fortnight of returning to England, I was crossing the Atlantic again with my children. 'I'm going to have to help Grandma oversee the packing up of the house, so you boys will have to occupy yourselves as best you can. You can spend most of the time up at the pool or with your cousins at the old Canadian High Commissioner's Residence,' I told them on the plane, preparing them for what I anticipated would be a busy time.

I could hardly believe my eyes when I arrived at the house to see practically everything Gloria had decided to take to Cayman already wrapped and packed away in crates. 'But I thought you wanted me to help you oversee things,' I said.

'Oh, it was easier to just let the professionals get on with it,' she said airily.

'But I thought you wanted me to help you,' I repeated, trying pleasantly to get across the message that she had nullified the purpose of my visit, which, I could now see, was just another way of tricking me into keeping her company.

'It's nice to have you and the boys here,' she said.

'At least we're here for the winding up of your old life,' I said, determined to keep things positive no matter what. I'd have to come up with some way of preventing her from trapping me day and night in the study, the only room still fully furnished. 'Boys, why don't you get changed and we'll go up to the pool and have a swim?' I suggested.

'They can't do that. I emptied the pool,' Gloria said.

'I don't understand,' I said, even more bemused. How could anyone empty a swimming pool when she knew her grandchildren were coming to stay? And to do so just before she was about to turn the house over to a new owner, when water cost a fortune in Jamaica and it took ages to get pools into tip-top condition?

'I really couldn't be bothered with the botheration of the damned pool anymore,' Gloria said.

I felt my blood pressure rise. 'But Mummy, you knew the children were coming out.'

'They'll just have to occupy themselves the way all children without the benefit of pools do,' she said so coldly that I decided then and there to take advantage of her selfishness to escape from a situation I had not envisaged and wanted no part of. It was one thing to travel thousands of miles to help someone, but quite another to be tricked into becoming a pair of ears by a woman who didn't even care about how my children would occupy themselves.

'Boys, don't worry,' I said, immediately returning the boomerang. 'I'll take you swimming. We'll go to Liguanea Club tomorrow. And I'm going to phone my cousin Maria and ask her if you can swim next door. I'll also take you to Silver Sands for a few days.'

'I see you've come to take a holiday instead of helping me,' Gloria said.

'No, Mummy,' I said in my 'I'm-not-going-to-take-any-of-your-nonsense-but-will remain-pleasant-and-cordial-if-you-let-me' tone of voice. 'I came out on the children's half term to help you with your move. I've arrived to see that you have taken matters into your own hands, which is of course your right and indeed what you should have been doing in the first place. But it means there's nothing for me to do. And you've made sure the children can't occupy themselves here by emptying the pool, so there's nothing for them to do either. As a mother, I have a duty of care to my children. I am sure you as a mother will understand that all mothers have to think of their children first and foremost and must do what is necessary to live up to that duty,' I said, making sure the boomerang would hit her where she was most vulnerable.

'The problem with your generation is that you think you must entertain *pickney*, when it's up to them to entertain themselves,' Gloria said disparagingly.

'That they would have been doing, had you not removed the one source of entertainment they had. But since you did, we'll just have to make the best of a bad deal,' I said decisively.

'If you want to make a fool of yourself over *pickney*, you go ahead and do so,' Gloria replied, intent on winning a struggle which should not have been taking place at all.

'If you wish to characterize responsibility as a mother as being foolish, you go right ahead and do so. The loss is yours, not mine. But I haven't travelled thousands of miles to have a row with you, so I will tell you yet again what my parameters are. I will have good and happy relationships or I will have none. That rule applies to everyone, including you. *Especially* you,' I said meaningfully. 'Now if you don't mind, I would like to telephone Maria. Do you have her number?'

As Gloria was fetching the number, the new owner dropped in. Mr Elliott was a black Jamaican of humble origin who had sold his businesses in London for £12,000,000 and had bought the house so that his 'English' children would have an inducement to come to Jamaica. Although he had already paid for it, he had agreed that Gloria could take several more months to vacate it if she felt so inclined. She was timing her departure for after Alex's death, and since no one knew when that would be, she was prepared to live in a no-longer-properly furnished house surrounded by packing crates. In the meantime, he was not allowed to require any changes inside or out.

Now Mr Elliott had arrived with a truck and a crew of workmen. 'Mrs Ziadie, would you mind if I stored some stuff in the pool house?' he asked.

'Go right ahead and do what you want,' Gloria said airily, her indifference patent.

'Your mother is quite a woman,' Mr Elliott said.

'Yes, she is,' I said.

We chatted for a few minutes, during which time I got the impression that he was a little sweet on Gloria. I became convinced of that fact when he said, 'Mrs Ziadie, you should be more like your daughter. She speaks to me like a person. To you I am just a rich black man who has bought your house.'

'But Mr Elliott, what else could you be to me?' Gloria said.

'You never know,' he said.

'I certainly do,' she said as neutrally as she could muster while making it absolutely clear from the set of her face that any idea of anything else was out of the question. I could tell she was seething underneath at his impertinence.

Afterwards, I said: 'Well, it looks as if you haven't lost your touch.'

'The idea! The idea that I could ever entertain the notion of a misalliance with that!' Gloria spat. 'That's the problem with Jamaica today.'

'I don't know,' I said conciliatorily. 'You're a good ten years older than Mr Elliott. You remind me of friends who are outraged when builders wolf-whistle. I always say: long may they appreciate. There's nothing wrong with appreciation. And he certainly wasn't disrespectful.'

'The very idea is disrespectful,' Gloria said hotly.

'You have it your way if you wish, but I still think there was no insult intended and none should be taken.'

A few days later, the boys and I set off for a four-day stay at Silver Sands: Jamaica's answer to Las Brisas, where the upper classes have their seaside cottages. Prior to going, I informed Gloria that I would photograph the garden when I returned. 'That way we'll always have a record of it, no matter what Mr Elliott does to it,' I said.

'I am not Lot's wife. I don't give a continental damn about the things I leave behind,' Gloria said.

I had good reason to see what she meant when I returned from Silver Sands. As I drove through the bottom gate, I saw in the distance a mound of plants, trees and branches which measured some sixty feet by forty feet by ten feet high.

'What in God's name is going on?' I spluttered to one of the workmen.

'Mrs Ziadie gave Mr Elliott permission to clear bush,' he said.

'Is Mr Elliott here?' I asked.

'Yes, ma'am. Him up by the pool.'

'Let's go, boys,' I said to the kids, surprise being my overriding emotion until I reached the pool and saw total devastation. Every orchid had been cut down, every tree, every plant surrounding the pool.

'Hello, Miss Ziadie, how you doing?' Mr Elliott said pleasantly.

'I'm not sure I know, Mr Elliott. I have just returned to photograph the garden, and now this,' I said, waving my arms at the abomination.

'We're just clearing bush,' Mr Elliott said.

'Mr Elliott,' I said as politely as I could, 'there is no bush here. Are you aware that this is a famous garden and that the plants in it would cost you at least US$300,000 if you had to replace them? And that's not the plants as they are now, mature, but as they would be as seedlings and saplings. This is a mature garden with valuable plants, and you are just chopping it down as if it was what you call "bush".'

'But what is the point of buying the Ziadie house if people can't see it from the road?' he asked as if I had missed the most obvious point of the whole enterprise.

I could hardly believe my ears. His pride in acquiring our family home was so great that he wanted every passer-by to see it. And if the price of doing so was to destroy a magnificent, mature garden, so be it.

I was also concerned that Mr Elliott was behaving in an insensitive manner by cutting down Gloria's life's work before her eyes and told him so. This evinced the second shock of the afternoon.

'But Miss Ziadie,' he said. 'Your mother gave me permission to cut down the bush.'

'And when did she do that?'

'Yesterday. I told her I wanted to clear out the bush,' he said, still insisting on misusing that word to describe the garden's contents, 'and she said I could start tomorrow for all she cared. I can even quote what she said. She said, "I'm not Lot's wife. You can do anything you want whenever you want as long as your men don't disturb me with any noise. None of it matters to me anymore." If I'd known you wanted me to wait, I'd have waited,' he said apologetically.

I was so stunned by Gloria's utter lack of care, not only for my wishes but also for the recording of her horticultural accomplishments, that I could have cried then and there.

'Can I ask you to hold off on cutting down anything else until we're out of the house?' I said.

'No problem,' he said.

When I got inside and asked my mother for her version of events, they accorded with Mr Elliott's. 'But Mummy,' I said, 'you knew I wanted to photograph the garden. He's cut down everything around the pool, and that was one of the most beautiful parts of the garden.'

'None of it matters. It's not mine anymore,' she said, driving home how utterly self-centred she was.

'Don't you care that he's destroying your life's work?'

'Why should I? It's his to do with as he pleases now that it's no longer mine.'

Stunned by Gloria's breathtaking response, I could not decide if it was positive or negative. Only with time would I come to see it for what it was. She was so entirely self-centred that she cared about things only as long as they were hers. She didn't even care about her handiwork. She took no pride in it. This was the antithesis of artistic accomplishment, when people care about their achievements as entities separate from themselves. Even her incontrovertible gift as a horticulturalist was of no significance to her except when it could bring her direct recompense. That degree of self-centredness, which allows for no importance outside of one's own being, was one of the characteristics which would ultimately lead me to conclude that she was not only a narcissist of the highest order but also an antisocial one. In her world, nothing counted except when it related directly to her and could benefit her directly. That applied across the board: parents, sibling, children, friends, possessions, even accomplishments, had no value to her except when they could be channelled into providing her with a return. That degree of self-concern is beyond sick.

Although I did not regret flying to Jamaica to help Gloria move, by the time I left I was so glad to be rid of my mother that I felt a great pressure lift off my shoulders as the JUTA cab taking us to the airport left the house behind. Of course, it was always going to be a difficult occasion, even if she had not reverted to type. That house had been the scene not only of some pleasure and privilege but also of a great deal of pain and punishment. It was our hellhole as well as our family home, and though I was sad to say goodbye to it for all time, I did so in the knowledge that it had been the site of so much unhappiness that one should have been relieved to see it leave our lives for all time. Yet I wasn't relieved; one peculiarity of humanity is, I daresay, a reluctance to say goodbye to one's past without a measure of nostalgia.

It was nevertheless the passing of an era, not only for me and also for many of my friends, whose teenage memories had been caught up with the Ziadie house and its swimming pool. In the days before my departure, they came one by one to say goodbye to the house, each with their own reminiscences. The only person, indeed, who seemed to have no nostalgia about saying goodbye was Gloria.

No sooner had I returned to England than I had to turn tail and cross the Atlantic yet again. Alex died and I had to go to Cayman to support Marjorie.

Gloria and Anthony met me at the airport. Were they or weren't they an item? If they weren't an item yet, were they planning to become one? I couldn't tell from their demeanour, but Libby agreed with me when she arrived for the funeral that there was a spark there.

I, however, knew something Gloria didn't. Once Marjorie had realized that Alex was dying, they had tried to get me to convince her to live anywhere else but Cayman. 'I can't do that,' I said. 'You're the ones who wanted her here. You're the ones who've convinced her to sell the house. It's now sold. Where would she live?'

'What's wrong with Florida?' Marjorie piped up hopefully.

'She doesn't want to live in Florida, and even if she did, I for one would do all in my power to talk her out of it. She can't drink and drive in Florida the way she does in Jamaica or Cayman. And you can't live in Florida without driving. Can you imagine the drama it would be if the police picked her up for driving under the influence? No thank you,' I said. 'I have quite enough problems without having to bail Mummy out of an American jail.'

After putting forth various other suggestions, Marjorie said, 'Having your mother here will kill me. I can't cope with her.'

'Auntie, I don't mean to be heartless, but this was your and Alex's idea. You can't look to me to rescue you from a mess of your own creation. Even if I had the influence with Mummy – which I don't – it would be a bit much to expect me to find another place for her to live in a matter of weeks. You seem to forget, I have two young children to think of.'

'Actually, Gloria living here was never my idea. It was always his. He seemed to think we could be the Caymanian version of *Seven Brides for Seven*

Brothers,' she said, giggling girlishly.

'Well, I'm afraid you'll just have to reap what you've sown, for I think it would be the ultimate in cruelty to tell her that you don't want her living near you. Not after you've convinced her to sell the house and you've charged her up with hope of another future,' I said. 'Personally, I always thought it was misguided to encourage anyone to change her life so radically after the age of seventy. If you want to tell her that you don't want her here, you're going to have to do it yourself, though I must implore you not to. It would be too, too cruel.'

Weeks later, Alex was dead, and we all congregated in Cayman for his funeral. This was organized by Anthony, who did his brother justice. It was as elegant, stylish and glamorous as Alex had been in life.

Behind the scenes, however, Alex's passing was not as sad as it could have been, for he had gone out as nastily and spitefully as anyone could engineer. In the weeks before his death, he had even refused to speak to Marjorie. To rub her nose in the dirt, he – who was a racist *par excellence* – claimed to have developed a childlike devotion to a new helper, a fat black former street-vendor named Vilma, through whom he directed all his comments to the wife he was now spurning. She had the 'honour' of doing everything for him, while Marjorie, who enjoyed being needed, was not allowed to do anything. 'It's as if he hates me,' she said to me when she telephoned me in some distress to complain about this latest development.

'Mickey was also very angry before he died,' I reminded her. 'Try not to take it personally.'

'Mickey never looked at any of us with hatred, nor did he curl his lip at us when we entered his room,' Marjorie said.

Later I would hear from other people, including the hospice nurses, that Alex did indeed give every indication of hating Marjorie. This was obviously devastating for her. She had dedicated the last thirty-four years of her life to him. But by the time he died, he had made his feelings so clear to everyone who knew them well, that she was torn between relief at no longer being the repository of such loathing, and grief mingled with humiliation at her loss. There was also, of course, the matter of the millions of dollars he had deliberately gone through in an attempt to leave her impoverished, and though he hadn't quite succeeded in his objective, he had been successful enough for her to worry that she would run out of money if she lived too long.

In the days after the funeral, I talked Marjorie through her predicament while helping her answer letters of condolence. I pointed out that she could maintain her lifestyle in exactly the same way for a good ten years without suffering financially. 'But if you're worried,' I then said, 'why not simply hive off the guest flat and rent it out? You'll still have space in the main house for guests, and if you get a nice tenant, you'll actually have someone around who is a breath of fresh air.'

'I would never have thought of that myself,' she said. 'I think it's a fabulous idea.' And she did exactly that, finding herself a nice young man as a tenant who became a good friend.

A few weeks after Alex's burial, Gloria became her second tenant, when she moved to Cayman that spring of 2001. She was renting the house my grandmother had left me. Although the rental was a nominal amount, and Marjorie would happily have allowed her to live there rent-free, the competitive Gloria was determined not to give her sibling the satisfaction of being her benefactress, so she paid a peppercorn rent, and in so doing, managed to derive the conflicting benefits of living virtually rent-free without the need for appreciation.

As this new arrangement unfolded, I remained quiet even though the situation was completely antithetical to my interests or to my grandmother's game plan. She had left my aunt a life interest in the house as a way of protecting me while I was young enough for people to take advantage of my inexperience, not as a means of further enriching a woman who was already rich. Though I was not happy about Marjorie receiving the income from my property, I was not prepared to make an issue of it. I saw that my aunt could hardly have reversed the position her late and now unlamented husband had adopted in effectively seizing my property, without making the tacit admission that he had been wrong to pocket the rent for all the years he had done so, with the corollary being that she had been weak or remiss in letting him do so. That admission, I knew, she would never make, if only because it would have made a mockery of all the decades of loyalty and devotion she had shown him. So I let sleeping dogs lie as my financial situation declined sharply, consoling myself that you have to make sacrifices for those you love. I would have been shallow indeed if I had let something as mundane as money come between my adored aunt and me.

To her credit, Marjorie took steps, in her own way, to rectify the matter. She 'rescued' me financially on more than one occasion, giving me sums of money which showed me that, left to her own devices, she would have turned over the proceeds of the house to me years ago, had Alex not wanted the income from it for himself.

If my situation was not ideal, neither was Gloria's. She was making the transition from an environment where she was well known and had stature, to one where she was not known and had no status save as a relation of someone of stature with whom she had an intense sibling rivalry. Of course she found adjusting difficult, which is hardly surprising, for it was a well-nigh impossible situation in which there was no real prospect of a positive outcome. 'I tried my very best,' she later said, 'I really did.' She was always asking people out for luncheon or dinner parties, and always picking up the bills, but as many another single woman has discovered, most married couples will take all the hospitality single people have to offer, but when it comes to reciprocity, they usually prefer the safety of couples rather than running the risk of having an unattached woman around. Whether that is because they fear unattached individuals, or simply find it easier to issue one invitation to a couple instead of going to the trouble of issuing two invitations to a single woman and a single man, is not something upon which I would care to speculate, though I suspect both motives come into play in social life.

Never having tasted the bitter draught of failure before, Gloria simply could not comprehend how the world hadn't received her with the open arms to which she had hitherto been accustomed. I tried to take the sting away by explaining as best as I could that the odds had been stacked against her, without adding that being as egocentric and difficult as she was made what little chance there was of success impossible. 'You have to realize, Mummy, that most people have their settled lives and settled circles after a certain age. And many of them regard it as rocking the boat to have to include a newcomer. And you are a newcomer. I think you've done pretty well for someone of your age, for this was never going to be an easy transition.' Then, trying to inject a dose of reality, I said, 'Maybe you should consider returning to Jamaica if you and Anthony don't get together. How's that going?'

'He comes and pays all my bills, but I don't see much of him otherwise,' she said, and I could see why. I had been out to dinner with them before my departure from Cayman following Alex's funeral, and it was obvious to me that they were fundamentally incompatible. Anthony was a socially driven butterfly who thrived on chitchat. He was very easy company and took pride in being a popular and humorous 'spare man'. His whole world was socializing, and you could tell that he was thrilled by his success socially, especially as in his youth he had not been lionized nor had he had the social access he now did.

Gloria, on the other hand, suffered from the sneering disenchantment typical of the celebrated socialite whose popularity had never been able to assuage her underlying discontent. With the passage of the years and the loss of her youth, she had become an overt misanthrope. This lack of regard for humanity extended even to Society, the one segment of human affairs she regarded as being worthy of her attention. She therefore had a fundamental if paradoxical contempt for anyone who prized – as opposed to merely possessing – social success, and she was always disparaging anyone who enjoyed their social success too much by dismissing them as 'social climbers'.

Another reason why Gloria and Anthony could never have worked as a couple was that, like all narcissists, she wanted the world to revolve around her; and, now that she no longer possessed youthful beauty and glamour, she preferred the non-competitive world of her own environment to the world at large, where she was sure to be eclipsed by someone younger and prettier. Far from relishing the forum for self-promoting display that is an intrinsic appeal of Society – and which Anthony clearly both relished and needed – now that time had eroded her distinctiveness, she had turned her back on it and was always going on and on about how she was a 'private' person.

It was clear to me, as Anthony chitchatted, that he was not impressing Gloria with his popularity or social activities any more than she was impressing him with her provocativeness. She seemed to think that it was as sexy at seventy-three as it had been in her twenties, thirties and even forties to turn each and every comment into a bone of contention over which she and her swain would tussle dramatically as they flexed their sexual muscles. I could tell that Anthony found that way of relating a real turn-off.

Later on, after Gloria had settled the bill and Anthony had headed off home into the night, her comments also told me that the primary reason for her move to Cayman was likely to end in frustration. 'Those Stantons are such social climbers, they make me want to puke. All they ever want to do is show themselves off. At least Alex was generous, even if it turned out that half the time it was at Marjorie's and my expense. But Anthony's so tight he makes constipation look like diarrhoea,' Gloria said, going on to inform me how she always paid when she and Anthony were out together.

'I thought he doesn't have any money,' I said.

'Everyone has enough to push their hand in their pocket occasionally,' she said.

I left Cayman convinced that their relationship would go nowhere, though for the next three years the signs were sufficiently mixed that one could never completely write it off. Sometimes, when you telephoned, Gloria was clearly hopeful, while at other times she was so down about the lack of progress and his inattentiveness that I would jolly her along with such consoling words as, 'Everyone in love is a perennial adolescent, whether they're fifteen or seventy-five.'

While Gloria's relationship with Anthony lurched like a Jane Austen novel from one non-event to another, her relationship with Marjorie was now more antagonistic than ever. Over the next two years, Libby, Kitty and I were constant buffers between the two sisters.

Knowing that Gloria would suck her dry if she allowed her to, Marjorie took steps a few days after her sister had definitively moved to Cayman to establish some boundaries. 'I am going to take you and show you how to get everywhere. I'm going to do it once more. Then it's up to you. I can't have you coming here day and night wanting me to chauffeur you around or chat a load of rubbish about nothing. I have my own life to lead, and you'll just have to develop yours or go back to Jamaica,' Marjorie informed her in an attempt to stop Gloria from just plugging in.

Gloria was mortally offended, complaining about how Marjorie was being unhelpful and how 'she has no time for her only sister but can't do enough for her friends'. Marjorie never made any secret of how important her friends were to her, while Gloria was equally frank about how little value she placed upon friendship. But Marjorie stuck to her guns. 'Your mother wants to take over my life and have me dancing attendance on her. I'm sorry, but I can't have her wreaking havoc in my life. I will not let her,' Marjorie, ordinarily so generous, said determinedly.

'All of you children and everyone else think that your aunt is so sweet,' Gloria was saying in the meantime, 'but she isn't. I'm her sister and I've known her better and longer than anyone else. I'm here to tell you she is one selfish cow who will trample anyone into the ground who gets in the way of what she wants.'

Thereafter, there would be periodic eruptions. Marjorie was the one who usually telephoned to complain about Gloria's latest antic. 'I don't know how anyone can stand your mother. How did you all put up with her and turn out so well?' gradually gave way to, 'Your mother is going to be the death of me. I'm sure she's bringing back my cancer. I can feel it. You have to convince her to go and live somewhere else. I tell you, she is going to kill me if she stays here.'

Of course, all of us sympathized with Marjorie, but there was very little we could do beyond sympathizing and trying to encourage Gloria to live elsewhere, which she was determined not to do.

Fortunately, Marjorie had a great sense of humour, and often a conversation that had begun painfully would end with us killing ourselves with laughter, such as the time she telephoned me to complain about a luncheon party of hers that Gloria had ruined. 'She never gave anyone else around the table a chance to even breathe in fresh air. Every time anyone opened up their mouth, she silenced them with, "Give me a chance. I haven't finished yet", then proceeded to bore everyone rigid with her preoccupations. I'm going to get a sign made and hang it outside of your grandmother's house. It will say: "Dr Gloria Ziadie, Specialist in Opthalmology. She is a true "eye" specialist. Everything with her is "I", "I", "I", "I", "I".'

I couldn't help laughing, which made Marjorie start to laugh as well, though we both knew that she had only spoken the truth.

'You know, Auntie,' I finally said, 'anyone listening to you speak about Mummy would think you'd didn't know her at all. Yet you only ever tell Libby, Kitty and me what we've been telling you for years.'

'I know, darling,' she agreed. 'But you must remember that I haven't lived in the same house as your mother since before any of you were born. And we haven't lived in the same country for nearly forty years. It was easy to forget what she's really like. But having her here has brought it all back and made me realize why I kept such a wide berth when your Uncle Ric was alive. I really don't know how you children have stood her all these years.'

On another occasion, Marjorie telephoned me in a state. 'I'm ringing you to tell you I never want to see your mother again. I've told her just now. She is so awful, she is beyond belief.'

'What do you want me to do?' I asked.

'Tell her to leave Cayman. I don't want her living here. I cannot stand it any longer. Please, I beg of you, get her to leave.'

Marjorie then launched into one of those typical Gloria stories which always started simply and ended with the victim being so upset she was barely sensible. If the details varied, the emotions never did, and I decided that maybe the time had come to insist that my mother find somewhere else to reside since Cayman evidently wasn't working out.

When I telephoned her, however, Gloria played the innocent and made out that Marjorie was being selfish and unreasonable.

'She can always bestir herself to show herself off to the general public, but she never has time for her one and only sister,' she said.

'So why stay in Cayman?' I said.

'Cayman doesn't belong to Marjorie and the Stantons, even though they seem to think it does. I'm perfectly happy here, and here is where I plan to stay,' Gloria said airily, always a sign that she was concealing something.

'But you're not happy there. You're always saying so yourself. There's a charming disused coaching-station at the beginning of the domain which we could do up for you,' I said. 'It has the most magnificent view of Villefranche and Albi. It would make the most charming dower house. You could spend summers there with us in France. Albi is near Gaillac, which is the original wine-producing region of France from the days of Ancient Rome. They have lovely wines which you'll enjoy. You could return to the West Indies for winter and maybe also visit Libby and Kitty, sharing yourself with us, so to speak. We'd all be pleased to have you with us,' I continued, knowing this wasn't strictly true but that we would all have done our duty and put a good face on it. 'Why restrict yourself to a place you're always saying is boring, when you can go back and forth between more interesting places?' I asked, hoping to find a solution to the problem that my aunt and mother had landed me with.

'Living with *pickney* has never been my idea of a life,' Gloria said.

'Think about it,' I said. 'Although you're only two years younger than Auntie, physically you're more like twenty years younger. You're still a relatively young and vigorous woman, while she's become an old lady. We have to face the fact that she will most likely die long before you. Then what will be the point of living in Cayman?'

'I don't see anything much of her now, so whether she's alive or dead won't make that much difference to me,' Gloria said.

'All the more reason to get out of what you call "that Godforsaken hole", if not permanently, then for a few months of the year at least,' I cajoled.

'I'll think about it,' Gloria said in a tone of voice that left me in no doubt that she was brushing me off.

Frankly, the prospect of having my nightmare of a mother staying near me for extended periods was hardly welcome. However, it was my duty as a daughter to recommend the best option for her. If she didn't take it, that was fine by me. If she did, which I hoped she would for her sake and my aunt's though not mine, I would just have to dig deep within my soul and find the resources to cope with having that ton of trouble around.

That November, Marjorie's beach house was damaged by a northwester with waves eighty feet high and a sea surge of nearly forty feet. The sea actually came into the house, which was ordinarily some thirty feet above sea level. The sea even moved Alex's car from the driveway at the side of the house onto the front veranda. The air-conditioning unit beneath the house was completely ripped out, and of course the furniture was damaged. Gloria telephoned me to inform me that 'your aunt's house has been destroyed. Destroyed.'

Having bought a house from a well-known bank at a £200,000 discount because they were told that it needed that amount of structural repairs, which I then had done for £16,000, I knew the importance of not exaggerating structural damage. So I said to my mother, 'The house is made of reinforced concrete. It can't be destroyed. How bad is the damage?'

'Child, I have just been wading through the house. The water is up to our knees. Alex's car is in the drawing room,' she alleged, even though it was not. 'The house is completely destroyed. Destroyed. D.E.S.T.R.O.Y.E.D,' she spelled out the word with so much relish that I could not help wondering if she wasn't secretly pleased that Marjorie had lost her Park Avenue palace by the Caribbean Sea and would now have to live in a more ordinary house, such as the one Gloria was occupying.

When Marjorie received the hundreds of thousands of dollars which the insurance company paid out to repair Blue Horizon, Gloria encouraged her to bank the money instead of repairing it. 'I so miss my house,' Marjorie thereafter complained time and again. 'I hate living inland. I loved living beside the sea. There's no point in living on an island like Cayman and being anywhere else but by the sea.'

'So get the house fixed,' I used to encourage her.

'I don't have the strength to do it on my own,' she would reply.

'If I could afford to, I would come out and help you. But I really can't for now.' I was too busy litigating against the Norwich Union. 'If I get a decent award, I'll come out when the case is concluded.'

By the time it did conclude in May 2003, and I was once more in a position to make myself available to help her, Marjorie was in the hospital. Over the previous eighteen months, her health had been deteriorating steadily. Libby's husband Ben, who is a gifted diagnostician, had agreed with her that her cancer was most likely back and had suggested over the Christmas season of 2002 that she return to her oncologist as soon as possible. Unfortunately, he either missed the signs or then realized that things were hopeless and did not tell Marjorie. Whatever, she returned from the States in January 2003 telling everyone she had been given a clean bill of health, but by May was being given six months maximum. The cancer was in her liver, amongst other places.

The news that our beloved Auntie was going to die catapulted my sisters and me into paroxysms of grief. I offered to fly out to Cayman immediately but Marjorie, who had always loved children, told me what she also told Kitty. 'Don't come now. Wait until the summer, when the children are on holiday. Bring them out to see me. I want to see them as well.' Because our birthdays were three days apart, we agreed that we would celebrate both birthdays together in Cayman. It would be, we all knew, her last birthday.

Thereafter, I spoke to Marjorie at least twice a week, usually more often. I also telephoned Gloria more frequently than I had done hitherto, thinking that she would need my support now that she was losing her only sibling.

By June, I started to get a sense that things were going badly wrong far more quickly than anyone had envisaged. 'I'm getting very forgetful,' Marjorie said, and when I interrogated the maids, they confirmed that she was not in good shape. Then she lost her mind overnight, and it looked as if death would be a better option than an insensible twilight, until Ben located a drug which kick-started her brain again, and she was back in command of her faculties.

By this time, I was becoming seriously worried that Marjorie would die before I had a chance to see her, so I started telephoning her every day to monitor her deterioration. I would speak to her and to the maids, trying to gauge the situation accurately. Trying to get anything sensible out of Gloria on the subject was, of course, impossible. On the last Friday in June, I returned to my London house from a party at the Ritz Hotel and decided to stop mucking around speaking to Marjorie and the maids. I got Monica, her housekeeper, to give me the doctor's number and telephoned him directly. 'I'm worried that Auntie won't last until August and I won't get the chance to see her,' I said.

'You're right to be worried,' John Addleson, her doctor, said. 'Her cancer has spread like wildfire. In the last week alone her deterioration has been tremendous. That often happens when patients have been in remission with Hodgkin's and it comes back as lymphoma. If you want to see her, you have to come right now.'

'Right now?' I echoed. 'It's three o'clock in the morning in London. I can't come right now.'

'If you don't come right now, you might well not see her alive. She'll be dead in a day or two, three maybe…five if you're incredibly lucky, though I doubt it,' he said, and I could have kissed him for giving me such precise information.

As soon as I hung up, I telephoned Delta, American and Virgin Airlines and organized flights for the boys and me. I then attended to the chore of getting Dima and Misha out of school and flying them to London as unaccompanied minors – an onerous task if ever there was one in these security conscious days, when the airlines make what used to be a simple exercise as complex as possible. This alone ate up two days which we might well not have to spare.

Having made the arrangements, I telephoned Gloria that last Saturday of Marjorie's life. 'Mummy, you do realize Auntie is dying, don't you?'

'I'm not a fool, you know,' she said waspishly.

'No one is implying that you are. It's just that you might not be aware of how imminent her death is,' I said. 'For your sake it's important that you say anything that you have to say before she dies.'

'I don't have anything to say to her. What would I have to say to her? She's my only sister, and we've always been closer than close,' she said, already rewriting history.

'Just as long as you don't leave unsaid anything that needs to be said,' I said.

'There's nothing I need to say to your aunt,' she said acidly, making it obvious that she regarded it as an impertinence that I would even suggest that they had had anything less than the perfect relationship. How do you deal with people like that?

That day, and on Sunday, I spoke to Auntie briefly. Although she knew it was me and made a valiant effort to speak normally, I could tell she was very weak, so kept the necessity for her to respond to a minimum. I had planned to speak to her on the Monday afternoon after returning from the bank with the boys, but I was mugged by a gang of three Chilean thieves who followed us from the Nat West bank in Sloane Square into one of London's best bookshops, John Sandoe Books in Chelsea, where I had gone to stock up on reading material for the weeks ahead in the West Indies. By the time the police and the police doctor were through with me – I had been injured during the mugging – it was four o'clock in the morning, and I only had enough time to crawl home, throw our clothes into some suitcases and head for the airport in my race against time before Marjorie died.

For no particular reason, as the plane was taking off at Gatwick, I did something I had never done before and have never done since. I looked at my watch. It was five minutes past ten. When we got to Miami, my cousin Enrique met us with the news that my beloved aunt had died at the exact moment I was looking at my watch.

The following morning, Dima, Misha and I flew to Cayman. Anthony and Gloria met us at the airport and took us back to Marjorie's rental, where we three sisters were meant to be staying. On the way, we had a superficially civil conversation, even if underlying currents from Gloria were significantly less friendly than they had been for years.

Anthony more than Gloria filled me in with details of Auntie's death, after which the boys and I told them about the mugging. Dima and Misha were especially proud of the part they had played in capturing one of the thieves, and I couldn't help being captivated by their account, which was full of charm, lucidity and the rapture of childhood. Tellingly, as Gloria listened to the children and heard how they caught one of the muggers – the trial judge would later call them into the witness box and praise them for their 'bravery', 'character' and tell them 'you are truly exceptional boys and your mother must be justly proud of you' – I could not help noticing that her response contained a greater degree of polite disinterest than usual. Normally, she would have made a meal of just this sort of sensation. I also noticed that she did not even display polite interest in the physical injuries I had suffered, leaving it up to

Anthony to ask how I was feeling and to provide me with the recommendation that I get John Addleson to give the police the medical report they required for the forthcoming trial of the captured mugger, who had been charged with aggravated assault as well as mugging.

Mistakenly, I marked Gloria's coolness down to shock at Marjorie's death. Later on, I would realize that the real reason lay in her need to create the distance necessary to assume the mantle of aggressive self-justification she always employed when she was cloaking herself in the disguise of 'persecutor-as-victim'. Unbeknownst to me, Gloria already possessed knowledge I lacked. Marjorie had either not left a valid will, or if she had, it was nowhere to be found, which meant that Gloria was going to try to seize Marjorie's estate for herself.

It was not beyond the realms of possibility that Gloria had located the will and ripped it up. With her, it was never a case of right or wrong, so much as what she could get away with. At that point in time, though, I did not yet realize that her ruthlessness actually extended to financial matters. Like many other children of narcissists with antisocial tendencies, I found it impossible to actually envisage each new arena of deceit and dishonesty until I found myself in the middle of it. That is because people with scruples always find it difficult to put themselves in the shoes of the unscrupulous. It is virtually impossible for someone with a heart and a conscience to imagine how they would behave if they lacked a heart and a conscience. This inability to relate to dehumanization is what invariably gives the narcissistic, antisocial personality an advantage over a social personality. We can never envisage the next horror until it takes place. On the other hand, they have the ability to imagine how we will behave and usually use that imagination to manipulate us into situations which they find self-aggrandizing.

Right after we arrived at Marjorie's house, her Canadian lawyer friend Myrna, Anthony, Gloria, her cousin by marriage Pam, and I sat down to discuss the funeral details at Anthony's behest. He was concerned that the printers, priests, choir, florists and undertakers would all run out of time unless we came to certain decisions for the funeral that Saturday July 5. Now that one of Marjorie's 'children' – in the shape of me – had arrived, he wanted some decisions, as Libby and Kitty were arriving after the deadlines had expired. I would have felt better waiting for my sisters but understood the urgency, so took the seat they suggested at the head of the dining table, Pam having quieted my misgivings of feeling like the chairman of the board.

'We all know that Marjorie lived for you children. That's right, isn't it Gloria?' she said.

'She certainly laid claim to them as being her own,' my jealous mother replied in apparent agreement,

Although everyone in the family always took it for granted that Gloria didn't mind in the least that we children were commonly regarded more as Marjorie's progeny than her own, I was not so sure. So I took care during the ensuing discussion to be as tactful as possible, including Gloria in all decisions. After all, she was Marjorie's sister and our mother, even if the reality, openly acknowledged by all, was that we had been closer to Marjorie than she had been.

During the discussion, Pam asked if anyone had found Marjorie's will. This was the first pointer to the trouble that lay ahead. While Myrna confirmed that she knew what Marjorie's wishes were – they had discussed the contents of her will over the previous months, but she had never seen the will itself and did not know which Caymanian lawyer Marjorie had used to draw it up – I looked down the length of the table to where Gloria was sitting beside Anthony. She had a tight little smile on her face which was supposed to convey innocence and cooperativeness but which I knew invariably presaged something underhand. Anthony then drew out of his pocket an unsigned copy of the will Libby's attorney daughter Elizabeth had drafted and Fed-Exed to Cayman shortly after Marjorie had regained her senses the month beforehand, when we had all first learned that Marjorie's signed will could not be located.

At that time, Libby had asked Anthony to arrange for Marjorie to sign it in front of a notary, in keeping with Cayman Islands law. Marjorie was saying she could not remember where she had put the signed will or indeed if one reflecting her wishes actually existed, hence the need for a replacement. 'I've had this in my pocket ever since Libby sent it,' Anthony said. 'I never got around to having her sign it.' Everyone except Gloria looked aghast. 'The moment never seemed right,' he quickly said by way of explanation, marking his inaction down to sensitivity for Marjorie's feelings.

'You girls might still find the signed will when you go through her things,' said the ever optimistic Pam, who was clearly as surprised as I by this turn of events but envisaged me or my sisters running across it.

'I doubt it,' Gloria said. Somewhere in the recesses of my being, I felt my hackles rise. But, as so often happened with my mother, before you had time to think through the ramifications of one development, she had diverted your attention with another. This now happened as she refocused the conversation with, 'but we have more pressing matters to deal with than wills,' as if a signed will involving a substantial estate were a mere *bagatelle*, while the funeral arrangements were of overriding importance. Then she switched the conversation back to Marjorie's funeral service, affecting to know what her sister's favourite hymns were.

Afterwards, as she was leaving to return home with Anthony, she brought up the subject of rent for Grandma's house. 'I'll give you what I was giving Marjorie,' she said, as if she were being magnanimous.

'I need enough to cover my basic French expenses,' I said.

'And how much is that?' she asked acerbically.

'Another three hundred or so dollars,' I said, never envisaging that my well-off mother would resent giving me such a paltry increase when she knew only too well that I needed the money while she did not.

In the days to come, relations in the family degenerated for no apparent reason. My brother-in-law Ben then supplied one by informing me that Gloria was justifying her hostility towards me on the grounds that I was trying to 'raise the rent', as if I were a greedy witch who was trying to drive a poor old widow to penury. The fact that she would still be paying only a percentage of the market value, that she had over seven figures more money than I did, and that she had fewer expenses and responsibilities, did not even enter into her reckoning. As far as she was concerned, all benefits should still accrue to her and I should regard myself as fortunate that she was being generous in giving me anything at all.

On the day of my arrival, however, I did not know that Gloria 'had it in' for me. We parted company in ostensibly friendly fashion, and I went to bed to rest. The muggers had ripped my breast tissue and damaged the musculature in the surrounding area when they had torn the handbag I was clinging onto for dear life away from me. I was in so much pain that I could no longer function.

Then Kitty, and later Libby, arrived. Their attitudes were openly and uncharacteristically hostile, even though absolutely nothing but friendliness and sisterliness had been emanating from me. When the children and I tried telling them about my mugging and the part the boys had played in catching one of the thieves, they didn't even bother to listen and cut us off midsentence, even though this incident was of sufficient interest for BBC TV to interview the children and me upon our return to England.

I was stunned by their attitudes, which had the unwelcome effect of alerting me to the fact that something was afoot. What or why was a mystery. At first I genuinely had no idea what it might be. As I floundered about trying to figure out what was happening, I wondered if Gloria might be up to her old tricks, plotting, scheming and manoeuvring. Time would reveal my mother's central role in what was a truly diabolic plan, but in the meantime I was left in the dark.

Libby, who takes great pride in being as straight as an arrow, was first to pull off the gloves. When I informed her that I had tentatively done – at Anthony's suggestion – a rough draft of the Nieces' Tribute, which would form part of Marjorie's funeral service, she reacted as if I were trying to usurp her rightful role. Nothing could have been further from the truth. Aside from the fact that I just don't function like that, I was in so much pain that it had been a real sacrifice for me to do even a rough draft of the entire tribute. I was therefore happy to reduce my contribution by two-thirds. This, however, was not good enough for Libby, who announced that she couldn't face sharing the same tribute or house with me, and promptly took herself and her family off to a hotel. Kitty then hopped on the bandwagon, undergoing a complete personality change and acting as if we had always been sworn enemies, when in fact we had always been the best of friends and had supported each other throughout the whole of our lives.

For the few days that my two sisters were in Cayman, their attitudes could not have been clearer. They stuck to Gloria like deodorant to an armpit, acting as if I were their adversary and the trio had to close ranks against me. They came and went with Gloria like identical triplets, pointedly excluding me from all their plans, conversations and activities, including going through Auntie's jewellery, This I especially resented, for I had as much right to be there as any of them. They passed belittling comments about me and my children within my earshot, yet never once did either of them ask how I was recovering from my injuries or indeed display even the slightest concern for me or my children. This did not stop Kitty from having me babysit her daughter Gabriela on several occasions while she, Libby and Gloria gadded about in triplicate, as if they had always been the adoring daughters of an adoring mother.

I cannot deny being bitterly hurt by my sisters' attitudes, though I could well understand, given the lack of closeness neither had enjoyed with our mother while growing up, why they were basking in her ostensibly loving attentions. I could tell by now that she was using them, though quite what for I did not yet know. 'I suppose, if you were a prisoner and had the chance to soak up sunshine for ten minutes every few years, you'd take it,' I said by way of explanation to our cousin after we had spoken about my sisters.

One evening, after Gloria and Libby had left Marjorie's house, things came to a head between Kitty and me. 'The three of you are clearly trying to give me the message that I am to be excluded from your magic circle,' I said. 'Well, I have to inform you, I am as much a member of this family as both you and Libby, and I have as many rights as each of you. I don't know what the game is, but I will warn you: be careful, for united we stand, and divided we fall. Mummy cannot be trusted and, as your interests and Libby's coincide absolutely with mine, it does not behove you to close ranks with her against me.'

Kitty's unresponsiveness indicated that there was no reaching her, so I decided then and there to leave them to their own devices. Time, I knew, would tell the tale. In the meantime, I would simply prick up my ears and wait to hear what it was. Then, when I knew what I was dealing with, I would see whether the breach between my sisters and me was reparable.

It was against this rather disturbing backdrop that Marjorie was buried. I have never been so grateful to have had my children with me as I was on that occasion, for they, by their loving presences, gave me all the emotional support anyone needed at such a sad time. After the funeral, there was the inevitable reception back at the house. None of the guests would have detected the divisions within the family, for we were now all so adept at concealing the vituperation that passed for family life that we all should have been getting Oscars 365 days a year.

After all the guests had left, Gloria, Libby, her husband and daughter, Kitty, her husband and daughter, and my boys and I gathered in the drawing room to discuss what to do with Marjorie's chattels. We were all agreed that, until a signed will could be found, the only correct approach would be to respect her wishes as we knew them to have been.

Using the unsigned will as a guide, those wishes were that her property would be divided between her sister and three nieces. What I did not know, however, was that Marjorie had discussed some months before with Libby her intention of leaving everything to the three of us sisters alone. She had not wanted to include Gloria, I suspect partly because she knew Gloria did not need the money but also partly because she wanted her will to reflect her feelings about the sister who had been nothing but a plague to her.

However, in an act of compassion that certainly did not spring from our mother's maternal deserts, Libby had argued with Marjorie to include Gloria, pointing out how hurt she would be if she were to be excluded. Marjorie had not communicated either agreement or rejection to Libby, so none of us knew whether she had included Gloria or not. But Libby had taken it upon herself to include Gloria in the draft she had Elizabeth prepare a few weeks before Marjorie's death.

As none of us wanted to bother Auntie with awkward matters at such a sensitive time, and because Libby was perfectly happy with a four-way split, even if it should have been three ways, no one broached the subject with Marjorie of whether she did want Gloria included.

I knew nothing about any of this at that time. Nor was there any possibility, with the open rupture in the family, that I would find such important information out until it was too late. Whether Gloria herself knew about Marjorie's intentions and had orchestrated this whole rupture to ensure that she received a quarter-share to which she was not morally entitled, is something upon which I can only speculate. What I can say with absolute certainty, though, is that this is just the sort of ploy she would have pulled, had Marjorie mentioned her intentions of cutting her out to her will. Someone who worshipped at the altar of Mammon the way Gloria did, and who was as resourceful and conniving as she was, would definitely not have stood by meekly and let us inherit everything – not when she could sow division and reap a rich harvest that included both malice and money.

Indeed, I will go further and say that it would have been well within Gloria's scope of operation to hide or destroy Marjorie's will if it did not include her. Certainly, she had access to the house and could easily have gone through her sister's papers without any of the staff even noticing, as West Indian servants simply do not hover when family members are in attendance. There was every possibility that Marjorie had indeed signed her will earlier that year, then forgotten what she had done with it once she became befuddled when the cancer spread to her brain.

Whatever the truth behind Gloria's actions, we now had to contend with the undesirable situation of dividing up an estate without a signed will. On the grounds of being the only family member resident in Grand Cayman, Gloria offered to apply for the Letters of Administration under an intestacy, which meant that she would be declared the lawful inheritor. Then she would divide the estate up between the four of us. We all agreed that this seemed the most practical way ahead, never imagining for a second what we were letting ourselves in for.

In fact the best way forward would have been to instruct a solicitor to apply for probate using the unsigned will as Marjorie's Letter of Intent. That would have enshrined all our rights equally. However, by agreeing to Gloria's offer, we were actually agreeing to the wolf standing guard over the henhouse, and in so doing stripping ourselves of our rights under the law. Talk about folly.

With the practical matter of probating the estate dispensed with, we next turned our attention to Marjorie's jewellery.

'Where is it?' Gloria asked. Upon being told by Kitty that it was in its usual place, she marched right into Marjorie's bedroom, opened up the drawer where it was kept and came outside clutching the bag holding it all. 'I will be taking this home with me. I will be inspecting it and after I have done so, you can all have your pick,' she decreed. As all of us had our own, superior jewels, we all ignored Gloria's aggressive stance. But it served the purpose she intended, which was to assert her authority, for we had all meekly accepted her dictat: a gross mistake when dealing with someone as unscrupulous and Machiavellian as Gloria.

Next up for discussion was the furniture. Marjorie had quite a lot of nice antique pieces, some of which she had inherited and some of which she had bought through a connection of mine in 1976. At that time, she had declared that all of those purchases were to go to me when she died: a declaration she renewed to Myrna her lawyer friend shortly before her death and which Myrna had already confirmed to the family. 'I don't want any of it,' Gloria, Libby and Kitty each echoed about those pieces of furniture that fell outside my remit. 'I already have more than I need.'

'In that case, I'll select from whatever you don't want and ship everything to France along with the furniture she specifically left me. If any of you or your children want any of it in the future, I'll be happy to give it to you. Please remember to tell that to Andrew and Elizabeth,' I said to my niece Melanie for her to convey to her brother and sister.

'So you want everything?' Gloria rasped nastily.

'What do you mean?' I said.

'Exactly what I said,' Gloria replied.

'Aunt Gloria, she hasn't said she wants everything,' Ben said, hopping to my defence and trying to use his position as favoured son-in-law to protect me. 'She's said she'll take whatever you all don't want, plus what Auntie left her.'

'If she gets the furniture, she can't get anything else,' Gloria said, reverting back to the bitchy attitude that had culminated in her trying to burn my face.

'By the time she's paid to ship the stuff to France and paid duty on it there, she could have bought it all over there for less. This isn't about money, Aunt Gloria. She's trying to preserve the family heritage,' Ben said, putting my position into words that even Gloria ought to be able to understand.

This monster of self-regard, however, was not about to have a little thing like reason – much less a triviality like family heritage – derail her from her objective. 'Marjorie left no one anything. There's no will, so everything's up for grabs,' she said.

'Actually not,' I said steadily. 'She was very clear about the furniture she wanted me to have. All of that is indisputably mine, and no one else has a claim to it. It can form no divisible part of the estate, and any attempt to set it off against anything else would be wrong. I am perfectly happy to let the others have what they want, now or in the future, from the rest. I see no merit in throwing away family property when one of us can house it and give it to later generations. So I will be shipping it to Europe, and that's all there is to that. Shall we therefore proceed to the next point, before this degenerates into yet another slanging match for which there is no necessity?'

Gloria jumped up and came to stand over me. 'You want everything. I said you want everything, and everything is what you want. I rule this roost, and that's all there is to that. It's my way or the highway, and don't you forget it.'

She moved in to me, forcing me to arch my back in the chair.

'Just remember who rules this roost,' she spat.

'Will you please get out of my face?' I said calmly, looking directly at her.

'I have a good mind to box you,' Gloria hissed, raising her hand as if she intended to hit me.

'If you dare to touch me, I will beat the shit out of you even worse than the time you tried to burn my face,' I said.

'Aunt Gloria, please,' Ben implored over and over again.

'Mummy, why don't you go and sit down and let's finish off the task at hand?' Libby chorussed.

'Mummy, go and sit down and don't upset yourself like this,' Kitty added. 'It isn't worth it.'

Gloria, however, was in the mood for a spat and was certainly not going to be placated, especially by one or both of the triumvirate. Ignoring them all but having the good sense to step back, she leaped onto the morally superior high ground to which she, of all people, had absolutely no entitlement.

'You are a whore,' she decreed apropos of nothing.

'I cannot be a whore when I have never sold myself to any man,' I said levelly, furious that she would dare to speak to me like that in front of my children.

'The number of men you have had march through you is legion,' she said as nastily and authoritatively as she could. 'I say you are a whore, and a whore is what you are.'

There was no way I was going to let my mother demean me in my children's presence. Aside from the fact that she was setting an appalling example, why should I allow their respect for me to be undermined by the lies of a vicious intriguer? I leaned forward in my chair, forcing Gloria to step back and therefore give ground, physically getting the message across that she was not in quite the imperviously ascendant position that she wished us to believe.

'My dear woman,' I said in as cool and measured but as sarcastic and cutting a tone as I could manage, 'the only whore around here is you. While I freely admit I have given my body to men, there certainly was no legion of them, nor did I ever sell my body to any.' I paused for dramatic effect before adding even more edge to my tone. 'Which is rather more than we can say for you.'

'I have only ever known one man in my life,' Gloria said, wrapping herself in the sanctimonious hypocrisy which was her speciality.

'Oh, come off it,' I snapped. 'We all know that you married Daddy for his money and stayed with him for it, which means that you sold your body to a man for money, and that is the definition of whore. Plus I know all about Tony Feanny and Frank Watson.'

'Frank Watson?' Gloria said incredulously. 'That ugly old man? He offered me £40,000 to marry him before I married your father, and I turned him down.'

'That *rich*, ugly old man,' I said, my voice laden with innuendo. 'According to his daughter Anne, you did a lot of turning of another sort later on.'

'Frank was nothing but a vain old fool who would have said anything to boost himself,' Gloria said.

'Except that Vida Macmillan told me, when she came to London shortly before she died, that you yourself told her how desperately in love with Tony Feanny you were.'

'Tony was in love with me,' Gloria said proudly.

'Whether he was or not is beside the point. You told Vida that you were in love with him and that you had an affair with him.'

'Everyone knows Vida was mad,' Gloria said dismissively.

'No one ever accused her of being a liar,' I said. 'Which is more than we can say about you.'

'You are a drug addict. You are on drugs. Everyone knows you are a drug addict,' Gloria said, as everyone's jaw dropped to the ground, for as anyone who has had even the most glancing acquaintanceship with me knows, I have never taken drugs and indeed drink alcohol sparingly and irregularly.

'I will not have you telling barefaced lies about me in front of my children and nieces, especially when you are the drug addict, not me,' I said.

'I have never taken drugs in my life,' Gloria declaimed sanctimoniously.

'What do you think alcohol is?' I said sneeringly.

'Alcohol is not a drug,' she said.

'It most certainly is, and everyone knows you are nothing but a drunken sod. So I'd suggest you don't throw bricks from a glasshouse at people who live behind brick walls.'

'You are nothing but a frea…' Gloria started to say, her face twisted with venomous frustration that I was winning yet another row. Before she managed to finish the sentence, however, I interrupted, for there was no way I was going to run the risk of her using my birth defect against me in front of my children – or worse, lying about it so that she could obtain an advantage.

'You will remember that my children are present,' I commanded in a tone that stopped her dead in her tracks. 'If you say one more word, you will live to regret it. That I promise you.'

Amidst a chorus of beseeching from Ben, Libby, Kitty and Melanie, who kept on repeating how surprised she was that my good intentions were being not recognized, Gloria backed off both verbally and literally, muttering under her breath while moving back towards her seat that she was now ready to be taken home.

After such a massive disruption, no one was in the mood to divide the remainder of what was 'up for grabs', to use Gloria's inelegant but revealing description, so Ben, Libby and Melanie agreed to drop Gloria home before heading to their hotel. Marjorie's possessions, however, still had to be dealt with, for Libby, Kitty and I were leaving Cayman in a few days, and if we didn't do it, no one else would. That meant we had to come to some sort of agreement and do so right now. Ben, stepping into the breach, suggested that Libby, Kitty and I go through the remainder of Marjorie's property the following day. Whatever we did not want, we could give away.

'I don't want any of Marjorie's *bangarangs* and "dust-gatherers",' Gloria announced as she approached the front door, using the pejorative Jamaican slang for knickknacks, and in so doing, expressed disdain for her late sister and rival.

Marjorie had extensive collections of porcelain and cut glass, as well as quantities of silver and linen, which certainly merited more than her narcissistic sister's belittlement. But Gloria had achieved her objective. She had created chaos; had denigrated Marjorie through her possessions, and, with no more incentive to stimulate her into further expressions of malice, sailed out of the house clutching the bag of jewellery with Ben, Libby and Melanie in tow, an expression of malignant satisfaction distorting her once-beautiful features.

Normally, Kitty and I would have discussed what had happened as soon as Gloria had departed, but this time, the best she could manage was a frosty goodnight uttered through gritted teeth. Clearly, she still had something against me, though quite what it was remained a mystery. Michael and Gabriela, however, managed perfectly friendly goodnights to the boys and me.

The following day Libby, Kitty and I went through generations of embroidery and linen, as well as a plenitude of silver, china and crystal, together with other chattels including paintings. I will say in their favour that neither sister displayed the slightest sign of avarice. The division was done with an underlying affection for our beloved Auntie, which surfaced time and again as we happened upon things that brought back memories of her or other deceased relations. It was sad to see how this rupture had blighted what would otherwise have been an affectionate occasion. But good manners did prevail, even if the events of the last few days had gone too far for the air to have anything but a definite chill to it.

It was against this background that I arranged to have lunch with Robby Hamaty, an old friend I had not seen for thirty-five years. There was, of course, no question of asking either sister to babysit my children, so I instructed the maids to watch over them till I returned. 'Now, you boys stay inside and watch television. Monica and Vilma will get you something to eat for lunch. I'll be back in about two hours,' I informed them.

I returned to an uproar. Gloria and Libby had come to Marjorie's house while I was out, and my crazy mother had launched one of the unprovoked physical assaults for which she was notorious against Dima. As he was crossing the drawing room from his bedroom to the kitchen, she slapped him across his face for no reason at all except her desire to strike out and 'box' someone: an old trick of hers when she was in the mood to be physically abusive.

One would have expected to return to find that the child's aunts had taken his side against his abusive grandmother, but not one bit of it. Both were outraged on Gloria's behalf because Dima had then written a note which he had pinned on her back. It said, in block capitals: 'YOU STINK, OLD WOMAN.'

'Look at this,' Kitty shrieked in high dudgeon as soon as I had set foot in the house. 'Look at what Dima wrote about Mummy. What sort of child writes about his grandmother in these terms?'

'What happened?' I asked.

'It doesn't matter what happened. What matters is how he could write something like this about his grandmother. Then pin it to her back so that she was walking around with it for everyone to read,' Kitty said accusingly, as she waved the offending missive in the air.

As I looked at the note and saw what it said, I am afraid I could not help laughing. Not only was the image of Gloria walking around with that note too funny for words, but there was absolutely no doubt in my mind that Dima would never have behaved as he had done without extraordinary provocation. Not only is he gentle and loving, but he was actually Gloria's favourite of the three younger grandchildren. Which explained why she had attacked him and not Misha or Gabriela: in Gloria's sick way of reckoning, by attacking her favourite she was showing that there was nothing personal in the attack.

'It's not funny,' Kitty scolded. 'There's nothing funny about a child pinning such an objectionable note to his grandmother's back.'

'Of course it matters what happened,' I said lightly, refusing to be drawn into this maelstrom of preposterous outrage. 'There is no way he would have done something like that without provocation. What happened?'

'Your child is the rudest child I have ever seen, and I will not stay in this house with you or them one minute longer,' Kitty said, announcing her intention to join Libby in a hotel rather than allow me and my children to pollute her and her daughter.

While Kitty gathered up her possessions, Dima told me what had happened, so when my two sisters were leaving, I was able to inform them that I was astonished that anyone could have taken the side of an abusive bitch like Gloria against a child she had physically abused.

'You're just trying to justify your child's unjustifiable behaviour,' Kitty said as she stormed into the car and slammed the door.

Neither sister, of course, condescended to say goodbye to me or my children prior to leaving Cayman. In fact, it would be months before I heard from either of them again.

Try as I might, I could not make head or tail of their attitudes. Patently, something was afoot. But what?

I got a clue the day after Libby and Kitty had left Cayman for their respective homes on the US mainland. Gloria dropped in to Marjorie's house and announced to no one in particular, though there was no doubt her comments were aimed at me, 'I'm here to see if there's anything I need to give away to the needy.'

Not for one second did I believe her. Not only had she already announced to all and sundry that she didn't give a fig where any of Marjorie's chattels ended up, but after marching into the kitchen as if nothing had happened between us and after pouring herself a tumbler full of scotch, she plopped down on one of the sofas in the drawing room and launched into an account, relayed in a superficially friendly and conspiratorial manner, of how Libby and Kitty had 'grabbed everything of value from your aunt's jewellery. Libby waltzed off with the pearls, even though I gave her mine years ago. And I don't know what anyone living in the wilds of Middle America needs with two separate pearl necklaces when there is never occasion to wear even one! And, of course, no surprise here, she seized the largest of Marjorie's diamond rings for Melanie. Kitty, not to be outdone, went through the jewellery as if she'd never before seen anything of value in her life. The way she scratched her way through the things reminded me of a chicken scratching for corn. Ever since she married Michael, she's become as obsessed with this world's goods as his money-mad family is. You've never seen such an unedifying spectacle in your life. There's not much of value left after those two scavengers picked their way through poor Marjorie's little trinkets, but you can come around and see if there's anything you want out of their leavings.'

'Thank you,' I said neutrally, not caring about the jewellery or even wanting to see her again, but knowing that I had to tread carefully until Auntie's estate was wound up and I had received my share. Only then could I throw caution to the wind and tell Gloria to take a hike. In the meantime I had to try to discern what was going on.

Why, I wondered, was Gloria behaving as she was? I suspected she wanted to normalize relations between us sufficiently so that I would not leave Cayman without us not speaking to each other. Whatever the underlying motivation for her machinations, she knew me well enough to be aware that a re-establishment of relations between us would be well-nigh impossible without an apology, if she took the chance of letting me leave the West Indies without mending fences sufficiently for the patina of civility to be reintroduced into relations between us. As she had never once in the whole of her life apologized to anyone for anything, nor indeed had she ever been known to acknowledge having ever done anything wrong or even made a mistake, she would be taking the chance of losing me entirely for the remainder of her life unless she mended fences enough for us to at least talk, albeit frostily. She knew only too well how I had frozen her out for over a decade in the 1980s and 1990s, and can have been in no doubt that I would have done the same again, especially as she had pulled her stunt in front of my children. And she clearly didn't want that door to be closed to her – at least not yet and certainly not upon my say-so.

Having delivered her message – whatever it was and whatever it meant – Gloria jumped up. 'Well, I must be off,' she said. 'Drop in before you leave. We can discuss the rent while you're looking through the jewellery.'

The evening before my departure, I duly went to my grandmother's house to see my mother. I took the precaution of leaving the children with the servants. 'I'm afraid I'll have to keep my eye on the clock,' I said, drawing the boundaries as soon as I entered the house, as was my wont when dealing with adversaries. 'Everything's taken much longer than I thought it would, and I have Anthony and Heather coming over to collect some stuff earmarked for them.'

'The jewellery is on my dressing table,' she said, meaning that I should go and fetch it.

I brought it out to the veranda, where she was sitting, and handed it to her.

'I'm not interested in any of Marjorie's *bangarangs*,' she reiterated disparagingly in case I had forgotten her previous declaration the evening of Marjorie's funeral. I knew her well enough to understand that her message was that her late sister's jewels were a very poor second to her own.

'Here,' she said pushing the side table forward. 'Spread them here. There's nothing of any merit left – not that there was ever much to begin with – but what there was has been cleaned out by your two sisters.'

I duly turned the case upside down and disgorged its contents.

'You see?' Gloria said gleefully. 'Very slim pickings.'

'But they've taken everything anyone would want,' I said.

'I told you so,' she said, malicious delight oozing through every pore.

'Who took Auntie's sapphires? I know Kitty wanted them. Did she get them?'

'Well, they aren't here, as you can see for yourself,' Gloria said. 'I needn't tell you what a hawk she's become since marrying Michael.'

'Kitty knew the only things I was interested in were the sapphire earrings and Auntie's pearls.'

'Which Libby made sure she took even though she already has my pearls,' Gloria interjected, repeating what she had said a day or two before.

'And the sapphire earrings?' I asked, mindful that my slippery mother had not actually stated whether Kitty had got them.

'The other vulture has scooped them up,' she said.

'The only reason why I wanted those two items,' I thought to myself as I looked through the remainder of the stuff, 'was that they were things which I would have worn a lot and thereby had Auntie's presence with me constantly.' So I chose a white sapphire Verdura ring and a pair of topaz earrings instead. Even though they were worth less in monetary terms, in wearable terms they were versatile, and would therefore fulfil the function, as effectively as the sapphire earrings and double strand pearl necklace, in keeping Auntie physically close to me.

I must have looked as pleased with my selections as I felt, for Gloria eyed me with a mixture of surprise and perplexity.

'Are you sure you don't want anything else?' she said. 'I can see the mileage you would've got out of the sapphires and pearls, but what use will those *bangarangs* be to you?'

'Oh, I'll be able to wear the ring all the time instead of this,' I said, flashing my left hand with its marquise cut sparkler at her. 'That way, I'll have a bit of Auntie with me on a daily basis. And though the topaz earrings aren't quite my thing, I'm sure I'll find many an occasion to bring them out and remember Auntie by.'

A look of disappointment flickered across Gloria's face. This perplexed me, for I could not understand why she would care one way or the other about jewellery that she had never wanted and meant nothing to her.

Only after she died and Libby, Kitty and I were in the bank looking through her safety deposit box did the pieces of the puzzle start to fall into place when we came across Auntie's pearls as well as Gloria's own. Libby had never had either Marjorie's or Gloria's pearls. Nor had Kitty got the sapphire earrings. The last Libby and Kitty had seen of those was the year before Gloria's death, when she had taken them up to America to have them repaired. Though both of them offered to deal with the repairs for her, Gloria, ordinarily so avid to shove responsibility for everything onto others, was adamant that she would deal with them herself. She duly collected the earrings from the jewellers, took them back to Cayman and either gave them away, threw them out, or left them in the house for someone to steal. Whatever happened to them, Gloria, knowing that each of us had wanted them, had made absolutely sure that none of us would ever possess them. Yet again, the great depriver had found a way to screw us.

That coup was still to come as Gloria and I sat in my grandmother's house with Marjorie's jewels strewn across the side table. Now she brought up the other means of screwing me.

'As far as the rent is concerned,' she said commandingly, 'I can only afford another two hundred dollars a month. You will just have to rub along with that.'

'I have a proposal that might satisfy honour all round,' I said. 'But I must run now. So I'll write and tell you what it is.'

'There's no way I'm going to have my own daughter gouge my eyes out financially,' Gloria said as if she were Hitler dictating to the Slavs. 'I am a poor woman with no one to help me in life, and there is no way I can afford more than I can afford.'

'I'm sure with a bit of good will on both sides, we can come to an agreement that answers both our needs,' I said, bending down to kiss her goodbye as I finished off the encounter. 'I'll write. Bye.' Then I dashed to the car and drove out before I choked on my mother's gall.

The following morning the kids and I left Cayman for Jamaica. When booking the tickets prior to Marjorie's death, I had scheduled a stop in Cayman on the way back to Europe so that we could offer Gloria the emotional support I had then felt she might need, having lost her only sibling. However, she had given not one indication of feeling sad about Marjorie's loss. She had shed not one tear. Furthermore, she had behaved so appallingly towards me that I really didn't want to see her again. Rather than incur the additional expense of rerouting the tickets, however, I kept quiet and simply stayed in a hotel.

By then, I had also discovered something from Anthony that helped me to come to the conclusion that my mother was a truly dangerous woman who would do anything to achieve her own ends. In the two years she had been living in Cayman, Gloria had gone around doing everything in her power to undermine the high regard in which Marjorie was held. Her worst offence, as far as I was concerned, was in telling various people, 'My sister Marjorie goes on and on about how much she loves children. She's always calling mine "her" children, and all of them have fallen for her act of being sweet and maternal. But Marjorie can be the most selfish bitch when she wants to be. Everyone feels sorry for her because she couldn't have children, but the reason why she didn't is her own fault. If she hadn't been so selfish and materialistic, she'd be a mother today. But when she became pregnant by her first husband Ric, she got rid of it rather than take a reduction in her standard of living. And having killed her own child, she couldn't have any more.'

This story, more than anything else that happened at that time, led me to conclude that my friend Kari, who had studied psychology, was right when she assessed Gloria as 'evil'. I vividly remember my mother telling me, when I was a teenager, how her sister had had to terminate an ectopic pregnancy that had very nearly killed her. This, rather than selfishness, was the true cause of Marjorie's infertility: a condition that had caused her tremendous distress. She had even gone to England in the 1950s and consulted the Queen's gynaecologist in the hope that something could be done.

I cannot convey how utterly distressing I found the turn events had taken. I had always imagined that Auntie's death would be an occasion for unity between the four of us; that Gloria would feel something more than inconvenience over such a substantial loss; and that the three of us siblings, all of whom had loved our aunt dearly, would at least share our grief together. In short, it would have been a re-bonding experience. Instead of which, Marjorie's death had turned into something utterly unexpected and rather ugly.

Because Libby and Kitty appeared to have joined forces with Gloria and had excluded me from their hallowed circle, I had no idea what was going on or why. It nevertheless took no genius to figure out that Gloria was not only a part of the whole scheme but most likely its prime mover. The motive was still a mystery, and since I knew nothing of Marjorie's desire to exclude Gloria from her estate, and since Libby and Kitty by their own actions had made it impossible for me to discover such a pertinent piece of information at a time when it could actually have been to our mutual benefit for me to know it, I was left to grope in the dark.

I returned to Europe and took to my bed for weeks, emotionally exhausted as well as grief stricken. Not only had I lost the aunt I loved like the good mother she was, but I had also lost the remainder of my immediate family. Although I was only marginally upset by Gloria's conduct, having long since learned not to expect very much positive from her, I was truly taken unawares by my sisters, especially Kitty, with whom I had enjoyed a close, trusting and supportive relationship throughout our whole lives. Her loss, more than Libby's, was devastating to me, and overnight I had gone from having a family with four loved ones to having none.

Why did this happen? I tried to work it out with various friends, but the person who knew all of us best, and whom I therefore relied upon the most, was our cousin Enrique. His branch of the family was closer to ours than any other, not only because our fathers were first cousins and good friends, but even more so because our mothers had been close since childhood. Helen was the one whose twenty-first birthday party had dictated the date of Gloria and Michael's wedding; and she and Gloria, rather surprisingly considering how volatile and difficult each of them was, had remained friends over the years, even sharing a box at the race track in the days when both women still condescended to go racing.

Enrique's side of the family was richer than ours and had rather more experience of lost wills and diverted funds than ours did. He was of the firm opinion that the underlying motive was monetary. 'Just be careful that Auntie's money doesn't get split three ways instead of four,' he warned me. 'It looks as if that's what will happen.'

'Kitty and Libby aren't like that,' I said. 'They'd never go along with anything like that.'

'Do you think they're going to give you your portion of their thirds if Aunt Gloria decides to cut you out?' he said. 'Give me a break.'

'I really don't think this is about money,' I said. 'Not even Mummy would sink that low.'

'There's no depth that bitch won't sink to. And she'll just love screwing you. Let me remind you I haven't spoken to her since I was twenty-one, over thirty years ago, when I went to your house to see her, and she spent the whole evening slagging you off with one lie after another. She is a total bitch, and if she can screw you out of your inheritance, she will. Maybe her motivation isn't money. Maybe it's malice. But you can bet your bottom dollar, if screwing you out of the money will hurt you, she'll do it just for the satisfaction. Personally, though, I bet her underlying reason is the money. Aunt Gloria has always loved money, and everyone knows it. Listen to me, Cuz. You've got to be really careful. You need this money, and Auntie wanted you to have your share. Everyone knows that.'

Everyone – that is, all those people whose opinion really mattered to Gloria – did indeed know that. This, I would see in the months to come, was an invaluable pressure point to apply upon Gloria in case Enrique was right about her motivation. Like many another unconscionable narcissist, Gloria didn't mind doing the dirty on you – and certainly had no objection to benefiting from it – but she never ever wanted either the world at large or the people she cared about to see her for the low-down skunk that she was.

The first three months after Marjorie's death were truly one of the lowest points of my life. My birthday came and went; and my sisters, for the first time in my life, both neglected to contact me. Neither did Gloria. I had been in touch with her prior to it, having written her with a most generous rental proposal, whereby I would give her a forty-percent reduction on the market value during her lifetime, and her estate would make up a twenty-percent difference between what she wanted to pay contemporaneously and what I required as the minimal amount once she was dead. But she had refused to sign the agreement, knowing very well that my sisters would not acknowledge anything that wasn't in writing. She didn't even bother to conceal her hope that this would cause trouble between us. 'For all I care, the three of you can tear each other's eyes out when I'm dead,' she said with a vicious little laugh. 'You get the difference from those two worshippers of Mammon you call your sisters if you can. And incidentally,' she continued, employing her favourite tactic of regulating conversation with sudden changes of topic, 'the fridge is broken. Anthony has ordered a new one for the house. It's about $1400 and there are other things that need to be done in the house as well, so you won't be getting any rent this month.'

'I'm not sure I'm following you,' I said, genuinely perplexed.

'You surely don't expect me to pay for a refrigerator for *your* house. Tenants never pay for things like that here.'

'I think I get your point,' I said, scarcely believing the bitch's brass neck. 'The landlord-tenant relationship takes precedence over the mother-daughter one when I'm paying, but not when you are.'

'Have it any way you want. I am not paying for any refrigerator when I'm only a tenant, and that's all there is to that,' she said coldly and slammed down the telephone.

It was therefore not much of a surprise when my birthday came and went, and I received silence instead of the usual five- or ten-dollar telephone call.

By the time Kitty's birthday rolled around in mid-September, I had talked through the ramifications of my predicament with enough friends to have arrived at the conclusion that my spiritual and emotional welfare, as well as my financial interests, dictated that I mend fences with my younger sister if I could. Something deeply ominous had been going on, and it simply didn't make sense to discount a lifetime of sisterly friendliness without giving us a chance to get to the bottom of it. So I telephoned Kitty to wish her a happy birthday.

Though that first conversation was rather stilted, in the months to come the conversations we had, while less frequent or unguarded than they had been beforehand, became a step in the right direction.

While this process of repair was taking place, my closest friends had joined my cousin Enrique in advising me to stay on my guard against the possibility that my mother would try to cut me out of my aunt's estate. 'What you need to come up with is what Basil always called "the big stick". When you've got an adversary, there's no point appealing to their better nature. They don't have one. But you can prevail against them as long as you have a bigger stick to beat them with than they have to use against you,' counselled Kari, through whom I had met the superb therapist Basil Panzer.

All my other close friends agreed with that advice. The difficulty was: what stick could I come up with? And against whom should it be directed? Gloria certainly. But should I have anyone else in my sights? My cousin Enrique was of the firm opinion that I should include my sisters in that number, but I was reluctant to, partly because I found it difficult to envisage either one being so treacherous when I had always found them to be honourable, and partly because I suspected the divisions in his family had influenced him to tar them with a brush that might apply against some of his own siblings, but did not necessarily apply against mine.

For months I remained preoccupied with finding the way out of the hole I was in. Despite the ever-present threat hanging over my head; despite turning over every alternative in my mind; despite countless suggestions from friends, not one practical or effective solution presented itself. Then, towards the end of the year, my sister Kitty informed me that Libby, who was still not talking to me, had informed her that Marjorie's estate was likely to be settled soon. Manna then fell from heaven during a conversation I was having with Enrique. 'What are you going to do? Wait until you're cut out, and your share has been distributed to Libby and Kitty, who will then refuse to hand it over to you on the grounds that they must respect your bitch mother's wishes, or risk losing out on the rest of the money when she dies, because they thwarted her wishes? You need to wise up and find a way to protect yourself,' he argued. 'It's a pity you can't find something to induce the three of them to join forces to keep you sweet.'

'What do you mean?' I said.

'Oh, I don't know…something…anything that will cause them to join forces not against you, but with you.' Then he laughed. 'You need to come up with some dire family skeleton they want kept in the closet. And if one doesn't exist, make one up. You don't actually have to use it. Just let them think you will. You're a writer. Put on your thinking cap. You must be able to come up with something.'

The one virtue I have always had is the ability to take good advice. Thanks to Enrique's comment, I saw that I had spent the last three months looking for a club where none existed. The challenge was now to find an inducement. And I could see that he was right. If one didn't exist – and one didn't, for I had spent the last three months trying to find it – I should invent one.

Enrique came up with the inducement a few days later. We were talking about the way our mothers had treated the servants while we were growing up. 'They wouldn't have done that if they'd had to walk through life in their servants' shoes,' he said. 'It's a pity God couldn't turn them black and poor and let them see what it's like to suck it instead of dishing it out.'

He laughed. I laughed. We rang off. I went downstairs to fix some lunch for the boys and myself, and in a blinding flash I started to connect the dots. I picked up the telephone and rang Enrique back. 'I think you've come up with the big stick,' I said. 'Hear me out and tell me what you think. You know how Mummy despises what she so charmingly calls "old *nayger*"? Well, maybe you didn't know it, but shortly after Mickey's death, Marina Salandy-Brown, a BBC producer who is a friend of a friend, telephoned me about a programme the BBC wanted to do on eminent white people who were descended from African slaves. She said she was approaching me because she knew that Mickey had been the Vice-President of the Association of Black Lawyers in Britain. I said that, while that was so, we actually didn't have any African blood and that our ancestors had actually owned rather than been slaves. I said she of all people must know that all white Jamaicans are honorary blacks and are happy to join any black organization in the Diaspora, and while I would be pleased to take part in a programme that was about honorary blacks, I didn't think it would be right to lay claim to antecedents I didn't actually have. I suggested she get in touch with George. Marquess of Milford Haven, the head of the Mountbatten family, or his cousin the Duchess of Abercorn, who were proud of their descent from the great Russian poet Alexander Pushkin, the great-grandson of an Abyssinian slave named Hannibal. Well, how do you think dear

Gloria would react if I spin things around a bit and get someone to ask me to participate in a programme like that on the basis that she is descended from black slaves? For a fat fee, of course. Which I will be forced to take unless I get Auntie's money.'

Enrique howled with laughter.

'Miss G, you are a genius. I only hope for your sake that her racism is stronger than her love of money.'

'Even if it's not, you can depend upon it, there's no way Libby or Kitty will go along with her depriving me of my share of Auntie's estate once the possibility exists that I'll appear on television tarring them – and their children and grandchildren – with that brush. Although you and I differ on whether they're capable of standing by silently while Mummy excludes me from Auntie's estate, I am sure we are as one on the fact that they will move heaven and earth to prevent Mummy from cutting me out once their and their children's racial asses are on the line.'

'I love it,' Enrique said. 'Do it.'

Before doing it, however, I had to refine the story and also get someone trustworthy in the television industry to make me the offer so that I would not actually be lying when I dropped my bombshell. Then my path was eased when a producer friend whom I approached to 'make me an offer' said, 'I think it's a great idea for a programme. If you ever change your mind and want to present it, let me know and I'll pitch it to some of the channels. You don't even have to lay claim to ancestors you don't have. Just being you and Jamaican will be great TV.'

With everything now in place, I telephoned Kitty.

'Oh, by the way,' I said after our initial chitchat, 'I've been offered a role as a presenter of a television programme. The figure of £50,000 has been mentioned, but I'm hoping to bump them up.'

'That's nice,' she said.

'It's more than nice. It's absolutely necessary, unless I get Auntie's money soon.'

'So what's it about?' she asked. 'Something else on Diana and the royals?'

'Not this time. It's about passing.'

'Passing?' Kitty echoed, clearly as much at a loss of what that meant as I would have been had I been in her shoes.

'Yes, passing. You know. About black people who are descended from slaves and pass for white.'

'That's interesting,' she said.

'Well, you know, there's a lot of interest in that sort of thing nowadays,' I said, realizing that she had not yet made the connection. 'And it's not as if to say it will have any impact upon my life. In England, no one cares who's descended from slaves – and people still regard you as white even if you have a black ancestor. It's not like America, where one drop of Negro blood makes you black. The original approach was made by a television producer who knew that Mickey was the Vice-President of the Association of Black Lawyers in Britain...'

'How could he have been when he wasn't black?' Kitty asked, plainly perplexed, as indeed I had been when Mickey had first told me he was joining the association.

'Oh,' I said rather more airily than I felt as I echoed Mickey's explanation to me, 'in England you don't have to be black to be a part of the black community or join black organizations. All Jamaicans, white, black, brown, yellow, pink or green, are regarded as fully paid up members of the black community, the only distinction being that some of us are honorary members while others are actual.'

'I see,' Kitty, who had finally got the message, said. 'But surely you're not going to let them think you have an African heritage everyone knows you don't have?'

'You know that. I know that. But the producers don't know that. Of course I'm going to lay claim to the whole bag of tricks if I have to. I'll have no choice. Unless I get Auntie's money and get it soon. I have to live too, you know, and unlike you and Libby, I have no husband supporting me.'

'But how are you going to come up with an ancestor who doesn't exist?' Kitty said disbelievingly.

'Oh, that's easy. I'll simply say that one of Mummy's ancestors was a black slave. It will be plausible. Believe me. No one will doubt for a second that someone from an old Jamaican family has black slaves as ancestors.'

'I see,' Kitty said, so quietly that I knew she was now fully attentive and on her guard, for she, like me, goes very still when she's concerned.

'Don't worry about me,' I then said brightly, taking advantage of the opportunity to achieve the necessary denouement in glorious Gloria-thinking-only-of-herself tradition. 'I'll be fine. It won't affect my position at all. Nor will it affect my children's, because they have no genetic link to me. It's not as if to say any prospective in-laws will be able to object to them on racial grounds, because they remain white no matter what I say in the programme. So I don't have to concern myself about affecting their futures. Of course, I won't enjoy doing the programme, and won't unless I absolutely have to. I've told the people who approached me that I need some time to think about it. Hopefully Auntie's money will have come through before I have to make up my mind. Otherwise I'll have no choice but to present it. One good thing that will come out of it, aside from my fat fee, is that Mummy thereafter will be known to the whole world as "*Nayger* Gloria". Let's see how that sits with that loathsome black-baiter.' I laughed ghoulishly but genuinely at the thought of that paragon of egotistical snobbery being knocked down a peg or three. Kitty, who ordinarily would have laughed as well, did not, which was all the confirmation I needed that my message had been received loud and clear.

No sooner had I hung up than I telephoned Enrique.

'Just you wait, Miss G,' he said when I had finished my verbatim account of our conversation. 'Kitty and Libby will be batting on your team from now on.'

'Let me put it this way. Even though I've always believed that they'll stand up for me if Mummy tries to pull a fast one, this gives them a strong personal incentive to strong-arm that bitch into doing the right thing. And not for me either. Not even for themselves necessarily, for neither of them leads a public life, and there's no reason for the periphery of their circles to know that we're sisters, so they can always kid themselves into thinking that they're inured from an injurious link. But now that Elizabeth has produced the heir to a presidential dynasty, Libby will be alert to the danger of one of the supermarket scandal sheets making the connection between me and her grandchildren. Do you remember the meal they made of Jefferson's illegitimate slave descendents? Well, you can depend upon it, Libby will be only too aware what the headlines would be like, if a TV programme I presented gave those rags the opportunity to declare that the legitimate heirs of presidents and signatories to the Declaration of Independence are the descendents of African slaves.'

Enrique laughed. 'You bet she will. Somehow, Miss G, I suspect you're over the worst now.'

'That's exactly what I'm hoping. Somehow I don't see Kitty wanting her beautiful blue-eyed, blonde treasure, who was too precious to associate with my children unless it was convenient for her to offload her on me, to be categorized as the descendent of slaves either,' I said, my bitterness about the way she had behaved towards me in Cayman surfacing. 'I could be wrong, but I don't see her being thrilled if her grand, aristocratic mother-in-law has cause to look down on Gabriela instead of taking pride in her.'

I don't know if my bombshell had anything to do with it, but the tone of my relationship with Kitty, which had already been normalizing, quickly fell back into its old place. Libby, who had hitherto been as silent as the grave, now started to speak to me again, albeit without any real warmth; and more as if she were doing me a favour than as if she were fond of me. But speaking nevertheless. And Gloria, whose lust for news was so great that she would sooner have stuck her head down a horse's mouth, while it was eating, than forgo the possibility of missing out on even the slightest morsel, telephoned me to ask me what I was up to.

'Oh, I'm *very* well,' I trilled, my tone, in evocation of my ruthless mother, as airy as it had been when I had spoken to Kitty. 'I've been discussing a most fascinating offer to present a television programme, and I'm just waiting to see if it goes ahead. The fee mentioned is £50,000, but I'm intent on bumping it up if I can. For something as controversial as that, I don't see why £100,000 or even £150,000 won't be equally acceptable.' This time I had no pangs of guilt at all. Not only did I owe my treacherous mother no loyalty – in the first place it was thanks to her that I was actually having to resort to such methods to ensure that my rights were protected – but I was actually patting myself on the back with glee as I used my god-given gift with words to misinform her while staying within the bounds of truth.

I waited expectantly for the woman who never displayed any interest in my professional accomplishments, or indeed any other area of my life, to grill me for news, knowing that if she did, the reason why she had decided to spend her beloved money on a telephone call was that she wanted to 'pick my brain', as she used to describe her intelligence gathering.

'That's nice,' she said pleasantly but in such a neutral tone of voice that I knew she was being canny.

I had not been brought up by Gloria for nothing. Superb though she was at psychological gamesmanship, she was not the only one who had antennae. While she used her skills for destructive purposes, I either did not use mine at all or did so only for productive or protective purposes. This meant that in a situation such as this, I had the advantage. Having learned the art of obfuscation from her and how it worked only if others did not know you were employing it, I now emulated her example and, using a psychological mirror on her, gave away nothing.

'It is, isn't it?' I said, then, utilizing the diversionary tactics I had learned from her, I continued. 'God really isn't sleeping. This opportunity has fallen into my lap like manna from heaven. It might not be ideal, but it is the answer to many of my most pressing problems.'

I could tell I had succeeded in depriving her of the information she sought when Gloria said sweetly, 'So what's the programme about?'

This, from the mother who had never once alluded to anything I was working upon, nor indeed anything that I had published, or indeed anything that had been written about me professionally, was all the confirmation I needed that the international telephone wires had been burning. Should I answer or shouldn't I? I decided that freezing her out would be a more effective technique than telling her anything.

'Oh, nothing that wouldn't bore you to tears,' I said. 'How is Anthony?'

'He's okay,' she said, playing her cards equally close to her chest.

'And Pam and John?' I said, driving the conversation further away from where she wanted it to be.

'They're fine,' she said with just enough annoyance in her voice for me to see that I was succeeding in my quest.

'That's good,' I said, giving her no time to grasp the nettle from me. 'They're so nice. You're really lucky to have them there. Incidentally, how is the refrigerator? Because you've never told me if it works or not – and I wouldn't want you to be inconvenienced in any way. Not when we have a landlord-tenant relationship.'

At this point I couldn't help myself. I started to laugh, and had to cough and splutter to conceal my amusement. Gloria, always quick on the uptake, cannot have been in any doubt that I was taking the Mickey out of her. But so superb were her gamesmanship skills that she never missed a beat as she said, 'It's working as any other new fridge works.' Then, she let her annoyance show again. 'But I didn't call you to talk about fridges.'

That was the perfect opening for the question: just what did she phone me for? But that question would have been a tactical error. I was never going to get the truth out of her, nor, thanks to her example, was she going to get it out of me.

'No, of course you didn't,' I said, sending her hurtling down another blind alley as I pretended that ours was a proper mother-daughter relationship and she was interested in my children. So I wittered on about what Dima and Misha were up to.

Although one could never predict what awful stunt Gloria would pull out of her glad-bag of tricks, I knew that she was utterly predictable once the die was cast. I would have staked my life that she would terminate this conversation at my first pause for breath, and intent on dragging it out for as long as I could, if only to annoy her and rub her nose in it, I – who normally speak rather slowly, pausing for thought or dramatic effect as well as to give conversational partners their chance to interject – now did a Gloria on Gloria and didn't even give the air time to enter my nostrils much less leave my lungs.

After about five minutes of this, I could keep up the pace no longer and was forced to take my first real pause. No sooner did I than Gloria, who never listened to what anyone said unless she was picking their brain for information, confirmed my suspicions. 'That's all very good and well,' she said in a real non-sequitur, 'but I have to go now before the Cayman Telephone Company bankrupts me. Love to the children. Bye.' And she hung up before I even had a chance to say goodbye.

For the first time since my aunt had died, I felt I was back in the loop. If I was still not in control of my destiny, at least I had re-established a connection with the forces surrounding it. Once more I now had a feeling of manageability and predictability if not of security. After the chilling exclusion to which I had been subjected, this was like the sun coming out after months of fog and rainfall. In short, life was getting back to normal. Or, at any rate, what passed for normal in our family.

Chapter Twenty-Five

With a person like Gloria, normality was a purely relative thing, to be measured according to her whims and needs. While she could be flagrant about her motivation, she could also couch it in the deepest, darkest mystery when that suited her purposes, with the result that one might suspect what she was up to or why, but until one had the proof, one couldn't be sure. Up to this point, she had been careful not to provide me with any proof of what her objective might be regarding Marjorie's estate. From her point of view, that was a very effective technique for keeping others on the hop. But from my point of view, it caused uncertainty, especially as no child wants to condemn a parent until all the proof is in.

In January 2004, she asked me how I proposed to pay Libby back the money she had lent me a year and a half before to keep the roof over my head. 'I'll pay her back out of Auntie's money when the estate is probated,' I replied, deciding that the best policy lay with assuming that she would not do the dirty.

I immediately knew that Gloria was springing her trap when she said, in that ice-cold tone she adopted when letting people know that she had neither heart nor scruples, 'My suggestion to you is that you get yourself a job. Marjorie left no will, and so everything of hers is mine.'

'What are you talking about?' I said angrily. 'You know as well as I do that she intended at the very least for Libby, Kitty and me to have an equal share with you.'

'And where is that written?' Gloria said icily, fulfilling the dread I had felt ever since I had set foot in Cayman for Marjorie's funeral and found myself at the centre of an inexplicable maelstrom.

'Actually, it's written in her will,' I said, on rather firmer ground than Gloria realized. Some years before, I had been a witness in the Eric Hopton case, when the remainder of his family and his other beneficiaries had proceeded against his nephew Christopher. I had learned, as a result, that an unsigned will can, in certain instances, be put forward for probate as a letter of intent and can be recognized by the court as being a valid instrument *in lieu* of a properly executed will. There were certainly enough witnesses as to what Marjorie's intent had been, including Myrna, her lawyer friend.

'What will?' Gloria snapped irritably. 'She didn't leave a will.'

'Oh really? And what was that document that Anthony pulled out of his pocket the day after Auntie died, when we were all sitting around her dining table?'

'That was an unsigned will,' Gloria said triumphantly.

'You might not know it,' I said equally triumphantly, matching power with power, 'but an unsigned will can be probated as a letter of intent. That was always an option we had. We didn't take it because you promised to get the letters of administration and split the estate four ways.'

'That was then. This is now,' Gloria said with finality, as if by doing so she could close the subject forever.

She should have known better than that.

'Are you saying that you will not be turning over my quarter share to me?' I asked in a matter-of-fact way.

'That's about the size of it,' she trilled, triumph reverberating down the telephone lines.

'I cannot believe that my own mother would try to rip me off. It's bad enough that I've had a publisher, solicitors and a financial advisor do so,' I said with as much fury as I felt, 'but for *you, my own mother,* to join their number is beyond belief.'

'Marjorie was my sister. I am her next of kin. The law is clear on that point. Because she died intestate, all is mine,' Gloria trilled again.

'You entered into an agreement with us,' I reminded her.

'Do you have anything in writing?' she asked in the smart-arse way she had when she was crowing about having outsmarted people.

'Ah, so are you now saying that your word is meaningless?' I countered.

'What word? I never agreed to anything with any of you,' Gloria declared in that tone of voice which meant she was fully prepared to brazen it out.

Nevertheless, I was relived to hear her lump me into the same category as my sisters. It was the first clue she had so far provided that she intended to cut the others out as well. That knowledge thrilled me, not because misery loves company but because I could see that her greed was getting the better of her judgement. I was far more likely to get my share if she alienated the three of us than if she froze only me out.

If my two sisters now shared my undesirable fate, there was a beautiful symmetry to them doing so after having joined the crow's team in Cayman and hurt me the way they had.

'You might not be aware of it, but an agreement doesn't have to be in writing to be valid and enforceable legally,' I said.

'I made no agreement with any of you,' said Gloria hotly, always ready to tell the boldest lie to your face if it served her purpose.

Yet again she had lumped all three of us together.

'You know, Mummy,' I said, emboldened by that observation, 'you've pulled some filthy tricks in your time, but this beats them all. You know as well as I do what you agreed with the three of us. I've known for many years that you're a devious, vicious, malicious piece of shit, but even I never had you pegged as a thief.'

'I can't steal what is mine,' she said.

'But you can steal what isn't yours, and that's precisely what you're trying to do. You know it, and I know it; but what you might not know is that Auntie didn't even intend you to have anything. The only reason why you got a look-in at all was that Libby twisted her arm to include you. That more than anything is the reason why Auntie didn't sign the will originally – if indeed, she didn't. For all we know, she signed it, and it's gone walkies.'

'Are you accusing me of purloining her will?' Gloria said, picking up on my innuendo.

'I haven't said so, but since you've brought the prospect out into the open, you are the only one of us who had means, opportunity and motive. You tell me.'

'I'm not going to listen to any more of your ravings, you nutty buddy,' Gloria barked, slamming down the phone.

I rang her right back. As soon as she answered, I launched right in.

'I know Grandpa and Grandma taught you how to behave, so you don't have the excuse of lack of breeding for behaving in an ill-bred manner. I would suggest you remember that you're supposed to be a lady and behave accordingly. If you don't want to listen to unpopular truths, don't embark upon ignoble behaviour. You know, Mummy, you are my mother and therefore there are sacred aspects to our relationship beyond our control. I can assure you, were it not for that fact, there is no way I would be speaking to you now or ever again. And, for what it's worth, I've suspected since Auntie's funeral that you were planning to pull the stunt you've just pulled.'

'I have pulled no stunts,' said Gloria, the past-mistress of denial, trying to disclaim the obvious with a display of dignity.

'Well, I am no fortune-teller, and either you are as transparent as glass, or I am sufficiently perceptive to have seen through your machinations. Either way, the fact remains that you are trying to con me out of money that Auntie intended me to have. You know, Mummy, you are going to die sooner rather than later. If you believe in God, as you claim to, you can have no doubt that Auntie and Daddy and Mickey and Grandma and Grandpa and Uncle Ric, and everyone else who does and doesn't matter to you who is dead, can see what you're doing right now, God included. I know you think you have Him wrapped around your little finger and that He'll forgive you any sin as long as you believe in Him, but just how do you think you're going to explain away stealing my share of Auntie's money to her and to our other loved ones? They're not God, and they won't forgive you.'

I paused. Deafening silence on the other end of the telephone. But I could hear her breathing and so I knew she was listening.

'And,' I said, picking up back the beat again, 'it's not only the dead who will soon know what you're up to. Believe me, if you hang onto my money, I will make it my business to go around to everyone who knows us and let them know that you are no better than a common thief.'

With that, Gloria came back to life.

'If you think people will believe you over me…' she began.

'Come off it, you deluded drunkard,' I snapped. 'You're not speaking about one of the servants. Everyone will believe me because they already know what Auntie's intentions were. It's the truth, and the truth has a ring to it that falsehood doesn't. And they know I have no reason to lie.'

'I'm not listening to another second of this,' Gloria said.

'That's fine by me. Hang up if you want. Just remember: if you try to steal my money, you will be stealing a lot more than just my money. You'll be stealing the regard everyone you know, living or dead, has for you. Everyone already knows you're a vicious, deluded bitch. Do you really want to add thief to the list? Bye!' I trilled, knowing that no matter the outcome, I had got the better of her, even if it should only prove to be for the duration of this conversation.

Sick with worry now that the very situation I had feared and tried to head off had materialized, I decided to purge my troubled soul and throbbing head of the pollution. So I rounded up the dogs for a walk.

As I headed towards the front door, I wondered what Enrique's reaction would be now that we had finally discovered that Gloria's love of money outstripped her contempt for the black race. Just then the telephone rang. I rushed to pick it up, wondering if it was my cousin. It was Kitty.

'You will never believe what just happened! Mummy telephoned me and complained that you'd been dunning her for Auntie's money. She said she had a good mind not to give you any when it comes through, which should be any moment now that the letters of administration have been granted. I told her that she had no right to hold onto your share, and she says she's going to cut me out as well for being rude to her on your behalf.'

Jubilation reared its beautiful head. The saga was unravelling just as I had hoped, albeit rather more quickly than I had dared to imagine. With luck, everything would be all right. Gloria was making the same mistake Hitler had made, fighting a war on too many fronts. Hopefully she would realize sooner rather than later that her position was unsustainable, especially as she had no army of followers backing her up and no real likelihood of any meaningful allies either. I could not see Libby selling out herself or her sisters. Not only did her sense of honour preclude such a possibility, but she also didn't need the money. So, after I set Kitty straight about how my conversation with our Dearest Mama had really gone, I asked what she was going to do.

'I'm waiting for Libby to phone me back. She's speaking to Mummy right now,' Kitty said. So she had already been in touch with our other sister, who was stepping into the breech to see what influence she could wield over the recalcitrant Gloria.

I know one should never say 'I told you so', but I fear I have not yet evolved to the stage where I can resist doing so in certain situations. This was one of them. I had endured three months of the most wretched anxiety and undeserved isolation, followed by another three months of uncertainty when neither sister had openly batted for me, but had managed instead to convey the message that I had somehow been deserving of the treatment they had dished out. And truth be told, I felt that Kitty was getting off lightly if you compared what I was about to do with all that had preceded it in the past six months. 'Did I not warn you at Auntie's house,' I said, indulging my petty streak, 'United we stand, divided we fall? You and Libby froze me out and lay down with the asp in her basket, drinking her venom as if it were honey. So you really shouldn't be so surprised that she's rounded on you and bitten you too. Not so painless now that the teeth are sinking into your flesh, is it?'

'We didn't really intend to freeze you out. Mummy…' she said, starting to explain.

'Don't even bother,' I said, cutting her off to spare her the discomfiture of an explanation that would only confirm what I already knew in substance if not in detail. 'I don't need to hear it.'

'We didn't mean for you to feel bad,' she said.

'Maybe not, but you succeeded with a brilliance beyond your intentions. Anyway, that's all water under the bridge now. United we stand, divided we fall. Unless we form a solid phalanx to defeat Mummy, you do realize that we're never going to see one penny of Auntie's money until she's dead, don't you? If we do even then,' I said, little realizing how close I had inadvertently come to the facts as they stood. Unbeknownst to us, Gloria had set up her affairs in such a way that if she had dropped down dead right then, Libby, Kitty and I would have inherited practically nothing from her – and every penny she had was money which our loved ones had left her with the understanding that she pass it on to us.

'Have no fear. She's not going to defeat us. Not if I can help it,' Kitty said. 'I need that money almost as much as you.'

No sooner had I hung up from her than Libby, who had up to that point had remained frostily distant with me, telephoned. Her normal self for the first time in months, she recounted Gloria's heavily slanted and self-serving account of the conversations with Kitty and me.

'I told her she has no right to withhold either of your bequests. Once she saw the three of us are batting on the same side, she quickly realized she had a choice. Mummy is no fool. She doesn't want to spend the rest of her life with none of us speaking to her. I was careful not to give her any reason to do to me what she's done to you.'

Irritated by the possible implication that we were somehow responsible for triggering what Libby had avoided, I snapped, 'We didn't give her any reason. She attacked both of us out of the blue, as you know only too well she is capable of. I needn't remind you of the countless times she victimized you.'

'None of that matters now. What matters is that she didn't attack me. That means the penny's dropped. She's now got to find a way back to giving you two your share. You know her. She can never admit she's wrong.'

'She's a debased bitch.'

'Listen to me,' Libby said. 'Don't take her on. You know how she loves a fight and can never back down once she has the bit between her teeth. I did my best to placate her. I told her I'll fly out to Cayman as soon as I can, to help her sort things out. She hasn't actually told me that she won't give either of you the money.'

'She certainly told both of us.'

'But not me. Let's take advantage of that. I'm sure I can massage things so that she does give you both your share. She now realizes the consequences if she doesn't, and I honestly don't think that's a price she wants to pay. But you've both got to lie low and let me deal with her.'

'I tell you what,' I said. 'You deal with her in your way. And I'll deal with her in mine.'

'No, Georgie, no. If you take her on, that might give her the excuse she's looking for to cut us all…'

'Don't worry. I'm not going to take her on. I agree with you about not getting roped into a fight with her. Don't forget, she's my mother as well. I know her too.'

This was a fine kettle of fish, as Queen Mary used to say. If Libby thought I was going to leave my fate exclusively in her hands, however, she had another thought coming. Although I was careful to keep my counsel, at least with either sister in case their mouths slipped and word got back to Gloria, I came up with my own fallback plan in case Libby's amelioration didn't work.

It was the essence of simplicity. If Gloria didn't cough up the money, I was going to have her declared mentally incompetent. As her eldest child, I would be her next of kin and would assume responsibility for her affairs. That would give me absolute control over her finances.

If that happened, I would respect Marjorie's expressed wish and divide her estate in three ways only, after which I would set up a system whereby Gloria's money continued to be managed in such a way that her lifestyle remained the same. She would still have her servants, her liberty, even as much money as she wanted to spend, on whatever she wanted, and none of the three of us would utilise any of her funds for ourselves until she was dead. She could even continue drinking if she wanted to, for I regarded it as no part of my duty to deprive her of the means to abuse herself. But – and here was the rub – the control freak, who had spent her whole life controlling everyone, would no longer have control over her own affairs. That fact alone would drive her up the wall.

There was ample medical justification for such a course of action. Indeed, she should have been declared incompetent years ago. Certainly Marjorie's doctor was of the opinion that she was 'out of touch with reality' and 'mentally incompetent', a view he had expressed to me at the time of Marjorie's funeral when he displayed concern over what would become of Gloria now that her sister was not there to look out for her.

'I wouldn't worry about her if I were you,' I had said then. 'She's a lot less helpless than she looks. The one person who always profits from her antics is herself. She may be as mad as a march hare, but she has the canniness of a fox, and is utterly sane in furthering her self-perceived interests. It's not her I worry about. It's everyone she comes into contact with.'

'She shouldn't be left in charge of herself,' he had said.

'Aside from the fact that she is very adept at playing the sane and sensible goody-two-shoes role when it suits her, and would therefore be difficult to nail down if we tried to take over her affairs, she would die if anyone tried to grasp the nettle from her. Can't you see that she is the one who must always be in the driving seat?' I asked him. 'She's determined to continue living here in Cayman and has always said she will never live with anyone but herself. I'm sure she'll manage. She always does. As I said, it's not her I worry about, but everyone she comes into contact with.'

'If ever you need me to help you, let me know,' he had said that summer in 2003. The time had now come, and I telephoned him and asked him if he would be prepared to provide a sworn statement to the effect of what he had said to me the year before. The answer was yes.

Next I telephoned Charles Thesiger, the psychiatrist who had dealt with Gloria in the 1970s. I explained that there was a possibility that I might have to have her declared incompetent. He said that while he would be happy to see her and give his considered opinion as to her present mental state, there was too large a gap between the time when he had treated her and the present for that treatment to be relevant now. While this response was not as helpful as John Addleson's, he did agree to provide a statement of her condition then. I had little doubt that if push came to shove and Dr. Thesiger was called upon to commit pen to paper, anything he had to say would contribute to her ultimate detention owing to the longstanding and intractable nature of her behaviour.

I am nothing if not thorough. By this time in my life, I had run across too many Glorias for me to commit the cardinal and fundamental error of providing her with any chance of escape. I knew only too well that this type of personality will slither through the tiniest crack if you are not careful enough to block all avenues of escape. So I telephoned her current GP, a woman I had never met but who I understood from Libby was responsible. She agreed that Gloria was usually drunk by midmorning, and I put her on notice that I might have to ask her to provide evidence as to Gloria's competence in the event that we had to 'intervene'. She agreed to assist. Next on my list was the lawyer who was supposed to have been acting for all of us. She stated that she 'could smell the liquor on your mother's breath' every time she saw her and had reservations about just how mentally competent she was. She too was prepared to say so for the purposes of a 'medical intervention'.

Once I had the medical and legal figures lined up, I felt far better than I had hitherto. Although I would have loathed having to declare Gloria incompetent – I knew from my own teenage experience how soul-destroying the loss of your personal autonomy can be, and could certainly have done without the prospect of the newspaper publicity that such a course of action would result in– now that the chips looked as if they might be down, there was no way she was walking off with my part of the pot. Either I got it, or she would have to accept the disagreeable consequences of her actions. If she didn't like them, so be it. I'd sooner see her suffer than do so with my children. She at least would deserve it, while none of us did.

One of the virtues of having survived as turbulent a life as mine is that you acquire a sense of proportion and an appreciation of the consequences of actions: your own as well as other people's. In the process, I have also acquired a solid core of good friends, whom I support and who have supported me throughout much of my adult life. Once more, they proved to be irreplaceable as I talked through the best way of dealing with Gloria. The easiest thing, of course, would have been to stop speaking to her. But I was hoping to get her on tape making her typically insane statements, such as the time she told me that she was behaving in a 'Christ-like' manner. 'Mark you, I didn't say Christian. I said Christ-like,' she trilled, making it clear that she regarded herself on a par with the Father and the Son. Comments such as these, I realized, would be extremely helpful in any legal process, so I duly hitched up my taping equipment and lay in wait for Gloria's Gloriaisms.

My mother, however, was no fool. She knew that I had trapped my crooked solicitor, publisher and financial advisor in just that way, and that there was every likelihood I was taping her as well now that we were in opposing camps. So she cannily started to sound the soul of reason.

Nevertheless, I kept on telephoning her, making my dutiful daughter calls, because it was crucial to my interests to keep the channels of communication open. How else could I judge for myself what was going on? This was where having been her favourite as a child came in handy. I knew her like the back of my hand, even if I didn't always want to acknowledge what I did know. As long as I spoke to her, I could, to use one of her hackneyed expressions, 'read between the lines'. This had always been one of her favourite ways of information gathering, and now it became mine too.

By making it clear to my mother that I was speaking to her only through a sense of duty, I was also dangling both a carrot and a stick before her. The one thing narcissists cannot stand is people who don't give them the feedback they require, so as I drove home the stake of duty with icy politeness, I was letting her know that her powers of persuasion had failed to illicit the affection or admiration she desired. On the other hand, I said only the things I would have ordinarily said if our relationship had been better. By doing that, I was giving her a taste of what she could have, but was missing, and would continue to miss, unless she shaped up and deserved to be treated with greater warmth.

One day Gloria, who hated being on the outside of anything, could no longer stand the chill of being out of the loop.

'I know you're up to something,' she suddenly said apropos of nothing,

'I don't know what you're speaking about,' I said with *faux* innocence, taking a leaf out of her book and thereby using her own technique against her.

'Oh, yes, you do. I gave birth to you. I know you're up to something. What is it?'

'Why would I need to be up to anything?' I said, still the innocent.

I didn't expect her to say: Because of Marjorie's money. She might have been evil, but she wasn't stupid. I suspected that she suspected she was being taped, so she wasn't going to make a compromising admission.

'You're up to something. You're getting ready to sue me, aren't you?' she said, and I took my hat off to her. She was still adept at ferreting out information.

'Now why would I do that, Mummy?' I said, still on the innocent kick which, I surmised, was maddening to her.

'You know as well as I do why,' she snapped.

Realizing that she would never actually compromise herself, I decided to teach her a lesson that she should have learned long ago.

'Listen, Mummy,' I said. 'I have told you time and again, there are sacred aspects to our relationship. I'm really surprised that someone who thinks she's a part of the Holy Trinity, along with the God the Father and God the Son, would miss the obvious spiritual ramifications. Is your much-vaunted belief in God nothing but the noise of an empty spiritual vessel making an almighty clatter to justify your roll through life? You act as if you aren't aware that if God, in His infinite wisdom, anointed us mother and daughter, the divine aspects of that relationship have to be respected as well as the temporal ones.'

Silence. I knew I had reached her yet again, for the one entity she regarded as her equal was God, and I had presented her with a thought that no one else ever had. Well, I can outwait anyone if I have to, especially when the silence is to my advantage, so I let time drag on into an uncomfortably long pause while Gloria went doggo on the other end of the line.

Finally, when she could stand the void no longer, she picked the conversational thread back up and said, rather more lamely than before, 'Are you going to sue me?'

'No, I'm not.'

'It's just that you're always suing people, and I thought you might sue me.'

'I'm not always suing people. I sue only people who wrongly injure me, which of course is precisely what you've done. But you're not people. You're my mother. And frankly, Mummy, there's no way I'd give you the platform to go around drumming up sympathy for yourself at my expense. I've seen you play "persecutor-as-victim" too many times over the years not to be alert to the dangers you pose as you cravenly grasp everything you want, irrespective of whether you are entitled to it or not. Then you pretend that the people you are taking advantage of, are taking advantage of you. Nor am I stupid enough to allow you to hop on the bandwagon of my celebrity to satisfy your lust for attention, admiration, sympathy and our money, especially as the press would get involved, and all of a sudden I'd find myself the centre of unwanted publicity yet again. I can well see why you'd love me to sue you. It would give you the opportunity to dress your dirty deeds up as something they're not, while you con the public with what a noble victim you are of an ungrateful daughter, after all you've done for her. I can just see you now, bemoaning all the press attention as you wallow in it, like a pig stuck in muck. No, my dear, there's no way I'll be suing you. Of that you can be sure. There are many ways to skin a cat, and I for one would never give a cat who wanted to pose as a victim the satisfaction of mewling furless.'

Then, pulling a Gloria on Gloria, I suddenly changed tack to let her know that it wasn't only the dead who would revile her but the living as well. I did so by introducing the subject of the very people whose approbation she would want to keep whether she ripped us off or not. So I said sweetly, 'Incidentally, isn't Pam a delight? We're so lucky to have her in the family. So kind and decent. Truthful and fair too. I was speaking to her yesterday, and she repeated word for word exactly what she said that Wednesday afternoon around Auntie's dining table about Auntie's intentions. Amazing how many people Auntie told. But I have to go now. You take care. Bye!' I trilled brightly, yet again conveying the message through the tone of my voice that I did indeed have something up my sleeve.

Gloria, however, also had something up her sleeve. Unbeknownst to us, she had decided to ingratiate herself with Anthony, who worked as a part-time estate agent when he wasn't enlivening dinner tables with his wit and charm. She had agreed behind our backs to sell Marjorie's beach house for US$250,000, and the docking rights to the only slipway on that part of the island for a further US$5,000, to a client he had found. This, despite the fact that the house, in its damaged condition, was worth at least seven figures in US dollars and the docking rights, being unique, were almost unquantifiable.

Moreover, her cousin John – one of Cayman's leading property developers – had told Libby at Marjorie's funeral that the area was earmarked for development and the prices, already astronomical in English or American terms, were about to go through the roof. So by any interpretation, Gloria's sale of the house was at best an act of insane selfishness, the proof of which was that the new owner promptly put up the house alone for sale, asking over US$1 million for it without changing even one pane of broken glass.

On the face of it, Gloria's conduct might have seemed inexplicable, but it wasn't. The treacherous aspect about the conduct of people with personality disorders like Gloria's is that no matter how off-the-wall it seems, if you examine it from their point of view and consider their expected pay-off according to their priorities, it always makes sound sense. Not good sense, mark you. Sound sense.

Although she never admitted her game plan in bald terms, she ultimately did so obliquely enough for me to see that she had hoped that, if she gave Anthony – whom she assessed as being very motivated by money – a significant enough sum of money by way of commission to whet his financial appetite, she would rope him in to become the foil in her final romantic drama.

With her warped sense of proportion, it was preferable to give him a commission of $50,000 and take a minimal loss of several hundred thousand dollars, than to come clean and just barter money for affection, for in so doing, she would have destroyed the illusion of romanticism that was one of the driving forces of her personality.

Once she provided me with the clue to her motivation, it wasn't so hard to understand. Like most narcissists, Gloria felt most alive when she was involved in a romantic drama. While Anthony was definitely miscast, he had captured her imagination, and once central casting had decreed that she wanted him in that role, the ever-persistent Gloria must have her way – irrespective of the price and irrespective of the mixed messages he had given her over the past three years. It is that disconnection with reality that makes narcissists so dangerous to others as well as to themselves.

'Of all my mother's children, I love myself the most,' was Gloria's guiding principle and oft-repeated mantra. She would baldly announce this fact several times a day, every day, to friend, foe and anyone in between. I suspect that she did so partly because the prevailing notion for the last thirty years has been that people judge us by our estimate of our own worth, hence high self-regard is judged to be admirable; and partly because this message neatly amalgamated her self-adoration with the underlying contempt she felt for others. The mixture of self-love, disdain for others and persistence had been a remarkably successful vehicle for achieving whatever she wanted in life, so why give up on it when it, plus the lure of money, might bring Anthony to heel? So she intermingled irreconcilable opposites and doubtless sat back confidently waiting for her latest little wheeze to pay her the dividends for which she hoped.

Anthony was not as easily manipulated as that. A few weeks after Gloria handed him the exorbitant twenty percent commission that she had agreed to give him, plus another 'bribe' hidden as something else (more about which in awhile), he announced that he had been having a relationship with another woman for the last few years and would be marrying her that summer. With that, Gloria's fantasy came crashing down with an almighty clatter. It really was a case of one woman's ceiling being another's floor, for the demise of Gloria's romantic hopes is the only thing that prevented her from turning over all the money she was supposed to be handing on to us to Anthony.

Hearing Gloria bitterly recount how her plans had gone awry would have been satisfying if we hadn't already lost so much money. But, with every word of recrimination against Anthony, she hanged herself for treachery towards our interests. 'He encouraged me to sell Blue Horizon. I'd never have sold it if he hadn't. But I knew he needed the money and thought it would be more elegant to give him the $50,000 by way of a commission than give him an outright gift,' she said, berating him for having manipulated her. 'I could kick myself for allowing myself to be led like that. There really is no fool like an old fool, as I used to tell Uncle Frank,' she continued, referring to her old beau Frank Watson. 'And look who's turned out to be the fool now!'

Of course, I knew that Gloria's ostensible admission of being an old fool was not really humility, but a way of mauling Anthony and accusing him of having taken advantage of her. 'If she thinks I'm going to sympathize with her when she conned us and betrayed us in that transaction, she can think again,' I said to myself, transfixed at my mother's ability to shift responsibility at the very time she was seeking sympathy from her victims.

Even more than the loss of all that money, what made Gloria's conduct noteworthy was the fact that she had sold the property behind our backs in the full knowledge that she had no right to do so. Before the sale went through, I had gone through Marjorie's papers and discovered, tucked away amongst a welter of unrelated items, a signed will that cut her out entirely, leaving everything to my sisters and me. Although the three of us were willing to let her have the agreed-upon portion of our aunt's estate, by any interpretation, she no longer had a right to any of Marjorie's property. Therefore, selling Blue Horizon and the docking rights was inexcusable and little short of formalized theft.

Although she would later lay the blame at Anthony's doorstep, saying that he had deliberately 'played me like a fish on the line', I suspect that his combination of charm and helpfulness kept her romantic hopes up, while his elusiveness compelled this woman who had to conquer all challenges to plumb new depths to have her own way. Whether through kindness or some other more human motive, Anthony had not indicated to Gloria that he was actively pursuing a relationship with another woman. Although the personal side of his relationship with Gloria had stalled long ago, he was still sufficiently courtly and attentive for her to have hopes for the future, especially as she thought he had no other romantic interests. Since they were at the age when most unions are more of a *mariage blanche* than a red-blooded affair, her hopes were not entirely unrealistic.

Nebulousness was not a state to which any of Gloria's children was a stranger. She had purposely kept us in limbo from early childhood, but none of us had any means of knowing that her proclivity for functioning in the dark was going to backfire not only on us but on her in the big way it now did.

The first inkling occurred when Libby flew down to Cayman to divide up Marjorie's estate. Because Gloria had, in the intervening months, come to realize that she would destroy her relationship with all her daughters and grandchildren, and ruin her reputation within the family and social circles that mattered to her, unless she honoured her agreement with us to share Marjorie's estate four ways, she now put as good a face on things as she could, announcing to each of us that she was going to give us 'something' out of Marjorie's estate.

'Something', Libby discovered, was significantly less than the third Marjorie had wanted us to have, or even the quarter Gloria had agreed with us the night of her sister's burial. Although she had decided to keep a quarter-share for herself, because she still did not know about Anthony's 'other woman,' she also wanted Libby, Kitty and me to share the remainder of the estate with Anthony. 'Absolutely not. Auntie didn't even like him,' said Libby, our rights strengthened by the discovery of Auntie's will. She therefore refused to agree to the split.

Using all her diplomatic skills and the sheer force of her character, Libby then wrung a concession out of Gloria. He could have the Cayman Water Company Shares, which were worth about US$120,000. No sooner did Gloria magnanimously agree to that than she informed Libby that this 'gift' had to come out of our quarter shares, not hers. Once more Gloria's generosity had proved to be more illusory than real, though, in typical Gloria fashion, she made sure she took the credit for our financial sacrifice by letting Anthony believe the money had come from her and not from us.

No sooner had Libby dispensed with the fraught business of dividing up the estate than she had another problem to contend with. Gloria had made Anthony a signatory on all her accounts and was adamant that he stay on them, even though the consequence was that he, and not we, would own all that money if she died. Libby, however, was having none of it. Fortunately for us, Gloria had respect for her, not because of her undoubted strength of character but because of the size of her husband's fortune. So when she refused to allow Anthony to remain as a signatory on the larger accounts, Gloria, faced with a breakdown in relations between her and her children, had little choice but to agree to her approaching Anthony about removing him from them.

'He was mortally offended,' Libby said. 'I had to point out to him that no one was impugning his honour. I simply wanted the legal position made clear. Our money was our money, and no one else's.'

What did Gloria do as soon as Libby's plane had taken off? Curried favour with Anthony by agreeing to put him back on the very accounts from which he had just been removed, though once she discovered that the great romance would never come to pass, Gloria made sure 'that leech isn't on one of my accounts'.

By this time I was speaking to Gloria with marginally more warmth than before, though hardly with the degree I had endowed her with in the second half of the 1990s. I had been truly appalled by her attempt to steal Auntie's money from me, especially as she had no need of it while I did. I didn't know when, if ever, I would forgive her. Certainly, I now knew I would never again trust her. She had blotted her copybook irretrievably, and there were only three reasons why I still spoke to her: the sacred aspect, the poor example I would set my own children if I severed ties totally with her, and my determination to see that she would hand on to me my share of the money that was due upon her death. As I could monitor this situation only by remaining in touch with her, my weekly duty calls became as regular as they had once been, though I was under no illusions about my reasons for making them. My attentions, when not spiritual, were like a jailer's. As I telephoned her regularly and 'read between the lines', I was ever vigilant for the one false step that would require me to call out the men in white coats and have her declared mentally incompetent.

To ensure success in the event that such a course of action was necessary, I kept my mouth tightly shut to my sisters. The element of surprise, I had learned only too painfully over the last months, was crucial when dealing with my mother, and I could not take the chance of their mouths slipping. One of Gloria's guiding mottoes had always been 'forewarned is forearmed', and I was hereafter adopting this effective adversarial technique which she had recently used so brilliantly against us. I only hoped Gloria wouldn't give me cause to have her sectioned, for I really didn't want to do so, though I would if I had to.

Within weeks of Anthony receiving his commission from Gloria and the $120,000 gift from my sisters and me, he telephoned me. 'I'm getting married,' he said. 'I wanted you to know.'

'To whom?' I asked, collecting myself but not so quickly that my surprise wasn't obvious.

'Helen. You've met her. I brought her to Marjorie's funeral reception,' he said.

'Oh, yes,' I said, as the face of a pretty, gracious, elegant older southern American lady sprang up before my eyes.

We chatted for a while, then he asked me not to break the news to Mummy until he had had a chance to do so. This was kind and gentlemanly of him, as well as informative, for it provided incontrovertible proof that he was fully aware of Gloria's feelings for him and had indeed kept knowledge of this additional interest from her.

Anthony dropped the axe on Gloria a few days later. She immediately telephoned me in a terrible state. Although her pride prevented her from admitting how hurt she was, the rage with which she informed me that he had 'found someone richer, having first made sure that he strung me along until he'd milked me for all he could without putting a wedding ring on my finger' gave sufficient indication of her sentiments.

Gloria's dream of a final romantic production had died, and with it, her desire to live. Because she had never ever had a deep and abiding interest in any of us, or indeed in anyone or anything except as it impacted upon her requirements, she was now confronted with the reality of how empty her life was. Having run out of alternatives, she was about to discover as never before that the love you feel for others is the wealth you have in life. Without it, you have nothing, no matter how much else you may appear to possess.

However, even a narcissist has feelings. Though Gloria had a severely restricted capacity for caring about others, like all narcissists she had a pronounced need to receive positive feedback from them, with a commensurate sensitivity towards her own shallow feelings. She seems to have now accepted with frightening speed that she had reached the stage in life when her most reliable feeding grounds would be her three surviving children. Although earlier that year, when she was trying to rip us off, she had threatened to pull the plug on visits that Libby and Kitty had been encouraging her to make to them, she now effected a complete *volte face* and suddenly became so reliant upon them, and upon me, for emotional sustenance that one felt like one was dealing with a baby. Aside from the telephone calls which she initiated frequently, instead of parsimoniously waiting for us to ring her, she now declared a need to see us, and not only encouraged me to come and visit her, but also decided to go ahead with her visits to Libby and Kitty.

Gloria being Gloria, however, she pulled the infirmity card out of her pack and suddenly decided that she was too old and frail to travel on her own and made them and her granddaughter Melanie accompany her on each leg of her trip, thereby causing them much unnecessary travel back and forth. I have to admit, I no longer had any sympathy whatsoever for my mother and thought that my sisters were being misguided in facilitating her.

'She's just using you to dance attendance on her now that she can't have Anthony,' I said. 'How she must count herself lucky not to have burned her bridges with us over Auntie's money. Personally speaking, I think you're making a big mistake in indulging her. I've learned with Mummy that an inch of concession becomes a mile of exploitation, and I question the wisdom of giving in to her on anything at all.'

For once, however, the proverbial little boy who had cried wolf was in danger of being eaten alive. As soon as Libby and Ben saw Gloria, they realized that Anthony's forthcoming marriage had triggered the most tremendous downward spiral. Gloria was in the grip of a genuine depression, and the rapidity of her decline was frightening. 'She's aged twenty years in only a few weeks,' Libby said.

I fear I reacted exactly as the villagers who had heard wolf cried once too often: I didn't believe a word of it. 'Mummy's always been a sympathy-seeker when she doesn't get her way,' I said. 'You let her dupe you into giving her sympathy because we thwarted her from stealing our money. I won't be giving that bitch one iota of sympathy. Any I have, I reserve for myself and her other victims.'

Ben, concerned about her, had a battery of tests done and discovered that she had cirrhosis of the liver. She had eighteen months at the most to live, unless she gave up alcohol. She didn't want to, and with good reason. Like most narcissists, alcohol was not her problem but a solution that dulled the icy emptiness of her inability to care about anyone or anything but herself.

When Libby telephoned me with the news, Gloria had driven me to the edge once too often for me to care very much whether she lived or died. While I wished her well, I was too distrustful of her manipulative propensities to be anything but sceptical. I remained dubious when Gloria transferred from the Midwest to Florida, and Kitty called to say how low our mother was. I was still out of sympathy with this Machiavellian who had misused my sympathies once too often over a lifetime of self-aggrandizing manoeuvrings. 'Let her dupe you if you want. She's not going to dupe me again. Not ever,' I said decisively.

Gloria returned to Cayman. By now she was wallowing in self-pity when she wasn't lambasting Anthony for having convinced her to 'give Marjorie's house away just so he could get his commission'. Having run out of sympathy for her, I found that I could quite dispassionately stand back and think: everything you've got, you deserve; the only thing is that it's a fraction of what you really deserve. I said as much to Libby, Kitty, Enrique and my friends.

'You really don't have any pity for her any more, do you?' Libby once said.

'Why should I? She has more than enough for both of us. I say let her flounder in the mess of her own creation. She's only getting some of her just deserts – which is more than I can say for any of the many victims whose lives she's blighted over the years.'

Gloria, of course, had no clue as to how I truly felt. Without being hypocritical, I was pleasant and civilized, indeed nurturing, when we spoke. This I accomplished by allowing myself to be guided by my spiritual beliefs rather than my feelings towards her. After all, she still remained my mother and, as I had often told her over the years, I want all my relationships to be as good and happy as they can possibly be. An honest expression of feeling would certainly have been counterproductive, not only in emotional terms but also in practical and spiritual ones.

It is not possible to have anything approaching a positive relationship with the Glorias of this world without disjointing the present from the past and wrapping it up in a spiritual cocoon, thereby doing an awful lot of 'moving on' from yesterday's treachery to today's intended goal of positivity. In so doing, one tempers one's actions and attitudes with lashings of kindness, compassion and patience, which are seldom deserved. It really is about behaving lovingly, even when the person patently does not deserve it and one does not really feel anything approaching love for him or her.

I now did something that I could never have done had I known the truth of how Gloria had lied to the three of us about her pearls and Marjorie's. When I had been in Cayman for Marjorie's funeral, Gloria had admired my nine-strand matinee-length pearl necklace. Thinking that she had no pearls, I had offered to get her a similar necklace: an offer I now renewed. Partly, I felt compassion for her, for she functioned in a world where all ladies have good pearls even if they don't wear them, but also there were calculating considerations to my supposed generosity. I wanted to lull her into believing that all was forgiven, not because I had forgiven her or wanted to let her off the hook, but because I discerned that this would be an effective way of keeping an eye on her. I duly went to the well-known London market, Portobello, and, seeing the price of the nine strands, thought: Why should I waste such a large amount of money on that bitch? So I bought only five strands instead. Then I telephoned her to tell her that I had got her the pearls. I agreed to bring them out to her that October along with the children during their half-term holidays, for the visit she was so eager for me to make.

'Why do the children have to come?' she wanted to know.

'Because they're my children, and now that I no longer have a nanny, I can't very well leave them to fend for themselves,' I said, careful to keep the annoyance her selfishness engendered out of my voice.

'You know I can't stand *pickney*,' she said, clearly hoping to blackmail me emotionally into leaving them in England with a friend or employee.

'And you know I take my responsibilities as a mother seriously,' I said, knowing that by resorting to moral precepts I would silence her.

As things turned out, I could not have chosen a more propitious time to visit Gloria. Hurricane Ivan, one of the worst hurricanes in recorded history, hit Grand Cayman a few weeks before our arrival. Satellite photographs showed the sea levels rising on the north and south coast to such heights that the water flooded inland and buried whole parts of the island for several hours. When the hurricane moved on and the sea retreated, it left devastation in its wake that was hard to believe. Most of the island's trees were blown down. Of those that remained standing, the foliage on all of them – without exaggeration – pointed in the same direction, blown there by the tremendous force of the wind. The sea had brought in so much sand that there were white hills inland, some obscuring roads entirely. Power cables were scattered across streets, like matches from a box dropped on a kitchen floor. Most houses had no roof, but those were often the lucky ones, for many others had whole walls blown away as well. There was the ludicrous sight at South Sound of two large, multimillion-dollar houses that had been lifted off their foundations by the sea: one onto the road, the other onto an adjoining plot of land. This was marginally better than the houses that had been washed out to sea in their entirety or then blown to such bits that nothing was left of them but their foundations. Few buildings of any description had glass in their windows.

Fortunately, Maisie had chosen the site of her house wisely. It was built on one of the few parts of the island that is sheltered from the elements. So it had sustained only limited damage, considering the force nature had unleashed on an island that is barely a few feet above sea level at its highest point. Nevertheless, I would ultimately have to get the roof retiled and the eaves replaced.

Grand Cayman had not had a bad hurricane in living memory, so no one was prepared for what happened. Satellite masts, telephone cables, electrical pylons and power lines having been destroyed along with everything else, all the amenities that people take for granted nowadays ceased to work. Telephones, televisions, fax machines, the internet and electricity having been blown to bits along with petrol stations and most vehicles, people had to pull together to survive. Most cars had either been washed out to sea or had their computers destroyed by being underwater, especially around the airport, where the sea level rose by twenty feet, poured inland and destroyed every computerized vehicle in its wake. Many boats, whether of a few feet or over a hundred feet in length, had either been severely or slightly damaged, and some had sunk altogether. Only aeroplanes had been spared, most airlines and private aeroplane owners flying out their crafts as a precaution before the hurricane hit.

The aftermath showed how people are often at their best in a crisis. My boys and I flew into Cayman before anything had been repaired or restored, with the exception of the electrical supply in Gloria's area – most of the island then having to wait several weeks, and in some cases months, for theirs. Although the Cayman Islands Government had imposed a ban on nonessential visits, owing to the difficulty they were having in feeding the people who were already there – drinking water as well as food was scarce – we were allowed in under a special permit. It was truly inspiring to see how cooperation reigned where once selfishness would have been the driving force.

Gloria was more fortunate than most for two reasons. She was one of the few people on the island to have slept through the whole hurricane; and she had one of the few cars on the island that still worked. Although there was a shortage of petrol, I managed to get hold of some, thanks to the generosity of strangers. This enabled me to offer lifts to all and sundry as I set about getting the insurance company to agree the damages and organize the contractors to undertake repairs.

In some ways, I was glad to have something to do. Shorn of all the contemporary sources of entertainment we take for granted, everyone had to rely on the old- fashioned tools of talk and self-generated activities. One was really at the mercy of the people surrounding one; and while I had the odd cousin or friend whom I could see, ultimately I was forced back onto the company of my mother. She was as selfish and self-centred as ever. No one and nothing mattered to her except herself. She made it as plain as day that she had no interest in anyone or anything except what she wanted – and that was to die as quickly as possible now that she would never be the star in another romantic drama again. In the meantime I was supposed to make myself available as an obliging pair of ears to listen to whatever bile she wanted to spew forth.

I was absolutely stunned when I first saw her. The vigorous powerhouse I had left behind two years before, with the energy and looks of a well-preserved sixty-year-old, had been replaced by a frail, wizened old lady of seventy-five who was grossly underweight and frail beyond belief. I took one look at her and burst out crying. Nor could I stop until I had repaired to my bedroom to compose myself, all the while thinking: my God, she's dying. She really looked as if she was hurtling to death's door, and I would dearly have loved to speak to my brother-in-law to find out if this was what one should expect from cirrhosis of the liver. With the telephone system knocked out, however, I couldn't even call him for guidance. Gloria also refused to let me take her to a doctor.

Confronted with my mother's mortality – always a profound moment for any individual – I decided to keep the past in the past and be as kind and loving as I could be. Let's give her a good send-off, I thought, and when I wasn't out and about dealing with chores and trying to ferret out the few supplies that one could still buy (for extortionate prices), I dedicated myself to sitting with her. Once more the obliging pair of ears of old, I listened as she reviled Anthony and bemoaned how dreadful the human race was. Everyone and everything was still to blame for her lot, she being the only perfect person in the world. Because consideration required me to remain silent rather than point out that she bore some responsibility for her own actions, I would merely listen silently and look at the clock, consoling myself that it was only a matter of time before I was released from this barrage of self-centred bitterness. In the meantime, I took my satisfaction from being a good daughter and giving my mother a loving send-off, even if my reward for doing so was to become aware, as I had not experienced since my youth, of how very long a minute can be when you have to listen to diatribes you would much rather not hear.

At least thirty times a day, Gloria complained of feeling queasy. I knew, from a friend's experience with her cirrhotic boyfriend, that this was a symptom of the condition. In my opinion, she was making matters worse for herself by refusing to eat anything, so I tried to reason with her, pointing out that hunger also makes one queasy. 'I'm not hungry. I'll eat as and when I want. You know I've always picked like a bird,' she would say proudly, turning alcoholic anorexia into a virtue.

Her determination aside, I could tell that for once Gloria wasn't faking: her alcohol consumption had declined to about a half a glass of white wine a day. She would have the servants bring her a drink, take two sips, leave it for an hour, then order them to put it in the refrigerator until later. I had no idea of the farce that was being played out until I went to get a glass of coconut water for myself and was confronted by about a dozen partially empty glasses taking up space in an overcrowded fridge.

The maids, concerned to establish their honesty and obedience, had not dared to throw out even one of the beverages. 'Mummy, the refrigerator is full of glasses of wine,' I shouted to her from the kitchen. 'Since they must all be stale, I'm going to get Paulette to throw them out.'

'You do that,' she said, clearly having never given one thought to the accumulation of alcohol in a household appliance she never went into.

I cannot pretend that this was either an easy or a pleasurable period. Whenever Gloria wasn't lambasting Anthony or the world at large, she would repeat the mantra, 'Death can't come soon enough for me. I'm sick of living. Mark you I didn't say life, I said living.' This told me something important, for she was making philosophic distinctions that elude most people. Whatever her problems, they certainly weren't intellectually based, so I decided to involve her in conversations that would capture her imagination in the hope that they would stimulate her interest. Gently leading her back into those parts of her past which I surmised would be happiest, or at any rate most interesting to her, by the judicious mention of a name or two, I would then sit back and let her talk. To my profound surprise, I discovered that, for all her moaning and groaning and complaining and sympathy-seeking over the years, she regarded herself as having had a most fortunate and fascinating life. I learned that the woman who had never had a nice word to say about the Ziadie family, and few about the Burkes, thought 'it was wonderful being a part of three large families', the Smedmores being the third. Why, I asked myself, had she always been so negative? So bitter? So hateful? It made no sense.

As I was effectively dedicating myself wholeheartedly to Gloria, I had to obtain the cooperation of my children to entertain themselves. This was no problem. They happily agreed to stay outside and play, and struck up immediate friendships with all the other children in the neighbourhood. All the schools had been closed due to hurricane damage, and since all the children on the island had nothing to do all day except swim and play, class distinctions had been suspended and everyone was mixing together happily.

After a day or two, I could tell Gloria was flourishing under my ministrations. She started to spend longer periods sitting in a recliner in the drawing room instead of lying in bed. And, although one would never have accused her of being selfless or easy company even now, she was certainly a lot less aloof, aggressive, critical and sarcastic towards me than she had been since my teenage years.

One afternoon I was sitting down listening to her talk about her glory days, when one of the maids signalled to me that the boys wanted me. 'I'll be right back,' I said to Gloria as I rose.

'Where are you off to now?' she asked in exasperation, as if I had been up and down like a jack-in-the-box, rather than this being the first time.

'I'm going to check on the boys.'

'They're perfectly all right. If they weren't, you'd hear soon enough,' she said.

'Be that as it may,' I responded, refusing to let her selfishness and irresponsibility annoy me.

'You can't pander to children all the time. If you do, you'll never have a life of your own,' she said, giving me the benefit of her 'wisdom'.

'Mummy, I haven't checked on them since lunchtime. I'll be right back,' I said firmly but pleasantly.

The boys wanted to come inside. They were sick and tired of being outside. They were completely swum and played out, and wanted to play on their PlayStations. 'Come,' I said, even though I knew she didn't want them in the house. 'Just tiptoe behind her and keep very quiet, even when you're in the bedroom, so she doesn't realize you're in the house.'

'We'll whisper,' they said.

I knew that I could trust them to be as good as their word. They had literally been whispering whenever they were in their bedroom – the only room in the house Gloria allowed them to be – ever since the afternoon of our arrival, for Gloria had announced, when they were speaking at a normal pitch, that she couldn't stand any noise and they must either be quiet or go outside. So they had obliged her by never speaking at anything but a whisper, even when they said good morning and good night to her.

This level of unnecessary and unreasonable tension took me right back to my own childhood, and as I watched the boys stealthily sneak past their grandmother on their way to their bedroom to play their electronic games, I saw a reflection of what my siblings and I had been through when we were their age.

Because of the position of her chair, Gloria would not have realized that the boys had even entered the house, much less walked behind her, had she not coincidentally shifted position just as they were turning the corner from the passage towards their bedroom. As soon as she saw them, she erupted. 'Children were made to play outside. What are you doing in the house?'

'They're fed up with being outside. They won't make any noise,' I said.

'I can't take all the traffic in and out of the house. This is not Grand Central Station,' she snarled. 'I don't know why you had to bring them.'

It's a good thing I have self-control. If I did not, I would have exploded then and there. 'I think they're exceptionally well-behaved eleven-year-olds,' I said firmly. 'They have not bothered you once and have gone out of their way to be considerate above and beyond the call of duty. What difference does it make to you whether they're in their bedroom or outside, as long as they don't disturb you?'

The answer to that question, as I would realize in the days to come, had nothing to do with whether they behaved badly or not. Any child, person, animal or thing that commanded even one second of her attention was something to be eliminated, unless she was in the mood to endow it with recognition. Her attitude had always been indicative of a determination to have absolute control over her environment and everyone within it. More than a mere control freak, she was a tyrant who could not tolerate any external entity that did not exactly accord with her requirements. I could see so clearly that, as far as she was concerned, she was the only person in the world who had a right to anything. Everyone else had to coexist as an acolyte.

Later that afternoon, a very nice English lady called Katrina, who used to live next door, dropped in to see how Gloria was. She, Gloria and I chatted for a while, and when she got up to leave, I accompanied her to her car, as good manners dictate. 'I'm so glad you've come,' she said. 'We were getting worried about her.'

Gloria had led everyone to believe she was dying of cancer.

'I can see why,' I replied.

'I know how difficult old people can be,' she said. 'We have to make allowances for them.'

I laughed. 'The joke is that Mummy is easier now than she's ever been.'

'You've just answered the question my mother raised when she came to visit. She said, "Katrina, mark my words, there's a reason why that lady is on her own so much. People like her don't end up on their own unless there's a good reason." I wondered what it was. Now I know,' Katrina said. 'But she is bright and interesting.'

'Absolutely,' I agreed, and clung to that thought, as I focused on keeping this stay argument-free until its end.

Finally, the day of our departure dawned. That morning, I went out and bought a mobile telephone. None of the landlines was working yet, and no one knew when they would be, but mobile service was due to be restored shortly. 'Let me show you how this works,' I said to Gloria.

'Give it to the servants. They're all experts where anything called "a telephone" is concerned. They live on them,' she said.

So I duly handed over the mobile to the maids with the instruction that they were to keep it at all times, so my sisters and I could reach our mother whenever service was restored. I also gave them our respective telephone numbers and told them to use them if they ever felt that Gloria needed anything.

The time then came to take our leave of Gloria. The boys said goodbye first. While they were doing so, I burst into tears, thinking I might never see my mother again. Even if she had been a pill, she was still my mother; and I defy anyone with a heart to say that they don't have some love for their mother, no matter how awful she has been.

'You will come again soon, won't you?' Gloria said plaintively.

'I'll be back in December,' I said, which was about five weeks away.

'I'm not sure I'll be alive then,' she said and presented me with a bony but still elegant cheek to brush past mine.

'Well, if you are, I'll definitely see you then,' I said, tears blinding me, for she had lent words to the thought that was also in my mind.

Upon getting back to England, I telephoned my sisters to update them. We compared notes and agreed that it would be a miracle if she lasted as long as eighteen months. They also said that she had been terribly frail when they had seen her in summer, thereby making me believe that her deterioration hadn't been as rapid as it actually had been.

Early in December, I duly flew back to Grand Cayman. As soon as I entered Gloria's bedroom and saw her huddled under several blankets, despite the searing heat outside, I knew her condition had declined further. She was even thinner than before, if that were possible. In fact, she was reminiscent of Mickey and Daddy, who looked as if they had been inmates of concentration camps before their deaths. If she weighed more than sixty-five pounds, I would have been surprised. Spontaneously, I burst into tears.

As soon as Gloria was resting, I telephoned my sister and brother-in-law the doctor.

'You've got to come out this weekend,' I said to Ben. 'Mummy looks as if she'll be dead in a few weeks. She refuses to see a doctor, but she can't stop you from arriving at an accurate assessment of her condition. You'vr got to come. I can't deal with this on my own when I have no medical training.'

Ben duly arrived that weekend with Libby and his medical expertise. They were as frightened as I had been when they saw her. She was so emaciated, her stomach so distended that he was convinced she had terminal liver cancer. Amidst her protestations of not wanting medical attention, Ben arranged with Marjorie's doctor John Addleson, to do a battery of tests.

When they came back, all became clear. Gloria had been starving herself. She was literally dying of starvation. She did not have cancer, though she definitely had cirrhosis which had entered its irreversible phase and which would kill her sooner rather than later, though not quite as quickly as starvation was doing.

'You've got to eat something. Anything,' I insisted, and went out and bought everything the servants thought she might like.

Although my concern was genuine, it was also coloured by financial considerations. Gloria had let slip one day while we were talking that she had an account in Jamaica containing nearly a million US dollars which neither my sisters nor I had hitherto known about. This was something of a disaster, for if the money remained in Jamaica, Gloria's estate would be liable for death duties. On the other hand, if the money were safely in Grand Cayman, where there is no inheritance or income tax, we would inherit the whole sum.

By this time, I had lost all the unfounded optimism which had, over the years, blinded me to the true awfulness of my mother's character. I knew that the only reason she had that money in Jamaica was because the Bank of Jamaica gave a higher rate of interest to foreign currency deposits than banks in the US or Cayman Islands. I also knew that she was selfish enough to insist that the money stay there, earning her the tens of thousands it did, until her death, at which time we would then be liable for hundreds of thousands of dollars in inheritance tax. I was not prepared to take a chance on losing out on yet another significant sum just so my selfish mother could benefit, in this instance lining her pockets to the tune of a few paltry thousand dollars.

While the year before, I would have given her the chance to do the responsible thing by pointing out to her how invidious a position her actions were creating for us, now there was no way I was going to give her even an outside chance of putting her immediate interests before our long-term ones. I therefore had to come up with some way of getting her to move that money to Cayman without her ever knowing I was doing it more for my sisters and myself rather than for her.

I am not an intriguer by nature, and it took me three days of round-the-clock pondering before I could come up with a plan that would most likely have taken Gloria all of ten minutes to invent. Throughout that interval, I kept on telling myself that it had to be something that appealed to her selfish interests. If she even got a whiff that we might benefit, she could well take the view that we should be made to suffer, so whatever I came up with, had to exclude the three of us.

At dawn on the fourth morning of almost total preoccupation, the pieces fell into place. Charles Hanna, the millionaire socialite whose mother Olga had been a friend of Gloria's and whose father Eddie had been a friend of Michael's, was due to attend a gala at Covent Garden to celebrate the Queen's Jubilee. I had actually been asked to it but had to decline as I was going to be abroad, so I telephoned Charles (using the mobile while I was at the supermarket) and asked him if I could link the two things and use them, and his name, to manipulate my mother into moving the money to Cayman. He agreed. I then telephoned another friend and got her to agree to telephone me on the landline, whose service had been restored a few days beforehand, pretending to be Charles's secretary. 'Mummy will answer,' I told her. 'She monitors everything that goes on here. After you've identified yourself to her as Charles Hanna's secretary, either listen and laugh as I rattle on and on or hang up if you prefer. I'll ring you using the mobile from the bathroom once Mummy's awake and in the drawing room. Then phone me back two minutes later. The timing is important, so please don't delay.'

When the time was ripe, I excused myself saying I needed to go to the loo, rang my friend on the mobile, then sauntered back to Gloria as if I didn't have a care in the world. The landline rang. She answered it. 'It's Charles Hanna's secretary for you,' she said, and I could tell from her tone of voice that she did not suspect a thing.

Maybe I should have been an actress. I didn't miss a beat as I chatted to 'Charles', declining his invitation with just the right amount of regret to make it convincing. Then I changed tack, my voice suddenly filling with horrified surprise. 'No. They wouldn't. Are they crazy?' I said, as Gloria's ears perked up and her eyes opened wide as if to say, 'What's happening now?'

I let 'Charles' talk for a while before saying, 'Those bastards are really something else. Don't they realize that they'll ruin the economy if they do that?'

On the word 'economy', Gloria forgot all about dying and sat bolt upright in her easy chair. 'What's going on?' she mouthed as I put up my hand to tell her to be quiet.

'You'd have thought they'd learned their lesson the last time around,' I said. 'But you know what some of these politicians are like. All I can say is, thank God I don't have any money in Jamaica.'

'Charles' talked a bit more, and then I brought the conversation to a close by saying, 'Enjoy yourself with the Queen, and if by any chance you see Princess Alexandra, you can remind her of that thing we all attended at Windsor Castle. And thanks again for thinking of me, Charles. It really was very sweet of you.'

While I had been speaking, I had been wondering if those magical words 'royalty', 'politicians', 'economy', and 'money in Jamaica' were gilding the lily, or if I was pressing the right buttons. I got an answer of sorts before I could even replace the receiver on the arm of Gloria's chair.

'What's that about the Queen and money in Jamaica and the politicians?' she asked, her eyes ablaze with interest.

The adrenaline was coursing through my veins as I slapped what I hoped was a convincing look of innocence on my face, steadied my voice so it would seem normal, and said chattily, 'Isn't Charles sweet? He's going to a gala at Covent Garden to celebrate the Queen's Jubilee and wanted to know if I'll be back in time. The tickets are several thousand pounds apiece, so it's really generous of him to have thought of me.'

'He always was such a nice young man,' Gloria said. 'It's good you children have remained friends. But what was he saying about money in Jamaica?'

'Oh that,' I said dismissively. Gloria's short-term memory was now affected by the cirrhosis, and there was every possibility that she would not remember what she had told me about her bank account in Jamaica days ago, so I took advantage of that by being as obtuse as I could be. 'Nothing to do with us. Thank God you got all your money out of Jamaica when you did, is all I can say.'

Now coiled as tightly as a panther about to strike at its prey, before she even said another word, I could tell that she was annoyed at having to extract from me the very information I was avid to impart despite all appearances to the contrary. 'Just tell me what he said,' she rasped irritably.

'There's evidently a power struggle going on right now in Jamaica between the left and right wings of the PNP. One part of the government wants to turn the country into an offshore banking centre like Cayman, while the other wants to reintroduce foreign exchange controls and trap the foreign exchange deposits that people have been incautious enough to place with the banks there,' I said in a tone of voice that was almost bored.

The words weren't even properly out of my mouth before a suddenly invigorated Gloria, at death's door only a few minutes before, said with all the energy of a whirling dervish, 'My address book is in my bedside table. Get it right this instant.'

'This can't be so easy,' I thought to myself as I executed her instructions and returned with the book.

'Phone the bank manager right now. Tell him that he's to take immediate steps to transfer the US dollars I have on deposit with him to my account here. And when I say now, I mean N-O-W,' she ordered, providing me with the details of her accounts which, in testament to her organizational skills, were readily available. 'I want that money here, safe and sound, by the close of business tomorrow.'

'I can't tell your bank manager what to do. I can dial the number for you. But you have to give him your own instructions,' I said.

'Nonsense,' Gloria decreed. 'I'll tell him to take your instructions, and you will make all the arrangements. His name is Mr Richards. He's a very nice man. Now do as I say. And child, you will do it right now. Do I make myself clear?' she said haughtily.

'Very,' I said, my heart in my mouth from the joy I hoped I was concealing.

Unfortunately, Gloria's money was more tightly tied up than we had thought. Ultimately, the Bank of Jamaica could not give its permission to a premature release of the funds, which were not due to mature for some months. So Jocelyn Richards came up with the brilliant scheme whereby the bank would loan her the entire sum on deposit, in return for which we would pay National Commercial Bank a substantial arrangement fee and interest of several thousand dollars. That way, the money would be out of Jamaica and, if she died, what was on deposit would be a debt and therefore not liable to death duties.

Such an elaborate mechanism, of course, took several weeks to organize. Ben agreed with me that Gloria could well die before it was done. So, unless Gloria started to eat enough to prevent irreversible organ failure due to starvation, there was an uncomfortably high chance that the money would never reach Cayman intact. I was determined that I would do whatever it took to keep her alive until those funds came through, and therefore started to cajole her into eating anything that caught her fancy. I told myself it was one thing to respect my mother's right to dispose of her life as she saw fit, but it was also my right to protect my – and my children's – inheritance. If disrespecting her right to kill herself by starvation meant that I was selfishly putting my own rights before hers, so be it. I saw no reason to allow her to screw up our heritage any more than she had already done, though I was careful to dress my encouragement up in such a way that I wasn't actually pitting myself against her, for then she would have stopped eating altogether just to be cussed.

Lo and behold, Gloria now started to lap up all the attention I was giving her and, as her mood lightened, she actually started to 'peck' – always one of her favourite words to describe how she ate. Could I dare hope that she might survive long enough to see the money arrive safely?

Hope without execution doesn't usually get anyone anywhere, so prior to returning to England, I took the maids to the supermarket and stocked up on everything that could tempt her birdlike appetite. I also bought essentials, such as liquid nutritional supplements for old people, which I managed to get Gloria to agree to take on a daily basis. 'I don't want her living on the supplements,' I told the maids, knowing only too well the predilection many Jamaican servants have for avoiding labour. 'She needs to eat. You will cook her nourishing things like chicken soup as well as proper meals with one meat dish, two vegetables, and two starches. I don't care if she eats only morsels, but make sure she eats. Don't wait for her to be hungry. She needs to eat without being hungry. Offer. Keep on telling her I've left you specific instructions to see that she eats something – anything – no matter how little it is. And make sure you do exactly as I say otherwise she will die. And then you'll be out of a job.'

Paulette and Vilma, doubtless motivated to keep their cushy jobs going as long as possible, not only agreed to carry out my instructions but executed them so well that when I returned to Cayman in February, Gloria was stronger than she had been in December. Although still painfully thin, with the awful abdominal distension that is a product of cirrhotic water-retention, she was obviously no longer in danger of dying imminently. This, of course, should not have been a surprise. The money had now safely arrived from Jamaica and, with the danger of death duties removed, the ever-contrary Gloria was daily becoming stronger even as she took to her bed and professed a heartfelt desire to die as quickly as possible. 'Well, Mummy,' I said with what I hoped was a suitable mixture of kindness and humour, 'we can't very well shoot you, so you'll just have to accept God's gift of life until He decides that it is time to take it away from you.'

'Christ, how I wish He would hurry up and do it. I feel so empty. Empty. Empty,' she said.

I looked at Gloria, lying on her bed, the windows shut, the blinds drawn, and the heat stifling. I realized she was giving me an insight into what her underlying problem had always been: emptiness. At her core there was a real void. This was why she had always needed praise and admiration. That was why she had always drunk. The alcohol gave her a feeling of wellbeing that she otherwise did not have except through the approbation of others. Unlike normal people, who have their emotions – their hopes and fears and concerns and loves to fill them up – she had these only in a reduced capacity. Whenever people didn't provide her with what she regarded as her just deserts, she reacted with anger and resentment, failing to understand that others were not her feeding ground, but individuals with their own points of view and needs.

The trouble with narcissists is that their internal emptiness is allied to their firm belief that they are perfect and deserving at all times of everything, not because they have earned it but because they are entitled to it by virtue of being themselves. This dichotomy sets up an irreconcilable conflict that only gets worse with the passage of time, and it feeds what is most likely at the root of their problem, namely their essential vacuity.

Without the positive emotions that sustain the healthy individual's link to other people at the same time that it fosters impersonal interests elsewhere, the Glorias of this world occupy a world where all is ultimately barren. No one and nothing is real to people like them except the uses to which they can put others.

I tried to imagine what it must be like to live a life without all the emotional wealth that both joy and pain bring as a result of caring for others and about one's impersonal interests. I couldn't; though I could see how chillingly dreadful it must be to go through life without the ordinary level of feelings that make most of us human.

I realized, possibly for the first time ever, how very lucky I was to have had both anguish and joy as a result of caring about others and things aside from myself. I had a life. Gloria, on the other hand, had nothing. Despite, on the face of it, having every blessing that life had to offer in the shape of beauty, brains, breeding and bread, she had never been in a position to benefit from any of those gifts because she ultimately had a reduced capacity for caring. She was, by her own admission, empty and, I could see, had always been.

Adoration of self hadn't left much room for anything else, including personal growth. No wonder she had sought refuge in drink from an early age. If you have only limited emotional capacity, it makes sense that you will opt for sensation. That way, you are at least feeling something and thereby escaping from the void within yourself. What you feel might not cut very deeply, but anything is better than nothing. On that basis, it made sound sense for her to drink, and showed why she had always regarded alcohol as a solution to a problem and not as the problem itself. She had been right.

Thereafter, the emptiness drum was one that Gloria beat constantly. Whether I was sitting beside her in the hospital while she lay on a gurney having the fluid drained from her abdominal cavity, or I was suffocating in the airless bedroom, or even on the rare occasions the action moved to the drawing room, she returned time and again to how empty she felt. She no longer had the steady diet of admirers who had surrounded her all her life and drowned out the stark silence of her absent inner life. Nor did she have the mood-altering delights of alcohol to mask that emptiness within. While she still drank, it was no more than a few sips of white wine or whiskey *per diem*. To all intents and purposes, she was well and truly off the bottle now, certainly for the first time since the 1980s, and bearing in mind her proclivity for deceptiveness, possibly before then. Looking into the mirror of her heart and soul without the mood-altering drug of alcohol to mask the absence within, she was confronting, possibly for the first time in her life, the fact that there was nothing there except vanity. Now that there was no escape from that nothingness, I could well see why life had been rendered pointless for her, and felt compassion for her.

But Gloria, ever resourceful as only a fully-blown narcissist can be, now found a way to resort to old tricks. Now that Anthony had well and truly bitten the dust, she utilised her belief in an afterlife to set up for herself a source of all the adoration and attention she would require once she had left this earth. Her attention therefore returned to her old co-star Michael.

Throughout the years of her interest in her sister's brother-in-law, Michael had been deader than dead. Now, however, he became a latter-day Lazarus. Whenever Gloria wasn't going on about how empty she was, she kept on saying how 'lonesome' she was; how much she missed Michael, and how she was looking forward to seeing him again.

The lack of a masculine foil might have been a killer for her, but the fact was that the only time she had actually been a halfway tolerable human being since her twenties had been in the early days of her widowhood when she had lacked a definite masculine interest. The prospect of Gloria on an eternal diet of enablement by Michael would have been funny had it not been so grotesque.

Trying to figure out what had made her tick, I decided that what she called 'lonesomeness' was really alienation. Because she cared for no one, she couldn't relate to people on a profound level. Sure, she was bright and canny enough to read them well and play them as and when it suited her. But such skills didn't actually profit her emotionally. If you feel nothing, nothing is what you feel.

As for missing Michael, I had no doubt that she missed the perpetual and silently compliant audience he had provided her with for the last eight years of his life. I would have put good money on the fact that, now that she expected to die soon, she was resurrecting the idea of the obliging Michael solely for the use he would provide as a romantic foil for the eternal drama she would be directing, producing and starring in throughout infinity, only because her desired co-star, Anthony, had moved his production elsewhere. Affection for poor Daddy didn't even enter into the equation.

Truthfully, Gloria's self-centredness remained so flagrant that one almost had to laugh at it. Yet, despite it, she was now evolving into a more pleasant person. Even though she could still come out with jaw-droppingly awful admissions, such as 'I'm so glad you came without the children. Kitty will insist on bringing Gabriela every time she comes, which is a real bore. I wish she'd leave her behind,' – ignoring the fact that Kitty had nowhere to park her daughter as if she were an inconvenient vehicle – Gloria did start to tell each of her three children, 'I love you.' And not once in a while either: two, three, four times a day, she would say it when we took turns to visit her. When we telephoned, we were liable to hear it at least once in a conversation.

This was a drastic change for a woman who had never shown her children any affection. Of course, Libby, Kitty and I commented upon it amongst ourselves. While it was welcome, Libby summarized all our sentiments when she said, more from regret than joyousness, 'It's taken over fifty years for me to hear my mother tell me something I've told my children all their lives.'

The question I had to ask myself was: is Gloria being sincere? I formed the view that she had decided that, now she was well and truly dying, and no longer stood to gain from the emotional terrorism with which she had plagued us for most of our lives, she wanted to die surrounded by love. At the time, of course, I didn't realize that all narcissists are motivated by love of self, and they require that fact to be confirmed from external sources. So this 'love' wasn't quite as sincere was it was cooked up to be. Without understanding that fact, I regarded this 'love' as a new and welcome sentiment. It was certainly a lot more agreeable than anything that had preceded it. What I didn't realize were the self-aggrandizing mechanics which motivate all narcissists. Since we three 'children' were the only people who still mattered to Gloria – not because she cared about us as individuals (she continued to offer us constant reminders that disinterestedness was still as alien to her as ever), but because we were living extensions of herself – she was functioning on the basis that if she told us she loved us, we would give it back to her.

Without appreciating that my mother had simply found another way to use her children to fulfil her emotional needs – and believing even at that late stage of my life that all love is good - I responded in kind, telling Gloria 'I love you too', whenever she repeated the three words which are often so magical to most of us.

In the countdown to death, there is no room for pettiness, and while I was delighted that Gloria had surrendered her loathsomeness for 'love', I also hoped that she would adopt some humility before it was too late. After all, she was facing eternity, and as a believing Catholic, I considered the state of her soul to be of overriding importance. But she was still acting as if she were the third part of the Holy Trinity, the only perfect person on earth. I had actually been seriously concerned since December, when I had asked her if she would like me to get in touch with a priest 'to prepare yourself for your Maker'. 'God and I are on perfectly good enough terms, thank you very much,' she had said dismissively, flicking my suggestion off as if it were a dead fly on a larder board.

Not realizing that Gloria's conversion to love was not 'love' as you and I would understand it, but was just the narcissist's need to be surrounded by the glow of love, I now brought up the subject of her immortal soul again. 'Priests only confuse things,' she said, but this time without being dismissive.

Her response, I felt, indicated a softening in attitude, so I laughed.

'You'd have liked *If You See the Buddha On the Road, Kill Him*,' I said. 'It's a very good book I read many years ago, which says that each soul has to find his or her own way to God. That's a view I share, but there are times when a priest can be a help. If you feel the need for one, please let me know and I'll find one. One must always prepare for important things, and I can't think of anything more important than meeting one's Maker.'

Whether that had any effect, or was merely coincidental, I will never know, but she now started to show an awareness that she might actually be less than perfect. The first clue I had was on the same day as that conversation. She was once more lying on the bed, and I was stifling in a chair by the one window she allowed me to open a crack. To my surprise, she shifted the conversation off herself and asked, 'Who does the children's laundry when you're not there?'

'They do.'

'They can do laundry,' she exclaimed as if such a talent were beyond belief, which, I suppose to someone who couldn't even boil water, it was.

'Ever since I got rid of the nannies, they've been doing their laundry themselves. I don't mean to imply any criticism, but the one thing I've been absolutely determined to do is bring them up to be independent. I think one of the cruellest things parents can do in this day and age is bring children up to be reliant on staff. I'll never forget being in New York aged eighteen and not knowing how to make a cup of instant coffee. You become such a prisoner of your own dependency that your staff are as much your gaolers as your helpers, and I vowed years ago that my children would never be placed in such an invidious position. Privilege without independence is nothing but a gilded prison,' I said.

Gloria looked at me, her eyes wide open, her mind clearly receptive to a concept that had never occurred to her before.

'I can see what you mean,' she said slowly, the wheels visibly turning. 'Yes, I think you're right. The way we were all brought up, uh...yes, I think where you children were concerned, it might have been a blunder.'

I could hardly believe my ears. For the first – and possibly only – time in her life, Gloria had admitted that something she had done had been less than perfect. Having opened that door, she now started making fence-mending comments. One day we were sitting outside in the drawing room, and she said, apropos of nothing, as if she had never noticed before, 'You know, you really are a very pretty girl.'

Although I immediately appreciated where she was coming from and what she was trying to accomplish, I also could not help observing that this was very little, very late. I felt like saying, 'All those years that people were raving about my looks and the newspapers seldom mentioned my name without the prefix "beautiful", you studiously ignored everything favourable and even tried to destroy my face. Now you're acting as if you've discovered something that no one else was privy to. This really is too rich. If you want to apologize, come clean and do so.'

However, I did not want to sully the moment with such a churlish observation. Nor did I want to accept a crumb delivered past its sell-by date as if it were a leg of lamb being fed to the starving. Opting instead for something more neutral which was nevertheless hinged in reality, I said lightly, with a little laugh which would hopefully take the sting out of any implied criticism, 'The way you say that, anyone would think this is the first time you've noticed.'

Quick as a flash, the Gloria of old re-emerged.

'You must admit,' she said, shifting blame, 'you're not getting any younger. But you do look damned good for your age.' Then she started comparing how Libby, Kitty and I were aging in relation to herself, who remained, of course, the paragon of perfection.

The following morning, however, she returned to her theme, this time making sure the compliment was delivered in sufficiently straightforward fashion as to invite no misunderstanding. After complimenting me on my sandals and attire, she said, 'You still have a very good figure. It's nice to see how well you're aging.'

'I could lose a few pounds,' I said.

'No, no, no. Men like women who have a little something on them. You don't need to lose an ounce, though you might not want to gain any more weight either,' she said.

I could hardly believe my ears. Gloria was trying to be positive: to get messages across that possibly should have been delivered decades before, but which she was nevertheless intent on delivering before it was too late. I must admit I was to an extent pleased, though rather less so than when my father had done something similar, possibly because he had managed to convey his regret for the past, even making an apology of sorts, while she could not bring herself to even hint at an apology. Nevertheless I was also aware that in the very act of saying what she had said, she was conveying regret of sorts for the past.

Nor was this change in attitude limited to compliments. On this visit, she signed all sorts of documents adding my name as a signatory to her various bank and trust accounts. Libby and Kitty, being American citizens, could not by law be on them; but I, as a British subject, had no such constraints. She therefore insisted that, since I was now dealing on a daily basis with the administrative details of her way of life, whether I was in Cayman or abroad, I become a cosignatory. I could hereafter transfer funds as and when they were needed, without her having to bother to do so.

As I had already set up standing orders to pay all her bills, there was really no necessity for me to be on any of the accounts, so this meant that she had given me all the financial leverage I would ever need to protect my sisters and myself against any antics she could come up with in the future. In so doing, she had also wordlessly informed me that we would be having no more trouble out of her. After the hell she had put us through the year before, this was quite a relief, I can tell you.

Only too soon, the day of my departure arrived. We said fond goodbyes; once more I wondered, as I looked back at my mother lying on the bed, if this would be the last time I saw her alive. 'Come again soon,' she said, and I promised to do so in May. In the meantime, my sisters would visit, for we had a rota system going where no more than a week or two elapsed without one of us being in Cayman with her.

At that time, Prince Charles was due to marry Camilla Parker-Bowles, and CNN wanted to interview me for a series of programmes they planned to run during the week of the wedding. So early in March I flew from London to New York. This visit would have a decisive effect in more ways than one, for without it, I would never have written this book.

I was staying with Nina Lerner Judson, who asked over a mutual friend, the eminent psychoanalyst Dr Erika Freeman. We were talking about how people cope with adversity, sometimes recovering from it and sometimes moving on despite wounds which never truly heal, when Erika, who knew that I have never got over some of my marital experiences, said, 'I think it's important for you to realize that you married a true sociopath.'

Erika was a great friend of my sister-in-law Jeanie Campbell, so she knew a lot about the Argyll family from her. She now went into some detail about how 'dark' Jeanie thought her two brothers and their father had been, expressing sentiments Jeanie had also conveyed to me. Then she told Nina how she admired the way I had developed other aspects of my personality once Colin Campbell and Ian Argyll had well and truly destroyed the ones they did.

Erika's comment had been calculated to drive home the point to me that I was blameless for the way my marriage had turned out. Her message was simple and true: no matter who my ex-husband had married, the outcome would have been the same. Her implication was also that nothing that had happened to me throughout my marriage had been personal. She actually gave voice to something I had long felt, which was that I was purely incidental to much that had happened during that union. In much the same way that a shark doesn't differentiate between a human swimmer and a sea lion, a sociopath consumes irrespective of the merits or deserts of his target.

Erika's comments started me thinking. Nina and I went out and bought Harvard Professor of Psychiatry Dr Martha Stout's seminal work, *The Sociopath Next Door.* I took it back to England and had the oddest experience while reading it. The truth bells were ringing not only about my ex-husband but also about my mother.

This was not an altogether welcome thought to have just as Gloria was dying. It muddied the waters and provided me with labels to things it would have been better for me to keep nameless and uncategorized until after I had seen her safely and lovingly off to the Other Side.

No matter how inconvenient the timing was, the fact nevertheless remained that I had stumbled upon a big clue as to why my mother could behave so unconscionably. Although I did not then know that people who suffer from one personality disorder often overlap with other personality disorders as well, what I was learning would start me on the road to recognising what my mother's personality flaws were. This would ultimately assist me to realize that unchecked narcissists must inevitably develop characteristics of sociopathy; that their narcissism grows with the passage of time and with this extension comes an ever-increasing disconnection with reality. This causes their rage to increase, for they go through life feeling evermore 'cheated' by others who fail to recognize them as justly deserving the admiration and respect that is at all times their due as perfect beings.

Dr Stout's basic recommendations for dealing with sociopaths can ultimately be summed up in one word: avoidance. This I had actually instinctively exercised with both Gloria and Conning, severing relations with the two of them at various times for various periods, even if the only one I had actually kept at bay permanently had been the latter.

It would have been a more comfortable experience if I had not read Dr Stout's book until after Gloria was dead. Having done so, however, I now had to reconcile the conflict between her advice of avoidance and my chosen path of lovingly seeing off my clearly disordered mother. I decided that while the advice, which incidentally should also be applied to narcissists, is sound when applied to spouses, friends, working colleagues and business partners – in other words, elective relationships – with God-ordained relationships such as parents and children, one does not always have the luxury of avoidance. Even if it is the most practical solution to the problem, it is not always the most spiritually-enlightened one.

Possibly I might have had a different attitude if Gloria and I had been younger, and I was facing a lifetime of ups and downs; but she was at death's door. Even if she had not been, she was the only grandmother my children had, and I would not have knowingly deprived them of the experience of extended family life just to make things easier for myself.

Although such financial considerations as had once prevailed had been taken care of, there were still the spiritual and familial dimensions to consider, so for those reasons, what God had ordained, I was not about to overturn.

As I saw it, I also had duties as a daughter, irrespective of what sort of mother Gloria had been. Maybe she had trained me too well, to be of use to users, but I nevertheless felt it is up to each of us whether we choose to be a good person or not. Goodness is an elective that is not dependent upon others. It is not a question of just deserts, for if that were the case, an eye for an eye would be the more evolved aim spiritually rather than loving thine enemies.

In the light of those facts, I did not think I would have been much of a person if I decided to duck my duty of being a loving daughter, even if my mother had been for most of her life unloving and undeserving of love. So I resolved to continue flying back and forth between the West Indies and Europe until such time as she was dead.

When I returned to Cayman in May, however, I could not escape making connections between Gloria's conduct and attitudes, and those in Dr Stout's book. It is just as well that I was still largely ignorant about narcissistic personality disorder, otherwise I would definitely have had too much to reconcile in too short a space of time. As it was, before I had even set foot in the house, I was forcibly reminded of how my mother, in true personality disordered fashion, always set up situations which caused maximum inconvenience for others, while answering her petty needs and prejudices.

'I know you told me to make sure I started the car once a week so the battery wouldn't run down the way it has each time you've been away,' Paulette informed me, 'but Ma'am refused to give me the keys.'

I walked straight into Gloria's bedroom and, after kissing her hello, said, 'Didn't you agree, the last time I was here, that you would let Paulette start the car once a week so I wouldn't have to deal with the inconvenience of a flat battery every time I come? I gather you refused to let her. Why would you do that, when I went to the trouble of teaching her how to start the car, and you agreed to let her?'

'I'm not giving any servant access to any vehicle. If you've forgotten what they're like, I haven't,' she said with her typical lack of repentance.

'If you felt that way, what's been stopping you from starting the car yourself?' I asked curtly.

'Ha,' Gloria harrumphed, as if such a ridiculous idea was beyond contemplation.

'Consider this: what sort of woman doesn't give a shit about putting people to the trouble of having to deal with *problems of her own creation*, after they've left their own, busy lives and flown halfway across the world to see her? I have to tell you, Mummy, I will be really peed off if, yet again, your refusal to consider any desires except your own, results in me having to get *this totally unnecessary problem* sorted out *yet again*.'

Sure enough, when I turned the key in the ignition, it had all the life of Lenin's corpse. I was absolutely fuming but decided not to allow the anger I was feeling to spoil the overall, loving tone that I wished my stay to have. After the battery had been recharged, as it had had to be on each of my prior visits, I went inside and sat with Gloria. She was, I noticed, no nearer death than on my previous visit. If anything, she looked even better. This was not a welcome observation, neither for me nor for her. She quickly proved the veracity of that observation by launching into a self-pitying diatribe about how cruel God was not to have taken her yet.

I could see that she was partly sincere and partly manipulating me, so that I would feel sorry for her and do whatever she wanted, which actually involved sitting with her all day in her musty, airless bedroom. When she was awake, I was supposed to lodge myself there, like a heavy meal on one's stomach, responding on cue to whatever it was she wanted to talk about. Only when she grew tired and wanted to sleep could I then go out and take care of whatever business it was that I had to perform on her behalf. It was still all about Gloria, Gloria, Gloria.

According to Dr Stout, sympathy seeking is one of the fundamental keys to diagnosing sociopathy. When it is allied to unconscionable self-centredness and ruthless inconsideration such as Gloria had evinced all her life, it is a slam-dunk as to what you're dealing with.

'My God,' I thought, startled. 'Mummy really is a sociopath.'

'You know, Mummy,' I said, promptly trying to crush the thought, 'you really ought to give thought to the fact that God gave you the gift of life and it is your Christian duty to appreciate it. The way you carry on, anyone would think that gift is a terrible burden. If you believe in Him and eternal life, why are you so keen to escape from this life into the next one? Whether you're here or there, you're still stuck with two inescapable things: life and yourself. Just what makes you think that when you die, you'll somehow be magically released from yourself and life? If I were you, I'd begin to focus on what's really important, instead of bemoaning your fate, as if somehow life, God and everyone else short-changed you by giving you the odd hurdle to leap over. A hurdle, incidentally, that is a hell of a lot lower than those with which ninety-nine point nine percent of this world's population have to contend. Just count yourself lucky not to have been born a Somali or a peasant in Jamaica and start to appreciate what God gave you.'

By this time, Gloria had taken to having her Bible beside her on the bed. Although I do not actually recall seeing her reading from it, I did not think it was just there for show. I do think the one sincere thing about her was her belief in the Almighty, so the presence of the Scriptures struck me as a welcome development: an indication that she was on the right track at this most crucial juncture in her life.

Bible or no, this was one leopard whose spots remained unchanged. 'I thank God for your visit,' she took to telling me once or twice a day. 'I've been so lonesome. God is really good to let you come.'

'Mummy is showing gratitude and appreciation for the first time ever,' I thought at first. But, as she kept on saying it, I realized that even here, her disorder had kicked in; she was intent on preserving her inviolability and maintaining her refusal to have any obligation to anyone. Far from being grateful to me, she had shunted any appreciation she should have had towards me, her daughter, onto God. It was Jehovah, not Georgie, to whom she was grateful; and once I picked up on this, I felt my blood pressure rising until I could remain silent no longer. When she next praised God for my trip, I said with just enough bite in my tone for her to know I was put out, 'It would be more appropriate if you thanked me instead of God. As far as I can recall, He didn't fly halfway across the world at His own expense to see you. I did.'

'He put the idea in your head,' she said. 'So it's Him I must be grateful to.'

'You really find it impossible to give credit where it's due, don't you?' I snapped.

'Are you going to pick me up on every little thing?' Gloria said.

'No. If I did that, I would be on your case every other sentence. But I will pick you up on what I regard as important.'

'Sometimes you can be waspish, you know,' she said, clearly reluctant to concede the point, while making one of her own.

'And you always manage to be unappreciative of anything anyone does for you. Cogitate upon that one,' I said, so much angrier than I had anticipated that I decided to go for a drive.

Relieved to be out of my oppressive mother's presence for a while, I set myself the simple task of buying the quintessential Jamaican snack – beef patties. However, I had to pass Blue Horizon to get to the patty shop. As I drove past the house that Gloria had sold for seven figures less than it was worth – and that doesn't even factor in the inestimable docking rights – I felt my blood pressure rise even more. I had to admit that she wasn't the only person who was yearning to be released from her existence. Gloria's death couldn't come one minute too soon for me either. No matter how hard one tried to keep things sweet – no matter how hard she was trying to depart on a good note – the fact remained that there was always a sting in her tail. She could no more help injuring and poisoning than a scorpion can help stinging or a rabid dog biting. This was her character, her destiny – and our fate.

If I needed further proof of this fact, by the end of the third day I had caught her out in a game that was anything but life enhancing. As I said earlier, she wanted to be surrounded by love before dying. This might have been commendable had she not shown her hand rather more clearly than she intended, with the result that I was left in no doubt that it was her egotism at play rather than anything so profoundly spiritual as actual love. I realized this because of two incidents that now happened.

The first took place the night after my arrival. I was sitting with her in her bedroom, dying of boredom, owing to her practice of making sure that she led all conversations and curtailed any that were introduced by others. Desperate for anyone or anything to relieve not only the tedium but also the unpleasantness and tension of having to be a pair of ears, I invited Vilma to sit with us for a few minutes when she brought Gloria a glass of water. Of course, West Indian servants are seldom so educated or sophisticated as to appreciate all the nuances of 'upstairs' conversation, and after a few minutes of the usual awkwardness that passed for conversation *à deux* or *à trois* with Gloria, Vilma's ignorance led her into bringing up the one subject of conversation she naïvely thought would be of interest to the three of us: Marjorie. As she launched into fond memories of her former employer, I saw Gloria purse her lips irritably. I was almost amused that Vilma had inadvertently committed the cardinal offence of diverting the conversation away from the only subject Gloria felt it should have been about, namely herself. I perked up, wondering how this would end. To my entertained horror, Gloria waited about three minutes before cutting Vilma off in the middle of a sentence as she was recounting something Marjorie had said by saying sharply, 'Let the dead bury their dead. You may go now, Vilma.'

Vilma looked surprised, as indeed most people would have been, at so sudden a dismissal.

'Do you want me to get you something to eat or drink, Ma'am?' she asked, clearly trying to rectify whatever offence she might have inadvertently committed.

'No thanks, Vilma, you go and watch television,' Gloria said in her mistress-to-servant tone of voice, before suddenly changing tack and continuing in more humane fashion, 'You're a good girl, and I love you.'

Vilma beamed with delight, but, as soon as she was out of the room, Gloria said, 'That ugly nigger is one dominating piece of work who doesn't know her place. But, as your grandfather used to say, it's Hobson's choice. It's either them or nothing, when you children aren't here. So I have to keep them sweet.'

'They do treat you well, don't they?' I said, responding on one level while my mind raced on another.

'Oh yes. They're good girls like that. But that Vilma is one to watch. Paulette is a much nicer person.'

Two days later, she once more told Vilma she loved her and, as soon as her back was turned, launched into another diatribe revealing that she felt anything but love for her. The only thing that was more startling to me than the hypocrisy was the awareness that there was every possibility that her utterances of love to me, Libby and Kitty might be equally insincere. Could Gloria really be telling us she loved us, not because she did but because she felt vulnerable and wanted to keep us onside, running back and forth between our homes and hers, catering to her needs and providing her with the attention she required?

Although I didn't want to think the worst of my mother, I also didn't plan on allowing her to use me shamelessly. So the next time Gloria told me 'I love you' I felt my spine stiffen. I was in her bathroom getting something for her and decided I would act as if I hadn't heard her. She repeated herself, and this time I said, 'So do I,' meaning, 'I love me too', not 'I love you also'. From then on, until I left Cayman, I only told her 'I love you' once, and that was when I was leaving. I did it when I wanted to, not in response to her manoeuvrings.

Some of Gloria's conduct was so textbook that there were uncomfortably frequent times when she reminded me of some passage in Dr Stout's book. The medical research on sociopathy – limited though it is – indicates that, while disadvantaged women might develop antisocial tendencies as a result of their early life experiences, the upper-class female is usually born that way. They suspect there is some deformity in the amygdala, a part of the brain that affects emotions. While study on the subject is in its infancy, and I for one suspect that the indulged narcissist evolves into sociopathy as an inevitable consequence of her narcissism remaining unchecked, the fact remains that any possibility of Gloria's condition being inherent had ominous overtones for me as her descendant. Could I have inherited any of her antisocial tendencies, I now asked myself?

As I turned this question over and over in my mind, not looking for differences but for similarities, I came to the conclusion that such similarities as existed were superficial, and some were even welcome. One could hardly discount the fact that Gloria's tremendous social skills had enhanced all our lives superficially. Moreover I was also aware that tests have shown that sixty percent of the population, if provided with the right conditions, will display some signs of reduced conscience. In other words, none of us is perfect and many of us can, if the circumstances are conducive, justify our moral failings to such a degree that we dismiss our supposedly conscionable misconduct and exhibit antisocial behaviour to a lesser or greater degree.

If I found unwelcome resonances with some of my mother's imperfections within myself, I ceased to be bothered by them when Erika Freeman once more crystallized the issue by telling me, 'The mere fact that you ask yourself if you are like your mother means you aren't.' In other words, people of conscience are bothered by their failings, while people without a conscience aren't.

Whether I was like my mother or not – a great dread for most of my life, incidentally – the one thing I was confident about was that Gloria was indeed born impossible. 'There was always something wrong with her,' her Aunt Pauline said after Gloria's death. 'Even when she was a baby, it was obvious. I remember hearing her cry and cry and cry when she was put down to rest in the afternoon. She would be inconsolable. She also used to rip off her clothes and run around naked. The servants would try to get her to put them back on, and she would refuse. No one could control her. Because we were relatively close in age, I used to try to comfort her. As a result, I always had a soft spot for her. I sometimes wonder if her problems didn't start in the womb. Cissiemay didn't want her,' she went on, using her nickname for her elder sister May, 'and tried to get rid of her when she first discovered she was pregnant. Nothing worked, and once the baby was born, she loved her. But I wonder if Gloria didn't have some prenatal memory of her mother trying to do away with her. It would certainly account for why she was so bitter.'

Although Aunt Pauline might well have been onto something, I doubt it. Many survivors of abortion turn out to be normal. I cannot see the link between a failed abortion and a foetus growing into a callous individual with only the most superficial feelings for anyone but herself, though I can see a relationship between a spoilt individual evolving into a callous and bitter one.

Gloria's complete contempt for anyone whose opinion she didn't wish to cultivate was always absolute, and it was inevitable that people would ultimately become angry when being used and abused by her. That, in turn, would expose her to their anger, to which of course she always felt they had no right, because she was a perfect being who deserved reverence and admiration, not admonition and anger. This would cause her to feel denigrated, which would feed her feelings of paranoia and rage, and, as narcissistic antisocial personalities lack both empathy and insight but possess self-regard in overweening measure, her resentment at not being given the just deserts she, the pinnacle of self-perceived perfection felt entitled to, would increase along with the certainty that she was in the right and everyone else in the wrong: an ideal recipe – and justification – for bitterness.

Narcissism and sociopathy are often uncomfortably close conditions. Both disorders have many of the same personality defects, such as lack of empathy and insight, the main difference between them being that a narcissist can have a conscience while a sociopath never does. That does not mean that sociopaths don't know the difference between right and wrong. This they frequently do. Certainly Gloria did. But, like all other sociopaths, she simply didn't think that the rules applied to her: a trait also shared by narcissists, who have one set of rules for the imperfect others, who occupy the world, and another set for their perfect selves. As far as they are concerned, they have absolute liberty to act as they please. Lacking a moral compass where their conduct is concerned, they honestly believe that they are above such trivialities as right and wrong. Nor are they ever responsible for anything that can rebound unfavourably upon them, though they will always claim credit for anything self-enhancing even when it is not their due; pathological falsifying of events and self-aggrandizement being two of the characteristics which allow them to reshape facts to suit their own needs.

I had reason to see how accurate the scanty medical research is on the disordered personality when I had lunch with Gloria's friend Katrina on the last Monday of my stay in Cayman that May. As she recounted Gloria's version of history, telling me how much she admired my parents for having been the wonderful, kind, benevolent and generous people they were, I could hardly believe my ears. The way she recounted our childhood, it was magical from start to finish with nary a negative moment to spoil the perfection of it all. We had been spoiled and overindulged by two of the most munificent demigods of all time. Then she brought up the school that Gloria and Michael had built, and I saw the full horror of pathological lying with a clarity I had never before seen.

'There is no such school, nor was there ever,' I said. 'I have to tell you, my mother is truly perverse. She gets all the credit she wants from you without having to put in the effort of actually doing the things she says she's done. Sure, she and Daddy might have given a donation to a school and might even have helped to endow one in a very modest way. And certainly Daddy helped to educate many people. But build a school the way Auntie reroofed the church or air conditioned it? Never. I'll be damned if I'm going to let her get away with getting credit for something she never did – and would never have done in a month of Sundays. She's lying. Don't believe a word of it. Which doesn't mean that she hasn't done some good, for she has. She's raised loads of money for charity over the decades, and has given endowments to various institutions. But build a school. *Never.* I'm so sick and tired of Mummy always overegging the pudding that I could scream. With her, enough is never enough.'

As if to prove the point, on the way home, the telephone rang. It was Paulette. 'The notary is here, and Ma'am is refusing to sign the papers,' she said.

'What?' I said, genuinely surprised.

'Ma'am says she doesn't know anything about the deal,' Paulette said, her tone of voice indicating that she knew as well as I did that Mummy was up to some of her usual mischief.

'Put the notary on to me,' I said, giving Gloria the benefit of the doubt in case Paulette had got the wrong end of the stick.

Sure enough, he confirmed Paulette's story and said he had another appointment in fifteen minutes so would have to leave the house in five. We were ten minutes away. This was particularly annoying. The notary was at the house by appointment for Gloria to sign some papers regarding the sale of her land at Port Royal, once known as the wickedest city on earth when it was the pirate capital of the world until most of it sank in an earthquake in 1692. It was now a site of interest to both the Chinese and Japanese. For the last six years, Gloria had had me liaising on her behalf with a potential purchaser, who had bought Marjorie's land adjoining hers and now wanted hers. The problem was that Gloria had either never applied for title after the land was reserved for her and she had paid the deposit on it, or then the deeds had been lost along with a record of the money she had paid for it. Gloria had known about this problem for well over two decades, learning about it at a time when her uncle Julian had been the President of the Brotherhood of Port Royal and in a position to solve the problem without any trouble. God forbid, however, that the third part of the Trinity should ever have bothered herself with something as mundane as approaching her uncle to obtain the title deeds for her. The result was that, ever since the purchaser had appeared, I had been trying at Gloria's behest to unravel the mess. Finally, after all these years, Gloria's lawyer in Jamaica had drawn up the papers, and I had located just about the only notary in Cayman who was prepared to make a house call to notarize the documents.

'Put Mummy on to me,' I asked him. As soon as she had come on the line I said, 'Mummy, it's the Port Royal land. You know all about it. You've had me working on it since 1999. You're the one who wants it sold.'

'I don't know anything about the sale of any land,' Gloria said in her most pathetic voice – a tone I recognized only too well from the past. In adopting it, she had given her game away. She was taking the opportunity to obtain the sympathy of the notary, who, unbeknownst to me, was married to a cousin of my father's. She wanted him to think that I – doubtless with the connivance of my sisters – was trying to sell her land from under her.

'Mummy,' I snapped. 'You know as well as I do that you knew exactly what the papers were about when I left the house at twelve thirty. You may be getting forgetful about things like where you left keys ten minutes ago, but you've never had any problems remembering things like *land* and *money* before this. I really don't feel like rearranging the appointment, so I'd suggest you sign the papers, none of which need leave your possession unless you want them to.'

'I'm just an old lady who doesn't know what all of this is about,' she said, playing to her audience. 'He can come back when you've explained what this is all about to me.'

'That conniving bitch,' I said to Katrina as soon as I rang off. 'Wait until I get back to the house. I'm going to wipe the floor with her.'

Sure enough, as soon as I entered the house, I stormed straight into her bedroom. 'How dare you pull a stunt like that? How dare you seek to imply to strangers that I or my sisters have been trying to sell your land from under you? Let me remind you that the person who sold *our house* from under us is *you*.'

'I don't know what the papers are for,' Gloria bleated, still in character as the pathetic old lady in danger of being fleeced by her greedy children.

'Oh, yes you do. Don't think I can't see straight through you.'

The eyes of a perfect being, who could never do any wrong, blazed with fury that any member of that subsection of life called humanity, would have the temerity to accuse her of anything less than Godliness. She harrumphed and waved me away angrily. This was not the reaction of the classic sociopath, who wouldn't care less what you thought of him or her, but of classical narcissism: a condition I still knew very little about. Even in the heat of the moment, I noticed the disparity and wondered for a split second if Gloria could really be sociopathic when she cared so intensely what others thought of her.

The discordant note, however, was not enough to divert me from the matter at hand. 'Let me tell you once and for all, you conniving bitch, you don't fool me for one second, even if you fool everyone else. I know, as well as you do, that this is all an act. I know what you're up to. But I will not let you get away with it. You are a mischief-maker who has always loved having everyone jump around like grasshoppers while you pull the strings and extract whatever it is you want from them. Well, you can forget all that shit. If that fucking land sells or doesn't sell, it makes no difference to me. But I will not have you besmirching my reputation and motives after having had me spend six years working on something that you should have been working on yourself – and would've done, if you hadn't been such a fucking irresponsible, lazy, useless piece of shit.'

'I don't know what all of this is about,' wailed Gloria, ever the past-mistress of denial, now that she saw that her haughtiness had got her nowhere.

'Oh, yes you do. And while you're hearing the truth, let me tell you, I know that as soon as my back is turned and I am out of this house, you get your lazy arse out of your bed and sit in the drawing room, and sometimes you even walk in the garden or go to the gate to get some exercise. Don't think I can't see through your manipulations. Well, from now until I leave I will not be sitting in this hot, stuffy bedroom with you. If you want to speak to me, you will get your fucking arse out of bed and join me in the drawing room. You've played the sympathy card once too often, and from now until you're in your grave, I'll be reserving my sympathy for myself, you conniving, ungrateful, opportunistic cunt,' I shrieked.

Gloria, suddenly invigorated, followed me outside.

'If I had known you were going to be so upset,' she said, still playing the innocent, 'I would have signed the damned papers even though I'd forgotten what they're about.'

'Maybe you would have. Maybe you didn't calculate on me blowing my fuse when you've got one foot in the grave. You thought that would preserve you. Well, you can see for yourself, it didn't.' Then I in turn harrumphed, ostensibly to myself but really to my mother, 'Didn't remember? Ha! She must think I'm more stupid than I am.'

'I got confused,' she said.

'No, you didn't,' I said. 'I know you better than that. If you'd been confused, you would've said "I'm confused" or "I don't remember." You didn't. You denied all knowledge of the deal. I can see right through you. And lest we forget, my dear, someone who can make the philosophic distinction between being tired of life as opposed to living definitely knows the difference between forgetting and not knowing.'

I swear, if I had a photograph of her face at that moment, I would exhibit it as proof of how her expression betrayed the veracity of all I was saying. Her eyes shone with pride, as if to say, 'That's my girl. Sharp as a needle. You've found me out.' Realizing that I had read her expression, she waved me away.

'I don't know what you're talking about,' she said. 'And anyway, he said he'd be back later in the week.'

'What you do then is up to you,' I said. 'For my part, my involvement in the sale of your land is at an end. Now and forever.'

With that, I left the house and dropped in on some relations who lived nearby. I was upset that I had been reduced to speaking the truth, but consoled myself with the knowledge that I am a mere human being and therefore not perpetually immune from the worst effects of a wicked mother's machinations.

Two days later I got ready to leave Cayman, the breach papered over as so many others had been. I wish I could say that I didn't feel defiled and sullied by Gloria's treachery, but I did. When the car came to take me to the airport, I walked into her bedroom to say goodbye as the maids were taking my luggage out. She was sitting on her bed.

'The car's here. I've come to say goodbye,' I said, the reserve in my voice giving away the fact that, while I had moved on, I had neither forgiven nor forgotten this latest episode.

'God bless you for coming,' she said, taking a stab at appreciation.

Realizing I might never see her again, I said I was happy to have come, which was the truth, despite the downside.

I bent down, kissed her on her cheek. 'Take care of yourself till Kitty comes,' I said. Kitty was due a week or so later with her husband and daughter. With that, I turned to leave, looked at the wizened if still graceful woman who was my mother, and feeling that I would never see her again, went back to her, kissed her again, said, 'I love you, Mummy,' and was already by the door when she said, 'Bless you for coming.'

It was the last time I would ever see her or speak to her face to face.

Chapter Twenty-Six

On Saturday, June 4 2005, I received a call from Vilma to say that Gloria had fallen. Vilma thought she had broken her hip. 'Paulette and I dragged her into her bed, but she says we're not to call the doctor,' she informed me.

'Can't she walk?' I asked.

'No. That's why we think she's broken her hip.'

'Put me on to her.'

When Gloria came on the line, she said she was not in much pain and did not think she had broken her hip, although she could not walk. She said she had tripped, the toe of her sandal catching on the border of the Persian rug in her bedroom when she was returning from the bathroom. She had fallen onto the tiled floor on her side and lain there until Vilma came to pick her up.

'You have to ring the doctor,' I said.

'I've been watching it,' she said, obviously hoping that she would feel better.

'Mummy, you've got to telephone the doctor. If you've broken your hip, the sooner you're treated, the better,' I said, wondering if she might not be hoping that she'd now simply waft off to the afterlife.

'Let's see how it goes,' she said.

'Put me back on to Vilma,' I said. 'When did this happen?'

'This morning,' Vilma replied.

'You mean, Mummy's been laid up in bed all day and the doctor hasn't been called yet?' I said, incredulous.

'That's why I've called you,' Vilma said.

'You need to phone the doctor,' I said. 'Tell Mummy I'm authorizing you to and then call me back and let me know what he says.'

Instead of ringing the doctor, whom Gloria did not want informed, Vilma telephoned Libby and Kitty, who told her to telephone an ambulance and take Gloria to the hospital.

Gloria being Gloria, it wasn't until the following day that she would consent to the ambulance being called. She was taken to George Town Hospital, where she chose to have Vilma and Paulette attend to her rather than the nurses.

Sure enough, she had broken her hip. Now came the real problem. She was so weak that the doctors did not think she would survive the operation to mend it.

Providentially, Kitty had been due to fly in to Grand Cayman that Monday, so the doctors agreed to wait until her arrival before we came to any decision as to what to do.

Kitty, Michael and Gabriela went straight from the airport to George Town Hospital. After speaking to the doctor in charge, Kitty consulted with our brother-in-law Ben and Libby and me. We arrived at the decision to authorize the surgery, despite the risks, because by this time Gloria was in considerable pain, and not only would that continue until the hip was fixed, but this was her only chance to walk again.

This was a rather busy time for me, as my latest book, *Empress Bianca*, was due to be launched at Daunt Books in Marylebone, London, by the Jamaican High Commissioner on Tuesday June 7 2005 in front of over a hundred guests. I had taken my kids out of school for the occasion, and it turned out to be a happy one, despite the question mark over Gloria's health.

The mobile telephone I had bought for her now came into its own. I asked Kitty to juice it up with credit and, on the morning of the surgery, asked her to take it in to the hospital so that I could speak to Gloria for what, we had been warned, might be the last time. I cannot tell you how beside myself I was when one of those tropical downpours, which grinds traffic to a halt by making visibility impossible, put paid to that plan. By the time Kitty, Michael and Gabriela arrived at the hospital, Gloria was already in surgery.

For the next several hours, I was mindful that I might have missed the last chance I would ever have to say goodbye to my mother. That, coupled with the fact that the doctor and Ben had warned us that there was a real prospect that Gloria's constitution was so weakened that she might die on the operating table, made Thursday, June 9 2005 one of the most anxious days of my life.

Irrespective of how appalling a mother she had been, I had loved Gloria even when I had loathed her. I was so paralyzed with emotion that I was unable to function at all and took to my bed until I received word of the outcome.

Kitty telephoned as soon as the doctor told her the news. Gloria had come through the operation with flying colours. She was doing far better than anyone had expected. Her heart, which he had feared would give out under the strain, was beating strongly. 'Those Burkes really have strong hearts,' Kitty said, alluding to the fact that not one member of our maternal grandmother's family had ever been known to have their heart give out, with the result that, although Gloria was still not out of danger, it looked as if she would be living for awhile yet.

The following day, when I telephoned her, Gloria not only claimed to be fine (something of a first for a born complainer) but sounded as vigorous as an ox. Because the Burkes were also known for having strong voices that didn't desert them until the moment of death, I knew that I could not rely upon how she sounded and made her pass the telephone to Paulette, who confirmed in a voice suggestive of admiring relief, 'Ma'am is doing fine. She's surprised us all.'

Kitty spent the next few days visiting Gloria in the hospital and updating Libby and me on her progress. This was so remarkable that we had already started to discuss a schedule for forthcoming visits. Kitty then left Cayman on Sunday, June 12 but not before further juicing up the mobile so that I could communicate with Gloria, who, Kitty had agreed with the doctor, should stay in the hospital for two weeks. The danger with releasing her prior to that was that she would not want to do her physiotherapy, which was painful. Without it, she would become bedridden; her lungs would fill with water, and she could develop pneumonia and die. It was therefore imperative to get her over this dangerous phase.

Though Gloria was well-behaved while Kitty was in Cayman, once she had left, the antics started. I received a variety of telephone calls from the nurses to tell me that Gloria was either ripping the drip out of her arm or resisting their efforts when they tried to put it back in. Finally, I had had enough. 'Tell her I said that if she pulls it out once more, I am authorizing you to sedate her to prevent her doing so again,' I said. 'Now let me have a word with her before you hang up so that she knows I mean business.' At which point I read Gloria the riot act.

That put an end to that nonsense. Sadly, this seems to have coincided with some of the nurses deciding that this rather tiresome woman deserved some payback. If Vilma and Paulette are to be believed, once those nurses knew that the immediate family would be absent for the remainder of her stay in the hospital, they set out to make Gloria's life a misery. 'They treated Ma'am rough. Rough. She was never used to hard life, and they stopped us taking care of her. They used to pull her out of the bed with such force that she would cry out in pain. They would drop her in the chair like a breadfruit hitting the ground and make her sit up for hours and hours, even after she was bawling from pain. And if you ever saw the way they kicked her heel to make her walk with the stroller when they were doing her physiotherapy, you would cry. Ma'am used to say to them "You are so cruel", but to us she would say "The wicked have to suffer before they die." We think it's the hard treatment that killed her. She wasn't used to it,' Paulette said.

Of course, neither maid said anything to Libby, Kitty or me at the time. If they had, we would have taken steps to bring any harsh treatment to a halt. Indeed, the therapist told Kitty on Friday, June 17, 2005, that Gloria had finally had a 'change in attitude' and was doing her physiotherapy with unprecedented willingness. We therefore thought she was getting stronger by the day and were already planning for Libby to go out to Cayman as soon as Gloria was released from the hospital, with me to follow shortly afterwards.

Although I used to speak to Gloria every day, she – who had spent her whole life complaining, even though there was usually no cause to do so – never once complained about this mistreatment when apparently there was justification for complaint. I have often wondered why she did not, and suspect that she had finally faced the fact that she needed to prepare her immortal soul for her Maker. The way to do it was to accept that she was a mere mortal who had been a sinner and not one third of the Trinity. Therefore, her comment that 'the wicked have to suffer before they die' was, on the one hand, a knife through my heart and, on the other, a balm to my soul. She had given herself the opportunity for salvation by admitting her fallibility, without which I doubted there would be any possibility for Divine forgiveness.

No one knows what actually caused her death, but at around 5.05 on the morning of Saturday, June 18, 2005, Gloria's heart stopped beating. 'Her system simply shut down,' the doctor told Kitty. 'I decided not to resuscitate her because it would have been too painful for her, and I knew she didn't want to live.'

Her death was a tremendous shock to each of her children, because none of us expected it. While she was dying, I was sitting around a Gloucestershire brunch table with friends discussing the Beaufort Ball, which we had attended the night before, and the guests who had been there, including Prince William and his girlfriend Katherine Middleton. I did not even know Gloria was dead until I got home later that afternoon and picked up my messages. I promptly returned Kitty's call, and she filled me in on what had happened.

Naturally, we were both upset. I would have preferred to start to come to terms with our mother's death in the privacy of my own home, but that was not a luxury in which I could indulge. Dominick Dunne, the bestselling author and broadcaster, had arranged for me to meet Mike Griffith, the well-known American lawyer who was the subject of the movie *Midnight Express*. He was passing through London. Although I did toy with the idea of cancelling our meeting, I decided to put my emotions to one side and honour it, especially as it was professionally based. Gloria, after all, was already dead; and since I was hardly a baby and ours had not been the most trouble-free of relationships, I should be able to exercise sufficient self-restraint to keep myself in check for a few hours.

No matter how awful a mother Gloria had been, she had still been my mother, and there was no question that I was upset by her death. In fact, I was feeling so out of sorts that, within minutes of meeting him, I had to explain to Mike, 'If I seem a bit odd, it's because my mother died today.' Then, to prove just how discombobulated I was, when we went on to dinner and I was in the ladies' room washing my hands, somehow I managed, for the one and only time in my life, to catapult a diamond and ruby ring down the plug-hole along with the water. The restaurant staff then had to get in a plumber to undo the sink and recover the ring from the s-bend. Talk about ridiculous.

After dinner, I begged off going to Annabel's, the fashionable nightclub, and instead went back home to begin the grieving process. It was a decidedly mixed experience. Though I did feel sad, I was a lot less sad than I would otherwise have been if Gloria had not damaged our relationship over the years. I can even say that I did not feel as sad as I would have liked to. Although there was a measure of love there, that sentiment has been supplanted by too many others for it to be more than a fractional part of my response. In a very real sense, I had gone through the grieving process years ago, at the time when I had actually 'lost' the mother I had once loved and who, I had thought, loved me. Her death was not like any other deaths I had experienced, because in many ways she had died, at least to me, years before.

To my surprise, the overriding emotion I felt was calm. Not acceptance. Calm. Although there was a measure of relief intermingled with it, the two emotions were separate; and what settled over me was this tremendous sense of calm.

In the days and weeks to come, as this new feeling did not leave me, I began to understand its significance. As long as my treacherous and vicious mother had been alive, prodding and poking, causing trouble, concocting mischief, lying, cheating, deceiving and occasionally charming, I had on some level always been rattled. One simply could never predict what dreadful new thing she would come up with next, or when it might change to something marginally more pleasant. Though I had not been aware that her disturbing presence had kept me permanently unsettled to the very core of my being, as soon as she was dead, this sense of calm – a feeling which must always have been natural to me, even though I had not known it before – immediately replaced all the unsettled feelings that her very existence had engendered.

It is no exaggeration to say that I was as shocked as any stranger would be by such an unexpected reaction. Gloria and I hadn't lived in the same country for nearly four decades. We hadn't been close for thirty-five years. We had even been estranged, in varying degrees, for some twenty-five of the last thirty-five years. One couldn't say that I had any profound separating or detaching to do, because I had done it years before. And yet, for all the loosening of emotional ties, the fundamental effect of her death provided me with this deep-seated sensation of calm. This told me that, on a fundamental level, I must always have found her a deeply disturbing, possibly even horrifying, presence. Someone around whom one could never relax: someone one always had to be on one's guard against. While her manifestations of evil were not murderous in a physical sense, they were equally deadly emotionally and spiritually. Like the poison strychnine, such sweetness as she possessed masked a deadliness that it behoved one to beware of. Only when she was well and truly dead, and therefore no longer a threat to one's well-being, did I feel sufficiently released from the endlessly awful possibilities which she had created or could create, to actually become calm in keeping with my true nature.

This was an unexpected and wholly welcome gift, I can assure you, made all the more desirable by its total unexpectedness. Never in a month of Sundays would I ever have imagined that my mother's very existence could have been having the persistent and unsettling effect she had obviously had over me throughout my whole life. This, I can tell you, was a real eye-opener.

Chapter Twenty-Seven

Now that Gloria was dead, her daughters had to arrange her funeral. Libby was keen to do the honours, so Kitty and I let her.

It quickly emerged that the funeral could not be conducted in the conventional time of a few days or a week or two after her death. Libby's daughter was scheduled to give birth to the male heir to the presidential dynasty, and she was relying upon her mother to take care of her two-year-old daughter while she was in the hospital. Also, my children were in school till the end of the month of June, and there was no way their end-of-term schedules could be interrupted. Nor could they miss their grandmother's funeral. We therefore decided to keep Gloria on ice until July, at which time she could be buried.

While Libby was assisting Elizabeth to do her dynastic duty, I took advantage of the hiatus to attend the wedding in Jordan of another dynasty. Usama and Abir Tuqan's daughter Suha, niece of the late Queen Alia of Jordan, was marrying the son of the billionaire Nadmi Auchi. In keeping with traditional Middle Eastern hospitality, the groom's father treated the guests, who consisted of some of the richest and grandest people in the Western and Near Eastern worlds, to a weekend of unrivalled splendour. Clearly a man of impeccable taste, after flying us in two aeroplanes from London, Nadmi Auchi put us up at his five-star hotel in Amman, which has to be one of the most luxurious and tasteful hotels anywhere. On the Friday evening, he played host to the many hundreds of us guests at a rehearsal dinner dance at the club he owns, the Dunes, outside Amman, which is one of the chicest and most sumptuous clubs I have ever seen.

No one does hospitality like well-bred Middle Easterners. Possibly this is because they are the descendents of the creators of Western civilization as we know it. Whatever the reason, no European or American, no matter how hospitable, ever manages to approach the true magnificence of the Near East; by the time the rehearsal dinner ended with a spectacular fireworks display, the like of which I have not seen since the Duke of Edinburgh's seventieth birthday party celebrations at Windsor Castle, even I was moved to say to the writer Trevor Mostyn, 'This whole evening is straight out of the Arabian Nights.'

The following morning it was refreshing to wake up to see that the fairytale continued. All the guests were given a choice of a variety of activities. I chose to go to the Dead Sea along with our hostess, Abir Tuqan, and a few other guests. After we had floated on the water – you cannot swim properly, as there is so much salt that it prevents you from sinking your feet into the water – we went back to the hotel to dress for the wedding reception, which was being held downstairs in the ballroom.

For sheer magnificence, this occasion was unsurpassable; and I say it having been to events in various British and European royal palaces, as well as many super-upscale American ones. Everything, from the entertainers through the food and drink to the several bands that kept us dancing until the morning, was of the very highest standard. Nor did the Tuqans and Auchis forget to live up to the principle of *noblesse oblige*. While we were inside watching the descent of the bride and groom, the people of the Jordanian capital were being treated to an even more spectacular fireworks display than the amazing one we had seen the night before.

Of course, thirty years ago, it would have been unthinkable for someone like me to attend a wedding or any other sort of social event, while my mother lay unburied in a morgue in Grand Cayman. Times, however, had changed. Not only was it perfectly all right to attend, it was actually thoroughly desirable. Life must go on, especially when you have no real mourning to do.

Like all well-raised ladies of my generation, however, I did doff my hat to older and more restrictive mourning practices by wearing two mourning colours in the evening, grey and lavender, and black or white during the day.

While I was sitting around the brunch table late on the Sunday morning with a variety of chums (none of us got to bed before four a.m. and some of the younger guests not until seven or eight), my publisher, Gary Pulsifer, rang me to say that the *Sunday Telegraph* had run a huge story about my recently published book, *Empress Bianca*. 'Read it out to me,' I said.

To my astonishment, I then heard that 'friends' of the billionaire Edmond Safra's widow Lily were asserting that I had based the central character upon her. I could hardly believe my ears. Aside from the fact that I had not indicated who it was I had based my story upon, out of deference to the family of the double murderess who was its inspiration – and I had even gone to the length of asserting at the beginning of the book in a printed disclaimer that, notwithstanding it being inspired by a true story, it was a work of fiction – these unnamed 'friends' were now linking the widow's name to the book and claiming outrage on her behalf.

Of course, if there is one thing everyone in the public eye knows, it is that 'unnamed friends' or 'sources close to' are usually journalistic code for the person who has been named but wishes to be discreet. As I had been in the public eye for over thirty years, no one knew journalistic code better than me.

Nor was my knowledge of how the press works based solely upon my experience of being written about. I was in the rare position of being both poacher and gamekeeper, so to speak, for I had written two biographies of the greatest unnamed source of all: Diana, Princess of Wales, who leaked like a sieve not only to me and to Andrew Morton but also to Richard Kay, aside from tipping off several paparazzi whose cameras she availed herself of to ensure that daily 'snatched' photographs of herself would appear in the newspapers of her choice, alongside her planted stories.

Since neither my publisher nor I had planted the story with the *Sunday Telegraph*, I was left with no choice but to suspect the Lily Safra camp of being the culprit. This, of course, presented me with quite a dilemma, for I had to ask myself: why on earth would anyone wish to link their friend or themselves to a novel about a double murderess?

Admittedly, Bianca is a fascinating, attractive, intriguing, stylish character. But she nevertheless remains a double murderess, and since I had not identified Lily Safra as the central character in the novel, why had her 'friends' done so?

Experience teaches wisdom, which makes spotting the game easier. The question at this point now became: what was the game behind the publication of the *Sunday Telegraph* story?

Too little had happened for me to arrive at a considered conclusion at that juncture, save that, before I had buried one unbelievable woman, fate seemed to be lumbering me with another.

In the days and weeks to come, I would form the view, whether accurately or erroneously, that Lily Safra might well have been misled by her advisors: always a distinct possibility when someone is as rich as she is.

The advisors of the very rich invariably stand to make hundreds of thousands, if not millions, by 'rescuing' their clients from problems with which, often as not, they have saddled them.

Another possibility was that the lure of the 'problem' of 'having' a 'biography' written by the Princess of Wales's biographer in the form of an allegedly thinly-veiled work of fiction possessed too much snob-appeal for the ambitious culprit to resist. And, as all of us who have been born into the social world know, people who aspire to leave their mark often can resist anything but attention.

Although I did not know Mrs Safra, I soon learnt that she gave vast donations to charities, and that these somehow magically ended up being reported in the press. The word in royal circles was also that her generosity to the Prince of Wales's charities had been so marked that his advisors felt compelled to acknowledge her input by seating her beside him at public fund-raising dinners. A place this lady had taken, showing that, gilded or not, this was one lily who was no wilting wall-flower that shied away from the limelight.

Because the lady in question was not a friend of mine, I could not assess for myself whether her philanthropy was motivated by genuine charity or whether it sprang from the more usual motivation of vaingloriousness. However, having been a part of the charity world more or less for the same length of time as the Prince of Wales, I knew that the reality of philanthropy is seldom altruism. Although most philanthropists want everyone to believe that they are marvellous human beings who give out of the kindness of their hearts, charitable foundations, especially in America, are obliged by law to give away a certain percentage of their income every year. If they fail to do so, they lose their favourable tax status. In other words, charitable foundations are nothing but a massive tax break that allows the rich to pose as altruistic benefactors while actually saving themselves vast sums on tax.

If there was one lesson I had learned from Gloria and her kind, it is that Society (which now includes the super-rich as well as the Old Guard) teams with a greater number of narcissists than any other sphere of human activity. For them, the social world is the stage upon which they act out, and have reinforced, their specialness, their wonderfulness, their superiority. Half of them are really not special or wonderful or superior at all, except insofar as their bank accounts or privileged backgrounds are concerned. Some might be good-looking. Others might be charming. Some might even be entertaining. Many will live and die upon the altar of 'taste'. Some will even pillory everyone but themselves with their knowledge of 'correct behaviour'. What few have ever done, however, is accomplish anything noteworthy. It really is a world of smoke and mirrors where substance is frequently denigrated at the expense of illusion, where true accomplishment is dismissed in preference to the twin gods of appearance and riches, where vanity passes itself off as kindness, and altruism has all the hallmarks of self-promotion.

Armed with this knowledge, as I read the *Sunday Telegraph*, I tried to gleam what sort of people I was dealing with. The article and its quite extraordinary tone gave me a potential insight. Lily Safra's spokesman was Prince Charles's former press officer, Mark Bolland. I knew quite a lot about this gentleman's reputation from my Palace links. The Duke and Duchess of York and Earl and Countess of Wessex were said to loathe him because he used to horse-trade unfavourable stories about them in exchange for positive coverage of his employer and Camilla Parker-Bowles. Not only did this practice cause tremendous ill feeling within the Windsor family, but it was frighteningly effective in damaging the Yorks' and Wessexes' reputations while elevating Camilla's. Indeed, Mark Bolland was credited with having pulled off the coup of all time, making the unacceptable Camilla Parker-Bowles so acceptable that she had gone on to become the Duchess of Cornwall. This, of course, had not saved his skin when push came to shove. Once his purpose had been served, his services were expended with along with much of the trouble his tactics had caused within the family.

Now Mark Bolland was dealing with the press on behalf of the woman he was billing as 'the richest widow in the world'. That very sobriquet was enough to tell me that his objective was not to keep press attention away from Mrs Safra, but to burnish and elevate her reputation to the greatest heights. He would have had to be very inept indeed to seek to accomplish the goal of deflecting media attention away from his client when he was creating such a tantalizing reputation as 'the richest widow in the world' – and whatever Mark Bolland was, he was not ineffectual.

However, in elevated circles, it is considered inelegant to polish one's public profile too obviously. Indeed, the Old Guard frown upon anyone who seeks to acquire too public a reputation for anything, generosity or wonderfulness included. As far as they are concerned, such conduct is a Mark of Cain. This presents the socially-ambitious *arriviste* with a dilemma. How does the world get to know that a new, self-created and self-generated star is glittering away in the constellation without alienating the Old Guard, whose acceptance is needed as proof of their arrival in the Pantheon of the Worldly Gods?

This is where the public relations officer comes in. It is his duty to plant stories which raise the profile of his clients in such a way that no one can trace his efforts back to them. Denial is the name of the game; hence, a good press relations' officer on a retainer will often tell you with a straight face that his brief is to keep his client out of the papers, while all of us who are in the public eye know that he and the client are beavering away behind the scenes to achieve the very recognition to which they deny aspiring! And of course, they always claim that they are not responsible for leaking positive information about this donation or that act of kindness to the press – even though the press couldn't possibly find out about it were it not leaked by someone in the employer's camp!

With three decades of experience sharpening my perception, I cast a practiced eye over the *Empress Bianca* saga as it unfolded in the following months. Lily Safra was threatening to sue the publishers for defamation. Faced with the threat of being buried under the Safra billions, they took what they announced was a 'commercial decision' and agreed to her demand to pulp the book.

Now, the one thing the publishing industry loathes is anything that smacks of censorship. And the pulping of *Empress Bianca* not only smacked of that, but also reminded people of how the Nazis had burnt books. The result, not surprisingly, was that the pulping became an international *cause célèbre*. Journalists on both sides of the Atlantic were outraged that any individual could threaten to destroy a publisher if he did not pull a work of fiction which only she was proclaiming publicly was about her.

For my part, I was watching developments in an ever-increasing fury, determined that no one would prevent my work from seeing the light of day any more than Gloria had succeeded in any of her self-serving plots and schemes.

For nearly a year, my lawyers and I investigated the best way of proceeding. Then we issued proceedings against Lily Safra for libel and tortuous interference with my publishing contract.

English court proceedings are always slow, and in the months to come, I was in the dark until we exchanged witness statements, Then, and only then, did I discover that Lily Safra was claiming that she had not been behind the *Sunday Telegraph* story, and was in effect as much a victim of her 'friends" claims as I was. By contrast, Mark Bolland baldly asserted in his witness statement that the *Sunday Telegraph* had informed him that Lily Safra herself had placed the story through a Jewish banker when they had first approached him for her comments! The whole question of how Mrs Safra had come to be publicly linked with Empress Bianca was certainly getting curiouser and curiouser, as Alice in Wonderland might have put it, but as far as I was concerned, Mark Bolland's statement was all the vindication I needed, and when the case concluded, I set about finding another publisher.

This, of course, was no easy task. Few publishers have the means or the courage to stand up to the threats of billionaires, but eventually, I found one, and *Empress Bianca* was once more headed for the bookstores.

I might well have been at a loss of what to make of the bizarre scenario Lily Safra's 'unnamed friends' unleashed upon me while I was in Jordan, had I not been in the public eye for as long as I have been and had I not had that arch-manipulator, Gloria, for a mother. Between those two sets of experience, however, I had learned that there is 'nowt so queer as folk'.

I therefore returned from Jordan to England without giving any further thought to what might be coming next from the Bolland-Safra camp. Having written a work of fiction which was plainly declared as such, I took the view that if people were misguided enough to link themselves or their friends to my book, such problems as there were ought rightly to remain theirs and not become mine under any circumstances. My focus was in getting my children and myself to Grand Cayman for my mother's funeral.

This was scheduled for Saturday July 9, so we flew out on Wednesday July 6, 2005. My boys and I arrived in Cayman to be greeted by my two sisters. They had been there since earlier in the week. 'There's a hurricane heading straight for Cayman,' they informed me. 'It's due to hit on Saturday. We've had to change the funeral to tomorrow.'

'This is Wednesday. Hurricanes change direction all the time. There's very little likelihood that a hurricane that is heading this way today will hit us on Saturday,' I said. 'Everyone here has been traumatized by Ivan. I daresay for the next few years every time a hurricane starts up a thousand miles away, the Caymanians are going to be battening down the hatches, convinced that this latest one will hit them too. Perfectly understandable. And perfectly ludicrous too.'

'Nevertheless, the funeral's been changed,' Libby said.

'Even if the hurricane doesn't hit Cayman, it might hit Florida, and I can't afford to be trapped here when I have to go back home and prepare for a possible hit there,' Kitty said, only too reasonably. 'We're all going back on Friday before they shut down the airports.'

'But how will people know that the funeral's been changed if you only changed it today?' I asked.

'Announcements are being made on the radio,' Libby said.

'What a pig's ear,' I said. 'Now we won't have enough time to go through Mummy's things and allocate them or do whatever else we have to do.'

'Kitty and I have already been through Mummy's things. There's really nothing we want. Didn't you say there was cash in the house?' Libby said.

'Yes. I don't remember exactly how much. Maybe a thousand dollars or so,' I said.

'Well, it's missing. And we haven't been able to locate any of Auntie's good jewellery,' Libby said.

'But I thought it was in the cupboard where Mummy kept the money, under lock and key,' I said.

'Maybe it will be in the safety-deposit box,' Kitty said. This was where Gloria had housed her own jewels since the political troubles in Jamaica in the mid-1970s.

'We have an appointment with the lawyer tomorrow morning,' Libby informed me. 'It turns out Mummy's will can't be probated because she left Mickey as her executor, and you can't have a dead executor. So we'll have to apply for letters of administration the way we did with Auntie.'

After discussing the matter among ourselves, we agreed that Libby would be the best person to obtain the letters of administration. She would then divide up the estate in keeping with the terms of the will, which left everything to Gloria's children.

When I saw that the will had been made in the 1980s, at a time when I was not speaking to my mother, I thought: Maybe she did love me after all; she could have so easily not included me; but she did. It was only later that it occurred to me that love might have had very little to do with it. Convention required that one leave one's money to one's children. This Gloria, always conventional if iconoclastic at the same time, had done. But, if she had made off with Anthony, or indeed with anyone else, we would have been cut out of the lion's share, for she had found the ideal way of doing so by making him a signatory on her accounts so that at the time of death all that money became his lawfully, and we ceased to have a lawful right to it. The money our father, grandmother and brother had expected to be passed on to us would therefore have gone to someone they would never have regarded as having a right to one penny of their bequests – and we would have been left with the crumbs alone. Gloria had found the perfect way to screw us one last time without us being able to complain about this last manoeuvre of our malicious mother. Only the absence of someone more important in her life had allowed us to inherit. So we had really inherited only by default, and any other interpretation was only so much wishful thinking.

When I thought the whole thing through, somehow love no longer came into Gloria's bequests to us. At least that realization did not hit me until well after Gloria had been buried and I was out of Cayman.

On the Thursday morning following my arrival in Cayman, Libby and Kitty asked me if I wanted to see Gloria before going on to the lawyer. I declined to do so, though when I had been given the same opportunity to view my aunt Marjorie for one last time in the privacy of the funeral home, I had leapt at the opportunity. That, I think, says all that needs to be said about how I really felt about the woman who had given birth to me as opposed to the woman who had nurtured me.

After we had dispensed with visiting the lawyer, Libby, Kitty and I went to the bank. Strictly speaking, we did not have a right of entry to Gloria's safety-deposit box, but because we as a family were longstanding customers and had a copy of the will, which showed that we three sisters were her sole beneficiaries, they allowed us to look at the contents of the box. A member of staff stood guard the whole time, however, to ensure that we did not remove any items – presumably to preclude the possibility of any of us suing the bank in the event that items were missing after we had examined what Gloria had in the way of jewellery.

As with everything else involving our mother, these jewels were something which Gloria had managed to turn into a source of mystery, uncertainty and conflict. Her attitude had always been that she was accountable to no one, so she had never condescended to provide us with an accurate gauge of what she had. We had to go by memory as well as the information she had provided over the years, some of which was none too accurate. For instance, the supposed losses resulting from the burglary that had occurred when she was visiting me in England in 1998 had grown with the passage of time. What we could say with certainty was that she had not given away any of her important jewels to anyone with the exception of the ruby bracelet which she had promised me when I was married, then accused me of stealing when she needed to undermine my reputation. This she had given to Libby, presumably in the hope that I would become jealous and resent Libby as a result – which I did not. Indeed, I didn't even resent Gloria for having done such a puerile thing, though I did pity her for being so mean-spirited.

As we looked through Gloria's treasure trove, we recognized an array of diamonds, rubies, emeralds, sapphires and other stones, all set in either platinum or gold, many of which had not been worn in decades. None of Auntie's jewellery was there, except the double-strand pearl necklace with the diamond and sapphire clasp which Gloria had told me Libby had taken. And what should also be in the box, big as life, but Gloria's golden pearls which she had told me she had given to Libby years before?

'I don't believe it,' I said. 'Here are the pearls.'

Because we were in the presence of someone outside the family circle, we agreed by unspoken consent to say no more on the subject until we were out of earshot. In the meantime, we tried to figure out what else was missing. 'I remember she said that the only thing of any value stolen in the 1998 burglary was the diamond and ruby parure. Since the white gold one is here, that means it's the yellow gold one that was taken,' I said.

Working from memory, we came to the conclusion that only the diamond and emerald parure she got in Mexico in the 1950s, and possibly one or two other pieces which we had forgotten about, were also missing. The rest of her stuff was intact.

'But where's Auntie's good stuff?' Libby and Kitty wanted to know.

'Mummy said you got the diamond and sapphire earrings,' I said to Kitty.

'I certainly did not,' she said hotly.

'Not only didn't she get them, but I took Mummy myself to the jeweller to have them repaired the last time she was visiting me. You know how she could never do anything for herself. Well, this is one thing she insisted upon doing,' Libby said.

'I also offered to help her with getting them repaired, but she refused me as well,' Kitty added.

The message was clear: Gloria was intent on keeping them in her possession, possibly because she knew either Libby or Kitty or both might want them. And she had made damned sure that they would never have them. What Gloria did with them, and whatever other jewels Marjorie had of real value, will forever remain a mystery. Did the help 'help themselves' to them? Did Gloria give them away? Did she hide them then forget where she had hidden them? Did she throw them away, either deliberately or accidentally? Who knows? All we know with any certainty is that our mother made damned sure that she kept them out of our possession while she was alive as well as when she was dead. As with so much else involving our mother, we could speculate endlessly without arriving at any firm conclusions, save that her actions were not those of a loving or caring person.

What required no speculation was how beautiful Gloria looked in death. Her funeral was scheduled to start at four o'clock the afternoon of Thursday July 7, 2005, so her three surviving children, together with Kitty's and my children (Libby's having been marooned in the US), arrived at John Gray Memorial Church in West Bay at about a quarter to four. The hearse was already there, and Gloria's coffin had been taken out and placed on the catafalque. In keeping with West Indian tradition, the coffin was open. We duly went up to say our goodbyes. Naturally, we were weeping. Whatever her faults, Gloria had been our mother, and we had loved her, even if that emotion had, for most of the time, been crowded out by other less positive ones.

As we stood over Gloria, I could not resist quipping to my two sisters, 'Mummy would say, "You see. I still don't have a line on my face." She really looks so lovely.' Their laughter intermingled with their tears, and we then took our seats, waiting for the funeral to begin.

On the nose of four o'clock, the Reverend Doctor Yvette Bloomfield began the service. I thought it rather ironic that a female priest should be conducting the funeral service of a woman who had never liked her own sex. The priest of our cousin Pam, she had been to see Gloria once or twice shortly before her death, so at least knew her somewhat. This was salient, for so often nowadays, especially in fashionable circles, people are laid to rest by total strangers. This happened with my celebrated stepmother-in-law Margaret, Duchess of Argyll, whose funeral struck me as the saddest part of an amazing life, not because of what it celebrated, but what it didn't. The priest had even made it plain he didn't even know the deceased he was burying. At least this didn't happen with Gloria.

Libby had chosen well, and the order of service was just as Gloria would have liked it to be. However, aside from relations and staff, there were no more than two or three other mourners present. Partly, this was because people who were due to fly in – such as Gloria's grandchildren by Libby and her husband Ben – could not do so in time now that the funeral had been moved up. Partly, this was also due to the fact that the funeral was taking place in Cayman, where Gloria was not known, rather than in Jamaica, where she had lived her whole life and had a profile. But I suspected that even in Jamaica her funeral might have drawn a far smaller congregation than her late husband's or son's had done, largely because of her unpopularity. No matter how grand you are, you cannot go through life spreading trouble instead of joy then expect people to come and pay you a tribute they do not think you deserve.

Nevertheless, despite the difficult circumstances, Yvette Bloomfield gave a most appropriate sermon; and Michael, the son-in-law Gloria had once targeted but had softened towards by the time she died, delivered a touching eulogy which Libby had written. 'Believe me, it was the most difficult thing I've ever had to do,' she said. 'I wanted it to be truthful without being negative – and that combination was not easy to pull off. Not when you consider what sort of person Mummy was.'

From the church, we followed the hearse the mile or so to the cemetery. Gloria was being buried beside her mother on the Seven Mile Beach. I could not help being struck by the second irony of the occasion. Gloria, who disliked the sea and her mother, was being buried beside both – and had chosen to be. And, irony to end all ironies, she was also being buried beside Perez, the man whom she had made sure she distanced herself from when the questions of her paternity arose. She could easily have chosen to be repatriated to Jamaica, to be laid to rest beside Michael, but she had declined that suggestion. Was this the last roll of an uncaring dice, or the fitting resting place for a conflicted soul?

As the gravediggers started to shovel in the earth at the end of the interment, the skies, which had hitherto been sunny, opened with such unexpected force that we all had to flee to the cars before we were thoroughly soaked.

Slightly bedraggled, we repaired to Cousin John and Pam's house for the inevitable reception. Yvette Bloomfield could not have been nicer to Libby, Kitty or me and tried her best to sympathize in the midst of such difficult circumstances. 'I know you had a hard time with your mother,' she said, 'but you have the consolation of knowing that, whatever else she was, she was a great lady.'

Yes, I suppose she was. I concede that we owe some of the worldly success we have enjoyed to her influence. But I felt like asking the kind priest, 'How much of a consolation do you think it is that the only thing we have to hang onto is that our mother was a great lady?' I suppose a twig in an ocean is better than nothing, but I doubt if it is anywhere as useful as a raft.

After the reception, we sisters had one last chore to complete on behalf of our mother. We had to choose her tombstone. The following morning they picked me up, Libby driving, Kitty sitting beside her. I jumped into the back of the car, and we headed off across town to the other side of the island.

We had just passed Gloria's final resting place on the Seven Mile Beach when Libby said, 'We have to decide what to put on the tombstone. I've been giving it a lot of thought. I don't know what you both think, but I suggest we simply put, "Gloria Dey Ziadie. November 12 1927 to June 18 2005. Wife. Mother. Sister." I don't think we can stretch to "beloved". It would be too hypocritical. What do you think?'

Kitty and I both agreed. And that, simply and honestly, is what her tombstone says.

Later that afternoon, my two sisters left Grand Cayman to fly back with or to their families in the US. I was left with the task of going through our mother's possessions. 'Thank God this is the last time I will ever have to wind up anyone's life,' I said to both of them. 'I've had to deal with Mickey's, Auntie's and now Mummy's things There is something profoundly poignant about going through the possessions of a lifetime. It makes you realize how utterly futile many of our cares are. When you stop to think how much Mickey or Auntie or Mummy valued certain things, which none of us even wants, it really gives you pause for thought about what we all value.'

The question of priorities aside, I also had to get rid of Gloria's stuff because the house had to be rented out, and you cannot rent out a house which is crammed with a lifetime of acquisitions as well as generations of furniture. Few people who need to rent a house appreciate antiques. Many of them have never heard of Baccarat or Waterford, much less Spode or Wedgwood; even if they have, the idea of reclining on an nineteenth-century *chaise longue* is as antipathetic to them as sitting on a eighteenth-century *fauteuil.* They would much rather have contemporary items that are good-looking, and should you wish to inflict articles of value upon them, they will recoil in horror rather than react with appreciation.

In the days to come, I had to plough through a plethora of stuff while Cayman came to a halt for a second time in a week. Another hurricane was due to hit, and of course the whole island took off work to stock up on supplies and put up hurricane shutters, which they had only taken down days before. This one missed the island too. In between all of this activity, I had to arrange for the builders to come and give me quotes to repaint the interior and exterior of the house as well as upgrade the kitchen, which, in typical patrician style, hadn't been touched since the house was built. Having made the appointments, I then was left to twiddle my thumbs while everyone was several hours late – if they showed up at all.

To add insult to injury, Lily Safra's lawyer, Anthony Julius, now came to life and threatened to sue Gary Pulsifer and the publishing house Arcadia unless they pulped *Empress Bianca* for the injury it might cause his client's reputation!

Whenever I wasn't dealing with the builders and cleaners, I now had to be on the telephone to London to deal with the mess in which Lily Safra had now embroiled herself and me. I needed this latter distraction like a hole in the head, but I was also aware that lawyers like nothing better than applying pressure when they think you are vulnerable. As news of Gloria's death had been published in the English's papers, Anthony Julius might well have jumped to the mistaken conclusion that he was gaining an advantage by rattling the legal sabres before my mother's corpse had time to properly defrost in the grave. In case he thought I was one of those lily-livered women who would quiver and quake before his client's billions, I wrote and let him know that I would not prove to be a tame animal in a witness box. Not only did I know about him as a result of Diana's divorce from Prince Charles, but I was also privy to some of his late client's secret dealings, which had resulted in the heir to the throne borrowing £17 million to pay off the wife who threatened to embroil him in a homosexual scandal if he didn't play ball and give her what she wanted, even though the scandal did not involve him but rather two of his valets. Falstaff might have thought that discretion is the better part of valour, but I had learnt that in the real world it was an unblinking eye and information that usually gave people pause for thought. Let him and his client cogitate upon that fact.

In the months to come, he would find out just how impervious I am to pressure. In the meantime, I had no choice but to deal with the overload as best I could. Only too soon, it became apparent that there was no way I would ever be able to get through the task of winding up Gloria's life or fixing up the house in the time allotted. Even without the hassle Anthony Julius was causing, there was simply too much to do to finish the job in such a limited space of time. I would have to return at the end of the summer, when the children were in school and I had some time available.

So we left Grand Cayman and my grandmother's house pretty much as Gloria had left it. I picked up the threads of my life once more with ease, for I had done most of my grieving decades before, and truth be told, Gloria's death was less a loss than a relief.

The week after my boys and I returned to London, something happened which provided an uncanny comparable to the grief that I would have felt had Gloria not destroyed the love I had once felt for her. Our dog Philippe died of a massive infection four days after undergoing abdominal surgery. I was beside myself. The shock only compounded the horror of losing a healthy three-year-old so unexpectedly and unnecessarily. In the days after his death, I would find myself sobbing uncontrollably as I struggled to come to terms with a loss that was wholly preventable and would have been avoided if the vet had only listened to my daily warnings and prescribed a dose of stronger antibiotics. But the vet had failed to do so, and Philippe had died as Misha and I were taking him to another clinic – an emergency one chosen after I finally stopped listening to the reassurances of the incompetent and started listening to my concerns instead – at four o'clock in the morning.

Philippe's death put Gloria's into sharp relief. 'The way you've cried over

Philippe,' Misha observed, summing up the reality of the situation, 'I'd say you're sadder over his death than Grandma's.'

'That's true,' I admitted. 'But then Philippe was young and loving and wanted to live, and Grandma was old and unloving and didn't want to.'

'Did you love Philippe more than Grandma?' he asked.

'I suppose I did,' I said.

'I can see why. Grandma could be so mean to you,' he said.

'Did you love her?' I asked.

Misha shrugged his shoulders as if to say he did. 'She was okay with us,' he said. 'It was Gabriela she was mean to.' Dima, on the other hand, admitted that he did love his grandmother. He didn't even hold the 'box' he got against her, which told me I had done the right thing as a mother when I had reincorporated Gloria back into our lives once I had the children.

The saddest reaction of all, however, came from Gabriela. 'Why does Grandma hate me so much when I've never done anything to her?' she once asked her mother. Kitty tried her best to explain that Gloria did not hate her personally, soft-soaping the whole issue with palliatives about illness and old people etc. While the explanation made Gabriela feel better, the sad fact is she had picked up and given voice to the reality that her grandmother was consumed with hatred and spewed it forth left, right and centre, with nary a care as to the effect it would have on the recipient. There was also the prospect that she might have targeted Gabriela because her granddaughter was young, beautiful and female and Gloria not only hated competition but also 'couldn't abide the female sex,' as she used to put it.

And yet, in the weeks and months to come, I realized that, relieved as I was to have seen Gloria safely dispatched to the great party in the sky, where she could no longer wreak her particular brand of havoc and might even be learning to accept the error of her ways, I also missed having a mother to ring up and play the dutiful daughter for. Although I had long since ceased hoping that any lasting good would come out of anything I did for or with her, I was being true to what I regard as one of nature's strongest impulses: a child's need to love a parent.

Although I was only too aware that it was easy to make a strong case for how awful a mother she had been, I also recognized that her existence as our mother had not been a total downhill trip. Her social skills had served the four of her children well, not only while we were growing up in terms of bringing fascinating people into our lives, but also in having equipped us to function as adults with anyone from the Queen of England down to a dustman. That ability, believe me, has been a great gift, and it is one that we owe to Gloria more than anyone else.

Her sense of humour also gave us a fine sense of the ridiculous, even if her ridiculousness sometimes made a sense of humour a necessary tool for surviving sanely. Although the dreadful abusiveness to which she was prone was something we would have been happier living without, the sad but true fact of life is that, unless you are destined for a very narrow way of life, the sooner you learn to cope with the downside of life so that it does not interfere with the upside, the better able you are to function as a life-enhancing individual. And, in terms of the pressures and malignancies of worldly success, Gloria's awfulness was just about the best preparation any of us could have had. The very tools we developed to survive in that University of Hard Knocks have stood us in good stead in the world at large. For, make no mistake about it, in this world of ours, the greater a success you are, the more privileged your existence, the more varied are the devices you need to cope positively with the demands that are made upon you.

What a mother like Gloria gave her children above all else was the ability to pick and choose from a range of coping mechanisms, some of which might have been destructive when employed by her but which, in other hands, would preserve one against adversaries whose thinking one could never have otherwise even begun to understand, had one not had the experience of surviving a mother like Gloria. It truly is an ill wind that blows no good, and though Gloria was definitely no gentle breeze, what does not kill you certainly makes you stronger. The fact that it also causes you tremendous pain doesn't alter the reality: it equips you well for coping with others who share the malign characteristics of the very person who caused you such suffering.

Make no mistake about it, there are Glorias everywhere. I would go as far as saying that there is every chance that the highest percentage of narcissistic personalities is to be found in the upper and upper-middle classes. As the stakes get higher and the rewards of prosperity greater, so too does the temptation to believe yourself superior to less privileged beings and to cut moral corners, to achieve what you want or to hang onto what you've already got by any means that are expedient.

I have come to realize that possibly the best thing Gloria did for me, aside from providing me with the experience which allows me to recognize others of her kind, is that her existence forced me to develop the armour and the means of retaliation to deal with people like her.

In the months after Gloria's death, as I was coming to terms with the loss as well as the boon that being free of her brought in their wake, I could not help but feel that the damp squib of her death and burial was not entirely worthy of the potent force she had been during life. I felt I owed it to her, as well as to the many people to whom she had shown hospitality over the years, to give them an opportunity to say a proper goodbye. So I proposed to my sisters that we organize a memorial service for her in Jamaica. Although Libby and Kitty wished me well, they wanted to have nothing to do with the arrangements, nor were they prepared to attend it. I hoped that Libby's children might come, for Gloria had been pleasant enough to them when they had been children. At first, as I set about making the arrangements long-distance with the help of my dear friend Nicola Croswell Mair, it looked as if they might.

In the middle of these plans, I had to fly to Grand Cayman to straighten out the house. The sad fact was that Gloria had nothing any of us particularly wanted. Not only had she died when we were old enough to be well-established, with everything one could desire in the way of worldly possessions, but we had also inherited stuff from Mickey and Marjorie. There are only so many pictures you can hang on your walls or pieces of furniture you can absorb before the plethora of possessions becomes a burden and you say, 'Spare me'. I fear that is the stage we had reached. None of the three of us actually could house anything else.

Libby and Kitty were gracious enough to take some of the china, but neither of them wanted any of the crystal, nor did I. So, after giving away certain antiques to relations and shipping one or two important family pieces to England that would hinder a rental, along with Gloria's silver dinner, tea and coffee services, I left the remainder in the house along with one of her complete bone-china dinner services and Marjorie's Spode. Then I arranged a yard sale and put everything in except the Baccarat decanters, which a friend wanted. I doubt very much that the people who came and bought Baccarat and Waterford cut glasses for ten and twenty cents can have realized the deals they were getting. Nor do I suppose anyone who bought one of Gloria's

Lanvin dresses for a dollar or two can have appreciated how they had lucked out. But it was a way of spreading the wealth, so to speak, and I did it almost with relief.

It was while choosing what to discard and what to keep that I realized how well organized my mother had been. Her possessions were in perfect order. Not only was everything neatly packed away, but she had regularly updated her address books, filing away the old ones along with inspirational material, which she had needed from the days when she used to make speeches to various organizations. I kept one or two which I felt were representative of her for the memorial service, then turned to the boxes full of notebooks. I opened one and saw that it had notes going back years. I discarded the whole lot, thinking how nice it would be if one could just store everything, though of course lack of space prevented that. Then I noticed that one of the books had flipped open to a recipe for *meshie*, a Lebanese dish I like. 'I'll keep that,' I thought, 'not only for the recipe but to have as a memento of Mummy's handwriting.' I put it to one side without apprising myself of its contents, little realizing how important that notebook would prove to be.

Had I read it at that time, I suspect I might well have pulled the plug on the memorial service there and then. It covered the period in 2004, when Gloria was trying to diddle us out of our share of Marjorie's estate, and so it provided an invaluable insight not only into how she functioned, but what her state of mind was. On one page she writes that she has told me during a telephone conversation 'All IS MINE' (underlined three times and capitalized as indicated), while on another she confirms that I have informed her that I have found Auntie's signed will. Even though that made it impossible for her to justifiably claim that anything, much less all, was hers, this did not prevent her hatching plans to sell Blue Horizon from under us and writing about them too.

Reading that notebook, it was obvious that the only person whose feelings or opinion she cared about was Anthony. She mentions that 'he was looking forlorn when he came to see me. I must ask him whether it is because Ptolemy (his dog) has died and he's missing him, or if it's something I said or did to upset him.' As if she had been important enough to him for him to care about, save as a source for a real-estate commission – something she herself recognized once she had done the dirty deed and he had tripped off with both the commission and the 'gift' extracted so forcibly from us by the woman who had not ever really cared about us except as far as she could benefit from us.

However, I did not look at that notebook until the following year, shortly before I went to New York. When I saw it, any excuses I could make for Gloria finally evaporated. There, in black and white, was all the evidence anyone could need of her treachery, calculation, amorality and ruthless self-centredness.

As I looked at the pages and tried to steady my shaking hand, I could not help but feel that someone up there was looking out for me. Of the plethora of notebooks that I had thrown away, I had kept this one and this one alone. Without knowing its contents, I had happened upon something that was truly life-changing. This begged the question: was it the only one that was so highly incriminating? Could the others have also contained equally damaging revelations?

Whatever the other notebooks had held, I concluded, it was providential that they no longer existed. Did I really need others to hammer home the point when I had already got it?

It is just as well that I did not discover what was in that notebook until the following year, for the same day that I found it along with its many other companions in boxes at the bottom of the storage cupboard, I also happened upon another box whose contents unsettled me enough to give me pause for months of thought.

This box was made of wood and had plainly been constructed many years before to hold important documents. As soon as I opened it up and saw that it contained the letters patents of my grandfather's Templar Knighthood as well as those of two of his brothers, I suspected that it had once belonged to Lucius. I was intrigued to see that Gloria's stories about him being a Knight Templar had indeed been truthful. Because I had long since stopped believing anything she said and had discounted that claim along with many others, some of which might have been true – or at any rate held a kernel of truth – my conscience pricked me and I momentarily wondered if maybe I hadn't been too harsh on her.

Before I had time to hurtle down the well-trodden road of guilt which she and Michael had been so adept at instilling in us children, I alighted upon a thick envelope over which she had written, in her distinctive and elegant script, 'Georgia Arianna Ziadie'. I opened it up to find the certification of my college degree as well as two yellowing, age-blotched envelopes. 'Now what on earth can those be?' I thought, opening up the larger envelope, which had scrawled over it in my father's handwriting, 'To my adored and lovable darling

Gloria.' I found a birthday card obviously written in the 1970s. It was one of those grand and obviously fearfully expensive things which lovesick swains give to women they are courting, along with expensive presents like good pieces of jewellery. I read the rather touching sentiments, thinking how sweet it was, until I came to the end and saw that my father had signed off with the blood-curdling 'To the most wonderful wife in the world – from her devoted slave, Mike.'

I felt my stomach churn. How could Michael have abased himself like that? Although the overweening vanity that was at the root of her narcissistic personality always required the most fulsome praise – worship, in fact – I felt sad that a man, who knew how appalling a wife she had been, could have felt driven to write such flattery about wifely attributes she did not possess. The sting in the tail, however, was the admission that he was her 'devoted slave'. I could just see Gloria relishing that admission. No wonder she had kept the card – the only one she ever did keep, for she was no sentimentalist.

Sickening as the contents of that envelope were, they were nothing compared with those of the other, smaller envelope. This was a regularly sized envelope. There was no handwriting on it, but because of the 'devoted slave' card I knew it too would contain something that Gloria held close to what passed for her heart. As I removed the sheets of paper, I was about to discover just how right I was. When I unfolded them, I saw five photocopies of the letter the doctor who performed the corrective surgery on me in 1970 had written contemporaneously, confirming my physical state at the time of the operation. Worse, in front of them was a sixth, and smaller document. This was the original letter – that letter which I had needed so desperately when I was suing the newspapers in 1975 and in 1992 for stating that I was a transsexual - and which Gloria had insisted she had never had.

Although I did not want to believe that my own mother had wilfully withheld a document whose absence she knew could well have jeopardized expensive libel actions I had instituted against various newspapers, as well as calling into question my legal rights as a woman under British law as it then stood, it was obvious she had deliberately withheld it and kept it safe and sound in case she, and not I, ever needed it. The only question was: had she been malevolent or self-protective? Had she wilfully wanted to saddle me with a reputation she knew my medical history did not warrant, or had she simply been determined to protect her shocking lack of support for me during my teenage years? She was intelligent and cannot have doubted that, if the newspapers made it clear that I had indeed had valid medical reasons for wishing to live my life as the female nature intended, people would wonder how she and my father had been able to stand by idly, while I had suffered from an identifiable medical problem that required a medical solution.

Had Gloria's competitive nature got the better of whatever passed as a sorry excuse for a conscience? I did not put it past the woman, who had tried to eliminate the competition she thought I had become in the early 1970s by burning my face, to stand by deliberately and allow a vicious ex-husband and a callous press to destroy much of my feminine allure with false rumours. 'Well, nutty buddy,' I could just hear her saying to herself, 'you thought you'd prevailed over me, but I've prevailed over you. You may still have your face and figure, but you've lost your reputation for femininity and, along with it, most of the advantages that much-vaunted face and figure would have brought your way. And I'm making damn sure that the one document that can incontrovertibly restore that feminine reputation will never see the light of day – at least, not as long as I'm alive.' Yes. I could see her taking quiet satisfaction in having tied me up in invisible rope as I tried to participate in the race of life, and in so doing, ensured that she had prevented me from achieving what I might have done without the additional handicaps I was being saddled with.

Although I had no doubt that this was precisely why Gloria withheld that letter, I could not prove it. In the absence of absolute proof, I felt that the only moral alternative was to give her the benefit of the doubt and factor in some other possible and less malign, albeit equally irresponsible motivation, for her refusal to turn it over to me. So I shelved my thoughts, just as I had shelved so much else to do with her, and got on with the business of winding up her life.

When I returned to England I continued arranging her memorial service and tried not to think that I was wasting my time on a woman who did not deserve it. Used as I was to focusing on the positive, I consoled myself that even if Gloria personally did not warrant the effort I was making, the friends and relations who would want to pay their respects did.

The question of the 'Family Tribute' now arose. Because my feelings were so hopelessly conflicted after discovering those documents, I decided that it would be unsuitable for me to prepare anything. Not only would I find it difficult to remain both truthful and positive, but I also could not convince myself that Gloria would be worth the effort it would take to pull off that grand slam. I decided that I was already going to enough trouble and expense – far more than she would have endowed any of her four children with – so I rang up Libby and got her to fax me her funeral tribute.

Originally, I had envisaged that one of Gloria's adult grandchildren would deliver the tribute, but when it became apparent that none of the three of them could spare the time to fly to Jamaica for the service, I approached her great-nephew by marriage: 'Oh Toothless One'. They had possessed an affinity for one another, and he moreover had a sufficiently outgoing personality to deliver the tribute well. He agreed to do it, so I turned my attention to formulating a suitable group of readers of lessons. To their credit, everyone I approached agreed happily, although in my own defence I should say that I only approached her cousin the Honourable Danvers Williams and good friends of ours like the artist David Boxer and the socialite Charles Hanna or Gloria's fellow orchid expert, the authoress Cecily Tobisch, one of the few people who had had the patience and tolerance to maintain a friendship with Gloria over two decades and to ignore all the rubbish that went along with it.

That only left someone to deliver the eulogy. This was where I hit a real problem. No one wanted to give it – none of her friends or any of her relations. It was clear that no one who knew her well wanted to stand up and deliver a public address that would have to limit itself to praise, when everyone in the church would know that so much that was negative had to remain unspoken. Cecily, who had already kindly agreed to arrange the flowers at the church, now stepped into the breach and offered to try to find someone to fulfil the well-nigh impossible task. Within days, she telephoned me in England to say that Marigold Harding, a magistrate and fellow horticulturalist and socialite, had consented to do it. Although I didn't know the lady in question, I was well on my way to appreciating her talents even before Cecily explained what a charming and gracious person she was.

'The truth is, Georgie, your mother made herself so unpopular that I've had a warm time getting even an adequate complement of ladies to help with decorating the church. Several of the ones I approached refused to even attend the service,' Cecily said.

'What did they say?' I asked.

'I wouldn't want to distress you with their comments,' she said embarrassedly.

I laughed, hoping to make light of the situation. 'I can just imagine. I bet at least one of them used the "B-word".'

Cecily laughed. 'Yes, they did. And there was also the social issue…'

'Oh God,' I groaned. 'Don't tell me Mummy was still riding her high horse and letting people feel inadequate.'

'You know what she could be like,' Cecily said gently.

I sure did.

'Well, Cecily, I can't really say I blame people whom Mummy denigrated for not wanting to attend her memorial service. The chickens, I daresay, have come home to roost. It will be interesting to see if *anyone* comes.'

'I'm sure there will be a respectable turnout. Some people did like her.'

Forewarned is forearmed. Because I had finally received confirmation from an independent and trustworthy source that Gloria's gift for turning people off had not been reserved for her immediate family, I arrived in Jamaica three days before the event on 20th November 2005 knowing I would have my work cut out for me in drumming up attendance. Since I dared not rely upon people reading the newspaper announcements and wanting to attend, I opened up her address book and telephoned people I had not seen or spoken to in years. Some, such as Madge and Pauline Seaga, were as true as they had been twenty years before. Others, who shall remain nameless, proved to me that Gloria's adage, 'Show me your friends and I will tell you who you are', was only too true. 'She's dead now, 'their attitude seemed to say. 'She can't be of any use to me socially and frankly, I really only have time for myself and people who can be of use to me in the here and now.' The problem with having false values is you have false friends who mirror those values – and behave accordingly. The futility of failing to keep in touch with true friends just so that she could surround herself with effete panderers to her vanity had never been plainer.

Meanwhile, Nicola and Randy Mair laid on a reception for me that was covered in the social columns, and another following the memorial service at which there was no press. This was just as well, for though everyone said the service was beautiful, and the church was decorated magnificently in floral arrangements which doffed a hat to the orchids which Gloria and so many of the other horticulturalists loved, there could have been no more than sixty or so people in attendance. Contrasted with the multitude who had attended both Michael's and Mickey's funeral services, the poor showing graphically demonstrated how few people had respects to pay.

And yet, for all her faults, Gloria did have her virtues. Possibly it is best to leave the final word to Marigold Harding, who said, 'As one writer puts it, "A good friend will joyfully sing with you when you are on the mountain top and silently walk beside you through the valley." Gloria Ziadie can be easily described as a good friend of mine personally and a good friend of the St Andrew Flower Arrangement and Garden Club.

'My relationship with Gloria goes back before I became a member of the club. As a matter of fact, Gloria was the one who persuaded me and the late Alice Jones to become members of the club and later to form the Jamaica National Council of Accredited Flower Show Judges. Persuasive she was, determined she was, kindness was her second nature, and generosity abounded in her giving, whether it was of her time, her talents or in offering her home for meetings and club socials.

'She brought to the club a new energy. Her ideas always stirred response. Sometimes not necessarily positive. But she stimulated new ideas, new approaches. She was creative, organized, methodical and hardworking. She was a lady of action. Gloria had a great sense of humour and quite often the way she expressed her opinion could be rather colourful. With all of these attributes one could easily describe Gloria as a palette of "Best Colour Harmony".

'Although she was most active in the St Andrew Flower Arrangement and Garden Club, her love for flowers and nature took her into other related organizations – the Orchid Society, and the Jamaica Horticultural Society where she made her mark and will always be remembered by all.

'The club will always remember Gloria as an exceptional member who carried out her responsibilities with great zeal and with pride. She was never satisfied unless everyone else was satisfied. She was always eager to learn more which led her to many parts of the world attending flower shows, symposiums and workshops. She was the recipient of many awards of excellence for floral designs and horticultural exhibits. Not only did she receive awards, but with her very generous nature she also gave awards to various organizations of which she was a member.

'When she decided to leave for Cayman she donated all her books on floral designs and her containers to the club for which the club was very grateful.

'Her memory will live on in the St Andrew Flower Arrangement and

Garden Club. Gloria my friend, our friend, you will be surely missed.

'May her soul rest in peace.'

Yes, I hope my mother's soul rests in peace. I also hope her life will be a salutary lesson to others, as it has been to me. Had she accepted the fundamental dichotomy of life – that each of us is unique and overwhelmingly important but also only one of billions of other similar beings and therefore unimportant – she might have been able to achieve the degree of balance she needed to lead a fulfilled and productive life.

'It profiteth not a man to gain the whole world and to lose his soul,' Gloria used to love to warn, thinking that, by believing in God, all would be forgiven her as she missed the point that a soul which is in good shape doesn't spew forth venom from morning till night. Ultimately, our truest value – as much to ourselves as to others – lies not in our attributes or possessions, or even in our achievements, but in our inner qualities. Each of us, whether queen regnant, powerful president or insignificant and anonymous peasant, is expendable. That is the nature of life. Each of us will live and die, and the world will go on without us, so no matter how important we or our accomplishments have been in a worldly sense, our actual importance is limited. The void created by our death is filled as absolutely as if we had been of no more importance than the billions of anonymous souls who have lived and died with only a handful of individuals being aware of their existence.

Worldly approbation, for all its merits, does not actually satisfy human beings on a fundamental level. For that, we need to be capable of enjoying genuine happiness and true fulfilment – a capability we might all possess naturally as children but which, as adults, we retain only if we keep ourselves spiritually healthy. Irrespective of how important and privileged we may be, we lose that ability unless we respect the fundamental rules of life and our place in the scheme of things. No one, no matter how privileged or fortunate, is any more entitled to happiness or fulfilment than the less privileged or fortunate, and those who feel they are, lose the ability to enjoy happiness and fulfilment along with their links to quantum rules which govern all our lives.

The laws of the spirit being the greatest leveller of all, we can only achieve and maintain happiness or fulfilment through being the sort of people we ought to be. That, and not wealth or privilege, is where life really is at, and it does not behove any of us to forget it, for all else is folly or vanity – which does not mean that folly and vanity can't be entertaining or amusing, for they too have their merits. But they are not profound. And a life frittered away on superficialities can never have the merit or rewards of one that is focused upon profundity.

Bibliography

This bibliography is limited to some of the academic works that were researched for Narcissistic Personality Disorder, Histrionic Personality Disorder and Antisocial Personality Disorder:

AKTAR, Salman, MD, *Broken Structures: Severe Personality Disorders and Their Treatment* (Jason Aronson, 1992)

Quest for Answers: A Primer of Understanding and Treating Severe Personality Disorders (Jason Aronson, 1995)

BECK, Aaron, MD with FREEMAN, Arthur, *Cognitive Therapy of Personality Disorders* (Guildford Press, 1990)

BECK, Aaron, MD with WRIGHT, F D, NEWMAN, C F, and LIESE, B S, *Cognitive Therapy of Substance Abuse* (Guildford Press, 1993)

BENJAMIN, Lorna, *An Interpersonal Theory of Personality Disorders*: Major Theories of Personality Disorder (Guildford Press, 1996)

BIRTCHNELL, John, COSTELLO, Charles (eds.), *Detachment*, Personality Characteristics of the Disordered Personality (John Wiley and Sons, 1996)

COHEN, Irving, MD, *Addiction*: The High-Low Trap (Health Press, 1995)

Diagnostic And Statistical Manual Of Mental Disorders, Fourth Edition (American Psychiatric Association, 1994)

DOWEIKO, Harold, *Concepts of Chemical Dependency* (Cole Publishing, 1996)

DOWSON, Jonathan and GROUNDS, Adrian, *Personality Disorders*: Recognition and Clinical Management (Cambridge University Press, 1995)

FENIGSTEIN, Alan, COSTELLO, Charles (eds.), *Paranoia*: Personality Characteristics of the Personality Disordered (John Wiley & Sons, 1996)

FIRST, Michael, MD, FRANCES, Allen, MD and PINCUS, Harold, MD, *DSM-IV Handbook of Differential Diagnosis* (American Psychiatric Press, 1995)

FORREST, Gary, D (ed.) *Alcoholism, Narcissism and Psychopathology* (Jason Aronson 1983)

FRANCES, Allen, MD, FIRST, Michael, MD and PINCUS, Harold, MD, *DSM-IV Guidebook* (American Psychiatric Press, 1995)

GOLOMB, Elan, PhD, *Trapped in the Mirror*: Adult Children of Narcissists in Their Struggle for Self (Quill – William Morrow, 1992)

HARE, Robert, PhD, *Without Conscience*: The Disturbing World of the Psychopaths Among Us (Guildford Press, 1993)

HOROWITZ, Mardi, MD, *Hysterical Personality Style and the Histrionic Personality Disorder* (Jason Aronson, 1991)

KANTOR, Martin, MD, *Diagnosis and Treatment of the Personality Disorders* (Ishiyaku EuroAmerica, 1992)

KERNBERG, Otto, MD, *Severe Personality Disorders, Psychotherapeutic Strategies* (Yale University Press, 1984)

Aggression in Personality Disorders and Perversions (Yale University Press, 1992)

MASTERSON, James, MD, *The Narcissistic and Borderline Disorders*: An Integrated Developmental Approach (Brunner, Mazel 1981)

MILLON, Theodore and DAVIS, Roger, *Disorders of Personality DSM-IV and Beyond* (John Wiley & Sons, 1996)

MILLON, Theodore and DAVIS, Roger, *An Evolutionary Theory of Personality Disorders*: Major Theories of Personality Disorder (Guildford Press, 1996)

OLDHAM, John, M.D. and MORRIS, Lois, *The Personality Self-Portrait*: Why You Think, Work, Love and Act the Way You Do (Bantam Books, 1990)

RICHARDS, Henry, PhD, *Therapy of the Substance Abuse Syndromes* (Jason, Aronson, 1993)

RODIN, Gary, IZENBURG, Sam, ROSENBLUTH, Michael and YALOM, Irvin (eds.), *Treating Difficult Personality Disorders, Treating the Narcissistic Personality Disorder* (Jossey-Bass, Publishers, 1997)

SALZMAN, Leon, MULE, Joseph (eds.), *Behaviour In Excess*: An Examination of the Volitional Disorder (The Press Press – MacMillan Publishing, 1981)

SPERRY, Len, MD, PhD and CARLSON, Jon, D Psych, *Psychopathology and Psychotherapy*: From Diagnosis to Treatment (Accelerated Development, 1993)

SPERRY, Len, MD, PdD, *Handbook of Diagnosis and Treatment of the DSM-IV Personality Disorders* (Brunner, Mazel, 1995)

STOUT, Martha, PhD, *The Sociopath Next Door* (Broadway Books, 2005)

WIDIGER, Thomas and CORBITT, Elizabeth, *Antisocial Personality Disorder*: The DSM-IV Personality Disorders (Guildford Press, 1995)

WINK, Paul, COSTELLO, Paul (eds.), *Narcissism*: Personality Characteristics of the Disordered Personality (John Wiley & Sons, 1995)

WURMSER, Leon, MD, LION, John, MD (eds.), *Addictive Personalities*: Personality Disorders, Diagnosis and Management (Williams & Wilkins, 1981)

ZUCKERMAN, Marvin, COSTELLO, Charles (eds.), *Sensation Seeking*: Personality Characteristics of the Disordered Personality (John Wiley & Sons, 1996)

Printed in Great Britain
by Amazon

40489261R00364